Antenatal and neonatal screening

Second edition

Edited by

Nicholas Wald

Professor, Wolfson Institute of Preventive Medicine,
St Bartholomew's and The Royal London School of Medicine and Dentistry,
University of London

and

Ian Leck

Professor Emeritus, University of Manchester

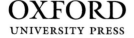

OXFORD
UNIVERSITY PRESS

OXFORD
UNIVERSITY PRESS

Great Clarendon Street, Oxford OX2 6DP

Oxford University Press is a department of the University of Oxford.
It furthers the University's objective of excellence in research, scholarship,
and education by publishing worldwide in

Oxford   New York
Athens   Auckland   Bangkok   Bogotá   Buenos Aires   Calcutta
Cape Town   Chennai   Dar es Salaam   Delhi   Florence   Hong Kong   Istanbul
Karachi   Kuala Lumpur   Madrid   Melbourne   Mexico City   Mumbai
Nairobi   Paris   São Paulo   Singapore   Taipei   Tokyo   Toronto   Warsaw

with associated companies in
Berlin   Ibadan

Oxford is a registered trade mark of Oxford University Press
in the UK and in certain other countries

Published in the United States
by Oxford University Press, Inc., New York

First edition (Edited by Nicholas Wald) published 1984
Second edition published 2000

Reprinted 2004

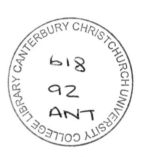

British Library Cataloguing in Publication Data
Data available

Library of Congress Cataloging in Publication Data

Antenatal and neonatal screening/edited by Nicholas Wald and Ian Leck.—2nd.ed.
    p.   cm.
  Includes bibliographical references and index.
  1. Prenatal diagnosis.   2. Infants (Newborn)—Diseases—Diagnosis.
  3. Pregnancy—Complications—Diagnosis.   I. Wald, Nicholas J.   II. Leck, Ian.
  RG628 .A54 2000   618.3'2075—dc21   00–035659

3 5 7 9 10 8 6 4 2

ISBN 0 19 262826 7

Typeset by J&L Composition Ltd, Filey, North Yorkshire

Printed in Great Britain by Biddles Ltd., King's Lynn, Norfolk

Contents

Foreword

Sir Richard Doll F. R. S.

In the 16 years that have passed since the publication of the first edition of this book, birth rates in developed countries have continued to fall until they are now down to or below those required to maintain the population at its present level and death rates have continued to decline, not only in infancy and childhood, when they were already low, but also in middle and old age. The expectation of life at birth consequently now exceeds 80 years in several countries and is likely to do so before long in many others. In these circumstances it is more than ever important that every new born child should be both wanted and able to enjoy a full life unhampered by physical or mental disability.

Advances in knowledge of the means to control fertility have gone a long way to ensure that every pregnancy is wanted. The same knowledge, however, combined with the social changes that have provided women with equal opportunities for higher education and, in an increasing number of countries, equal opportunities for a professional or business career, has led many women to postpone pregnancy to their late thirties, when the fetus is at greater risk of intra-uterine death or of having some serious congenital abnormality. Knowledge of how to ensure a successful outcome to pregnancy and how to avoid the birth of a child with a major physical or mental defect has, consequently, become of even greater importance than it was 16 years ago. Sadly, it is still far from complete.

What we do know has, in a few instances, justified the adoption of national policies that affect the whole population, irrespective of whether or not the individual members are at risk of pregnancy, such as the fortification of flour with folic acid in some countries and of salt with iodide in others to reduce, respectively, the risks of neural tube defects and hypothyroidism in the developing fetus. More often, however, it has justified the screening of selected populations to see whether special investigations or special treatments are required.

Developments in molecular biology have increased the number of situations in which intervention might be productive, but the possibility of effective intervention is not, in itself, an adequate reason for screening; for it may cause anxiety, can, in some instances, have adverse effects, may not be 100 per cent effective, and almost always costs money that is urgently required for other medical purposes. These issues have to be faced fairly and squarely and are so faced by the contributors to this book in relation to the various scientific possibilities. For some types of screening, the balance of evidence weighs strongly in their favour. They are not, however, offered equally everywhere within those countries that have adopted them and it is much to be hoped that those responsible for the provision of prevention services will read this book and reassess their priorities in the light of the evidence it presents.

Preface to the second edition

Although much has changed since 1984, when the first edition of this book appeared, the approach of the book remains the same. The focus is on the prevention of disease and the reduction of serious morbidity and mortality. Specific disorders for which screening can make a reasonable claim were identified, and the chapters on these disorders have a common structure: each disorder is first described, with its birth prevalence, and the relevant screening and diagnostic tests are then considered, including quantitative estimates of their performance whenever possible. There are also a few chapters which focus not on specific disorders but on specific procedures which are either relevant to the detection of more than one disorder (e.g. amniocentesis) or of doubtful value (e.g. continuous electronic fetal monitoring in labour).

Although these features of the first edition have been retained, all but one of the chapters are new or have been substantially revised. The exception is the first chapter on principles of screening. This only needed minor editorial changes, because the principles it discusses are the same as they were when the first edition appeared. A second chapter has been added to cover the principles of screening in which several screening markers are used simultaneously.

Some procedures which were discussed in the first edition have been omitted from the second, for example screening for cervical cancer, because although cervical smears are often performed in pregnancy it was felt on reflection that this was not an example of antenatal screening.

Also, there is no longer a chapter entitled 'Needs of the community'. Bearing in mind that these needs are no more and no less than the collective needs of the individuals who form the community, we have chosen in this edition to substitute a chapter on 'The ethics of antenatal and neonatal screening', which examines the responsibilities which providers of screening services have both to individuals and to communities. This chapter expresses the personal reflections of its three authors, and differs from the other chapters in not making specific references to published work.

Another difference between the first and second editions of this book is in how the term 'screening' is defined. The definition given in the first edition was 'The identification, among apparently healthy individuals, of those who are sufficiently at risk of a specific disorder to justify a subsequent diagnostic test or procedure, or in certain circumstances, direct preventive action.' In the current edition we use a modified definition which was first proposed in 1994 (Wald N. J. Guidance on terminology, *J. Med. Screen.* **1**, 76). This reads:

Screening is the systematic application of a test or inquiry, to identify individuals at sufficient risk of a specific disorder to benefit from further investigation or direct preventive action, among persons who have not sought medical attention on account of symptoms of that disorder.

This definition was substituted for the earlier one for two reasons:

1. Screening, like other medical interventions, is intended to benefit the individuals to whom it is offered. It does not include procedures to identify people at high risk of disease which are undertaken primarily in order that other people may benefit (e.g. by being protected from infection), whereas the earlier definition implied that if such measures were justified they could be classified as screening.

2. Screening for a disorder can be offered to all 'who have not sought medical attention on account of symptoms of that disorder', including people with other disorders as well as the 'apparently healthy' who were the only candidates for screening identified in the earlier definition.

This second edition has had a long incubation period. We are grateful for the generous forbearance of the authors, particularly those who delivered their manuscripts promptly. It will be for others to judge whether the result is a product that was worth waiting for.

The first edition of this book was stimulated by Professor Tom Whitehead nearly 20 years ago and produced with the help of many others. During the preparation of the second edition we were saddened by the death of one of our contributors, Sarah Bundey. We would like to thank Eva Alberman, David Clayton, Mike Conner, Christopher Frost, James Haddow, Wayne Huttly, Simon Rish, Robert Robinson, Karen Wald and Hilary Watt for reading and criticizing parts of the text of this edition, and for other helpful advice. We would also like to thank Luba Mumford for her attentive help as our editorial assistant, and Margaret Allison, Janette Clarke, Rachel Lynch, and Jaine Melbourne for other assistance with preparing the manuscript for publication. As before, the staff of Oxford University Press have been most helpful and tolerated our late schedule with courtesy and understanding. Most of all we thank our contributors, who dealt with our editorial strictures so patiently and constructively.

Nicholas Wald and Ian Leck
August 2000

Preface to the first edition

Screening represents a radical departure from traditional medicine, for it is usually concerned with the detection of disorders at an asymptomatic stage which cannot, therefore, have prompted the patient to seek medical attention; indeed it often involves seeking out such asymptomatic individuals among people who are not receiving any type of medical attention. It is tempting to believe that the early detection of disease is a good thing and an end in itself, forgetting that the identification of either trivial or untreatable conditions may cause anxiety with no useful result. Screening must, therefore, be concerned with the prevention of disease and the recognition that it is only worthwhile screening for disorders which lend themselves to effective intervention. In this book we have given priority to the screening of diseases which fall into this category.

Prevention is used in two senses: first the prevention of the occurrence of a disorder by removing the cause ('primary prevention'), such as the prevention of rhesus haemolytic disease, and secondly the prevention of overt cases through early detection and appropriate intervention ('secondary prevention'). The latter includes the prevention of the birth of an affected fetus through selective abortion, and although the use of the term 'prevention' in this way is sometimes questioned, it is convenient, and the distinction between the two uses is invariably clear from the context.

Screening, particularly during the antenatal and neonatal period, increasingly relies upon the use of complex technology such as detailed biochemical analyses and electronic equipment. Indeed, screening is an area of medicine where such technology has made an important contribution. But there is a danger that the technology, once introduced, will take on a momentum of its own; it may be difficult to change direction, and the needs of patients may become obscured. The aim of this book has been to consider each screening procedure critically and, wherever possible, quantitatively—keeping in mind that the technology must be the servant of screening and not its master.

Some screening tests are so simple that they are often not regarded as such. For example, the 'test' which separates an at-risk group from the general population may involve no more than asking a woman her age, such as when screening for Down syndrome. Another example is the detection of carriers of certain genetic disorders, such as haemophilia or cystic fibrosis, in which the initial screening test or procedure usually involves the identification of an affected close relative.

The timing of screening tests is often critical, either because the discriminatory value of the test depends on when it is done or because the institution of therapy in affected cases must not be delayed. Sometimes when a single specimen, such as the spot of blood collected in the neonatal period, is used for several screening tests (phenylketonuria, galactosaemia, and hypothyroidism) no one time is best for all tests and a compromise must be found. Some antenatal screening tests, such as those for the detection of carriers of genetic disorders, are best done before rather than during pregnancy.

The approach adopted in the development of the book was to identify specific disorders for which screening can make a reasonable claim, or for which screening might be of value in future. Disorders for which screening is already established and are regarded as an important part of medical practice are dealt with in detail, while others for which screening is of little or uncertain value are dealt with more briefly. The chapter lengths vary accordingly and reflect the public health priorities.

It was convenient to consider the field under three headings: (i) screening for disorders primarily affecting the fetus (e.g. chromosome abnormalities); (ii) screening for disorders affecting the mother which can have adverse effects on the fetus or neonate (e.g. diabetes); (iii) screening for disorders which affect only the mother, of which screening for cancer of the cervix is the only example. The contributing authors have shown great patience in following, wherever possible, a similar chapter structure. This usually consists of a brief introduction, a description of the disorder being screened for, a summary of the treatment or remedy available following early detection, and a description of the available screening and diagnostic methods, citing examples from existing screening programmes. Most chapters include a discussion of problem areas and research needs besides an assessment on the value of screening for the specific disorder being described. A few chapters are devoted to the procedures or tests themselves rather than to the effectiveness of screening for specific disorders. This is either because of their broad application (e.g. ultrasound), or the concern that they may be hazardous (e.g. amniocentesis) or because of their uncertain value (e.g. placental function tests). The book does not consider screening for certain personal habits which can adversely affect the development of the fetus, such as cigarette smoking and alcohol consumption.

An attempt has been made to avoid the unnecessary use of jargon, but some screening terms are useful, and to help the reader a short glossary is given at the end of the book. Throughout the book estimates are given as to how commonly the various disorders occur, and in this connection it was apparent that the terms 'prevalence' and 'incidence' could cause confusion. I have followed epidemiological usage and taken *incidence* to be the frequency with which *new* cases of a condition arise in a given period, and *prevalence* the proportion of a population that is affected by the condition at a particular time or during a particular period. Down syndrome represents an illustrative example. It is a disorder caused by the presence of an extra chromosome No. 21 and necessarily arises around the time of conception. By definition, therefore, the lifetime incidence is the number of conceptions with an extra '21 chromosome' divided by the total number of conceptions. After conception, any assessment of the proportion of fetuses or individuals affected by Down syndrome is a measure of its prevalence, the figure always being less than the lifetime incidence on account of the selective mortality of affected fetuses. The frequency at birth is then referred to as the birth prevalence rather than the incidence. If a condition can arise only after birth (for example, respiratory distress syndrome) we are usually concerned with the incidence. The importance of making a distinction between incidence and prevalence, particularly in perinatal medicine, relates to aetiology and prevention. Incidence can be decreased only by preventing the development of new cases, whereas prevalence can be decreased by increasing the mortality (e.g. termination of pregnancy) of affected individuals as well as by reducing the incidence. For example, an effective screening programme for open neural-tube defects might reduce the birth prevalence of this defect by 90 per cent, but it will obviously not influence the incidence.

For some disorders, such as rhesus haemolytic disease, the birth prevalence is a good estimate of the incidence because there is a low rate of fetal loss, whether through miscarriage or termination of pregnancy. For disorders such as Down syndrome this is not the case, making birth prevalence a poor estimate of the incidence.

A screening test may itself be effective while the screening service which uses the test may not. For example, screening for cancer of the cervix has been shown to be an effective method of reducing the incidence of invasive cervix cancer but in Britain, in spite of many cervical smear examinations, the screening programme has been a failure. The distinction between whether screening for a particular disorder is worthwhile and whether screening programmes for that disorder are in practice effective is an important one, and one which is made throughout the book.

Assembling a list of disorders for which screening is now, or may in the near future be, useful, necessarily involves being selective, and no two people are likely to agree completely on the disorders which should be included. I hope readers will, none the less, let me know of any omissions or unnecessary inclusions which they think exist in this book, so that appropriate revisions can be made in any future edition.

The initiative for this book first came from Professor T. Whitehead, who has encouraged me in my attempts at bringing together the fields of epidemiology and clinical chemistry. I thank him for his encouragement. I also thank Mr R. Barlow, Dr J. Boreham, Mr A. Bron, Dr I. Chalmers, Mr M. Gillmer, Dr I. Grant, Dr J. E. Haddow, Mrs P. Haddow, Professor W. Holland, Dr E. Ilgren, Professor G. Knox, Dr A. MacFarlane, Dr J. I. Mann, and Mr P. Vickers who read and criticized parts of the text, Professor I. Leck and Dr C. Redman for their helpful advice, Miss A. Balkwill for assisting me in the editorial work, and Mrs C. Harwood for skilfully reconstructing edited chapters suitable for the Publishers. The staff of Oxford University Press have been most helpful and it has been a pleasure working with them. Finally, I would like to thank the authors themselves who, in spite of their heavy professional commitments, agreed to contribute to this book.

N.W.

Oxford
October 1982

Contributors

Zarko Alfirevic
Senior Lecturer
Department of Obstetrics and Gynaecology
University of Liverpool
Liverpool L69 9BX
England

John M. Bowman
Distinguished Professor Emeritus, Department of Pediatrics and Child Health
University of Manitoba
Women's Hospital, 5th Floor
735 Notre Dame Avenue
Winnipeg, Manitoba R3E 0L8
Canada

David J. H. Brock
Formerly Professor of Human Genetics, University of Edinburgh
Craigden
Glenfoot, Abernethy
Perthshire PH2 9LT
Scotland

Sarah Bundey (deceased)
Formerly Professor in Clinical Genetics,
University of Birmingham
England

Howard S. Cuckle
Professor of Reproductive Epidemiology
Centre for Reproduction, Growth and Development
School of Medicine
University of Leeds
26 Clarendon Road
Leeds LS2 9NZ
England

George C. Cunningham
Chief, Genetic Diseases Branch
Department of Health Services
2151 Berkeley Avenue
Annex 4
Berkeley, CA 94704
USA

Alan Donnenfeld
Director of Prenatal Diagnosis
Section of Genetics
Pennsylvania Hospital
3rd Floor Cathcart Building
Eighth and Spruce Streets
Philadelphia, PA 19107
USA

Christine Gosden
Professor of Medical Genetics, University of Liverpool
Departments of Biological Sciences and Medicine
Liverpool Women's Hospital
Crown Street
Liverpool L8 7SS
England

Adrian Grant
Professor of Health Services
Health Services Research Unit
Department of Public Health
University of Aberdeen
Polworth Building
Foresterhill
Aberdeen AB25 2ZD
Scotland

J. A. Muir Gray
Director of the Institute of Health Sciences, University of Oxford, and Director of the National Screening Committee
Institute of Health Sciences
Old Road
Headington
Oxford OX3 7LF
England

Allan Hackshaw
Lecturer in Epidemiology and Medical Statistics

Department of Environmental and Preventive Medicine
Wolfson Institute of Preventive Medicine
St Bartholomew's and The Royal London School of Medicine and Dentistry
University of London
Charterhouse Square
London EC1M 6BQ
England

W. Harry Hannon
Chief, Clinical Biochemistry Branch
National Center for Environmental Health
Centers for Disease Control and Prevention
4770 Buford Highway
Atlanta, GA 30341
USA

Joseph G. Hollowell
Chief, Environmental Health Services Branch
National Center for Environmental Health
Centers for Disease Control and Prevention
4770 Buford Highway
Atlanta, GA 30341
USA

Pauline A. Hurley
Consultant in Obstetrics and Fetal Medicine
Women's Centre
John Radcliffe Hospital
Headley Way
Headington, Oxford OX3 9DU
England

R. J. Jarrett
Formerly Professor of Clinical Epidemiology, University of London
45 Bishopsthorpe Road
London SE26 4PA
England

Feige Kaplan
Associate Professor
Departments of Human Genetics and Pediatrics, McGill University
Director, Montreal Tay-Sachs Disease Screening Programme
McGill University-Montreal Children's Hospital Research Institute
2300 Tupper Street
Montréal, Québec H3H 1P3
Canada

Anne Kennard
Lecturer
Department of Environmental and Preventive Medicine
Wolfson Institute of Preventive Medicine
St Bartholomew's and The Royal London School of Medicine and Dentistry
University of London
Charterhouse Square
London EC1M 6BQ
England

Ian Leck
Formerly Professor of Epidemiology, University of Manchester
18 Cadogan Park
Woodstock, Oxon OX20 1UW
England

Elizabeth A. Letsky
Consultant Perinatal Haematologist
Department of Haematology
Queen Charlotte's and Chelsea Hospital
Goldhawk Road
London W6 0XG
England

Amy B. Levine
Assistant Professor
Department of Obstetrics and Gynecology
Thomas Jefferson Medical College
834 Chestnut Street
Suite 400
Philadelphia, PA 19107–5088
USA

Charles J. Lockwood
Professor of Obstetrics and Gynecology
New York University School of Medicine
550 First Avenue
New York, NY 10016
USA

Marie-Louise Newell
Reader in Epidemiology
Department of Epidemiology and Public Health
Institute of Child Health
University of London
30 Guilford Street

London WC1N 1EH
England

Catherine S. Peckham
Professor of Paediatric Epidemiology
Department of Epidemiology and Public Health
Institute of Child Health
University of London
30 Guilford Street
London WC1N 1EH
England

Charles H. Rodeck
Professor of Obstetrics and Gynaecology
University College London Medical School
University of London
86–96 Chenies Mews
London WC1E 6HX
England

Charles R. Scriver
Alva Professor of Human Genetics, and Director Emeritus, Charles R. Scriver Laboratory for Biochemical Genetics
McGill University-Montreal Children's Hospital Research Institute
2300 Tupper Street
Montréal, Québec H3H 1P3
Canada

Michael de Swiet
Consultant Physician
Queen Charlotte's and Chelsea Hospital
Goldhawk Road
London W6 0XG
England

Ann Tabor
Consultant in Obstetrics and Gynaecology
Hvidovre Hospital
University of Copenhagen
Kettegaard Allé 30
DK-2650 Hvidovre
Denmark

Stephen B. Thacker
Director, Epidemiology Program Office
Centers for Disease Control and Prevention

1600 Clifton Road, NE
Building 1, 5th Floor
Atlanta, GA 30333
USA

Bradford L. Therrell
Professor, Department of Pediatrics
University of Texas Health Science Center at San Antonio
Director, National Newborn Screening and Genetics Resource Center
1912 W Anderson Lane #210
Austin, TX 78757
USA

Nicholas Wald
Professor of Environmental and Preventive Medicine
Wolfson Institute of Preventive Medicine
St Bartholomew's and The Royal London School of Medicine and Dentistry
University of London
Charterhouse Square
London EC1M 6BQ
England

Sir David Weatherall
Regius Professor of Medicine, University of Oxford, and Director, Institute of Molecular Medicine
John Radcliffe Hospital
Headington
Oxford OX3 9DS
England

Dose schedules are being continually revised and new side effects recognized. Oxford University Press makes no representation, express or implied, that the drug dosages in this book are correct. For these reasons the reader is strongly urged to consult the pharmaceutical company's printed instructions before administering any of the drugs recommended in this book.

To our wives and children,
Nancy Wald, Karen, David, Richard
and Jonathan,
and
Ann Leck, Sue, Chris, Patsy, and John

I

Principles of screening

1 *Tests using single markers*

Howard S. Cuckle and Nicholas Wald

INTRODUCTION

Screening large populations offers the possibility of being able to make deep inroads into the prevention of certain diseases but it is important to recognize that screening may also cause harm. A screening procedure may lead to unnecessary anxiety by yielding positive results in unaffected individuals or it may engender a false sense of security by yielding negative results in affected individuals. The large scale of screening may mean that the absolute number of errors can be great even if the proportion is small.

There are special ethical considerations which apply to screening. In ordinary clinical practice, investigations are done on individuals with symptoms who seek medical help; the physician's obligation is to treat the patient in the best way he can, even if there is incomplete knowledge about the disease or its remedy. In screening the position is somewhat different; apparently healthy individuals are approached for investigation, and there is therefore a special obligation not to initiate any action unless the full consequences of doing so are known and there is, of course, an effective remedy available.

For the enthusiast screening can become almost an end in itself. To avoid this, it is important to define the objectives of screening and in doing so it is useful to pose a number of specific questions. In this chapter we try to define these questions, indicate the data needed to answer them, and outline the methods used for the statistical analysis of the data so that the value of a screening procedure can be properly assessed. The subject is mainly dealt with by reference to screening in the antenatal and neonatal period.

The screening procedure may take the form of a simple enquiry (e.g. determining ethnicity when screening for cystic fibrosis) or a special test (e.g. maternal serum alphafetoprotein (AFP) estimation when screening for open neural tube defects). It differs from a diagnostic procedure in that there is no intention to offer *therapeutic* intervention solely on the basis of a positive screening result.

When screening leads to direct *preventive* action the aim is to remove a cause of the disease (e.g. treatment of urinary tract infection when screening for pyelonephritis) rather than being able to detect the disease at an early stage and offer therapeutic intervention. Sometimes tests may be carried out on apparently healthy individuals to identify 'high-risk groups' for research purposes without intending to make a diagnosis or offer any therapeutic or preventive action. From the point of view of this book such activity is not regarded as screening.

Screening enquiries or tests (for simplicity we shall refer hereafter to all screening procedures as 'tests') are often offered in steps. For example, when screening for Tay–Sachs disease Ashkenazi Jews (who have a tenfold increased carrier risk) are first identified by, say, approaching the members of synagogues and then a biochemical or DNA test offered. Although the latter is often regarded as the screening test it in fact represents the second step of the screening process—determining ethnic origin is the first step. In this way a screening process may involve two or three screening tests or enquiries performed and interpreted in sequence before a diagnostic test is offered.

The way in which a test is provided determines whether it is a screening test. If Ashkenazi Jewish couples request a biochemical investigation to see whether they are carriers of Tay–Sachs disease then the test is not a screening test. If they are systematically approached and offered the test, then it is a screening test. There are two reasons for making this distinction. Firstly, as indicated above, different ethical considerations apply and secondly selective referral of patients may distort the evaluation of the screening test—the prevalence of the disorder may not be representative of the population as a whole.

In this chapter we consider screening tests based on single variables, such as AFP, which can also be referred to as markers of the disorder that is being screened for. The diversity of screening procedures makes it difficult to specify a single set of criteria needed for their assessment but some have been published,[1-4] and a simple list is given at the end of this chapter which we will refer to again later (Table 1.2). Before considering in detail the screening test (and also subsequent tests which form part of a screening process) it is necessary to consider the disorder for which screening is being carried out, its definition, its prevalence, its natural history, and the efficacy of its treatment or prevention.

THE DISORDER

The disorder for which screening is being carried out should be well-defined but there can be difficulties. For example, there may be disagreement over whether a given individual is actually affected. Intrauterine growth retardation assessed by ultrasound examination of the fetus is such a disorder (see Chapter 17). Theoretically each fetus is regarded as having its own 'correct' rate of growth and an individual whose actual growth is less than this might be said to be growth retarded. However, it is not possible to know an individual's correct rate of growth; all one can do is to relate the actual rate to the population average and the usual variation in this rate (a specified deviation from the average rate being regarded as a positive test result) and this may be quite misleading. Also there is no independent way of assessing the merits of the test. Even an attempt to assess the results of the test by relating them to neonatal development will be of little value unless it can be established that retarded postnatal development is actually a manifestation of 'intrauterine growth retardation'.

Screening for neonatal hypothyroidism provides another example of such circular reasoning, in which the disorder, though relatively well-defined and understood is none the less diagnosed largely by the results of the screening test itself (see Chapter 15). The clinical disease is the mental and physical retardation called cretinism caused by lack of thyroxine in early life, but the screening test detects only the hormone abnormality. How do we know that an individual born with the hormone abnormality will necessarily have the clinical disease—a problem not easily solved since the detection of the hormone abnormality is sufficient grounds for treatment. Is there a 'hypothyroidism' which does not result in cretinism? Those responsible for introducing screening are aware of the problem and have suggested that 'transient hypothyroidism' can be detected by temporarily stopping treatment after one year and reassessing thyroid function.

A similar circular argument applies to the use of blood-pressure measurement in the detection of hypertension, and blood-glucose assay in the detection of diabetes mellitus. The problem is essentially one of definition. If hypertension were not itself regarded as a medical disorder, but simply as a cause of disorders such as stroke or heart disease, and similarly blood-glucose levels were not used to define the disease diabetes mellitus but merely used as a method of estimating a person's risk of developing certain associated disorders, much of the circularity would be avoided. The argument is more than a semantic quibble, because only when the definition of the disease is made independently of the screening test can the performance of the test be properly assessed.

Being a carrier for a recessive genetic disorder (i.e. being a heterozygote) is sometimes regarded as a 'disorder', but the individuals are invariably healthy and their recognition is usually only a means of screening those at risk of bearing homozygous infants who will have the disorder. Identifying carriers can be difficult; usually a carrier can be recognized only after he or she has had an affected child, and even this is not completely reliable since a proportion of affected cases arise as *de novo* mutations.

Even if the disorder is well defined, there may still be problems in defining the particular form of the disease which screening aims to detect. Screening may detect only a certain subgroup of a general disorder (e.g. only spina bifida with open lesions), and it is then necessary to evaluate screening as a method of detecting this particular subgroup.

Prevalence

The prevalence of the disorder being screened for needs to be known for two main reasons. First, screening is likely to be acceptable only if the prevalence exceeds a certain rate, which will depend on various factors such as the seriousness of the disorder and the nature of the screening test; even a very rare abnormality may justify screening if it is serious and the test very unobtrusive. Secondly, once a decision to screen has been taken, the choice of screening policy will depend on the prevalence since this will influence the chance of being affected if the test is positive (see p. 12).

Data on the birth prevalence of non-fatal congenital malformations are often sparse. In the United Kingdom, congenital malformations are notified only on a voluntary basis, and reporting is therefore not complete. Dividing the numbers of notifications of a particular malformation by the total number of births (published by the Office of National Statistics) provides an initial estimate of the birth prevalence, which needs to be adjusted to take account of under-reporting. One way of doing this which in certain circumstances is valid, would be to apply a correction factor derived from data relating to anencephaly which, being a malformation that is always fatal at or shortly after birth, is recorded through death certification as well as through malformation notification. Since death certification is compulsory, it is complete and so for anencephaly the ratio of malformation notifications to death certifications estimates the degree of under-reporting. This ratio when applied to the notified rate of another malformation yields the corrected rate but, of course, such a correction is valid only if the tendency to under-report the other malformation is similar to that for anencephaly.

Ad hoc studies designed to estimate the birth prevalence by searching hospital birth records may be inaccurate, especially if the disorder is uncommon; a few special referrals of high-risk women to specialist centres could exaggerate the estimate drastically. Also records on affected individuals are more likely to be missing because they have been removed on account of some special clinical or research interest in the disorder concerned. It is important to bear in mind that an estimate based on a hospital source may not reflect the overall population prevalence on account of selective referral patterns or variation in diagnosis.

The problems of estimating birth prevalence are further complicated in disorders which are either difficult to diagnose (e.g. congenital heart disease) or are over-diagnosed (e.g. congenital dislocation of the hip). It may be necessary to estimate the prevalence at some time after birth when the clinical state is more clear.

A problem can arise if the estimate of the birth prevalence of a disorder is higher after the introduction of screening than it was before. One example of this is the greater number of chromosomal defects diagnosed by amniocentesis than would have been expected from the birth prevalence. This difference is partly explained by a high spontaneous fetal loss rate of affected pregnancies in the second half of pregnancy, but it is also possible that the birth prevalence had been under-estimated prior to the introduction of antenatal diagnosis. Another example is congenital hypothyroidism. The number of cases diagnosed through screening is approximately double that previously seen at birth. This may have occurred because cases were missed before the start of screening (so the expected birth prevalence is an under-estimate) or because screening generates false-positives who have abnormal hormone levels but will not develop cretinism.

The prevalence of a disease among individuals actually screened may be different from that in the general population in ways which were not anticipated. For example, women of lower socioeconomic classes and those of advanced parity tend to attend their first antenatal visit late in pregnancy. If the screening test needs to be performed early in pregnancy and if the disorder being screened for is more prevalent in the lower classes or in women of advanced parity, then the prevalence among those actually screened (at the correct time) will be lower than in the general population.

Natural history and the efficacy of treatment or prevention

It is obvious that the disorder being screened for should be serious and there must be an effective way to treat or prevent it which could not be similarly achieved without screening. For this to be known it will be necessary to study both the natural history of the disorder and the efficacy of the actions which follow a positive screening test (including the efficacy of the treatment or remedy) *before* screening programmes are started. This is not always straightforward, since it is difficult to carry out a screening test without also offering subsequent intervention to those with positive results. However, it is important to resist this temptation because otherwise it may be impossible to assess the effect of screening on the natural history of the disease; affected individuals with positive screening tests may have a different natural history from affected individuals with negative results, or they may respond in a different way to treatment. For example, maternal serum alphafetoprotein levels used to screen for open spina bifida tend to be higher in the most severely affected cases that die at or shortly after birth. The impact of screening on the extent of handicap is therefore somewhat less than would otherwise be expected.

THE SCREENING TEST

To assess the effect of a screening test two important questions need to be asked:

1. To what extent can the test discriminate affected from unaffected individuals?

2. What is the chance that those who have positive results are affected?

To answer the first question we need to know the separate relative frequency distributions of test values for both affected and unaffected individuals. To answer the second question we need to know the answer to the first and also the prevalence of the disorder.

Relative frequency distributions may be estimated by direct observation using large series of results or by fitting a known statistical frequency distribution (such as the Gaussian distribution) to smaller series after ensuring that the data fit the distribution satisfactorily. The test results may be expressed as values of a continuous variable (e.g. maternal age or a quantitative biochemical measurement) or simply as qualitative categories (e.g. positive or negative).

Discrimination between affected and unaffected individuals
Values for unaffected individuals

Unaffected individuals are those who do not have the disorder being screened for. In deriving their distribution of values, data on all unaffected individuals (or a random sample) should, in general, be included. Exclusions can be made for conditions associated with positive results which are recognizable at the time of the test—for example, multiple pregnancy—provided the exclusion is specified. Otherwise there should be no exclusions.

False-positives can be associated with a fetal death or a disorder other than the one being screened for (e.g. a fetal death can yield positive AFP results). For some conditions the identification of such disorders might be considered desirable, and it would therefore be misleading to classify them as false-positives. In these circumstances it would be advantageous to regard them as another type of affected pregnancy and to omit them when calculating false-positive rates. It may also be helpful to derive a separate distribution of results relating to such a disorder which is not the subject of screening.

Values for affected individuals

Affected individuals are those who have the disorder being screened for. A problem in accumulating data from affected individuals arises because the prevalence of the disorder is usually low. Often no single centre will have sufficient data to describe the distribution of values reliably, and it will be necessary to combine results from many centres. Even data collected in a large referral centre may be insufficient and possibly subject to bias on account of the inclusion of data from samples sent to that centre for the confirmation of positive results.

The combining of data from many centres will be satisfactory if it can be shown that on average the same specimen would have been assigned a similar value at each centre. In the United Kingdom Collaborative AFP Study (see Chapter 3) a fourfold range of maternal serum AFP values was obtained for specimens with the same expected concentrations tested in different centres, but it was found that the results from different centres varied by a constant multiple of each centre's median value found for unaffected pregnancies. The data could therefore be combined by expressing all results for a given centre in multiples of the median.

The use of percentiles or standard deviations from the mean for unaffected individuals is a less satisfactory method of combining data; the actual concentration of the screening variable corresponding to a given percentile or standard deviation from the mean will be different from centre to centre depending on, among other things, the degree of assay imprecision experienced there. This is illustrated in Fig. 1.1. Improving assay precision will reduce the standard deviation of the distribution of the screening variable and 'move' the percentiles in the tail of the distribution towards the centre of the distribution. In Fig. 1.1(i) (imprecise assay) the 95th percentile is equivalent to a value of 6.77; in Fig. 1.1(ii) (precise assay) the same percentile is equivalent to a value of 6.26. The use of percentiles (or standard deviations from the mean) will thus tend to make the false-positive rate similar at different centres but will make the detection rate extremely variable. This is a disadvantage because once screening has begun the former can be readily determined locally, but the latter cannot because of the rarity of the disorder, and will, therefore, remain unknown.

When data from affected individuals are collected prospectively those with positive test results are likely to be recognized earlier than those with negative results; for example, a positive antenatal test might lead to the termination of pregnancy while an affected individual with a negative result will not be identified until birth. Hence at any point in time a greater number of affected individuals will appear to have positive results than is in fact the case. It is therefore necessary to allow a lapse of time after collecting the last result before reaching any firm conclusions so that 'missed' (i.e. false-negative) cases can be identified.

It may be that we are really interested only in detecting a particular subgroup of affected individuals—for example, those with a severe form of the disorder or those who are likely to survive for a long time with severe handicap. It would then be necessary to construct the distribution of values in that particular subgroup.

Possible bias in estimating distribution of values for a biochemical test

In constructing the distribution of test values for affected or unaffected individuals it is important to use only the first technically satisfactory result from each individual.

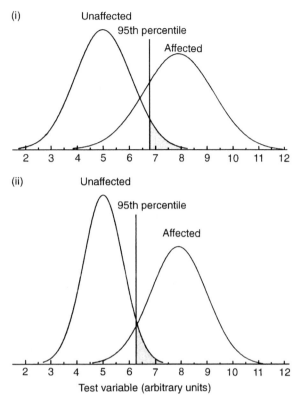

Fig. 1.1 Hypothetical relative frequency distributions of a screening test variable in affected and unaffected individuals, showing the 95th percentile associated with an imprecise and a precise assay. Although by definition the proportion of unaffected individuals with positive results is fixed (5 per cent) the cut-off level (95th percentile) reflects a higher value for the screening variable with the imprecise assay than with the precise one. The proportion of affected individuals detected will therefore be lower with the imprecise assay than with the precise one.

The inclusion of results from fresh samples collected in order to obtain a second, or repeat value (with or without the exclusion of the original values), is likely to lead to bias. For example in clinical practice individuals with extreme values can often have a second test and only the second one used. In general the second results will tend to be less extreme (regression to the mean) so that the proportion of individuals with extreme values will be under-represented.

Bias can also be introduced if stored samples are retrieved and tested over a short period of time in order to construct the distribution of values for affected or unaffected individuals. In such circumstances the samples will be tested in a smaller number of analytical batches than would have occurred in usual practice. Between-batch assay imprecision will therefore exert a disproportionately small effect on the overall distribution of values leading to an under-estimate of their variance. It is therefore best to estimate the underlying distribution using data accumulated in the same way as would occur if screening were being carried out.

Detection rate and false-positive rate

The discriminating power of a test is expressed in terms of the detection rate* (the proportion of affected individuals with a positive result) and the false-positive rate* (the proportion of unaffected individuals with a positive result). For tests which yield only qualitative (or categorical) results (e.g. karyotype determination, gel acetyl-cholinesterase determination) the detection rate and false-positive rate are fixed proportions (see Table 1.1). For tests which yield results as a continuous variable (e.g. age, or serum AFP level) the detection rate and false-positive rate vary and are determined by the cut-off level (see Fig. 1.2). The rates can be estimated directly if sufficient data are available, in which case all the results are classified as positive or negative using a particular cut-off level and the calculation performed in the same way as for a qualitative test. Alternatively the detection rate and false-positive rate can be estimated indirectly if a known frequency distribution can be satisfactorily fitted to the data. The use of say cut-off level A in Fig. 1.2 illustrates the indirect method; here the detection rate is given by the area under the *affected* curve to the right of cut-off level A and the false-positive rate by the area under the *unaffected* curve to the right of the same cut-off level. The two areas can easily be determined for any cut-off level by referring to published tables of the relevant distribution—a worked example is given in Appendix 1 (p. 19).

No hard and fast rule can be adopted for whether the direct or indirect method should be used. In general the direct method is to be preferred and is less likely to result in serious error, although if the data fit a known distribution well the indirect method can reduce some of the random error associated with deriving the estimates.

There is often no 'natural' cut-off level since there is usually some overlap between the distribution of values for affected and unaffected individuals; moving the cut-off level to reduce the false-positive rate will automatically reduce the detection rate (see Fig. 1.2). Only if the overlap between the distributions is negligible will the cut-off level be obvious.

Sometimes it is not possible to determine the false-positive rate and the detection rate of a test directly because therapeutic intervention is automatically carried out before the disorder being screened for becomes manifest. However, indirect estimates are sometimes possible. For example, if the frequency of true-positives is likely to be much less than the frequency of false-positives (e.g. screening for avoidable perinatal death by electronic fetal monitoring) the overall positive rate (including both true- and false-positives) will be a reasonable estimate of the false-positive rate. Estimating the detection rate is, however, more difficult; if the intervention is effective, then overt cases which would otherwise occur will be prevented, falsely suggesting that the detection rate is less than it really is. There is unfortunately no completely satisfactory way of resolving the problem. One approximation is to estimate the risk of the disease in an unscreened population and also in a population which was screened and found to

---

* The alternative terms sensitivity (detection rate) and specificity (1—false-positive rate) are also used in texts on screening but, since these terms have different meanings when used in analytical biochemistry, we have avoided them. An advantage in using the term false-positive is that it focuses attention on the group that will be offered medical intervention. Also changes in the false-positive rate provide a better perception of the quantitative effects in screening than the corresponding change in specificity—for example, a 10% false-positive rate leads to twice the number of unaffected individuals being offered further intervention compared to a 5% false-positive rate whereas the corresponding change in specificity (from 95% to 90%) conceals this.

Table 1.1 Definition of detection rate and false-positive rate of a qualitative test

	Test Positive	Negative
Affected	a	b
Unaffected	c	d

Detection rate (sensitivity) $= \dfrac{a}{a + b}$

False-positive rate (1—specificity) $= \dfrac{c}{c + d}$

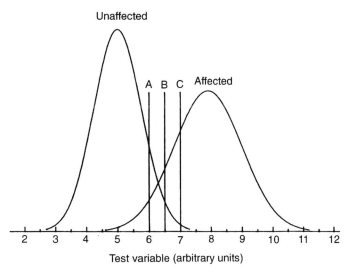

Fig. 1.2 Hypothetical example of the detection rate and false-positive rate of a screening test at three different cut-off levels, A, B, and C

Cut-off level	Detection rate (%)	False-positive rate (%)
A	96	10.0
B	90	2.5
C	79	0.5

have negative results. If these risks were r_1 and r_2 respectively, then the approximate detection rate is $(r_1 - r_2) \div r_1$. This approach does not, of course, exclude the possibility that those who are screened may be at lower risk of the disease than those not screened.

Chance that those who have positive results are affected

The second important question which needs to be asked to assess the effect of a screening test is 'what is the chance that those who have positive test results are affected?'. This can be expressed as a probability (e.g. 33 per cent if out of every three positive results one is affected) which is termed the predictive value of a positive test. The chance can also be expressed as the odds ratio of the number affected to the number unaffected among those with positive results (i.e. as an odds 1:2 in the last example).

There are two main advantages in using odds rather than probability—the calculations are simpler and, if most individuals with positive results are affected, the odds convey a better impression of the reliability of the test than the probability. For example, a new technique which increased the predictive value of a positive result from 95 to 98 per cent appears to be only a marginal improvement but the equivalent odds would be about 20:1 and 50:1 respectively—more than a doubling in the odds of being affected in those who have a positive result.

Odds of being affected in relation to test results

Those planning a screening programme need a summary estimate of the odds of being affected for all those with positive results, but when a particular individual is counselled a different estimate is required, namely the odds of being affected, given that individual's particular test result. We will consider the two calculations in turn.

(a) OVERALL ODDS OF BEING AFFECTED FOR THE GROUP OF IN-DIVIDUALS WITH POSITIVE RESULTS: The calculation involves only two steps. First, the birth prevalence is expressed as an odds ratio (e.g. prevalence of 4 per 1000 is 4:996). The next step is to apply the detection rate to the left-hand side of the ratio and apply the false-positive rate to the right-hand side of the ratio. For example, for a detection rate of 90 per cent, a false-positive rate of 2.5 per cent and a prevalence of 4:996, the new odds ratio would be $(90 \times 4):(2.5 \times 996)$ or 360:2490 which simplifies to 1:7. The calculation is equivalent to multiplying the birth prevalence expressed as an odds by the number of times the detection rate is greater than the false-positive rate (i.e. $90/2.5 \times 4:996$).

The odds of being affected, given a positive result, is critically dependent upon the prevalence of the disorder in the screened population as well as on the detection rate and false-positive rate of the test. For example, consider using the screening test in the example given above (detection rate 90 per cent and false-positive rate of 2.5 per cent) in two situations, one where the prevalence of the disorder being screened for is 10 per cent and the other where the prevalence is only 1 per cent. In the first situation the odds would be 4:1 [i.e. $(90 \times 1):(2.5 \times 9)$] and in the second the odds would be only 1:3 [i.e. $(90 \times 1):(2.5 \times 99)$].

The important influence which the prevalence of the disorder has on the odds of being affected is often not recognized. A frequent problem is that tests are introduced in centres where the disorder is more common than in the general population because of the referral of individuals suspected of having the disorder. In such situations the odds of being affected may be acceptably high, but the results will be less impressive in the community as a whole where the prevalence is lower. The problem is avoided by indicating the detection rate and the false-positive rate of a test and then indicating separately an estimate of the prevalence of the disorder in the area where the test will be used. These three figures can then easily be used together to calculate the appropriate odds of being affected given a positive result in the way we have described.

(b) ODDS OF BEING AFFECTED FOR AN INDIVIDUAL WITH A PARTIC-ULAR TEST RESULT: This calculation is similar to the one above except that the percentage of affected and unaffected individuals with the particular test result replace the detection rate and the false-positive rate. However, even in the largest studies the number of affected and unaffected individuals with any particular test result is likely to be very small, and it is usually not possible to perform the calculation directly. An indirect approach is therefore necessary, and this can be done by fitting a known statistical frequency distribution to the data.

If, as in Fig. 1.3 we wish to determine how many times greater the percentage of affected individuals is than the percentage of unaffected individuals for the arbitrary value of 6.75, this is given by the ratio of the heights of the distribution curves for affected and unaffected individuals respectively at that value (the likelihood ratio), i.e. y_2/y_1. Estimates of y_1 and y_2 can easily be calculated using the equation for the Gaussian distribution (see Appendix 2, p. 20).

The odds of being affected for an individual with a particular test result will usually be much less than the average odds of being affected for individuals with test results equal to or greater than the particular result. Both may need to be considered when deciding where to place a cut-off level. A possible but rather arbitrary approach might be to place it so that no-one with a positive test will have a risk of being affected which is less than, say, the risk of fetal loss due to amniocentesis, if this is the procedure which is to follow a positive result. As a rule of thumb, the risk of an individual being affected is equal to the background prevalence at the point where the relative frequency distributions for affected and unaffected individuals intersect—i.e. where the value of y_2/y_1 is exactly one. Thus, in Fig. 1.3 individuals with a test result of 6.25 have a risk of being affected which is exactly equal to the risk in the population as a whole.

When to screen

The extent of discrimination between affected and unaffected individuals provided by the test may vary according to when in pregnancy the test is done, or in the case of a

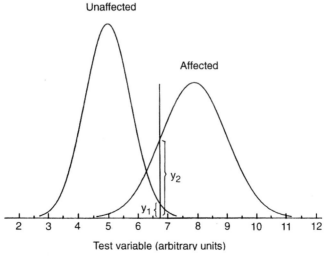

Fig. 1.3 Hypothetical relative frequency distribution of a screening test variable in affected and unaffected individuals. The likelihood ratio (y_2/y_1) for being affected at exactly 6.75 units is 5.4.

neonatal test, according to the time after birth. From the point of view of the screening test alone the optimal time to screen would be when the distributions of test results for affected and unaffected individuals had the smallest overlap. In practice though, other factors will be involved. For example, the optimal time to perform the secondary or diagnostic tests may be earlier than the optimal screening time. In such cases the best time to screen would be when the product of the false-positive rates for the various tests was minimized in relation to the product of the detection rates. Alternatively, it could be argued that it is more important to maximize the discrimination of the diagnostic test where an error might be considered less acceptable than one caused by the screening test. The timing of the test will, of course, also be influenced by the need to act on a positive result in good time, e.g. if pregnancy is to be terminated.

Other considerations applicable to tests involving quantitative measurement

Many different types of test involve quantitative measurement, such as the biochemical assay of a protein, the determination of maternal weight or estimating the biparietal diameter of a fetal skull. For simplicity the following description will relate principally to biochemical assay, but the arguments also apply to other sorts of quantitative measurement.

Estimating sources of error and other variation

The variance of screening values among unaffected and affected individuals is unlikely to be fixed, so that the discrimination between the two groups can be increased by reducing their variances. This could be achieved, for example, by performing repeat tests to reduce random measurement error and the effect of within-person fluctuations. In order to assess whether such policies are worthwhile it is necessary to know how much measurement error and within-person fluctuations contribute to the total variance of results (see, for example pp. 73–4). Another approach is to take account of specific biological factors, such as body weight, which contribute to the variance.

Random measurement error

Random measurement error (imprecision or lack of reproducibility) can be estimated by measuring the same sample in many analytical runs and calculating the variance. Ideally the specimens should be treated in the same way as those from screened individuals and the person performing the assay should not be able to identify them.

The degree of precision required of a test cannot be judged from an examination of its assay performance alone. The assay may be imprecise, producing results of, say, 10, 100, 80, 300, 82, 120, and 13 (in some arbitrary units) when a single specimen is tested on different occasions, but if unaffected individuals had values in the range 0–500 and affected ones in the range 10 000–100 000, the imprecision would be unimportant.

Within-person fluctuations

This component of variability due to the value of a screening variable changing over time in a given individual can be estimated by obtaining values for several samples taken from each of a group of individuals. (It should be noted that the variance of such values also includes a component due to assay imprecision, and an estimate of this needs to be subtracted in order to estimate the 'pure' within-person component.) The samples should be collected over the same interval of time as that over which repeat sampling would typically take place. It is important that the second and subsequent samples should not have been collected because the first yielded an extreme result. Because repeat sampling after obtaining extreme values will tend to yield less outlying ones (regression to the mean) the erroneous inclusion of these individuals would exaggerate the estimate of variance due to within-person fluctuations.

Repeat testing policies

It is often necessary to estimate the value of performing additional tests on freshly collected samples and deciding which groups should have such repeat tests. Should everyone have repeat tests or just those with positive tests? Should the second test alone be used, or the average of the two? Should a different cut-off level be adopted for the second test? These questions can be answered if (i) the components of variance due to assay imprecision and within-person fluctuations are known together with the parameters (mean and standard deviation) of the distributions of values for affected and unaffected individuals; and (ii) the overall distributions of results and the distribution of errors and fluctuations can be adequately described by a known statistical frequency distribution. Details of how this is done are outlined in Appendix 3.

Biological factors

If the values obtained in the screening test can be related to one or more biological factors it may be necessary to take account of these factors in the interpretation of results and so reduce the variance of screening results. An example comes from AFP screening, where maternal serum AFP levels increase by about 17 per cent a week in the second trimester of pregnancy. The distribution of values for affected and unaffected individuals should therefore be derived separately at each gestational week or period during which the test is to be performed.

Allowing for a biological factor may decrease the screening false-positive rate by reducing the contribution which that factor makes to the total variance of the screening test, but it is quite possible for this to be at the expense of a reduction in the detection rate. This will happen if affected individuals differ from unaffected ones with respect to this factor, and if adjusting for it will bring the distribution of values for the two groups closer together.

Judging the performance of a screening test

The performance of a screening test depends on the cut-off level chosen. Since the total number of positive results is principally determined by the cut-off level, the choice of cut-off level will be influenced by the resources which can be made available for the further investigation of individuals with positive results. The cut-off level also determines the chance of being affected for individuals with positive results and this should be chosen so that the odds of being affected if the result if above the cut-off level is high enough to justify further tests or procedures, some of which may be hazardous. Such decisions require value judgements and it is therefore impossible to produce a single formula suitable for choosing a cut-off level. Any choice will be a compromise based on several considerations, only some of which can be quantitatively measured.

After a cut-off level has been selected the performance of a test can be assessed quantitatively in terms of the detection rate and the false-positive rate and also when applied to a particular population, in terms of the odds of being affected given a positive result. It is not possible to specify a range of values for these three measures of test performance within which all screening tests might be regarded as worthwhile, because other relevant considerations need to be taken into account, such as the importance of preventing the abnormality and the cost involved in doing so. While it is relatively straightforward to specify how to estimate the performance of a test, it is impossible to lay down rules which will enable one to judge whether a particular test is worthwhile.

SUBSEQUENT SCREENING AND DIAGNOSTIC TESTS

The effectiveness of a screening programme will be determined by the detection rate and false-positive rate of all the individual screening and diagnostic tests. The same care is needed to estimate the detection rate and the false-positive rate for the subsequent tests as for the original test. The best way to proceed is to construct a 'flow diagram' in which a large number of individuals, say, 100 000, are screened. Figure 1.4 is such a diagram for a hypothetical screening programme. The first screening test has a detection rate of 90 per cent and a false-positive rate of 5 per cent. These rates are applied to a population where the birth prevalence of the defect in question is 2 per 1000. The second screening test has a detection rate of 95 per cent but the false-positive rate is 45 per cent, while the corresponding figures for the diagnostic test are 99 and 0.5 per cent respectively. From Fig. 1.4 the detection rate of both screening tests taken together is 86 per cent (171/200) and the false-positive rate is 2.3 per cent (2245/99 800). The odds of being affected in the group undergoing the diagnostic test is 1:13 (i.e. 171:2245). The overall detection rate is 85 per cent (169/200) and the overall false-positive rate 0.01 per cent (11/99 800). The odds of being affected given a positive diagnosis is 15:1 (169:11).

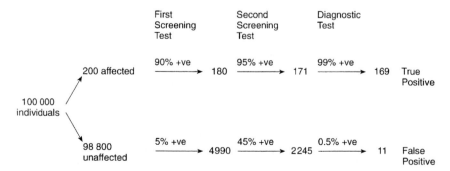

Fig. 1.4 Hypothetical flow diagram used to estimate the consequences of a screening programme.

In constructing the flow diagram shown in Fig. 1.4, we have assumed that each of the three tests provides independent information on the risk of being affected. It is important to be sure that this is a reasonably valid assumption to make. Ideally it should be investigated directly by checking that the detection rate and false-positive rate of a given test are not influenced by whether a prior test is positive or not. It is not always feasible to investigate a sequence of tests in this way because the data can soon become very sparse. In this event an indirect approach can be used to see whether the individual results of a first and second test show any sign of being correlated, either among affected individuals or among unaffected ones. If there is no sign of a correlation the tests can, in practice, be regarded as independent and combined in the way shown in Fig. 1.4. When there is any suggestion of substantial correlation, however, account must be taken of this. The degree of extra discrimination can be calculated by a generalization of the method for repeat testing given in Appendix 2.

Subsequent screening tests which are performed on those with positive first screening tests decrease the false-positive rate, but this will always be at the cost of a loss in detection. No new true positives can be generated, but some true positives will be reclassified as negative. It is possible that the apparent gain from using an additional test might be illusory, since the same final discrimination between affected and unaffected individuals might have been achieved simply by changing the cut-off level of the first test.

MONITORING

The discriminating ability of the test, the prevalence of the disorder, and other factors may change over time. As experience with a screening procedure increases, fewer random measurement errors are likely to occur. This improvement in precision means that the distribution of values in both unaffected and affected individuals will become contracted. Such contractions of the distribution can affect the detection rate and the false-positive rate in various ways. Figure 1.5 illustrates three situations using a fixed cut-off level, where the detection rate is (i) less than 50 per cent, (ii) exactly 50 per cent, and (iii) greater than 50 per cent. In all cases shown, increased precision will lead to a decrease in the false-positive rate, but only in case (iii) is the detection rate increased; in case (i) it is decreased, and in case (ii) it is unchanged.

Changes in the prevalence of a particular disorder are often difficult to monitor once screening has begun since the process of screening may itself influence the prevalence. This is especially so if the consequence of a positive screening test is termination of pregnancy.

The natural history of the disease may also change because of the introduction of new treatments or interventions. If more infants with congenital malformations are actively treated the proportion with severe handicap may increase. On the other hand, as in the case of spina bifida, policies of non-intervention have reduced the numbers of handicapped survivors.

All these possible changes mean that it is necessary to monitor screening programmes effectively so that they can be modified, or if the disorder becomes less serious or much rarer, even abandoned.

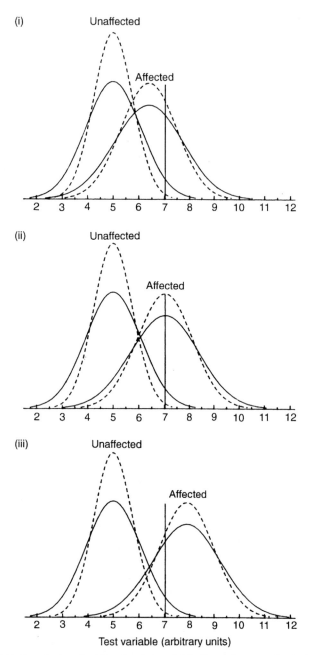

Fig. 1.5 Hypothetical examples of relative frequency distributions of a screening test variable in affected and unaffected individuals showing the influence of assay precision on the detection rate and false-positive rate, and how this depends on the relationship between the cut-off level and the distributions. The continuous lines represent the distributions of values associated with the imprecise assay; the interrupted lines are those associated with the precise assay.

COSTS AND BENEFITS

The large scale on which population screening is likely to be carried out means that the total cost can be high even if the cost per individual screened is only small. Because of this, screening raises the question of priorities more acutely than is the case with many other medical procedures and emphasizes the need to estimate the cost-effectiveness of a screening programme. This is conveniently done by drawing up a balance sheet of the financial costs of screening (including the costs of subsequent intervention) and the consequent savings arising from not having to treat affected cases. It is also sometimes helpful to see the results of a well reasoned cost–benefit analysis, which differs from an estimate of cost-effectiveness in that an attempt is made to place a value on the non-financial benefits.

There are, however, problems with cost–benefit analyses. They are usually based on broad assumptions and therefore need to be interpreted critically and cautiously. A cost–benefit analysis is only one method which can assist making a value judgement on whether a particular course of action should be taken.

CONCLUSION

Nine requirements for a worthwhile screening programme are summarized in Table 1.2. The first three relate to the disorder, its prevalence, and its natural history. The next five ensure that certain financial and ethical prerequisites will be fulfilled. Information on the overlap of test values from affected and unaffected individuals is necessary to determine detection rates and false-positive rates which, together with data on prevalence, permit the estimation of the risk of being affected. This information is also needed for subsequent screening or diagnostic tests with the additional requirement that the degree of independence between the different tests is known. While not a prerequisite for the introduction of a screening programme, the ability to monitor it simply and cheaply is important so that decisions can be made regarding the conduct or even the continuance of the programme. The purpose of these requirements is that screening should be carried out on the basis of quantitative considerations with adequate knowledge of the consequences.

APPENDIX 1: ESTIMATING THE DETECTION AND FALSE-POSITIVE RATES FOR FITTED KNOWN FREQUENCY DISTRIBUTIONS

The method will be demonstrated using the example illustrated in Fig. 1.2. The distribution of values for unaffected and affected individuals are both Gaussian with means of 5.00 and 7.90 and standard deviations of 0.77 and 1.09 respectively. The disorder concerned has a birth prevalence of 5 per 1000. We want to estimate the detection and false-positive rates for the cut-off level A which has a value of 6.0.

A is $\frac{6.0 - 7.90}{1.09}$ or -1.74 standard deviations from the mean for affected individuals. From tables of the Gaussian distribution the area to the right of this cut-off level is 96 per cent of the whole area under the curve for affected individuals. This is our estimate of the detection rate.

Table 1.2   Requirements for a worthwhile screening programme

Aspect	Requirement
1. Disorder	Well defined
2. Prevalence	Known
3. Natural history	Medically important disorder for which there is an effective remedy available
4. Financial	Cost-effective
5. Facilities	Available or easily installed
6. Acceptability	Procedures following a positive result are generally agreed and acceptable both to the screening authorities and to the patients
7. Equity	Equal access to screening services
8. Test	Simple and safe
9. Test performance	Distributions of test values in affected and unaffected individuals known, extent of overlap sufficiently small, and a suitable cut-off level defined

A is $\frac{6.0 - 5.0}{0.77}$, or 1.30 standard deviations from the mean for unaffected individuals. The area to the right of this cut-off level is 10 per cent of the whole area under the curve for unaffected individuals. This is our estimate of the false-positive rate.

APPENDIX 2: ESTIMATING THE ODDS OF BEING AFFECTED FOR AN INDIVIDUAL WITH A PARTICULAR TEST RESULT

The method will be demonstrated using the example illustrated in Fig. 1.3. The means and standard deviations are the same as those given in Appendix 1 for Fig. 1.2. The disorder concerned has a birth prevalence of 5 per 1000. We want to estimate the odds of being affected for an individual with a value of 6.75.

The equation of a Gaussian distribution is

$$y = \frac{1}{s\sqrt{(2\pi)}} \cdot e^{-\frac{1}{2}\left(\frac{x-m}{s}\right)^2}$$

where y is the height of the distribution for a given value, x, of the test variable; m is the mean and s the standard deviation.

$$\text{NB } e^{-\frac{1}{2}\left(\frac{x-m}{s}\right)^2} \equiv \text{antilog}_e\left[-\frac{1}{2}\left(\frac{x-m}{s}\right)^2\right]$$

Therefore, referring to Fig. 1.3

$$y_1 = \frac{1}{0.77\sqrt{6.28}} \cdot e^{-\frac{1}{2}\left(\frac{6.75-5.00}{0.77}\right)^2} = 0.0392$$

$$y_2 = \frac{1}{1.09\sqrt{6.28}} \cdot e^{-\frac{1}{2}\left(\frac{6.75-7.90}{1.09}\right)^2} = 0.2098$$

$$\frac{y_2}{y_1} = \frac{0.2098}{0.0392} = 5.35.$$

The birth prevalence is 5/1000 or 5:995.

The odds of being affected for an individual with a test result of 6.75 is therefore $(5.35 \times 5):(995)$ or about 1:37, equivalent to about 3 per cent.

APPENDIX 3: ESTIMATING THE EFFECT OF REPEAT TESTING

Prepared in collaboration with Julian Peto.

The effect on the detection rate and false-positive rate of repeat testing using a freshly collected sample is easy to estimate when every person has a repeat test and the average of the two values for each person is used. The components of variance due to assay imprecision and within-person fluctuations would be halved. If these components are known together with the total observed variance for affected and unaffected individuals, the new detection rate and false-positive rate of the test can be estimated from the Gaussian distributions for affected and unaffected subjects with the variance accordingly reduced. (This assumes the data satisfactorily fit the Gaussian distribution—if not, another distribution may need to be selected but the methods we outline here can still be applied using the alternative distribution instead of the Gaussian.)

The value of performing a second test will depend mainly on the extent of the association between the first and second tests. If the association is strong (e.g. the correlation coefficient, $r = 0.8$) a high (or low) first value will invariably be followed by a relatively high (or low) second value and the benefit of doing repeat tests will be small. If the association is weak (e.g. $r = 0.3$) a high (or low) first value will more often be followed by a relatively low (or high) second one (the effect of 'regression to the mean' will be more marked for a weak association and the value of doing repeat tests will be greater). The correlation coefficient between the first and second tests can be estimated using simple linear regression analysis. It can also be estimated by an analysis of variance. For example, if 30 per cent of the normal variance of a test variable is due to assay imprecision and within-person fluctuations then the remaining proportion (70 per cent) is the value of r^2 for the correlation between two sequential tests on the same person, so in this example r equals $\sqrt{0.70}$ or 0.84. (If there were no assay imprecision and no within-person fluctuations an individual's results would all be identical and r would be equal to 1.)

The value of performing second tests on only those who have high (or low) values for the first test can also be estimated. The proportion of individuals with a given first test result whose repeat tests yield results above a specified cut-off level is dependent on both r and the original result. For a bivariate Gaussian distribution with the same mean, m, and standard deviations, s, for both variates, the conditional distribution of the second variate, when the first equals x, is Gaussian with mean $\{m + r.(x-m)\}$ and standard deviation $s.\sqrt{(1-r^2)}$. Suppose, for example, that the correlation coefficient, r, between repeated tests is 0.8 and the standard deviation is 10 units. A group of individuals whose first test result is, say, 30 units above the mean will have on average, second results of 24 units (30×0.8) above the mean, and the second results will have a standard deviation of 6 units $[10.\sqrt{(1-0.8^2)}]$. From these parameters the proportion above a given cut-off level can be estimated using tables of the Gaussian distribution. To estimate the proportion of individuals with first results equal to or greater than a given cut-off level who also have as high repeat test results, it is necessary to perform this calculation repeatedly for increasing levels (numerical integration) taking account of the probability of being at each level. In practice this will be done by computer and a fuller treatment of the method is given in reference 5.

REFERENCES

1. Thorner, R.M. and Remein, Q.R. Principles and procedures in the evaluation of screening for disease. *Public Health Monograph* No. 67. US Department of Health Education and Welfare. Public Health Service Publication No. 846 (1961).
2. McKeown, T. Validation of screening procedures. In *Screening in medical care. Reviewing the evidence*. The Nuffield Provincial Hospital Trust, Oxford University Press (1968).
3. Cochrane, A.L. and Holland, W.W. Validation of screening procedures. *Br. Med. Bull.* **27**, 3 (1971).
4. Wilson, J.M.C. and Jungner, G. Principles and practice of screening for disease. *Publ. Hlth Pap. WHO* No. 34 (1968).
5. Fourth Report of the UK Collaborative Study on Alpha-fetoprotein in relation to neural tube defects. Estimating an individual's risk of having a fetus with open spina bifida and the value of repeat alpha-fetoprotein testing. *J. Epidemiol. Community Health* **36**, 87–95 (1982).

2 *Tests using multiple markers*

Nicholas Wald and Allan Hackshaw

INTRODUCTION

The previous chapter describes screening using a test that is based on the measurement of a single continuous variable. This chapter describes screening using a test that is based on the measurement of several continuous variables (also called markers) used simultaneously. We also cover various points on data handling that apply to tests based on one or more markers.

When more than one screening marker is measured the results of each measurement can be interpreted either in sequence or simultaneously. Interpreting measurements in sequence, so that individuals with positive first test results proceed to the next test, is only practical if the subsequent test has a very high detection rate, so that an individual identified as positive using an initial screening test will almost never become a false-negative as a result of the subsequent test. This is a severe limitation that can be avoided if all persons have both measurements interpreted simultaneously as a single test. Doing so would also maximize the detection rate for a specified false-positive rate.

MULTIVARIATE SCREENING: PRINCIPLES OF COMBINING SIMULTANEOUS MEASUREMENTS

In antenatal screening for open spina bifida by means of maternal serum alphafetoprotein (AFP) measurement, it is necessary only to identify an AFP cut-off level to define positive and negative results. If two or more markers are to be used simultaneously, such as AFP and unconjugated oestriol (uE_3) in screening for Down's syndrome, a method is needed to combine information from all the markers. This cannot be done while retaining the original units. They are not directly comparable insofar as a unit of uE_3 is not the same as a unit of AFP in predicting the presence of Down's syndrome. A common 'currency' is needed, and this is provided by the 'likelihood ratio'— a measure of the increased risk of having a disorder given a particular test result. Likelihood ratios for different *independent* markers (that is, where the value of one marker is unrelated to the value of another marker considered separately for affected and unaffected individuals) can be multiplied together and applied to the background risk to yield a test-specific risk of having the disorder for which the person is being tested. If they are not independent, a single likelihood ratio can still be calculated which allows for the correlations between them. The risk estimate itself then becomes the screening variable and a risk cut-off level can be used to determine screen-positive and screen-negative status in the same way as with single screening variables such as serum AFP in screening for open spina bifida.

'Risk' is here defined as the chance that an event will occur. Risk can be expressed numerically either as an odds $(1:n)$ or as a probability $(1/1 + n)$, where n is the number of unaffected individuals for every one affected individual. If the risk is low, it is of little practical consequence which is used because they are numerically similar (for example, $1:1000 = 1/1001$ which is approximately equal to $1/1000$) but if the risk is high, it is important to make the distinction (for example, $1:2 = 1/3$, which is very different from $1/2$).

In the previous chapter it was shown that the likelihood ratio (LR) for an individual is the ratio of the heights of the Gaussian distributions for affected and unaffected individuals at a particular value for a screening variable (see Fig. 1.3). If the background risk of the disorder is $1:n$ then the risk, given a test value of a, is $LR_a \times 1:n$ where LR_a is the likelihood ratio corresponding to a marker value of a.

In combining several markers into a single screening test it is necessary to see if they are independent predictors of the disorder of interest and, if not, to measure the correlations between them. Two screening markers, A and B, are independent of each other if there is no correlation between them among either affected or unaffected individuals. Figure 2.1 illustrates the importance of assessing correlations separately for individuals with and without the disorder. In the scatter plot, A and B are independent predictors of a disorder but if the presence or absence of the disorder were ignored, there would, of course, be an association because both A and B tend to be

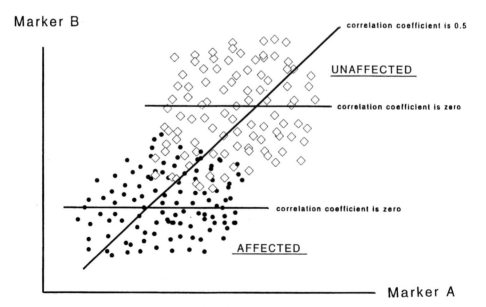

Fig. 2.1   The correlation between two markers calculated separately for affected (solid circles) and unaffected (open diamonds) individuals and over all individuals.

low in subjects with the disorder. The same would be true if A and B tended to be high in affected individuals, or one were high and the other low. If the correlations between A and B among affected and unaffected individuals were perfect (correlation coefficient of 1), then one effectively duplicates the other and no further information about the risk of the disorder is obtained using both instead of one. If A and B were independent (that is, with correlation coefficients of zero in affected and in unaffected individuals), the combined likelihood ratio relating to a given value *a* (for marker A) and a given value *b* (for marker B) is simply the product of the likelihood ratios corresponding to the values *a* and *b*. The combined likelihood ratio multiplied by the prevalence of the disorder expressed as an odds is the test-specific risk of having the disorder.

For example, if the prevalence of the disorder were 1:100 and the likelihood ratio for marker A at value *a* were 4, and the likelihood ratio for marker B at value *b* were 5 then the test-specific risk would be $(4 \times 5) \times 1{:}100$ or 20:100 which simplifies to 1:5. In practice the two screening markers are rarely completely independent; more severe cases of the disorder are likely to be associated with more extreme values for both of the markers. For example, in both Down's syndrome pregnancies and unaffected pregnancies, there is a degree of correlation between AFP and uE_3: the correlation coefficient is approximately 0.28 for each type of pregnancy. When two markers are related, the degree of dependence must be allowed for when calculating the likelihood ratio by looking at the *joint distribution* between the two.

The derivation of the joint distributions of the two markers is straightforward. Antenatal screening for Down's syndrome using the serum markers, AFP and uE_3, can illustrate the method. If AFP and uE_3 are each divided into, say, 10 groups according to concentration, we can derive a grid of 100 (10×10) cells in which each 'cell' contains the frequency or proportion of Down's syndrome pregnancies that has a particular combination of AFP and uE_3 results; a similar procedure is performed for unaffected pregnancies (Fig. 2.2). The likelihood ratio for a specified combination of AFP and uE_3 is then estimated from the ratio of the frequency of Down's syndrome and unaffected pregnancies in that cell. For example, a woman with an AFP level of 0.4 MoM (the fourth AFP group in Fig 2.2) and a uE_3 level of 0.6 MoM (the fourth uE_3 group) would have a likelihood ratio of 6 (36/6).

If a third marker is to be used, such as hCG (again divided into, say, 10 groups), each cell in Fig. 2.2 can be divided into 10 hCG groups. There are now effectively 10 (AFP) $\times$ 10 (uE_3) $\times$ 10 (hCG) cells or a total of 1000 cells for the Down's syndrome pregnancies and 1000 cells for the unaffected pregnancies.

In practice, a very large amount of data would be required to produce cells which contain enough observations to derive robust likelihood ratios by observation. This is avoided by using a model which estimates the numbers in each of these cells. With one marker, it is usually possible to fit a Gaussian distribution to the frequency distribution. This can also be done with two or more markers, using a *multivariate* Gaussian distribution (described in Appendix 1). Provided the data fit the model, the model can be used to estimate the frequencies in each cell. If many markers are used, however, it can be difficult to judge how well the data fit the model for extreme combinations of test values, because there are too few data points against which to compare observed and expected frequencies.

Down's syndrome pregnancies

AFP (MoM)	uE₃ (MoM) 1 ≤0.33	2 0.34-0.41	3 0.42-0.53	4 0.54-0.67	5 0.68-0.85	6 0.86-1.08	7 1.09-1.37	8 1.38-1.75	9 1.76-2.22	10 ≥2.23	Total
1 ≤0.23	1	0	3	3	0	0	0	0	0	0	7
2 0.24-0.29	1	1	3	8	2	4	0	0	0	0	19
3 0.30-0.37	5	3	6	13	22	5	1	1	0	0	56
4 0.36-0.47	2	5	23	36	32	5	10	2	0	0	115
5 0.48-0.60	1	8	36	35	43	19	8	4	1	0	155
6 0.61-0.76	5	13	22	50	59	41	19	6	0	0	215
7 0.77-0.97	1	8	28	59	57	40	22	2	2	0	179
8 0.98-1.23	0	3	14	31	36	25	9	8	0	0	126
9 1.24-1.56	0	1	1	15	22	24	14	6	4	0	87
10 ≥1.57	0	0	1	4	13	10	8	4	0	1	41
Total	16	42	137	234	266	173	91	33	7	1	1000

Unaffected pregnancies

AFP (MoM)	uE₃ (MoM)										Total
	1 ≤0.33	2 0.34-0.41	3 0.42-0.53	4 0.54-0.67	5 0.68-0.85	6 0.86-1.08	7 1.09-1.37	8 1.38-1.75	9 1.76-2.22	10 ≥2.23	
1 ≤0.23	0	0	0	0	0	0	0	0	0	0	
2 0.24-0.29	0	0	0	0	2	0	0	1	0	0	3
3 0.30-0.37	0	0	0	3	4	4	2	0	0	0	13
4 0.36-0.47	0	0	0	6	12	6	11	3	0	0	38
5 0.48-0.60	0	1	6	12	19	19	16	8	1	0	82
6 0.61-0.76	0	1	4	15	36	45	22	12	1	1	137
7 0.77-0.97	0	1	3	21	43	47	34	21	9	0	179
8 0.98-1.23	0	0	3	18	40	65	51	19	9	5	210
9 1.24-1.56	0	0	3	13	25	37	33	27	10	5	153
10 ≥1.57	0	1	1	3	27	49	52	33	18	1	185
Total	0	4	20	91	208	272	221	124	48	12	1000

For the fourth AFP group and fourth uE₃ group (as indicated by the bold cell outlines) the likelihood ratio is 36/6 = 6

Fig. 2.2 The joint distributions of AFP and uE₃ in 1000 Down's syndrome pregnancies and 1000 unaffected pregnancies. The range of AFP (on a log scale) has been divided into 10 groups of equal width; similarly for uE₃. Cells which contain 35 or more individuals have been highlighted to indicate where the larger proportion of the data lie (namely around the mean).

DEFINING THE STARTING RISK IN SCREENING USING MULTIPLE MARKERS

When screening is based on using several markers simultaneously, the principle is to start with an initial risk and then modify this on the basis of a combined likelihood ratio which incorporates the information from the various screening markers used. The starting risk is usually the prevalence of the disorder in the population being screened, for example, 1.3 per 1000 births for Down's syndrome for pregnant women in general, or the age-specific risk, say 1:900 at age 30.

ESTIMATING DETECTION RATES AND FALSE-POSITIVE RATES USING ANTENATAL SCREENING FOR DOWN'S SYNDROME AS AN EXAMPLE

The principle of estimating detection and false-positive rates is to 'generate' a large hypothetical population of women and, using the birth prevalence of the disorder and the distribution of the markers, allocate the appropriate numbers of affected and unaffected pregnancies to the various marker combination specific 'cells'. Each cell has a specific risk given by the numbers of affected and unaffected pregnancies in that cell. The number of affected pregnancies that exceed a specified risk cut-off (say, 1 in 250) can then be counted and expressed as a proportion of all affected pregnancies to give the detection rate. Similarly, the number of unaffected pregnancies that exceed the risk cut-off can be counted and expressed as a proportion of all unaffected pregnancies to give the false-positive rate. The method is valid if a woman's serum marker level is not materially affected by her age (that is, for example, age and AFP are independent of each other). In antenatal screening for Down's syndrome, maternal age-specific sets of marker cells are generated using published data on the age-specific prevalence of Down's syndrome and the age-specific distribution of pregnant women.

The procedure is illustrated in detail as follows, using maternal age and AFP in screening for Down's syndrome.

1. We first assume that we have a large hypothetical population of pregnant women aged 15–55 years, say 5 million. The number of affected and unaffected pregnancies at each age resulting in a livebirth can be estimated using the age distribution of births for a specified population and the age-specific risk. Table 2.1 illustrates this. We use the age distribution of births for England and Wales[1] to estimate the proportion of pregnancies at each age and apply this to our figure of 5 million. The age-specific risk of having an affected birth (expressed as an odds)[2] applied to the total number of births at each age gives the expected number of Down's syndrome births. By summing all the affected pregnancies estimated in this way there would be an expected birth prevalence of 1.3 per 1000.

2. Using the means and standard deviations of serum AFP obtained from a sample of Down's syndrome and unaffected pregnancies,[3] we can derive the distribution of AFP (Fig. 2.3(a)). The whole range of AFP values (on a log scale) is divided into a number of groups of equal width. For illustration, we have divided the range into 10 groups only, although in practice about 30 groups are used.

Table 2.1 Estimation of the number of Down's syndrome and unaffected pregnancies in 5 million pregnancies according to maternal age

Maternal age (years)	Percentage of births[1] (a)	Number of births[2] (b)	Age-specific risk[3] (1:c)	Number of pregnancies Down's syndrome $d = ([1/(c + 1)] \times b)$	Unaffected (b − d)
15	0.17	8418	1:1578	5	8413
16	0.66	32 993	1:1572	21	32 972
17	1.60	79 954	1:1565	51	79 903
18	2.60	129 824	1:1556	83	129 741
19	3.57	178 391	1:1544	115	178 276
20	4.33	216 512	1:1528	142	216 370
21	5.15	257 345	1:1507	171	257 174
22	5.92	295 813	1:1481	200	295 613
23	6.57	328 468	1:1447	227	328 241
24	7.07	353 652	1:1404	252	353 400
25	7.38	369 184	1:1351	273	368 911
26	7.40	369 839	1:1286	287	369 552
27	7.15	357 617	1:1208	296	357 321
28	6.69	334 448	1:1119	299	334 149
29	6.09	304 501	1:1018	299	304 202
30	5.43	271 631	1:909	298	271 333
31	4.61	230 294	1:796	289	230 005
32	3.85	192 387	1:683	281	192 106
33	3.17	158 387	1:574	275	158 112
34	2.60	129 815	1:474	273	129 542
35	2.11	105 658	1:384	274	105 384
36	1.69	84 269	1:307	274	83 995
37	1.32	66 161	1:242	272	65 889
38	0.98	49 149	1:189	259	48 890
39	0.70	34 975	1:146	238	34 737
40	0.48	24 021	1:112	213	23 808
41	0.30	14 973	1:85	174	14 799
42	0.18	8962	1:65	136	8826
43	0.10	5145	1:49	103	5042
44	0.06	3034	1:37	80	2954
45	0.03	1598	1:28	55	1543
46	0.02	921	1:21	42	879
47	0.01	535	1:15	34	501
48	0.01	380	1:11	32	348
49	<0.01	230	1:8	26	204
50	<0.01	159	1:6	23	136
51	<0.01	113	1:4	23	90
52	<0.01	87	1:3	22	65
53	<0.01	59	1:2	20	39
54	<0.01	40	1:1	21	19
55	<0.01	58	1:1	30	28
Total	100.00	5 million	1:770	6488	4 993 512

1. Estimated using OPCS Birth Statistics 1984–88[1] and rounded to two decimal places.
2. b = a (without rounding) × 5 million.
3. The odds of having an affected birth for a given maternal age.[2]

3. In each AFP group, the area under the curve for Down's syndrome represents the proportion of all affected pregnancies in that group and can be obtained from statistical Gaussian tables. This is illustrated using, as an example, the fourth group (see Fig. 2.3(b)). The fourth group has −0.4200 and −0.2456 (AFP log MoM) as the boundaries. For the distribution of Down's syndrome pregnancies, the number of standard deviations from the mean (usually called z-values) corresponding to these boundaries are

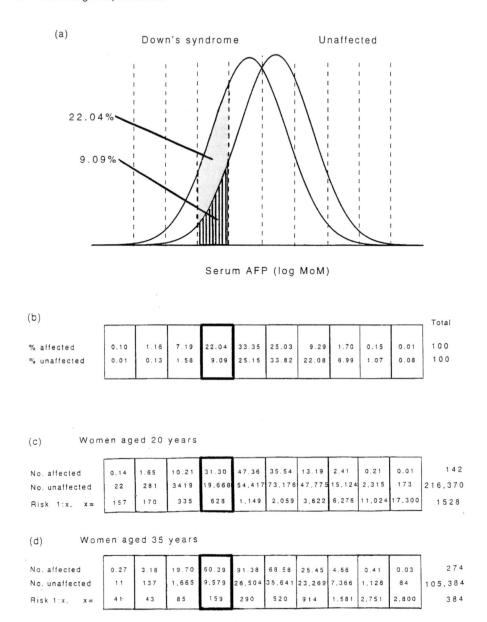

Fig. 2.3 Calculation of risk using maternal age and AFP: (a) the distribution of AFP in affected and unaffected pregnancies, (b) the proportion of pregnancies in each AFP group, (c) and (d) the number of pregnancies and corresponding risk according to AFP group in women aged 20 years and 35 years respectively.

−1.376 (calculated as $[-0.4200-(-0.1427)]/0.2015$) and −0.511 (calculated as $[-0.2456-(-0.1427)]/0.2015$) respectively, where −0.1427 and 0.2015 are the mean and standard deviation, respectively, of AFP (log MoM) in Down's syndrome pregnancies. From statistical tables, the proportion of Down's syndrome pregnancies that would be expected to lie below these z-values are 30.47 per cent and 8.43 per cent respectively, and so the estimated proportion *within* this AFP group is 22.04 per cent (30.47–8.43 per cent). Similarly, the proportion of unaffected pregnancies in this group is estimated as

9.09 per cent calculated using the same boundary points but the mean and standard deviation for unaffected pregnancies (mean 0, standard deviation 0.1986) instead of those relating to affected pregnancies. The fourth group is therefore expected to contain 22.04 per cent of all affected pregnancies and 9.09 per cent of all unaffected pregnancies.

4.   The next step is to estimate the number of women (with and without an affected pregnancy) across all combinations of age and AFP by taking each year of age in turn and observing how many Down's syndrome and unaffected pregnancies are in each serum AFP group. For example, among women aged 20 years, there are an expected 142 affected pregnancies and 216 370 unaffected pregnancies (from Table 2.1). In the fourth AFP group for example (highlighted in Fig 2.3(b)) we expect 31.30 affected pregnancies (22.04 per cent of 142) and 19 668 unaffected pregnancies (9.09 per cent of 216 370) as shown in Fig. 2.3(c). The risk of having an affected pregnancy in this group (that is, women aged 20 years in the fourth AFP group) is 1:628, simply the ratio of the number of Down's syndrome to the number of unaffected pregnancies (31.30:19 668) (Fig 2.3(c)). In the same way, we estimate the risk at age 20 in the other nine AFP groups. The risk increases from right to left indicating the higher risk associated with low levels of AFP.

5.   Step (4) is repeated for all ages. For example, at age 35, (an expected 274 Down's syndrome and 105 384 unaffected pregnancies) there are, in the fourth serum AFP group, 60.39 Down's syndrome pregnancies (22.04 per cent of 274) and 9579 unaffected pregnancies (9.09 per cent of 105 384). The risk of Down's syndrome in these women is 1:159 (60.39:9579) (Fig. 2.3(d)).

6.   The hypothetical sample of 5 million women created in step (1) has now been divided into groups according to their age and serum AFP level and for each group the risk of having a Down's syndrome pregnancy has been estimated. In our example, there are 410 groups (10 AFP groups × 41 age groups).

7.   To estimate detection and false-positive rates we first specify a risk cut-off level, say 1:250. The detection rate is then determined by examining all the groups of women (410) and counting the number of affected pregnancies in those groups (or cells) with a risk of 1:250 or greater. For example, in women aged 35 years (Fig. 2.3(d)) there are 83.54 (0.27 + 3.18 + 19.70 + 60.39) Down's syndrome pregnancies with a reported risk of 1:250 or more. Over all ages, the total number of Down's syndrome pregnancies with a risk of 1:250 or more is 2160; the detection rate is therefore, 33 per cent (2160/6488). The false-positive rate is determined in a similar way by counting the number of unaffected pregnancies in the same groups. For example in women aged 35 years (Fig. 2.3(d)) there are 11 392 (11 + 137 + 1665 + 9579) unaffected pregnancies with a risk of 1:250 or more. The total number of unaffected pregnancies with a risk of 1:250 or more is 215 350; the false-positive rate is therefore 4.3 per cent (215 350/(5 million − 6488)).

8.   Histograms can then be derived showing the distributions of risk for Down's syndrome pregnancies and for unaffected pregnancies. The entire range of risk is divided into risk intervals (say ⩾1:49, 1:50 to 1:99, 1:100 to 1:149, and so on) and the numbers of Down's syndrome and unaffected pregnancies in each risk group are counted and expressed as percentages of the total number of affected and unaffected pregnancies, respectively. These histograms (Fig. 2.4(a)) can then be plotted as smooth curves and the detection and false-positive rates can be found for any risk cut-off level as areas under the appropriate curve (Fig. 2.4(b)).

(a) Histograms

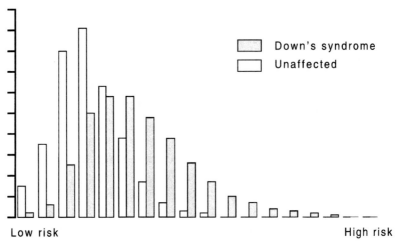

(b) Curves

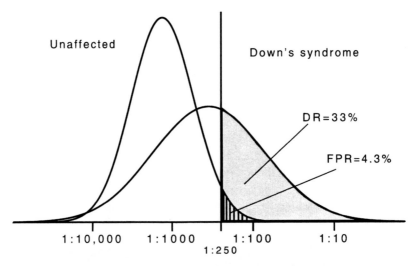

Risk of having an affected pregnancy

Fig. 2.4 Relative frequency distribution of the reported risk of having a Down's syndrome term pregnancy in affected and unaffected pregnancies: screening using maternal age and serum AFP. (DR = detection rate; FPR = false-positive rate).

Screening using maternal age with multiple markers

Estimating screening performance using more than one marker together with maternal age, (for example, the double test using AFP and total hCG) is simply an extension of step (5) above:

(a) Among, for example, women aged 35 years, it is known how the number of Down's syndrome pregnancies (274) and unaffected pregnancies (105 384) are distributed over the 10 AFP groups (Figs. 2.3(d) and 2 .5(a)).

(b) Each AFP group is taken in turn and subdivided into 10 hCG subgroups. For example, in the fourth group the 60.39 Down's syndrome and the 9579 unaffected pregnancies are allocated to each of 10 subgroups of hCG (Fig. 2.5(b)). The numbers of Down's syndrome pregnancies and unaffected pregnancies for each combination of AFP and hCG are estimated taking account of any association (quantified by the correlation coefficient) between AFP and hCG. This is done using a model called a multivariate Gaussian model. The risk in each subgroup is then calculated as before. The risk increases from left to right indicating that high hCG levels are associated with a higher risk. Carrying out this procedure for each AFP group results in 100 subgroups (10 AFP × 10 hCG) each containing the numbers of Down's syndrome and unaffected pregnancies and the corresponding risk.

(c) Step (b) is performed for each year of age (15–55). The population of women is thus divided into 4100 subgroups (41 × 10 × 10) according to all possible combinations of age (41), AFP (10), and hCG (10).

The detection and false-positive rates are found as before by specifying a risk cut-off, examining all the subgroups and counting the number of Down's syndrome and unaffected pregnancies in cells which exceed this risk cut-off.

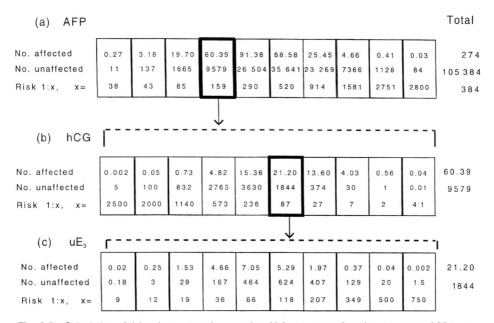

(a) AFP — Total

No. affected	0.27	3.18	19.70	60.39	91.38	68.58	25.45	4.66	0.41	0.03	274
No. unaffected	11	137	1665	9579	26 504	35 641	23 269	7366	1128	84	105 384
Risk 1:x, x=	38	43	85	159	290	520	914	1581	2751	2800	384

(b) hCG

No. affected	0.002	0.05	0.73	4.82	15.36	21.20	13.60	4.03	0.56	0.04	60.39
No. unaffected	5	100	832	2763	3630	1844	374	30	1	0.01	9579
Risk 1:x, x=	2500	2000	1140	573	236	87	27	7	2	4:1	

(c) uE₃

No. affected	0.02	0.25	1.53	4.66	7.05	5.29	1.97	0.37	0.04	0.002	21.20
No. unaffected	0.18	3	29	167	464	624	407	129	20	1.5	1844
Risk 1:x, x=	9	12	19	36	66	118	207	349	500	750	

Fig. 2.5 Calculation of risk using maternal age and multiple serum markers in women aged 35 years.

Similarly, the detection and false-positive rates for the triple test (uE_3 in addition to AFP and hCG) are estimated by counting, at each age, the number of Down's syndrome and unaffected pregnancies in *each* combination of AFP and hCG, spread over 10 groups of uE_3 (Fig. 2.5(c)). Histograms are derived, as before, and smoothed to yield overlapping risk curves relating to affected and unaffected pregnancies (Fig. 2.6). At a risk cut-off of 1:250, the detection rate is 58 per cent and the false-positive rate is 5 per cent as published.[3]

In practice, finer divisions are used to define the groups and subgroups. With the triple test, for example, 41 single-year age groups (15–55 years) are used and each serum marker is divided into about 30 groups resulting in over 1.1 million subgroups ($41 \times 30 \times 30 \times 30$). Estimation of screening performance therefore requires the use of a computer.

ALTERNATIVE METHODS OF ESTIMATING RISK AND DETERMINING DETECTION AND FALSE-POSITIVE RATES

Logistic regression

Using the multivariate Gaussian model to estimate the likelihood ratio is the method of choice when the markers are measured on a continuous scale and their underlying distribution in the population is reasonably Gaussian. This is often the case, but there are occasions when this model is not valid, for example if the data remain significantly skewed even after transformation into logarithms. Screening performance, and indeed risk, would then be incorrectly estimated if the Gaussian model were used.

An alternative approach that is not dependent on the data fitting a known distribution is to use logistic regression. This is similar to linear regression, but the dependent variable, instead of being continuous, is binary (that is, the outcome of interest is present or absent; for example, a pregnancy is either affected or unaffected) and is expressed as an odds.

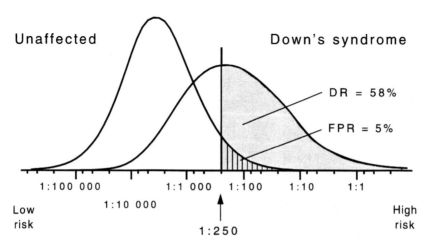

Fig. 2.6　Distribution of the reported risk of having a term Down's syndrome pregnancy in affected and unaffected pregnancies: screening using maternal age with serum AFP, uE_3, and hCG. (DR = detection rate; FPR = false-positive rate).

Figure 2.7 illustrates the principle of logistic regression using data based on 77 Down's syndrome and 385 unaffected pregnancies.[3] AFP and hCG are each divided into quintile groups based on the unaffected pregnancies alone. For each AFP group, the natural logarithm of the odds of being affected (often shortened to the 'log odds') is calculated. The log odds is useful because it provides a scale on which equal relative differences in risk are represented by equal quantities so a risk of 20:1 is as high as 1:20 is low (equivalent to plus or minus 3 on the $\log_e$ scale).

In the upper part of Fig. 2.7 the odds in the lowest quintile group are 38:77 and in the highest quintile group they are 6:77. Log odds ratios for each quintile group are calculated by taking the lowest quintile group as the reference group (odds of 1 or log odds of 0) and comparing the other quintile groups with the lowest. The log odds ratio

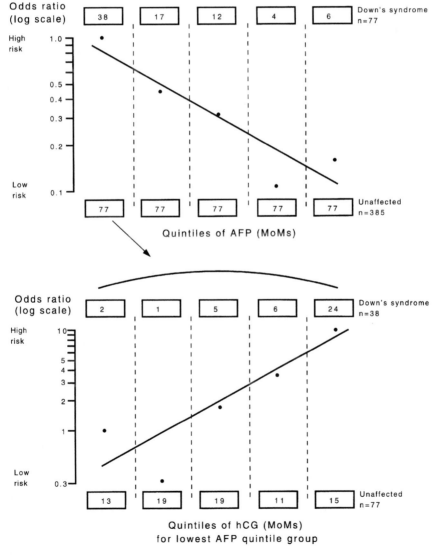

Fig. 2.7   Illustration of the principle of logistic regression.

(or the odds ratio plotted on a log scale as in Fig. 2.7) is regressed on AFP. To obtain the odds ratio for AFP and hCG together we observe how the Down's syndrome and unaffected pregnancies in each AFP group are distributed over the hCG quintile groups. The log odds ratios now take into account the effects both of AFP and hCG. A straight line is fitted to these points. For example, suppose we had the following regression model:

$$\log_e \text{ odds} = -2.773 - 5.850 \times \log_{10} \text{AFP} + 5.615 \times \log_{10} \text{hCG}$$

The regression coefficients -2.773, -5.850 and 5.615 are estimated using statistical techniques (usually performed with a computer package). So, for example, a woman with an AFP MoM of 0.75 and an hCG MoM of 1.25 would have a $\log_e$ odds of -1.50 (by substituting her $\log_{10}$ values into the above regression model), the antilog of which is approximately 0.22, that is an odds of being affected of 1:4.5 (that is, 1:1/0.22). Because the regression was based on 77 Down's syndrome pregnancies and 385 unaffected pregnancies the likelihood ratio at these AFP and hCG values is 1/4.5 $\div$ 77/385, approximately 1.11. If she were aged 30, her background risk would be 1 in 900, and so her overall risk is about 1 in 810 (1:900/likelihood ratio, 1:900/1.11).

In this simple example it is assumed that there is no correlation between AFP and hCG. In practice there is, and this is taken into account by including an 'interaction term' (AFP $\times$ hCG) so the regression model might become:

$$\log_e \text{ odds} = -2.91 - 6.98 \times \log_{10} \text{AFP} + 6.0 \times \log_{10} \text{hCG} + 5.17 \times \log_{10} \text{AFP} \times \log_{10} \text{hCG}$$

Detection rates and false-positive rates can then be calculated, as before, by defining a risk cut-off and counting the number of affected and unaffected pregnancies in a standard population that exceed this value.

These examples assume the same standard deviation for affected and unaffected pregnancies. If they differ, quadratic terms need to be included in the equations.

Empirical methods

If the result of the screening measurements were categorical (that is, not continuous) and a large dataset were available with a sufficient number of affected individuals, it would be possible to assess screening performance directly from the observed data. Risk is calculated in each category as the ratio of the proportion of affected to unaffected individuals. Again, summation of the appropriate proportions exceeding a given risk cut-off value will give detection and false-positive rates. In practice, markers used in antenatal screening are usually continuous variables that would have to be put into many small categories in order to apply this empirical method effectively. While this method has the theoretical advantage of reflecting the data directly and is not constrained by a model that relies on an underlying statistical distribution, it has the major disadvantage that it requires an impractically large amount of data to 'occupy' the necessary number of categories, particularly if there are many categories. Also, where an individual category is empty (that is, no observations for either affected or unaffected) the risk cannot be calculated. Although there are statistical techniques (which do not rely on any underlying distribution) to 'smooth' over categories in order to estimate data for empty categories, such techniques are complex and usually impractical.[4]

ADVANTAGES AND DISADVANTAGES OF THE MULTIVARIATE GAUSSIAN MODEL AND LOGISTIC REGRESSION AS METHODS OF RISK ESTIMATION

An advantage of using the multivariate Gaussian distribution is that it is modular. The different pieces of information which completely specify the Gaussian model (namely means, standard deviations, and correlation coefficients) can be derived from different sources and integrated into the screening model. It allows researchers to make comparisons between studies and check for consistency. For example, if a mean and standard deviation estimate from one study were regarded as being invalid or substantially different from estimates derived from other sources, the former estimates could be rejected in favour of better ones. In logistic regression the estimates of screening performance are entirely based on the analysis of a single dataset; although the regression coefficients for a marker can be compared between two data sets, different coefficients for different markers cannot readily be combined into a model to be used to calculate risk. Another advantage of the multivariate Gaussian model is that, provided parameters of the underlying distribution are determined appropriately (see the section 'Handling of Data'), the final model is likely to be robust, that is, not strongly dependent upon chance variations from one dataset to another. Outliers, for example, would not have an undue influence on the final risk estimation. A disadvantage of the multivariate Gaussian model is that it relies on the distribution being reasonably Gaussian and cannot easily incorporate markers which are measured on a categorical scale. If the data are not Gaussian, logistic regression may give a better estimate of performance. If the distributions are Gaussian, and affected and unaffected pregnancies have the same standard deviations and correlations, then the same results are obtained using the Gaussian model and logistic regression.

USING THE GAUSSIAN MODEL AND OBSERVED DATA TO ESTIMATE DETECTION AND FALSE-POSITIVE RATES

The first method we described to estimate detection rates and false-positive rates uses the Gaussian distribution to calculate both (i) the likelihood ratios to estimate risk and (ii) the proportions of affected and unaffected pregnancies at specified risk levels (found as areas under the Gaussian curves). This can be called the 'model-based' method of estimating screening performance.

A somewhat different approach is to use the Gaussian model to calculate the likelihood ratios in a sample of affected and unaffected pregnancies and then obtain the observed detection and false-positive rates in these women ('sample-based' method). Again taking Down's syndrome screening as an example, suppose there were a dataset of 100 random Down's syndrome pregnancies and 1000 random unaffected pregnancies. The age of each woman is known (and therefore her age-specific risk of having a Down's syndrome pregnancy) as well as her AFP, uE$_3$, and total hCG levels. Means, standard deviations, and correlation coefficients for the three serum markers can then be obtained to form a multivariate Gaussian distribution in affected and unaffected pregnancies (as described above). These distributions can be used to estimate the likelihood ratio for each woman which, when combined with her age-specific risk, gives an estimate of risk of having a Down's syndrome pregnancy. We then count the number of Down's syndrome and unaffected pregnancies that exceed a specified risk cut-off. The two numbers divided by 100 (the total number of affected pregnancies) and 1000 (the total number of unaffected pregnancies), respectively, yield the detection rate and the false-positive rate when expressed as percentages.

A disadvantage of the 'sample-based' method is that the estimates of the detection rate will be more subject to the random error arising from the relatively small number of observations likely to be found in a given dataset than if the 'model based' method were used.

This can be illustrated as follows. Suppose that in the example, 58 of the 100 Down's pregnancies had positive test results (that is, exceeded a specified risk cut-off). The detection rate is then 58 per cent. Now suppose that 10 further cases are added to the original 100 Down's syndrome pregnancies (that is, 110 in total), and by chance these have risk estimates below the cut-off. They are likely to have been missed by a small margin. If so, the means, standard deviations, and correlations estimated from all 110 women will not be very different from those estimated using the original 100 women, so that if the 'model-based' method to estimate performance is used, similar detection and false-positive rates will be obtained with the samples of 100 and 110 Down's syndrome pregnancies. If, however, we use the 'sample-based' method, which relies on observed data to estimate performance, we still have 58 women with positive test results, so the detection rate falls from 58 per cent to 53 per cent (58/110). The 'model-based' method of estimating the detection and false-positive rates for a given screening test is more stable than the 'sample-based' method. The 'sample-based' method will give good estimates if based on large numbers of affected and unaffected subjects, but this is usually impractical for rare disorders.

HANDLING OF DATA

Is the distribution Gaussian?

A convenient method of judging whether the distribution of a variable is Gaussian is to draw a probability plot. This involves arranging the data in rank order and estimating the centile position of each observation. A centile can be calculated from the following formula for n observations:

$$\text{centile} = (r \times 100)/(n + 1)$$

for the rth smallest observation. For example, with 250 observations the 25th value ($r = 25$) is the 10th centile [$(25 \times 100)/ (250 + 1)$]. (This corresponds to a z-value of 1.282, obtained from Gaussian statistical tables.) In a probability plot, each marker value (for example, log AFP MoM) is plotted on the vertical axis and its corresponding centile value (as a z-value) on the horizontal axis. The horizontal axis is labelled using the centile position. For example, the 10th centile corresponds to a z-value of -1.28 and the 50th centile corresponds to a z-value of zero. A full

Table 2.2   Calculation of the centile and *z*-value for 50 individuals with an AFP measurement

AFP MoM	log MoM	Rank	Centile (rank × 100)/51	Standardized (*z*) value (distance from mean measured in SD units)†
0.20	−0.6990	1	1.96	−2.06
0.45	−0.3468	2	3.92	−1.76
0.49	−0.3098	3	5.88	−1.56
0.52	−0.2840	4	7.84	−1.42
0.53	−0.2757	5	9.80	−1.29
0.59	−0.2291	6	11.76	−1.19
0.60	−0.2218	7	13.73	−1.09
0.61	−0.2147	8	15.69	−1.01
0.62	−0.2076	9	17.65	−0.93
0.64	−0.1938	10	19.61	−0.86
0.66	−0.1805	11	21.57	−0.79
0.67	−0.1739	12	23.53	−0.72
0.70	−0.1549	13	25.49	−0.66
0.71	−0.1487	14	27.45	−0.60
0.72	−0.1427	15	29.41	−0.54
0.73	−0.1367	16	31.37	−0.49
0.74	−0.1308	17	33.33	−0.43
0.75	−0.1249	18	35.29	−0.38
0.76	−0.1192	19	37.25	−0.33
0.77	−0.1135	20	39.22	−0.27
0.78	−0.1079	21	41.18	−0.22
0.79	−0.1024	22	43.14	−0.17
0.81	−0.0915	23	45.10	−0.12
0.85	−0.0706	24	47.06	−0.07
0.87	−0.0605	25	49.02	−0.02
0.88	−0.0555	26	50.98	0.02
0.89	−0.0506	27	52.94	0.07
0.96	−0.0177	28	54.90	0.12
0.97	−0.0132	29	56.86	0.17
0.98	−0.0088	30	58.82	0.22
0.99	−0.0044	31	60.78	0.27
1.01	0.0043	32	62.75	0.33
1.03	0.0128	33	64.71	0.38
1.05	0.0212	34	66.67	0.43
1.07	0.0294	35	68.63	0.49
1.08	0.0334	36	70.59	0.54
1.09	0.0374	37	72.55	0.60
1.16	0.0645	38	74.51	0.66
1.17	0.0682	39	76.47	0.72
1.20	0.0792	40	78.43	0.79
1.25	0.0969	41	80.39	0.86
1.31	0.1173	42	82.35	0.93
1.33	0.1239	43	84.31	1.01
1.39	0.1430	44	86.27	1.09
1.43	0.1553	45	88.24	1.19
1.54	0.1875	46	90.20	1.29
1.59	0.2014	47	92.16	1.42
1.89	0.2765	48	94.12	1.56
2.01	0.3032	49	96.08	1.76
2.56	0.4082	50	98.04	2.06

† Obtained from Gaussian tables using the centile value.
SD = standard deviation.

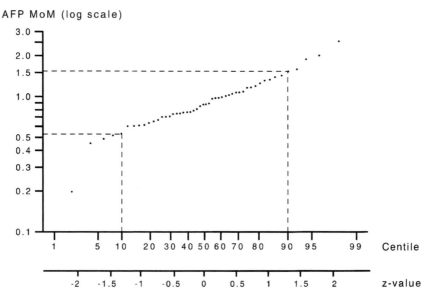

Fig. 2.8   Probability plot for AFP in 50 individuals (the 10th and 90th centiles are indicated).

worked example of estimating centiles based on 50 individuals with AFP measurements is shown in Table 2.2, and the result is plotted in Fig. 2.8.

The probability plot is constructed so that it yields a straight line if the distribution of the marker is perfectly Gaussian (see Fig. 2.9(a)). Effectively the horizontal axis is in standard deviation (z) units and so the slope of the line defines the standard deviation, that is, the slope is the increase in the value of the marker equivalent to a one standard deviation unit increase. The steeper the slope the larger the standard deviation. If the plot tends to be bowed upwards, the distribution is positively skewed; if it is bowed downwards it tends to be negatively skewed (Figs. 2.9(b) and 9(c)). Appropriate transformation of the data, for example, using logs, can sometimes linearize a plot that would otherwise be bowed upwards. The advantage of linearizing the data is that it can be summarized simply by the two parameters that define a Gaussian curve, namely the mean and standard deviation, which enables the calculations of risk estimation to be simplified.

If two or more markers are used it is necessary to check that they are *jointly* Gaussian. Usually, if each of the markers is Gaussian (as assessed by a straight line on a probability plot for each one) then they are jointly multivariate Gaussian. Other methods to assess joint normality include a formal statistical test called the Shapiro–Wilks test and a probability plot (based on the chi-squared distribution) for the combination of markers which is similar in principle to that for a single marker.[5]

Truncation

In practice, most markers will not follow a Gaussian distribution for the entire range of values. Observations at the extreme ends tend to deviate from the Gaussian distribution. A woman, therefore, with a value in either tail will tend to have her risk over-

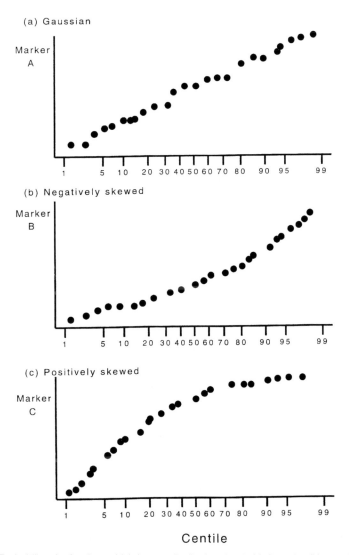

Fig. 2.9 Probability plot for data which have a distribution that is (a) Gaussian (b) negatively skewed, and (c) positively skewed.

or under-estimated using the Gaussian model. To overcome this, her marker value can be truncated to a value at which the distribution is reasonably Gaussian. For example, Fig. 2.10 shows a probability plot of the distribution of serum AFP in 385 unaffected pregnancies. Observations tend to deviate substantially from the Gaussian distribution below about 0.33 and above 3.0 MoM. If a woman's AFP MoM value is 3.5 the risk reported to her will be based on an AFP value of 3.0 MoM. Similarly, if a woman has an AFP of 0.2 MoM, the risk for an AFP of 0.33 MoM will be calculated. This process is done for each marker as necessary. The estimate of risk for the individual is then only specified as being either less than or greater than the risk at the truncation limit beyond which the distribution is judged to be materially non Gaussian.

AFP (MoM)

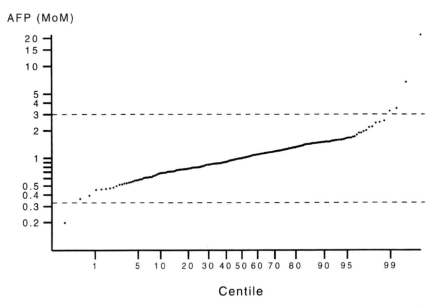

Fig. 2.10   Probability plot for AFP in 385 unaffected individuals illustrating where data deviates from the Gaussian distribution.

Measures of central tendency

The two most widely used measures of central tendency are the mean and the median. The mean is the sum of the values divided by the number of values. It uses all the values and so it can be influenced by outlying values. The median is the middle value if all the values are arranged in rank order (the mean of the two middle ones if there are an even number). The median has the advantage that it is not greatly influenced by outliers, which commonly occur in biological data. It therefore tends to be more stable than the mean. It is also unchanged by transformations such as converting the values into logarithms. The mean and median will coincide if the distribution is perfectly symmetrical.

Estimate of standard deviation

Using all the data to estimate the standard deviation is not robust if there are a number of outlying values.

A simple way of estimating the standard deviation is to identify the range over which the probability plot is linear, identify the percentile positions for which this holds true, and look up in statistical tables the number of z-values that spans this range; for example, between the 10th and 90th centiles, the distance in z-values is 2.56. The range of values covered by the 10th to 90th centiles can then be divided by 2.56 to determine the standard deviation. In the example shown in Fig. 2.8 the 10th centile is $\log_{10}(0.53)$ = -0.276 and the 90th centile is $\log_{10}(1.54) = 0.188$. An estimate of the standard deviation is therefore $[0.188-(-0.276)]/2.56$, which is 0.181 (in $\log_{10}$ MoM). An alternative to dividing the 10–90th centile range by 2.56 would be to perform a linear regression of the values (or log values) against the z-values, between say the 10th and 90th centiles; the standard deviation is then given by the slope (or regression coefficient).

Other statistical aspects of screening

Relationship between risk and screening performance

For a given combination of measurements and a fixed risk cut-off, it is of interest to examine how the detection rate and false-positive rate alter when the degree of separation between the distributions of a marker in affected and unaffected individuals changes, due, for example, to changes in assay or measurement error. For example, the standard deviation of unconjugated oestriol (uE₃) (in $\log_{10}$ MoM) in women with unaffected pregnancies is 0.14 at 15–24 weeks of pregnancy when gestational age is based on the date of the last menstrual period. When gestational age is based on an ultrasound scan examination there is less measurement error and the standard deviation reduces to 0.11, a 38% reduction in the variance. This decreases the overlap between the distributions of the marker in affected and unaffected pregnancies, which leads to improved screening performance—a higher detection rate for a given false-positive rate. To illustrate how screening performance changes when overlap decreases, it is convenient to assume a disease prevalence of 50 per cent (odds 1:1) and assume the standard deviations and correlation coefficients of the marker to be the same in affected and unaffected individuals.

The degree of separation between the two distributions can be specified in terms of the number of standard deviation units the two means are apart (D); this increases when the standard deviation is reduced. (See Appendix 2 for the calculation of D for multivariate distributions.) Figure 2.11 shows how the detection rate and false-positive rate change with increasing values of D in three situations: risk cut-off is (a) less than the background risk, (b) equal to the background risk, and (c) greater than the background risk. Intuitively one would expect the detection rate to increase and false-positive rate to decrease as the separation D increased. This is true in situation (b) when the risk cut-off is equivalent to the background risk, but not necessarily for other values of the risk cut-off. In situation (c) (where the risk cut-off is greater than the background risk so that the likelihood ratio at the cut-off is greater than one) it will hold only when the detection rate is *greater* than 50 per cent. In situation (a) (where the risk cut-off level is less than the background risk, so that the likelihood ratio at the cut-off is less than one), it will hold only when the false-positive rate is *less* than 50 per cent. Otherwise, both detection rate and false-positive rate will increase or decrease together, though each to a different extent so that discrimination still improves with increases in D.[6] Figure 2.11 illustrates how this arises, and Table 2.3 summarizes the effects.

Relationship between confidence interval of risk estimate and screening performance

As the ability of a screening marker to discriminate between affected and unaffected pregnancies (defined as the detection rate for a given false-positive rate) improves, the range of risk gets wider. Figure 2.12 illustrates this using the distribution of two markers (A and B) for Down's Syndrome, each with the same standard deviation but with different medians in affected pregnancies (0.7 MoM for A and 0.6 MoM for B). The range of risk between two specified marker values (0.5 and 2.0 MoMs in Fig. 2.12) is wider for B than for A, because the separation (quantified by D, as described above) between affected and unaffected pregnancies is greater for B. The risk estimates are given for a 35 year old woman. The confidence interval for risk is based

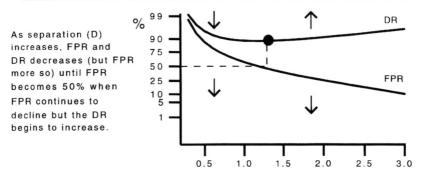

(a) Fixed risk cut-off less than background risk, ie LR < 1.0 (eg LR=0.5)

As separation (D) increases, FPR and DR decreases (but FPR more so) until FPR becomes 50% when FPR continues to decline but the DR begins to increase.

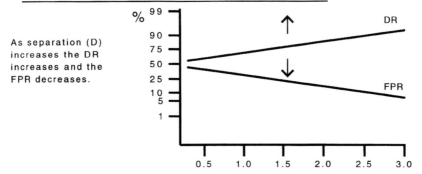

(b) Fixed risk cut-off equal to background risk, ie LR=1.0

As separation (D) increases the DR increases and the FPR decreases.

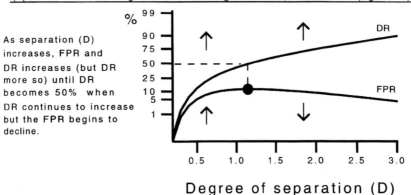

(c) Fixed risk cut-off greater than background risk, ie LR > 1.0 (eg LR=2)

As separation (D) increases, FPR and DR increases (but DR more so) until DR becomes 50% when DR continues to increase but the FPR begins to decline.

Degree of separation (D)

Fig. 2.11 Detection rate (DR) and false-positive rate (FPR) according to risk cut-off and degree of separation (D). LR = likelihood ratio. Full circle indicates the point of inflexion.

on the variance of the likelihood ratio (in $\log_e$), and because the variance is equal to D^2 the confidence interval range will increase as D increases. The mathematical basis of this is given in Appendix 3. At first sight this is counter-intuitive but precision (or reproducibility) is not the same as accuracy; that is, being on target. One can consistently obtain the wrong answer. The risk of a 30-year-old woman having a Down's syndrome pregnancy is about 1 in 1000 (based on her age alone) and will be so each time one

Table 2.3   Effect of increasing the separation of distributions of a screening marker in affected and unaffected individuals on the detection rate (DR) and the false-positive rate (FPR)

---

1. Risk cut–off less than the background risk (that is, LR of less than one). As separation increases at same risk cut–off:
If FPR >50%: DR ↓ FPR ↓↓
If FPR <50%: DR ↑ FPR ↓

2. Risk cut-off equal to the background risk (that is, LR of exactly one). As separation increases at same risk cut–off:
DR ↑ FPR ↓

3. Risk cut-off greater than background risk (that is, LR greater than one). As separation increases at same risk cut–off:
If DR >50%: DR ↑ FPR ↓
If DR <50%: DR ↑↑ FPR ↑

DR ↑↑ FPR ↑ indicates both increase, but DR increases at a faster rate

estimates it. Determining a woman's age is accurate and repeatable, but it is a poor means of discriminating affected from unaffected pregnancies. For this reason it may be misleading to quote confidence intervals on a person's risk of having a disorder— they will tend to be wider the better the marker.

Relationship between relative odds and screening performance

The extent to which screening performance (detection rate for a given false-positive rate) changes with the relative odds has been described before.[7] For a single continuous screening marker the RO_{10-90} is defined as the relative odds of being affected at the 90th centile for unaffected individuals compared with the 10th centile for unaffected individuals. The RO_{10-90} can be found using the Gaussian distribution by taking the ratio of the two likelihood ratios at the 90th and 10th centiles. The RO_{10-90} is a measure of relative risk used to describe the strength of a risk factor in relation to a disease. The detection rate, for a given false-positive rate, is a measure of screening performance. The two measures are directly related. A specific detection rate and false-positive rate corresponds to a specified RO_{10-90}. The latter can be calculated from the former. This is illustrated in the following example.

What is the RO_{10-90} that corresponds to a screening performance of a 50 per cent detection rate and 5 per cent false-positive rate?

First we need to know how far apart the distributions of the marker in affected and unaffected individuals are in standard deviation units (Fig. 2.13(a)). For affected individuals, the area of 50 per cent is associated with a z-value of 0 (from tables of the Gaussian distribution). For the unaffected individuals, the area of 5 per cent is associated with a z-value of 1.645. The two curves are thus 1.645 SD units apart (1.645 − 0). Figure 2.13(b) displays this together with the 10th and 90th centile positions in unaffected individuals.

For any z-value the height of the Gaussian curve is $[1/(2\pi)^{1/2}] \exp(-z^2/2)$ (where 'exp' is the antilog to the base e). At the 10th centile, the z-value for unaffected individuals is −1.282 (from tables of the Gaussian distribution). The z-value for affected individuals at this point is −2.927, the distance between the mean for affected individuals and the 10th centile (i.e. −1.282–1.645). The heights of the Gaussian curves for unaffected and affected individuals are, therefore, 0.1754 and 0.0055 respectively, yielding

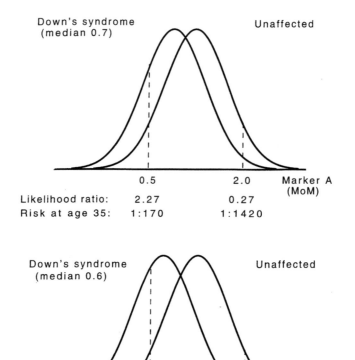

Fig. 2.12   Distribution of two markers (A and B) illustrating how the range of risk increases as discrimination improves. Risk = likelihood ratio × 1:384 (age-specific risk for women aged 35 years).

a likelihood ratio of 0.031 (0.0055/0.1754). Similarly, at the 90th centile, the z-value for unaffected individuals is 1.282 and that for affected individuals is −0.363 (that is, 1.282–1.645). The likelihood ratio at this point is therefore 2.129 (0.3735/0.1754). The relative odds, RO_{10-90}, is therefore 69 (2.129/0.031).

An RO_{10-90} of 69 is a high relative risk; few etiological factors yield odds ratios as high as this. Nonetheless, it corresponds to a screening test of only moderate performance. A risk factor must be very closely associated with a disease to be considered as a useful screening test.[7] Table 2.4 shows the relationship between RO_{10-90} and detection and false-positive rates.

Inversion of risk

When the distributions of a screening marker in affected and unaffected individuals have the same standard deviation there is only one point of intersection between the two distributions where, by definition, the likelihood ratio is one (Fig. 2.14(a)). On one side of this point the likelihood ratio is greater than one and on the other side it is less than one. There is a continuous gradation of risk with increasing values of the screening marker.

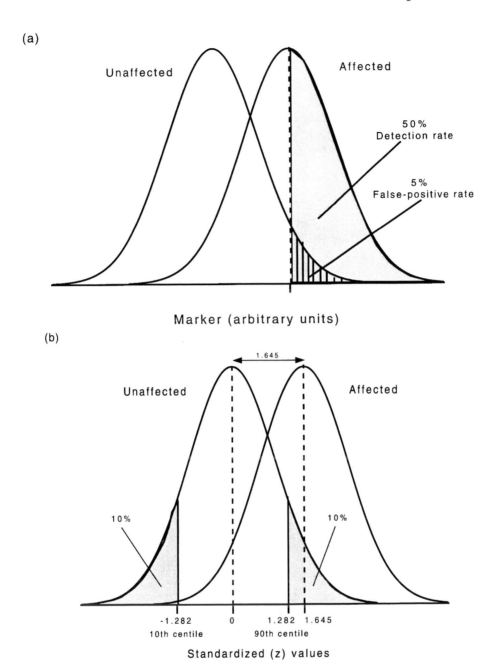

Fig. 2.13 The distribution of a screening marker illustrating (a) a detection rate of 50 per cent and a false-positive rate of 5 per cent and (b) the equivalent distributions measured in standard deviation units, showing the 10th and 90th centiles in unaffected individuals.

When the distributions of a screening marker in affected and unaffected individuals have different standard deviations, the distributions will cross at two places, so that there are two positions where the likelihood ratio is equal to one (Fig. 2.14(b)). This means that there is no longer a monotonic relationship between values of the screening

Table 2.4   Detection rate for a 5 per cent false-positive rate according to $RO_{10\text{-}90}$ (the relative odds of having the disease at the 90th centile of a distribution compared to the 10th centile)

$RO_{10\text{-}90}$	Detection rate (%) for a 5% false-positive rate
2	8
4	13
8	20
10	23
15	28
20	32
69	50

(a)

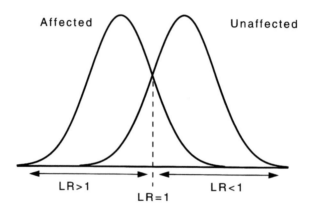

(b)

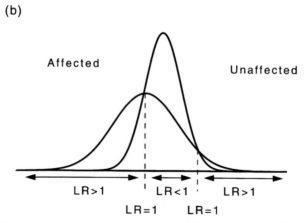

Fig. 2.14   The distribution of a screening marker in affected and unaffected individuals for which (a) the standard deviations are the same and (b) the standard deviation is greater in affected individuals. The vertical dashed lines indicate the points of intersection.

marker and risk. At some value between the two likelihood ratios of one, there will be a change in direction of risk in relation to increasing values of the screening variable. This may be counter-intuitive. For example, the distribution of the ultrasound marker nuchal translucency measurement is wider in affected than unaffected pregnancies (standard deviation of 0.235 compared to 0.12 $\log_{10}$MoM).[8] Over most values, the higher the nuchal translucency the higher the risk of having a Down's syndrome pregnancy, but there are two places where the likelihood ratio is one: at 1.44 and at 0.42 MoM. Therefore, at very low values (below 0.42 MoM) risk will actually increase again. Although this may seem surprizing, it is not a statistical artifact; if the dispersion of nuchal translucency values is, in fact, wider in affected pregnancies than in unaffected pregnancies, it is a genuine effect.

In practice one of the positions where the curves cross and the likelihood ratio is equal to one is usually far into the tails of the two distributions and so its influence will be small. (If, as can rarely occur, this point is close to the centre of one of the two distributions, the phenomenon will have a greater impact.) When the second cross point lies in the tails of the distributions, there will necessarily be considerably greater uncertainty over risk estimation, because there will be few empirical data with such extreme values. In such circumstances, it may be sensible to truncate the data over which risk estimation is performed, excluding the effect of extremely outlying values and so avoiding the risk inversion phenomenon.

CONCLUSION

In this chapter we have described how different screening or diagnostic markers for the same disorder can be used simultaneously in a single test. The method is based on estimating an individual's risk of having the disorder being screened for. It is the most efficient method of screening with multiple markers, in that it maximizes the detection rate for a given false-positive rate. Risk replaces the component markers as the screening variable. At the same time it gives an indication of the misclassification rate, or error, associated with the test. For example, a risk of 1 in 100 means that were this to be regarded as a negative result, individuals with the same result would be incorrectly classified 1 in 100 times (1 out of 100 such individuals would be affected in spite of being test-negative). Conversely if a risk of 1 in 100 were regarded as a positive result, individuals with the same result would be incorrectly classified 99 times in 100 (99 out of 100 such individuals would be unaffected in spite of being test-positive). The risk estimate is, in effect, the error associated with classifying an individual as either positive or negative.

Risk therefore has three important related qualities: it indicates the probability that an event will occur, it provides a quantitative measure that combines information on different markers of a disorder in the most efficient manner, and it specifies the error in predicting whether an individual has or does not have the disorder.

The use of risk as a screening variable is relatively new in medical practice. It tends to replace intuitive subjective interpretation with objective methods. It makes uncertainty explicit, while previously it was disguised or only implied. The uncertainty inherent in medical practice is now increasingly recognised and as this becomes quantified it is important that the estimation of risk and its application is understood if it is not to be misused. The theory set out in this chapter has been developed in relation to antenatal screening, but it applies to other areas of medicine in which combinations of markers are used together.

APPENDIX 1: THE MULTIVARIATE GAUSSIAN DISTRIBUTION: CALCULATING A LIKELIHOOD RATIO

This appendix is divided into three sections: a definition of the multivariate Gaussian distribution and the matrices which comprise it; a brief introduction to matrices; and matrix calculations which will show how the different parts of the model 'fit' together to produce the Gaussian height, and hence, a likelihood ratio.

An example from Down's syndrome screening using two markers, AFP and uE_3, is used to illustrate the calculations.

The multivariate Gaussian distribution

The height of a multivariate Gaussian distribution for a given set of values can be calculated from the following expression:

$$\text{Gaussian height for a particular woman} = \frac{1}{\text{product of SDs} \times (2\pi)^{P/2} \times \det(R)^{1/2}} \times \exp(-\tfrac{1}{2}Z^T R^{-1} Z)$$

where π is the number pi (approximately 22/7), p is the number of screening markers, the 'product of SDs' is the product of the standard deviations of each of the markers, R is a matrix containing the correlations between the markers, $\det(R)$ is called the determinant of the matrix R and is described later, Z is a matrix containing the woman's value for each screening marker each expressed in standard deviation units from the mean (namely [marker value-mean]/standard deviation). (Z^T is a transformation of the matrix Z and is described later.)

For each woman, two Gaussian heights are calculated—one assuming that she has an affected pregnancy and the other assuming that she has an unaffected pregnancy. Her likelihood ratio is the ratio of these two heights.

Introduction to matrices

With one screening marker the means for affected and unaffected individuals together with their standard deviations specify the two distributions. With several markers, there will be two means and SDs for each marker, and also correlation coefficients measuring the extent of association *between* the markers. The calculations thus require the use of 'matrices', commonly used in mathematics. A matrix is a way of incorporating all the relevant information we have about the markers into a manageable form.

A matrix consists of rows and columns of numbers. The number of rows and columns is called the 'size' or 'order' of the matrix. The numbers inside a matrix are called the 'elements'. For example, a matrix with three rows and two columns is called a '3 by 2 matrix'; it has 6 elements and size (3×2):

$$
\begin{array}{ccc}
 & \text{Column} & \\
 & 1 \quad\quad 2 & \\
\text{Row} \begin{array}{c} 1 \\ 2 \\ 3 \end{array} & \begin{pmatrix} 3 & 4 \\ 9 & 5 \\ 7 & 1 \end{pmatrix} &
\end{array}
$$

A single number is a matrix of size 1×1. A position on a graph which is defined by two coordinates (x, y) is a 1×2 matrix, and it represents two dimensions.

The multivariate Gaussian distribution as presented here is composed of two matrices—*Z* and *R* as follows:

Z: This is a matrix containing the results of each marker (expressed in units of one standard deviation) for the individual being screened. Each woman has an observed value for each screening marker. For example, she may have a $\log_{10}$ AFP level of 0.10 MoM and a $\log_{10}$ uE$_3$ level of 0.15 MoM. These values are expressed in standard deviation units assuming that she has a Down's syndrome pregnancy and assuming she has an unaffected pregnancy.

In Down's syndrome pregnancies the mean AFP and mean uE$_3$ in logged units are −0.1427 and −0.1411 respectively.[3] The corresponding standard deviations are 0.2015 and 0.1478.[3] For this example, the distances of the AFP and uE$_3$ values (in the screened woman) from the log means for these variables in Down's syndrome, expressed in units of a standard deviation, are 1.20 (that is, (0.10 − −0.1427)/0.2015) and 1.97 (that is, (0.15 − −0.1411)/0.1478) respectively. Then:

$$Z_{Down's} = \begin{pmatrix} 1.20 \\ 1.97 \end{pmatrix} \begin{matrix} AFP \\ uE_3 \end{matrix}$$

In unaffected pregnancies, the mean is zero for both AFP and uE$_3$ and the standard deviations are 0.1986 and 0.1391 respectively.[3] The standardized values assuming an unaffected pregnancy are therefore 0.50 for AFP [(0.10–0)/0.1986] and 1.08 for uE$_3$ [(0.15–0)/0.1391]. Then:

$$Z_{unaffected} = \begin{pmatrix} 0.50 \\ 1.08 \end{pmatrix} \begin{matrix} AFP \\ uE_3 \end{matrix}$$

R: This is a matrix containing the correlations (that is, the extent of association) between the tests. The correlations between AFP and itself and between uE$_3$ and itself will, of course, be one. In Down's syndrome pregnancies the correlation between AFP and uE$_3$ is 0.3359 and in unaffected pregnancies it is 0.2853.[3] Thus:

$$R_{Down's} = \begin{pmatrix} 1 & 0.3359 \\ 0.3359 & 1 \end{pmatrix} \begin{matrix} AFP \\ uE_3 \end{matrix}$$
$$\qquad\qquad AFP \qquad uE_3$$

$$R_{unaffected} = \begin{pmatrix} 1 & 0.2853 \\ 0.2853 & 1 \end{pmatrix} \begin{matrix} AFP \\ uE_3 \end{matrix}$$
$$\qquad\qquad AFP \qquad uE_3$$

A matrix can be thought of as a type of 'number' which we wish to use in a similar manner, namely add, subtract, multiply, and divide. Figure 2.15 summarizes how these calculations can be performed using matrices compared to the single number system. Furthermore, there are two key numbers in our normal number system, namely 0 and 1; the matrix equivalents are shown in Fig. 2.15. The matrix *I* is called the 'identity' matrix and only occurs for matrices for which the number of rows equals the number of columns. The pattern is the same for all such matrices—values of one along the centre diagonal and zeros elsewhere.

Single number system	Matrix system

Identity:

$$1$$

$$I = \begin{pmatrix} 1 & 0 \\ 0 & 1 \end{pmatrix}$$

$$3 \times 1 = 3$$

$$A \times I = A$$

Addition:

$$8 + 4 = 12$$

$$\begin{pmatrix} a & b \\ c & d \end{pmatrix} + \begin{pmatrix} e & f \\ g & h \end{pmatrix} = \begin{pmatrix} a+e & b+f \\ c+g & d+h \end{pmatrix}$$

$$\text{eg. } \begin{pmatrix} 1 & 2 \\ 3 & 4 \end{pmatrix} + \begin{pmatrix} 5 & 6 \\ 7 & 8 \end{pmatrix} = \begin{pmatrix} 6 & 8 \\ 10 & 12 \end{pmatrix}$$

Subtraction:

$$8 - 4 = 4$$

$$\begin{pmatrix} a & b \\ c & d \end{pmatrix} - \begin{pmatrix} e & f \\ g & h \end{pmatrix} = \begin{pmatrix} a-e & b-f \\ c-g & d-h \end{pmatrix}$$

$$\text{eg. } \begin{pmatrix} 5 & 6 \\ 7 & 8 \end{pmatrix} - \begin{pmatrix} 4 & 3 \\ 2 & 1 \end{pmatrix} = \begin{pmatrix} 1 & 3 \\ 5 & 7 \end{pmatrix}$$

Multiplication:

$$8 \times 4 = 32$$

$$\begin{pmatrix} a & b \\ c & d \end{pmatrix} \times \begin{pmatrix} e & f \\ g & h \end{pmatrix} = \begin{pmatrix} ae+bg & af+bh \\ ce+dg & cf+dh \end{pmatrix}$$

$$\text{eg. } \begin{pmatrix} 1 & 2 \\ 3 & 4 \end{pmatrix} \times \begin{pmatrix} 5 & 6 \\ 7 & 8 \end{pmatrix} = \begin{pmatrix} 19 & 22 \\ 43 & 50 \end{pmatrix}$$

Division:

$$8 / 4 = 2$$

does not exist in general

But $8 \times 4^{-1} = 2$

$$A \times B^{-1} = C \quad *$$

Fig. 2.15 Calculations using matrices; illustration using a 2 by 2 matrix A. Comparison of addition, subtraction, multiplication and division using single numbers and matrices. *Generally only possible when the matrix B is square (for example 2×2, 3×3) and the number of columns in A is the same as the number of rows in B.

Addition and *subtraction* are straightforward and can only be done for matrices of the same size.

Multiplication depends on the sizes of the matrices *and* the order in which they are being multiplied. For two matrices M and A, the result from $M \times A$ is not necessarily the same as that from $A \times M$.

Multiplication can only be performed if the number of columns of the first matrix is the same as the number of rows of the second matrix. This can easily be determined by writing the sizes of the matrices under the multiplications:

$$
\begin{array}{ccc}
M & \times & A \\
\text{size} \quad 3 \times 2 & & 2 \times 4
\end{array}
$$

The '2s' are adjacent to each other so multiplication is possible. The size of the resulting matrix is (number of rows of first matrix × number of columns of second matrix). So for the above multiplication of $M \times A$, the result is a 3 × 4 matrix.

For the following example, multiplication is not possible since the two adjacent numbers '4' and '3' are not the same:

$$
\begin{array}{ccc}
A & \times & M \\
\text{size} \quad 2 \times 4 & & 3 \times 2
\end{array}
$$

The multiplication process can be awkward to perform but with practice becomes straightforward. It involves the simultaneous multiplication and addition between the rows of the first matrix and columns of the second matrix as indicated in Fig. 2.15.

The procedure involves: (1) taking the first row of the first matrix (A) and multiplying the elements with those of the first column of the second matrix (B), and finding the sum ($ae + bg$); (2) doing the same with the first row of the first matrix and the second column of the second matrix ($af + bh$); (3) repeating both processes using the second row of the first matrix instead of the first.

The concept of *division*, as we normally understand, does not exist for matrices in general. Instead there is a calculation called *inversion*. Inversion is analogous to reciprocating in our normal number system in which any number multiplied by its inverse (or reciprocal) results in one. For example, the reciprocal of 3 is 1/3 and so 3 × 1/3 is 1. The inverse of a matrix is indicated by a superscript of –1: the inverse of M is M^{-1}. Generally, this is only possible when the matrix has the same number of rows as it does columns, i.e. of size 2 × 2, 3 × 3, 4 × 4, and so on. Any matrix multiplied by its inverse results in the identity matrix (I).

The method required to find the inverse can be complex and it uses a result called the 'determinant'. This is a unique number associated with a particular matrix which has various geometric properties. It is notated as $\det(M)$ or $|M|$. For a 2 × 2 matrix:

$$
\text{if } M = \begin{pmatrix} a & b \\ c & d \end{pmatrix} \text{ then } \det(M) = ad - bc.
$$

The inverse is given by:

$$
M^{-1} = \frac{1}{\det(M)} \begin{pmatrix} d & -b \\ -c & a \end{pmatrix}.
$$

In the Gaussian distribution model we have $\det(R)$ and R^{-1}. For Down's syndrome pregnancies:

$$
R_{\text{Down's}} = \begin{pmatrix} 1 & 0.3359 \\ 0.3359 & 1 \end{pmatrix}
$$

(where 0.3359 is the correlation between AFP and uE_3). Therefore $\det(R)$ is 0.89 (that is, $1 - 0.3359^2$). The inverse of $R_{\text{Down's}}$ is then:

$$R^{-1}_{\text{Down's}} = \frac{1}{0.89} \begin{pmatrix} 1 & -0.3359 \\ -0.3359 & 1 \end{pmatrix} = \begin{pmatrix} 1.12 & -0.38 \\ -0.38 & 1.12 \end{pmatrix}$$

This result can be checked by multiplying $R_{\text{Down's}}$ with $R^{-1}_{\text{Down's}}$:

$$\begin{pmatrix} 1 & 0.3359 \\ 0.3359 & 1 \end{pmatrix} \times \begin{pmatrix} 1.12 & -0.38 \\ -0.38 & 1.12 \end{pmatrix} = \begin{pmatrix} 1 & 0 \\ 0 & 1 \end{pmatrix}$$

The result is the identity matrix (I).

For unaffected pregnancies, we have:

$$R_{\text{unaffected}} = \begin{pmatrix} 1 & 0.2853 \\ 0.2853 & 1 \end{pmatrix}$$

Therefore $\det(R)$ is 0.92 (that is, $1 - 0.2853^2$). The inverse of $R_{\text{unaffected}}$ is then:

$$R^{-1}_{\text{unaffected}} = \frac{1}{0.92} \begin{pmatrix} 1 & -0.2853 \\ -0.2853 & 1 \end{pmatrix} = \begin{pmatrix} 1.09 & -0.31 \\ -0.31 & 1.09 \end{pmatrix}$$

The determinants and inverses which have been calculated here will be used in the next section to calculate the likelihood ratio.

Calculation of the likelihood ratio

Illustrated example

The Gaussian distribution model contains the term $Z^T R^{-1} Z$ that is, both multiplication and inversion. The 'T' superscript indicates that the first matrix Z has been 'transposed'. In the Down's syndrome screening example of AFP and uE_3, Z is a 2×1 matrix and R is a 2×2 matrix, so the product ZR is not possible. If, however, we swap the columns and rows in Z (that is, transpose them by making the first column become the first row and the second column become the second row) then Z^T is of size 1×2 which can be multiplied by R:

$$Z_{\text{Down's}} = \begin{pmatrix} 1.20 \\ 1.97 \end{pmatrix} \quad Z^T_{\text{Down's}} = (1.20,\ 1.97)$$

$$Z_{\text{unaffected}} = \begin{pmatrix} 0.50 \\ 1.08 \end{pmatrix} \quad Z^T_{\text{unaffected}} = (0.50,\ 1.08)$$

We now have the necessary information to calculate the two Gaussian heights for a woman with a logged AFP level of 0.10 MoM and a logged uE_3 level of 0.15 MoM:

$$\text{Gaussian height} = \frac{1}{\text{product of SDs} \times (2\pi)^{p/2} \times \det(R)^{1/2}} \times \exp(-\tfrac{1}{2} Z^T R^{-1} Z).$$

We can now fill in this expression using the parameters and matrices for AFP and uE_3 described above.

Assuming the woman has a Down's syndrome pregnancy:

$$\text{Gaussian height} = \frac{1}{0.2015 \times 0.1478 \times (2\pi)^{2/2} \times 0.89^{1/2}}$$

$$\times \exp\left[-\frac{1}{2}(1.20 \quad 1.97)\begin{pmatrix} 1.12 & -0.39 \\ -0.39 & 1.12 \end{pmatrix}\begin{pmatrix} 1.20 \\ 1.97 \end{pmatrix}\right]$$

$$= \frac{1}{0.1765} \times \exp\left(-\frac{1}{2} \times 4.1155\right)$$

$$= 0.7237$$

where the product of the three matrices in the exponential term can be calculated as described before, where

$$(a \ b)\begin{pmatrix} c\,d \\ e\,f \end{pmatrix}\begin{pmatrix} a \\ b \end{pmatrix} = (ac + be \quad bd + bf)\begin{pmatrix} a \\ b \end{pmatrix}$$

$$= a(ac + be) + (bd + bf)$$

that is, a single number.

Assuming the woman has an unaffected pregnancy:

$$\text{Gaussian height} = \frac{1}{0.1986 \times 0.1391 \times (2\pi)^{2/2} \times 0.92^{1/2}}$$

$$\times \exp\left[-\frac{1}{2}(0.50 \quad 1.08)\begin{pmatrix} 1.09 & -0.31 \\ -0.31 & 1.09 \end{pmatrix}\begin{pmatrix} 0.50 \\ 1.08 \end{pmatrix}\right]$$

$$= \frac{1}{0.1665} \times \exp\left(-\frac{1}{2} \times 1.2091\right)$$

$$= 3.2812.$$

Her likelihood ratio is therefore 0.221 (0.7273/3.2812). If she is aged 35 years, her risk of having a Down's syndrome pregnancy before being screened is 1:384. After her test results, her risk becomes 1:1737 (i.e. 0.221:384). In practice, estimation of risk requires a computer package.

APPENDIX 2: DEGREE OF SEPARATION BETWEEN TWO DISTRIBUTIONS

The degree of separation (D) between two distributions (affected and unaffected), when the variances and correlations are the same in the two groups, is calculated as follows:

$$D^2 = (\mu_1 - \mu_2)^\mathrm{T} V^{-1} (\mu_1 - \mu_2).$$

where μ_1 and μ_2 could be the matrices of the mean AFP and mean uE$_3$ in Down's syndrome and unaffected pregnancies respectively.

The matrix V contains the variances of AFP and uE$_3$ and covariances between AFP and uE$_3$ and can be derived from the correlation matrix and the standard deviations. A correlation coefficient is the covariance between two tests divided by the product of their standard deviations. If, for example, we assume the correlation matrix in Down's syndrome pregnancies to be the same as that in the unaffected pregnancies we have

$$R = \begin{pmatrix} 1 & 0.2853 \\ 0.2853 & 1 \end{pmatrix}$$

The standard deviation of AFP is 0.1986 and the standard deviation of uE$_3$ is 0.1391. Then

$$V = \begin{pmatrix} 1 \times 0.1986^2 & 0.2853 \times 0.1986 \times 0.1391 \\ 0.2853 \times 0.1986 \times 0.1391 & 1 \times 0.1391^2 \end{pmatrix} = \begin{pmatrix} 0.0394 & 0.00788 \\ 0.00788 & 0.0193 \end{pmatrix}$$

The distance (D^2) between pregnancies with and without Down's syndrome with respect to AFP and uE$_3$ is given by

$$\left[\begin{pmatrix} -0.1427 \\ -0.1411 \end{pmatrix} - \begin{pmatrix} 0 \\ 0 \end{pmatrix} \right]^{\mathrm{T}} \begin{pmatrix} 0.0394 & 0.00788 \\ 0.00788 & 0.0193 \end{pmatrix}^{-1} \left[\begin{pmatrix} -0.1427 \\ -0.1411 \end{pmatrix} - \begin{pmatrix} 0 \\ 0 \end{pmatrix} \right]$$

which simplifies to 1.23. This measure can also be called the Mahalanobis distance and D the Mahalanobis separation. The distinction between D and D^2 is analagous to that between standard deviation and variance. A distance of zero signifies no difference between the distributions and there exist statistical tests which tell us whether an observed D^2 is significantly greater than zero.

APPENDIX 3: CONFIDENCE INTERVAL ON AN ESTIMATE OF RISK

A confidence interval for a likelihood ratio (LR) for a particular individual can be given by the $\log_e$(LR) $\pm$ 2 $\times$ standard error of the LR, where the LR is based on the marker levels for the individual. These limits can then be combined with the prevalence or the age-specific risk to give the confidence interval for the risk estimate.

The LR for a single marker at a value x is the ratio of the Gaussian heights of affected and unaffected pregnancies, (see Appendix 1). If the standard deviation (SD) is the same in affected and unaffected pregnancies, the expression for the LR can be simplified to:

$$\log_e \text{ LR} = \tfrac{1}{2}\,[(m_u^2 - m_a^2)/\text{SD}^2] + (x \times \text{D})/\text{SD}$$
$$= \text{constant} + (x \times \text{D})/\text{SD}$$

$$\text{variance of } (\log_e \text{ LR}) = 0 + (D^2/\text{SD}^2) \times \text{variance of } (x)$$
$$= D^2$$

(since the variance of $(x) = \text{SD}^2$). Here x is the observed value of the screening marker for the individual, m_a and m_u are the means in affected and unaffected individuals respectively and D is the difference between the means of the two distributions in SD units (that is $[m_a - m_u]/\text{SD}$), the Mahalanobis separation from Appendix 2).

As screening performance (i.e. the detection rate for a given false-positive rate) increases, the degree of separation (D or D^2) between affected and unaffected individuals also increases, but so does the variance of the likelihood ratio. Since the standard error is the square root of the variance, the confidence interval for the likelihood ratio will widen as D increases.

REFERENCES

1. Office of Population Censuses and Surveys (1984–8). *Birth statistics*, Series FM1, nos. 11, 12, 15–17. HMSO, London.
2. Cuckle H. S., Wald N. J., and Thompson S. G. (1987). Estimating a woman's risk of having a pregnancy associated with Down's syndrome using her age and serum alpha-fetoprotein level. *Br J Obstet Gynaecol*, **94**, 387–402.
3. Wald N. J., Densem J. W., Smith D., and Klee G. G. (1994). Four-marker serum screening for Down's syndrome. *Prenat Diagn*, **14**, 707–16.
4. McLachlan G. J. (1992). *Discriminant analysis and statistical pattern recognition*. Wiley, New York.
5. Krzanowski W. J. (1990). *Principles of multivariate analysis—A user's perspective*. Oxford Statistical Science Series, vol. 3. Oxford University Press, Oxford.
6. Royston P. and Thompson S. G. (1992). Model based screening by risk with application to Down's syndrome. *Stat Med.*, **11**, 257–68.
7. Wald N. J., Hackshaw A.K., Frost C. D. (1999). When can a risk factor be used as a worthwhile screening test? *BMJ*, **319**, 1562–5.
8. Nicolaides K.H., Snijders R.J.M., Cuckle H.S. (1998) Correct estimation of parameters for ultrasound nuchal translucency screening. *Prenat Diagn*, **18**, 519–23.

II

Screening for specific disorders
(a) Antenatal screening

3 *Neural tube defects*

Nicholas Wald

INTRODUCTION

Antenatal screening and diagnosis for neural tube defects involves the application of two methods—maternal serum followed by amniotic fluid alphafetoprotein (AFP) measurement, and ultrasound examination of the fetus. Serum AFP is raised in pregnancies associated with anencephaly and open spina bifida, and this is used as an indication to perform a diagnostic ultrasound examination (which demonstrates the absence of the cranium in anencephaly or the presence of a spinal lesion in spina bifida) and usually also a diagnostic amniocentesis and amniotic fluid AFP test. Ultrasound is also used as a screening procedure in which certain cranial signs are identified that are usually associated with spina bifida. The present challenge in screening is to integrate the two screening and diagnostic methods into a coherent screening strategy. In the past, in AFP screening, a maternal serum AFP measurement was first carried out and if this was raised an ultrasound scan examination was performed to check the gestational age and revise the assessment of the AFP level if necessary. This is no longer the preferred approach. It is better to carry out the ultrasound examination before an AFP screening test is offered. The ultrasound examination will detect virtually all cases of anencephaly with sufficient certainty to be diagnostic, so an AFP screening test is then not needed. Prior dating of a pregnancy by ultrasound improves the performance of screening for spina bifida by AFP measurement and in some centres AFP screening for open spina bifida is not used because ultrasound screening alone is thought to be sufficient. This chapter examines the different methods of screening and diagnosis, and takes a view on how they should be integrated.

THE DISORDER

Description

Three main types of neural tube defect (NTD) can be identified, namely anencephaly, spina bifida, and encephalocele. The prevalence of anencephaly and spina bifida in the absence of screening and termination of affected pregnancies is approximately equal, and together they account for about 95 per cent of all NTDs. Encephalocele is rare, accounting for the remaining 5 per cent.

An important distinction, from the point of view of screening and antenatal diagnosis based on AFP measurement, is whether the neural tube defect lesion is open or closed. An open lesion is one in which neural tissue is exposed or covered by a thin transparent membrane. A closed lesion is one in which the neural tissue is completely covered by skin or a thick opaque membrane. The pathophysiologic basis of the screening test is leakage of AFP from the lesion into the amniotic fluid and then into the maternal circulation. In open lesions (anencephaly and about 85 per cent of spina bifida cystica) leakage occurs and can usually be detected. Closed lesions, which do not allow this leakage, are not associated with high AFP levels in amniotic fluid or maternal serum.

Natural history

Most open neural tube defects are the end results of defects in neurulation (the formation of the neural tube, which later develops into the brain and spinal cord). When a severe defect of this kind has occurred, the affected part of the neural tube does not become covered by the vertebral arches or calvarium, but remains inadequately protected and is affected by trauma and degeneration. This leads to anencephaly or to open spina bifida, depending on whether the initial defect of neurulation occurred in the cephalic part of the neural tube or in the part that forms the spinal cord.[1]

Anencephaly is a fatal condition. Infants born with open spina bifida have a poor prognosis, with a 5-year survival rate of 36 per cent when treated.[2] Among the group of 5-year survivors in this series, 82 per cent were severely handicapped and 10 per cent were moderately handicapped. On average, they had spent over half a year in hospital and had, on average, six surgical operations by the age of 5. Closed spina bifida has a somewhat better prognosis. The 5-year survival rate was 60 per cent, and among these survivors, about one-third were severely handicapped and another third moderately handicapped.

A recent case report suggests that in the future the prognosis in spina bifida may be improved by intra-uterine surgery. The report described a case of open thoraco-lumbo-sacral spina bifida in a 23 week fetus. This defect was closed with skin flaps to protect the spinal cord, and a cerebrospinal fluid shunt with a one-way valve was inserted as a precaution against hydrocephalus. The baby was later born without the paraplegia and hydrocephaly that usually occur in infants with thoracolumbar spina bifida.[3] If results like this were shown to be regularly attainable by intra-uterine surgery, antenatal screening for neural tube defects would have a part to play in identifying cases for surgery, as well as in its present role of detecting affected fetuses in order to offer a termination of pregnancy. The possibility is, however, too tentative to influence current screening practice.

Birth prevalence

The birth prevalence of NTDs in England and Wales in 1997 was 0.14 per 1000 births—less than 5 per cent of the rate 25 years previously. Most of this decline is due to screening which has been highly effective. Figure 3.1 shows the decline in the birth prevalence of neural tube defects in England and Wales from 1965 to 1997 and Table 3.1 shows the numbers and rates in selected years over this period. The decline has been dramatic. In 1997 there were fewer than 100 neural tube defect births compared with 2800 in 1965. This reduction has been due partly to antenatal screening, diagno-

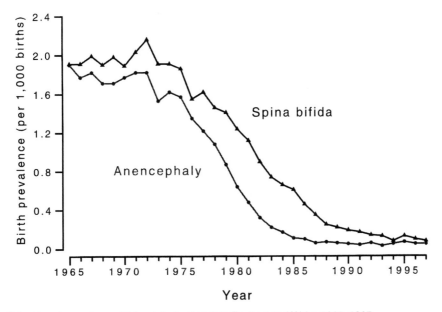

Fig. 3.1 Prevalence of neural tube defects at birth in England and Wales 1965–1997.

Table 3.1 Number and prevalence of neural tube defect births in England and Wales 1964–97

Year	Anencephaly		Spina bifida without anencephaly	
	Births[A]	Rate per 10 000 births[B]	Births[A]	Rate per 10 000 births[B]
1964	1335	18.5	1395	18.0
1965	1346	19.0	1454	19.1
1970	1137	17.7	1309	18.9
1975	775	15.7	986	18.6
1980	342	6.4	712	12.4
1985	59	1.1	352	6.1
1990	26	0.5	116	1.9
1995	35	0.6	72	1.3
1996	24	0.5	57	1.0
1997	30	0.6	40	0.8

[A] Data from notifications of birth defects to the Office of Population Censuses and Surveys (now the Office of National Statistics).[4,5,6] Separate data on spina bifida without anencephaly are not published for the period of 1986–1997 but were obtained as a personal communication from Mrs B. Botting at ONS (formerly OPCS).
[B] Rates were adjusted to take account of under-reporting as follows: anencephaly (adjusted) = anencephaly (observed)/0.81; spina bifida (adjusted) = spina bifida (observed)/0.87.[7]

sis, and selective abortion, and partly due to a decline in incidence arising from an improvement in diet and an increase in folate consumption. It is now known that folate deficiency is a cause of neural tube defects.[8,9] About 75 per cent of cases of neural tube defect can be prevented by taking extra folic acid before and during early pregnancy.[10] The consumption of folate rich and folic acid fortified foods has increased and with it the average intake of folate.

There are genetic as well as environmental determinants of neural tube defects. The risk of fetal neural tube defects is increased about 10-fold among women who have previously had one affected pregnancy, about 20-fold among women who have had two affected pregnancies, and about 40-fold among those who have had three.[11] Despite these high risks of recurrence, over 95 per cent of affected pregnancies arise in women who have not previously had a pregnancy with a neural tube defect. It is primarily to these women that screening for open neural tube defects is offered.

SCREENING AND DIAGNOSIS

Ultrasound

Ultrasound scanning for neural tube defects is used as both a screening test and a diagnostic test. It can diagnose anencephaly directly, and in some experienced centres, can also diagnose spina bifida directly by visualizing the spinal lesion. Even in centres where the expertise needed to diagnose spina bifida ultrasonographically is lacking, ultrasound scanning can contribute to the detection of neural tube defects in three ways: (1) immediate diagnosis of anencephaly, (2) assessment of length of gestation based on biparietal diameter, which improves the performance of AFP screening, and (3) identification of cranial signs of spina bifida. There are two such cranial signs: (i) the frontal region of the fetal skull is 'pinched' creating the so-called 'lemon' shape instead of the normal egg shape,[12] and (ii) the thickness of the cerebellum is diminished, so that typically the transverse diameter of the cerebellum is reduced, and sometimes the cerebellum is not seen at all. The changes can lead to the two cerebellar hemispheres adopting a bow shape—the so-called 'banana' sign.[12,13] These changes result from the Arnold–Chiari malformation (herniation of the cerebellum and brainstem through the foramen magnum), which arises in association with spina bifida.

Determining the performance of ultrasound scanning in the detection of spina bifida (whether as a screening or diagnostic test) is complicated for various reasons. Unlike the position with a biochemical test the detection rate of an ultrasound scan examination will depend on the skill of the operator and the prevalence of affected pregnancies since he or she is likely to look harder if the disorder is more likely to be present. The reported screening performance of the cranial ultrasound signs is summarized in Tables 3.2 and 3.3, Table 3.2 using data from Tables 18.7 and 18.8 in

Table 3.2   Ultrasound screening and diagnosis in the detection of spina bifida. Taken from Tables 18.3, 18.7, and 18.8. Figures based partly on women known to be at high risk of having an affected pregnancy

	Detection rate	False-positive rate
Screening (cranial signs)		
Lemon sign (pinching of frontal bones)	86% (497/577)	0.23% (23/9879)
Banana sign (bow shaped cerebellum)	93% (243/260)	0.05% (5/9455)
Diminished cerebellar diameter (≤ 85% of median)	68% (141/208)	1.4% (6/440)
Diagnosis (examination of spine)*	84% (146/173)	0.5%**

* Data collected after 1986.

** Determining false-positive rate is usually impossible due to destruction of fetus, 0.5% assumed; 5/141 571 is reported.

Table 3.3 Percentage of pregnancies with and without spina bifida according to transverse cerebellar diameter

Transverse cerebellar diameter (MoM)	Spina bifida pregnancies (n = 208)	Unaffected pregnancies (n = 440)
≤0.80	58.7	0.7
≤0.85	67.8	1.4
≤0.90	79.8	4.1
≤0.95	90.9	18.0
≤1.00	96.6	58.9

Taken from de Courcy Wheeler *et al.* (1994).[13]

chapter 18 (Ultrasound Screening for Congenital Abnormalities). The performance of ultrasound as a diagnostic test (visualizing the spina bifida) is also summarized in Table 3.2, using data from Table 18.3 in chapter 18.

Performance of screening by ultrasound

According to Table 3.2, the 'lemon' sign has a detection rate of 86 per cent for a false-positive rate of 0.2 per cent; the 'banana' sign has an 93 per cent detection rate for a 0.05 per cent false-positive rate. However, the detection rates in these studies are based almost entirely on tests performed in women known to be at high risk of having a neural tube defect pregnancy. These detection rates are therefore likely to be higher than would be obtained if all pregnancies were screened using the 'lemon' and 'banana' signs alone. The false-positive rates reported for these signs are also open to question. These rates were reported to be zero in many of the individual studies (listed in Table 18.7 and 18.8 in Chapter 18) on which Table 3.2 is based, but it is likely that in reality false-positive results will occur with both the 'lemon' and 'banana' signs, because there is bound to be a gradation in skull shapes in unaffected pregnancies. Also the quantitative results from de Courcy Wheeler and his colleagues[13] (Table 3.3) demonstrated a variation in cerebellar diameter in unaffected pregnancies which over-laps the distribution in affected pregnancies. Because this is an objective component of the 'banana' sign it suggests that the sign itself can occur in unaffected pregnancies. A possible explanation for the low false-positive rates associated with the 'lemon' and 'banana' signs is that the presence of either prompts the person performing the ultrasound examination to examine the spine, and this must also reveal spina bifida before the test is regarded as positive. In effect, three tests are being performed and all three, or at least two, must be positive for the overall result to be positive. This will yield a very low false-positive rate (if each of the three tests had a false-positive rate of 5 per cent and they were independent the overall false-positive rate would be 0.05 × 0.05 ×0.05, or about 1 in 10 000). The detection rate would be less than with one test alone, but the effect might be small if once a cranial sign were found substantial effort was put into finding the spinal lesion.

Performance of diagnostic ultrasound

The detection rate for diagnostic ultrasound (examination of the spine) given in Table 3.2 (84 per cent) does not appear to have been much affected by the inclusion of cases examined because they were known to be at high risk. The largest of the series[14] on which the rate is based included cases referred due to raised serum AFP, but the detection rate in the remaining studies (82 per cent) was only slightly lower than in all series combined. The false-positive rate for these series is surprisingly low (0.004 per cent for all series combined, which included more than 140 000 fetuses without spina bifida). This may be because a positive result would nearly always result in a termination of pregnancy and this would usually involve the destruction of the fetus, making it impossible to examine the fetus to see if it had spina bifida. In the circumstances it is probably more reasonable to assume a false-positive rate of, say, 0.5 per cent.

Biochemical screening

Alphafetoprotein

The marker measured in biochemical screening is maternal serum alphafetoprotein (AFP). AFP was identified in 1956.[15] Its function is not known. The association between raised amniotic fluid AFP levels and open neural tube defects was identified in 1972,[16] and this was followed by a report from Japan[17] of a raised serum AFP level in an anencephalic pregnancy. The association between raised serum AFP levels and open spina bifida was first demonstrated by two studies in 1974.[18,19] Following the discovery that serum AFP was raised in affected pregnancies, the UK Collaborative AFP Study group was formed, representing 19 centres (including one in Australia), to investigate whether maternal serum AFP measurement would be an effective and reliable screening test. Results were collected from 18 684 singleton and 163 twin pregnancies without fetal neural tube defects, and from 301 singleton pregnancies with fetal neural tube defects (146 with anencephaly, 142 with spina bifida, and 13 with encephalocele)[20] and confirmed the earlier findings. The study established the scientific and practical basis of antenatal screening for neural tube defects.

Figure 3.2 shows the source of AFP and how it enters the amniotic fluid and maternal serum. At about 17 weeks in unaffected pregnancies, the relative concentrations in fetal serum, amniotic fluid, and maternal serum are in the ratio 50 000:300:1. Figure 3.3 shows the rise in maternal serum AFP with gestation.

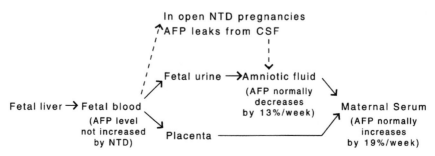

Fig. 3.2 Source of amniotic fluid AFP and maternal serum AFP in the early second trimester of pregnancy.

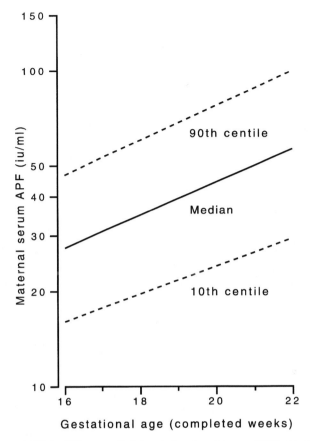

Fig. 3.3   Median and 10th to 90th percentile interval of maternal serum AFP for singleton pregnancies without neural tube defects (from Wald and Cuckle 1984).[21]

Distribution of maternal serum AFP in affected and unaffected pregnancies

AFP screening is intended for the detection of *open* spina bifida and should not be expected to detect *closed* spina bifida, which in most cases can be detected by ultrasound. AFP screening now has a minor role in the detection of anencephaly since this is readily diagnosed directly by ultrasound imaging examination. For this reason, this discussion of biochemical screening deals almost entirely with screening for open spina bifida. Nearly all cases of spina bifida will also be detected by ultrasound in centres with ultrasound experience.

To allow for the increase in the concentration of maternal serum AFP in the second trimester of pregnancy, it is convenient to express all AFP values as a multiple of the normal median (MoM) at the relevant gestational age. This also allows for systematic differences between laboratories in the measurement of AFP. An advantage in using the median (the middle value at a given week of pregnancy, when all the values are arranged in ascending order) rather than the mean as a measure of central tendency is that, unlike the mean, the median is not influenced by occasional outlying values. Maternal serum AFP values are therefore usually expressed in MoMs. A MoM value is simply the observed value divided by the expected value.

The separation between the distribution of maternal serum AFP levels in pregnancies with open spina bifida and in unaffected pregnancies is greatest at 16–18 weeks of pregnancy.[18] Table 3.4 shows the percentage of pregnancies with maternal serum AFP levels equal to or greater than different multiples of the normal median at 16–18 weeks of gestation. ('Normal' relates to unaffected pregnancies.) These percentages were derived by direct observation using data from the UK Collaborative AFP Study.[20] At 2.5 times the normal median 88 per cent of anencephalic pregnancies and 79 per cent of open spina bifida pregnancies are detected. At the same stage of pregnancy, 3.3 per cent of unaffected singleton pregnancies (or about 3.6 per cent of all unaffected pregnancies including twins) had AFP levels at or above this level.

In the original UK Collaborative AFP Study[20] and in the Fourth Report,[22] serum AFP data on pregnancies with and without neural tube defects were combined in 3-week groups, and separate estimates of the means and standard deviations of the distributions in these groups were calculated. This led to abrupt changes in the median MoM values for, say, open spina bifida, from one 3-week period to the next. This was artificial, and to avoid the problem revised parameters for each week of gestational age have been estimated and published.[23,24] Also, the standard deviation of AFP has decreased over time, due mainly to improvements in assay precision, and this has been allowed for[25] (Table 3.5).

Figure 3.4 illustrates the overlapping distribution of maternal serum AFP in pregnancies with and without open spina bifida at 17-weeks of pregnancy using the 17-week parameters in Table 3.5 based on dates (time since first day of last menstrual period). The detection rate (DR) and false-positive rate (FPR) are shown using three cut-offs, namely 2.0 MoM, 2.5 MoM, and 3.0 MoM. The DR and FPR corresponding to a cut-off of 2.5 are shaded. Figure 3.5 compares the distributions when gestation is based on dates and based on the ultrasound measurement of the biparietal diameter (BPD). The performance of screening improves when gestational age is estimated from a BPD measurement, for two reasons. First, there is a small effect because ultrasound imaging increases the precision of estimating gestational age and so reduces the variance of AFP at a given gestation. Second, because spina bifida fetuses tend to have small BPDs, they are, on average, credited with a less advanced gestational age than is the case (see Fig. 3.6). This error turns out to be advantageous, since it leads to AFP MoM values being higher when based on a BPD measurement than

Table 3.4 Percentage of singleton pregnancies with maternal serum AFP levels at 16–18 weeks of gestation equal to or greater than specified cut-off levels. (Adapted from UK Collaborative AFP Study Report 1977 based on direct observation (i.e. without modelling)).[20]

Pregnancy	Percentage ≥ cut-off level (MoM)*				
	2.0	2.5	3.0	3.5	4.0
Singleton NTD pregnancies					
Anencephaly	90.0	88.0	84.0	82.0	76.0
Open spina bifida	91.0	79.0	70.0	64.0	45.0
All spina bifida†	83.0	69.0	60.0	55.0	38.0
Singleton non-NTD pregnancies	7.2	3.3	1.4	0.6	0.3

* MoM = multiple of the median for unaffected singleton pregnancies of the same gestational age.
† Including closed lesions as well as those open or not known whether open or closed.

Table 3.5   Means and standard deviations of maternal serum AFP levels in singleton pregnancies (between 15 and 22 completed weeks of gestation) with and without specified neural tube defects. Taken from Wald *et al.* (2000)[24,25]

Pregnancy		AFP ($\log_{10}$ MoM), with gestation estimated by	
		Dates	BPD using ultrasound
Unaffected			
Mean		0.0000	0.0000
Standard deviation		0.1688 (0.1649)	0.1579 (0.1468)
Anencephaly			
Means	15 weeks	0.6412	na
	16 weeks	0.7469	na
	17 weeks	0.8110	na
	18 weeks	0.8335	na
	19 weeks	0.8144	na
	20 weeks	0.7537	na
	21 weeks	0.6514	na
	22 weeks	0.5075	na
Standard deviation		0.3335 (0.3316)	0.3282 (0.3230)
Open spina bifida			
Means	15 weeks	0.4554	0.6107
	16 weeks	0.5522	0.7075
	17 weeks	0.6024	0.7578
	18 weeks	0.6060	0.7613
	19 weeks	0.5630	0.7183
	20 weeks	0.4734	0.6287
	21 weeks	0.3372	0.4925
	22 weeks	0.1544	0.3097
Standard deviation		0.3378 (0.3358)	0.3324 (0.3272)
Closed spina bifida			
Mean		0.0000	0.1553
Standard deviation		0.1688 (0.1649)	0.1579 (0.1468)

Dates = from first day of last menstrual period.
BPD = biparietal diameter.
Values in parenthesis are adjusted for maternal weight.
na = not applicable.

when based on dates—on average, 43 per cent higher.[26] This has a large effect on increasing spina bifida detection rates and also, incidentally, leads to the detection of some cases of closed spina bifida because ultrasound imaging increases the MoM value in these cases as well. Figure 3.7 shows the application of a 2.5 MoM cut-off at 17 weeks using BPD to estimate gestation; the figure summarizes the performance of AFP screening for open spina bifida.

Table 3.6 summarizes the screening detection rate and false-positive rate for open spina bifida according to AFP cut-off level, gestational age, and method of determining gestational age (either dates or BPD).

The timing of screening is a compromise. The AFP test is usually part of the triple or quadruple screening test for Down's syndrome (see Chapter 4) which, if positive, can lead to an amniocentesis and a fetal karyotype, a test that can take 2 to 3 weeks to complete. To avoid creating a situation in which a woman may be offered a termination of pregnancy after 20 weeks, it may be best to aim to screen women at 16 weeks of gestation, even though the screening performance for open spina bifida may be marginally poorer at this time than at 17 or 18 weeks. At 17 weeks of gestation, using

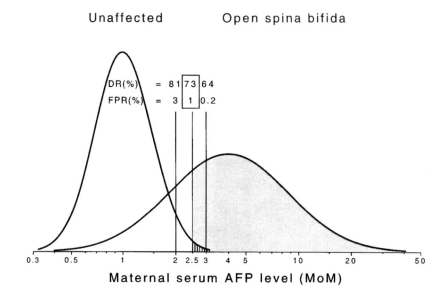

Fig. 3.4 Relative frequency distribution of maternal serum AFP in pregnancies with and without open spina bifida at 17 weeks of gestation according to dates and with maternal weight correction. Three cut-off levels are shown (2.0, 2.5, and 3.0 MoM) with the detection rates (DR) and false-positive rates (FPR) specified. The shaded areas show the DR and FPR using a 2.5 MoM cut -off level. (MoM = Multiple of the median for unaffected pregnancies of the same gestational age.)

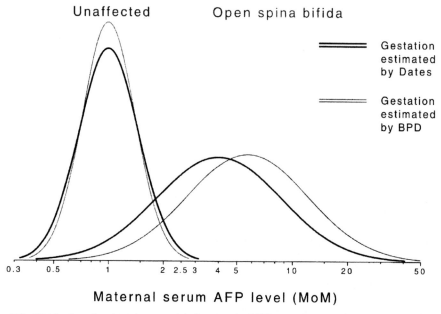

Fig. 3.5 Distribution of maternal serum alphafetoprotein (AFP) levels (corrected for maternal weight) in pregnancies with open spina bifida and pregnancies without neural tube defects (unaffected) at 16 weeks of gestation with gestational age estimated by dates (from first day of last menstrual period, LMP) and by ultrasound imaging (fetal biparietal diameter measurement, BPD).

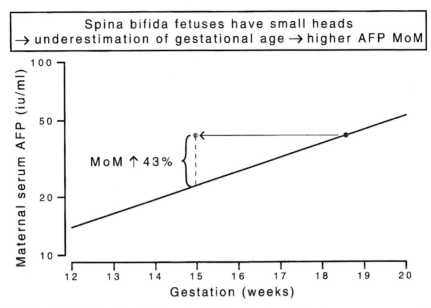

Fig. 3.6 The effect of using a biparietal diameter (BPD) to estimate gestational age on a pregnancy with spina bifida. Gestation is, on average, under-estimated by 16 days and this increases the AFP MoM value by 43 per cent.

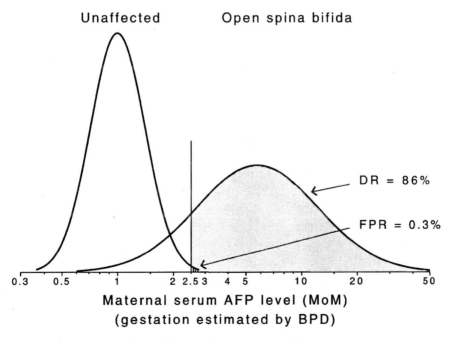

Fig. 3.7 The relative frequency distributions of maternal serum AFP in pregnancies with and without open spina bifida at 17 weeks of gestation using a biparietal diameter measurement to estimate gestational age. Using a cut-off level of 2.5 MoM the detection rate (DR) is 86 per cent and the false-positive rate (FPR) is 0.3% per cent. (MoM = Multiple of the median.)

Table 3.6 Maternal serum AFP screening at 15–20 weeks of gestation; detection rate for open spina bifida and false-positive rate according to method of estimating gestational age used to calculate MoM value and AFP cut-off level. Timing of test based on estimating gestational age from a woman's LMP. AFP MoM levels are adjusted for maternal weight. Based on Wald *et al.* (2000)[24,25]

Method used to estimate gestational age	AFP (MoM)	Detection rate (%)						False-positive rate (%)
		Gestation (completed weeks)						
		15	16	17	18	19	20	15–20 weeks
Dates	≥2.0	68	77	81	82	78	70	3.4
	≥2.5	57	68	73	73	69	59	0.8
	≥3.0	47	59	64	65	60	50	0.2
BPD	≥2.0	83	89	92	92	90	84	2.0
	≥2.5	74	83	86	87	84	76	0.3
	≥3.0	66	76	80	81	77	68	0.1

MoM = Multiple of the median for unaffected pregnancies of the same gestational age.
BPD = Biparietal diameter.

an AFP cut-off level of 2.5 MoM or greater, the detection rate for open spina bifida is 86 per cent with a false-positive rate of 0.3 per cent using the BPD to estimate gestational age and with AFP levels corrected for maternal weight. Using a cut-off level of 2.0 MoM the detection rate would be 92% and the false-positive rate 2.0%.

Screening performance is improved by correcting AFP levels for maternal weight because maternal serum AFP levels, on average, decrease with increasing maternal weight.[27,28] This is due to dilution of fetal AFP in the maternal circulation, the extent of dilution being greater in the larger plasma volume of heavier women than in that of lighter women. Adjusting AFP values for maternal weight will reduce the variance of maternal serum AFP in affected and unaffected pregnancies and so tend to reduce the extent of overlap in the distributions shown in Figures 3.4, 3.5, and 3.7. A simple method of adjusting AFP values for maternal weight is to divide the observed MoM value by the expected MoM value for a given maternal weight.

In addition to gestational age and maternal weight there are other factors that are associated with maternal serum AFP and can usefully be taken into account in screening by adjusting the AFP MoM value. These are:

1. Insulin-dependent diabetes mellitus. Serum AFP levels are, on average, lower in women with insulin-dependent diabetes mellitus. Table 4.10 in Chapter 4 (Screening for Down's syndrome) summarizes the published literature on studies. After weight correction, AFP is about 10 per cent lower in women with insulin-dependent diabetes; without weight correction it is 16 per cent lower. The differences are statistically highly significant and can therefore usefully be taken into account. Adjustment for diabetes is carried out by dividing the observed MoM for a woman with diabetes by the corresponding median MoM in diabetic women without neural tube defect pregnancies.

2. Twin pregnancies. AFP levels in women with twin pregnancies are about twice those in singleton pregnancies (2.23 MoM, see Table 4.11 in Chapter 4). As with diabetic women, the AFP MoM is adjusted by dividing the observed MoM value in a

twin pregnancy by the median MoM value in twin pregnancies without neural tube defects.

3. Ethnic group. Corrections for ethnic group can help allow for extraneous variation in serum AFP.[29] The median maternal serum AFP is raised in black women compared with white (1.17 MoM); (1.15 MoM after weight correction).[30] The effect in South Asian women is small: their median AFP value is 1.02 MoM (0.94 MoM after weight correction). It is worth adjusting AFP values in black women.

Tables 3.7 and 3.8 summarize factors (or conditions) associated with high and low serum AFP levels. The tables indicate the size of the effect and what action, if any, need be taken.

Refining the performance of AFP screening

An analysis of variance[21] has shown that about half (51 per cent) of the variance of AFP in any given week of pregnancy is due to differences between pregnancies (as opposed to differences between mothers). These differences must reflect the effect of

Table 3.7   Summary of factors associated with high serum AFP

Factor	Comment	Action	Reference
1 Under-estimated gestation	Moderate effect	Reduced by prior scan	
2 Low maternal weight	Small effect	Adjust MoM	23,27,28,31
3 Multiple pregnancy	Large effect	Identified by prior scan	20,30,32,33,34,35
4 Spontaneous fetal loss	Large effect	None practical	36,37,38,39,40,41,42,43,44
5 Raised AFP in previous pregnancy	Small effect	None	45,46
6 Male fetus (see Fig 3.8)	Small effect	None	21,37
7 Afro-Caribbean	Small effect	Adjust MoM	29,30,31
8 Low birth weight	Moderate effect	None	27,37,44,47,48,49,50,51,52
9 Abdominal wall defects	Large effect	Scan and amnio	53,54,55,56
10 Congenital nephrosis	Large effect	Amnio	57,58,59
11 Smoking	Small effect	None	60,61
12 Pre-eclampsia	Moderate effect	None	39,62,63
13 Preterm delivery*	Moderate effect	None	39,41,63,64

* This is probably due to the under-estimation of gestational age resulting in a high serum AFP MoM value and apparent early birth.

Table 3.8   Summary of factors associated with low serum AFP

Factor	Comment	Action	Reference
1 Over-estimated gestation	Moderate effect	Reduced by prior scan	
2 High maternal weight	Small effect	Adjust MoM	23,27,28,31
3 Down's syndrome	Small effect	Use AFP with multiple marker screening	7,30
4 Trisomy 18	Small effect	Use AFP with multiple marker screening	30,65,66,67
5 Insulin-dependent diabetes	Small effect	Adjust MoM	68,69,70
6 Iatrogenic low birth weight	Small effect	Avoid elective delivery of small infant in mistaken belief that pregnancy is post-mature	50

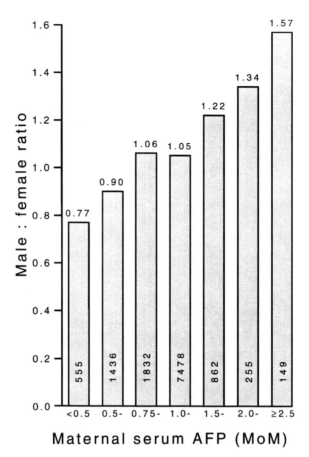

Fig. 3.8   Fetal sex ratio (male:female) according to maternal serum AFP level in 7367 singleton pregnancies at 16–18 weeks of gestation. (MoM = Multiple of the median.)

the fetal–placental unit, because maternal factors such as age and parity which change from pregnancy to pregnancy have negligible effects on AFP. A further 17 per cent of the variance is due to within-pregnancy fluctuations in serum AFP; about 14 per cent is due to assay error and about 10 per cent is due to gestational age error, leaving only 8 per cent to be accounted for by mother to mother differences, to which maternal weight and ethnic group contribute. An observation of biological interest but no screening importance is the association between maternal serum AFP and fetal sex (see Fig. 3.8).

Odds of being affected given a positive result

Table 3.9 shows the odds of having a singleton pregnancy with open spina bifida for groups of women with AFP levels equal to or greater than specified cut-off levels and for individual women with AFP levels equal to the specified levels.

Outcome of pregnancies with high serum AFP

Table 3.10 shows the outcome of pregnancies with high serum AFP in Oxford between 1975 and 1980;[21] 24 660 women were screened between 16 and 22 weeks of

Table 3.9 Odds of having a singleton pregnancy with open spina bifida at 17 weeks of pregnancy (using a scan estimate of gestation and maternal weight correction)

Serum AFP level (MoM)	Natural birth prevalence	
	1 per 1000	2 per 1000
Population odds:		
≥2.0	1:42	1:21
≥2.5	1:11	1:5
≥3.0	1:3	1:2
≥3.5	1:1	1:1
≥4.0	> 1:1	> 1:1
Individual odds:		
= 2.0	1:575	1:287
= 2.5	1:133	1:66
= 3.0	1:33	1:16
= 3.5	1:9	1:4
= 4.0	1:3	1:1

MoM = Multiple of the median.
Using the results in Table 3.4 and the parameters in Table 3.5.

Table 3.10 Outcome of pregnancies with maternal serum AFP levels equal to or greater than specified cut-off levels. Each specified outcome excludes those listed above it. (Oxford data 1975–1980, 24 660 women tested at 16 weeks of gestation by dates, without weight correction) (taken from Wald and Cuckle (1984)[21])

Outcome	Cut-off level							
	3.0 MoM*		3.5 MoM		4.0 MoM		4.5 MoM	
	No.	%	No.	%	No.	%	No.	%
Miscarriage	66	16.4	52	21.1	32	19.5	23	19.3
Multiple pregnancy †	49	12.2	28	11.4	15	9.1	12	10.1
Anencephaly	21	5.2	20	8.1	15	9.1	14	11.8
Open spina bifida	20	5.0	19	7.7	15	9.1	10	8.4
Abdominal wall defect	5	1.2	5	2.0	5	3.0	5	4.2
Non NTD, non-exomphalos termination of pregnancy	15	3.7	13	5.3	11	6.7	8	6.7
Stillbirth ≤ 2.5 kg	3	0.7	2	0.8	2	1.2	2	1.7
Stillbirth > 2.5 kg	1	0.2	0	0.0	0	0.0	0	0.0
Neonatal death:‡ 1st week	6	1.5	6	2.4	6	3.7	4	3.4
Neonatal death: 2nd–4th week	2	0.5	2	0.8	1	0.6	1	0.8
Birthweight ≤ 2.5 kg	31	7.7	12	4.9	8	4.9	7	5.9
'Healthy' singleton	183	45.5	87	35.4	54	32.9	33	27.7
Total	402	100.0	246	100.0	164	100.0	119	100.0

* MoM = multiple of the median.
† The proportion of multiple pregnancies among women with raised serum AFP levels has decreased in recent years since they are more often recognized by ultrasound scan before 16 weeks of gestation and as a result an AFP test is not performed.
‡ All ≤ 2.5 kg.

pregnancy, of whom 402 (1.6 per cent) had AFP values equal to or greater than 3 MoM. Of the 402 women 176 had a pregnancy with an open neural tube defect or anterior abdominal wall defect, a miscarriage, a termination for a reason unconnected with a raised AFP, or multiple pregnancy, leaving 226. Of these, four had stillbirths (1.8 per cent), eight had infants who died neonatally (3.5 per cent), and 31 others had infants born weighing 2.5 kg or less (13.7 per cent)—clearly a group at very high risk of an adverse outcome. Similar results were reported from Edinburgh.[71]

Biochemical diagnosis

The main biochemical diagnostic tests for open neural tube defects are amniotic fluid AFP measurement and amniotic fluid acetylcholinesterase (AChE) measurement. The AChE test is usually performed by polyacrylamide gel electrophoresis, a qualitative test. A result is positive if there is an AChE band in the gel that migrates to the same position as the AChE in cerebral spinal fluid, and the band is inhibited by the specific AChE inhibitor given the code name BW284C51. An alternative assay,[72] based on an immunoassay, performs well but has not been shown to perform better than gel electrophoresis. The Second Report of the Collaborative Acetylcholinesterase Study[73] showed that AChE measurement was a better diagnostic test than amniotic fluid AFP (Table 3.11). The study was based on 32 642 women with singleton pregnancies, including 428 with open spina bifida and 238 with anencephaly, who had an amnio-centesis at 13 to 24 weeks of gestation. The AChE test yielded a detection rate for open spina bifida of 99 per cent (95 per cent confidence interval: 98–100 per cent) at a false-positive rate of 0.34 per cent (95 per cent confidence interval: 0.28–0.40 per cent) excluding miscarriage, intrauterine death, and serious fetal abnormalities. Comparable rates for amniotic fluid AFP as a diagnostic test were less favourable, yielding a lower detection rate and a higher false-positive rate—90 per cent and 0.46 per cent respectively.

Although AChE is a better diagnostic test than AFP, almost as high a detection rate can be achieved by restricting AChE measurement to women with AFP levels exceeding 2 MoM (about 5 per cent) with the advantage of reducing the corresponding false-positive rate (see Table 3.11, column headed 'Any reason' for the amniocentesis: 0.14 per cent compared with 0.34 per cent with a small difference in detection—96 per cent compared with 99 per cent). Table 3.11 also shows the performance according to whether the amniocentesis is performed on account of a raised maternal serum AFP level or for other reasons, and whether the amniotic fluid sample was clear or blood stained to the naked eye. Blood contamination of amniotic fluid is an important cause of false-positive results. Fortunately, this is rare. Among clear samples, the selective AChE testing policy (row C in Table 3.11) yields a detection rate of 98 per cent with a false-positive rate of 2 in 1000 (0.19 per cent) among women having an amniocentesis on account of a high serum AFP screening test result.

The reason for the higher amniotic fluid AFP false-positive rate in women with a high serum AFP level is that there is an association between maternal serum and amniotic fluid AFP. The higher AChE false-positive rate is less easily explained, but may be due to an association between high amniotic fluid AFP and the presence of amniotic fluid AChE.

Table 3.11 Open spina bifida detection rates and false-positive rates according to reason for amniocentesis and whether amniotic fluid (AF) sample is blood stained. Taken from Wald et al. (1989)[73]

	Amniocentesis for high serum AFP				Amniocentesis for other reasons				Amniocentesis for any reason			
	All AF samples		Clear* AF samples		All AF samples		Clear* AF samples		All AF samples		Clear* AF samples	
Test policy	DR (%) $n = 344$	FPR (%) $n = 5557$	DR (%) $n = 298$	FPR (%) $n = 4785$	DR (%) $n = 84$	FPR (%) $n = 25\,896$	DR (%) $n = 76$	FPR (%) $n = 24\,223$	DR (%) $n = 428$	FPR (%) $n = 31\,453$	DR (%) $n = 374$	FPR (%) $n = 29\,008$
A. AChE alone	99	0.56	99	0.23	96	0.29	96	0.15	99	0.34	99	0.16
B. AFP alone **	90	1.5	91	1.3	92	0.23	92	0.11	90	0.46	91	0.30
C. AChE if AF-AFP ≥2.0 MoM	97	0.40	98	0.19	95	0.09	95	0.03	96	0.14	97	0.06

n = number of pregnancies; AFP = alphafetoprotein; AChE = acetylcholinesterase; AF = amniotic fluid .

* A clear sample is one which is not visibly blood stained.

** Using gestation-specific AF–AFP cut-off levels; 2.5 MoM (13–15 weeks); 3.0 (16–18 weeks); 3.5 (19–21 weeks); 4.0 (22–24 weeks).

MoM = Multiple of the median for unaffected pregnancies of the same gestational age.

CONCLUSIONS

The place of AFP screening

It is uncertain whether maternal serum AFP screening for spina bifida is necessary at centres that routinely offer an ultrasound examination designed to identify the ultrasound screening markers of spina bifida. Although the performance of ultrasound screening is not reliably known, it is undoubtedly high. AFP screening, however, does have a number of advantages. It is simple and easily applied to large numbers, not requiring the kind of operator training and vigilance necessary with ultrasound. AFP has a modest value in screening for Down's syndrome and is useful in the identification of other disorders such as trisomy 18. On balance, it is sensible for centres to retain AFP screening for the moment, recognizing that, if it can be reliably documented that it achieves no more than ultrasound screening, it could be abandoned in the future.

Combining biochemical and ultrasound diagnosis

The spina bifida detection rate using ultrasound has been estimated to be 84 per cent with a false-positive rate of 0.5 per cent (Table 3.12)—a performance somewhat less than that based on amniotic fluid biochemical analysis (97 per cent and 0.4 per cent respectively). The main disadvantage of an amniotic fluid biochemical diagnosis is the risk of fetal loss due to the amniocentesis. The best estimate of this is from the randomized trial of amniocentesis reported by Tabor and her colleagues (1986).[74] An excess risk of 1.0 per cent is cited. If the fetal loss rate in women randomized to the control group is subtracted from the rate in women allocated to the study group, the excess risk is 0.78 per cent (95 per cent per cent confidence interval: 0.04–1.53 per cent). If an adjustment is made for cytogenetically abnormal fetuses that were termi-

Table 3.12 Comparison of three policies in the diagnosis of open spina bifida among women with raised maternal serum alphafetoprotein (AFP) levels

Diagnostic policy	Detection rate (%)	False-positive rate (%)	Fetal loss rate per 1000 women with raised serum AFP but unaffected pregnancies due to:		
			Diagnostic error	Amniocentesis*	Both
Ultrasound only**	84	0.5	5	0	5
Amniocentesis only[†]	97	0.4	4	8	12
Ultrasound and amniocentesis[††]	94[‡]	<0.1[‡‡]	<1	8	8–9

* From the Copenhagen randomized study,[74] subtracting the fetal loss rate in women allocated to the control group from the rate in women allocated to the amniocentesis group.
** From Table 3.2.
† From Table 3.11.
†† Ultrasound examination is repeated if it is negative but the amniotic fluid results are positive; a final positive result is one in which both the ultrasound examination and amniotic fluid results are positive.
‡ Assumes four out of five of cases missed by ultrasound examination are detected upon re-examination after a positive amniotic fluid result is known (as found in Richards et al. (1988)[75] and Drugan et al. (1988)[76]).
‡‡ Assumes that at least three out of four of amniotic fluid false-positives will be corrected by ultrasound examination; in fact the proportion is likely to be greater, but data on this are lacking.

nated but would otherwise have miscarried, the estimate would be 0.87 per cent (95 per cent confidence interval 0.08–1.58 per cent).

If the indication for diagnostic testing was a serum AFP level greater than or equal to 2.5 MoMs at 17 weeks (with gestational age estimated from BPD on ultrasound), and if the natural birth prevalence of spina bifida was 1/1000, then, from Table 3.6, the odds of having an affected pregnancy for those selected for diagnostic testing would be 1:3.5 (i.e. 86/0.3 × 1:1000). According to Table 3.12, a *positive* diagnostic amniotic fluid analysis would increase the odds to 69:1 (i.e. 97/0.4 × 1:3.5) and a *negative* analysis would decrease the odds to 1:116 (i.e. 3/99.6 × 1:3.5), over eight times the odds before screening.

A *positive* ultrasound scan diagnosis would increase the odds to 48:1 (i.e. 84/0.5 × 1:3.5)—a substantial increase but not so high as to make a false-positive an extreme rarity: there would be one false-positive for every 48 true positives. These odds are critically dependent on the estimate of the *false-positive rate* for diagnostic ultrasound scan, and unfortunately this estimate is not secure. If the false-positive rate were 0.1 per cent instead of 0.5 per cent, there would be one false-positive pregnancy for every 240 true positives.

A *negative* ultrasound scan diagnosis would decrease the odds of having spina bifida to 1:22 (i.e. 16/99.5 × 1:3.5) which is 46 times greater than the odds before screening. In this case the odds are mainly dependent on the estimate of the *detection rate* of ultrasound. For example, if the detection rate were 5 per cent higher (89 per cent instead of 84 per cent), then the odds would be 1:32—one pregnancy would be affected and 32 would be unaffected in women with negative scan results.

Greater accuracy can be achieved by using both ultrasound and amniocentesis in all women with raised serum AFP. For the final result to be regarded as positive with this policy, positive results must have been obtained in both the amniotic fluid analysis and an ultrasound examination. Ultrasound examination is repeated if it is negative but the amniotic fluid results are positive; and when this is done, four-fifths of cases missed by the first examination are detected, according to the findings of Richards *et al.* (1988)[75] and Drugan *et al.* (1988).[76] When combined in this way, diagnostic ultrasound and amniocentesis yield a detection rate of 94 per cent, a false-positive rate of less than 0.1 per cent and an overall fetal loss rate (mainly due to amniocentesis) of 0.8–0.9 per cent (Table 3.12). If the natural birth prevalence of spina bifida is 1/1000, the odds of having an affected pregnancy when the serum AFP (corrected for maternal weight) is greater than or equal to 2.5 MoMs at 17 weeks are >269:1 (i.e. 94/<0.1 × 1:3.5) if the diagnostic ultrasound and amniocentesis are both positive and 1:58, (i.e. 6/>99.9 × 1:3.5) if they are not.

The best policy, therefore, is one in which amniocentesis and ultrasound are used as complementary diagnostic investigations. Only if a woman explicitly chooses to forego the extra accuracy from an amniotic fluid AFP and AChE test is it reasonable to abandon the amniocentesis.

Overall performance of screening and diagnosis

Figure 3.9 shows two flow diagrams of screening and diagnosis. The first diagram is applicable to centres using AFP as the method of screening with an ultrasound scan examination used to estimate gestational age routinely. It yields a detection rate of 81

(i) AFP screening at 17 completed weeks with prior routine ultrasound used to date the pregnancy and diagnose anencephaly

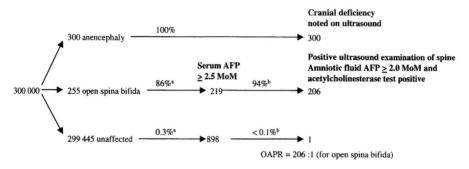

(ii) Ultrasound alone used (centres with specialist ultrasound facilities)

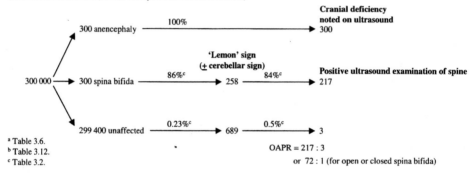

a Table 3.6.
b Table 3.12.
c Table 3.2.

Fig. 3.9   Flow diagrams illustrating screening for neural tube defects.

per cent for open spina bifida and a false-positive rate of 0.0003 per cent. The second diagram applies to centres with sufficient expertise in ultrasound to use this alone in screening and diagnosis. This model yields a detection rate of 72 per cent for all spina bifida and a false-positive rate of 0.001 per cent. These estimates are more uncertain than those for AFP screening; the detection rate for the lemon sign in Table 3.2 which is used in the diagram is likely to be higher and the false-positive rate lower than the true figures for all pregnancies, for the reasons indicated when Table 3.2 was discussed. These uncertainties strengthen the case for not abandoning serum AFP screening and amniotic fluid measurement in the diagnosis of neural tube defects unless and until there is firmer evidence that ultrasound is at least as reliable. Nonetheless many centres have abandoned it, with unknown consequences.

REFERENCES

1. Hunter A. G. W. (1993). Brain and spinal cord. In *Human malformations and related anomalies*) (Oxford monographs on medical genetics no. 27) vol. II, (ed. R. E. Stevenson, J. G. Hall, and R. M. Goodman), pp. 109–37. Oxford University Press, New York.

2. Althouse R. and Wald N. (1980). Survival and handicap of infants with spina bifida. *Arch. Dis. Child.*, **55**, 845–50.

3. Adzick N. S., Sutton L. N., Crombleholme T. M., and Flake A. W. (1998). Successful fetal surgery for spina bifida. *Lancet*, **352**, 1675–6.

4. Rogers S. C. and Weatherall J. A. C. (1976). *Anencephalus, spina bifida and congenital hydro-*

cephalus. England and Wales 1964–1972, (Office of Population Censuses and Surveys. Studies on Medical and Population Subjects No 32). HMSO, London.

5. Office of National Statistics (1996). *Congenital malformation statistics 1993 (notifications)* (Series M B 3, no 9). HMSO, London.
6. Office of National Statistics (1998). *Congenital anomaly statistics 1995 and 1996 (notifications)* (Series M B 3, no 11). The Stationery Office, London.
7. Cuckle H. and Wald N. (1987). The impact of screening for open neural tube defects in England and Wales. *Prenat. Diagn.*, **7**, 91–9.
8. MRC Vitamin Study Research Group (1991). Prevention of neural tube defects: results of the M. R.C Vitamin Study. *Lancet*, **338**, 132–7.
9. Czeizel A. E. and Dudas I. (1992). Prevention of the first occurrence of neural-tube defects by periconceptional vitamin supplementation. *N. Engl. J. Med.*, **327**, 1832–5.
10. Wald N. J.(1994). Folic acid and neural tube defects: the current evidence and implications for prevention. In *Neural tube defects*, CIBA Foundation Symposium 181, pp. 192–211. Chichester, Wiley.
11. Little J. (1992). Risks in siblings and other relatives. In *Epidemiology and control of neural tube defects*, (ed. J. M. Elwood, J. Little, and J. H. Elwood), pp. 604–76. Oxford University Press, Oxford.
12. Nicolaides K. H., Campbell S., Gabbe S. G., and Guidetti R. (1986). Ultrasound screening for spina bifida: Cranial and cerebellar signs. *Lancet*, **ii**, 72–4.
13. de Courcy-Wheeler R. H. B, Pomeranz M. M., Wald N. J., and Nicolaides K. H. (1994). Small fetal transverse cerebellar diameter: a screening test for spina bifida. *Br. J. Obstet. Gynaecol.*, **101**, 904–5.
14. Papp Z., Tóth-Pál E., Papp Cs., Tóth Z., Szabó M., Veress L., and Török O. (1995). Impact of prenatal mid-trimester screening on the prevalence of fetal structure anomalies: a prospective epidemiological study. *Ultrasound Obstet. Gynecol.*, **6**, 320–6.
15. Bergstrand C. G. and Czar B. (1956). Demonstration of a new protein fraction in serum from the human foetus. *Scand. J. Clin. Lab. Invest.*, **8**, 174.
16. Brock D. J. H. and Sutcliffe R. G. (1972). Alpha-fetoprotein in the antenatal diagnosis of anencephaly and spina bifida. *Lancet*, **ii**, 197–9.
17. Hino M., Koki Y., and Nishi S. (1972). Nimpu ketsu naka no alpha-fetoprotein. *Igaku No Ayumi*, **82**, 512.
18. Brock D. J. H, Bolton A. E., and Scrimgeour J. B. (1974). Prenatal diagnosis of spina bifida and anencephaly through maternal plasma alpha-fetoprotein measurement. *Lancet*, **i**, 767–9.
19. Wald N. J., Brock D. J. H, and Bonnar J. (1974). Prenatal diagnosis of spina bifida and anencephaly by maternal serum alpha-fetoprotein measurement. A controlled study. *Lancet*, **i**, 765–7.
20. Report of UK Collaborative Study on Alpha-fetoprotein in relation to neural tube defects. (1977). Maternal serum alpha-fetoprotein measurement in antenatal screening for anencephaly and spina bifida in early pregnancy. *Lancet*, **i**, 1323–32.
21. Wald N. J. and Cuckle H. S. (1984). Open neural-tube defects. In *Antenatal and Neonatal Screening* (1st edn), (ed. N. J. Wald), pp. 25–73. Oxford University Press, Oxford.
22. Wald N. J. and Cuckle H. S. (1982). Estimating an individual's risk of having a fetus with open spina bifida and the value of repeat alpha-fetaprotein testing. Fourth Report of the UK Collaborative Study on Alpha-Fetoprotein in Relation to Neural-tube Defects. *J. Epidemiol. Community Health*, **36**: 87–95.

23. Wald N. J., Cuckle H. S., Densem J. W., Kennard A., and Smith D. (1992). Maternal serum screening for Down's syndrome: the effect of routine ultrasound scan determination of gestational age and adjustment for maternal weight. *Br. J. Obstet. Gynaecol.*, **99**, 144–9.

24. Wald N. J., Hackshaw A.K., Cuckle H. S. (2000). Maternal serum alphafetoprotein screening for open neural tube defects: revised statistical parameters. *Br. J. Obstet. Gynaecol.*, **107**, 296–8.

25. Wald N. J., Hackshaw A. K., George L. Assay precision of serum alpha-fetoprotein in antenatal screening for neural tube defects and Down's syndrome. *J. Med. Screen.*, In press.

26. Wald N., Cuckle H., Boreham J., and Stirrat G. (1980). Small biparietal diameter of fetuses with spina bifida: implications for antenatal screening. *Br. J. Obstet. Gynaecol.*, **87**, 219–21.

27. Haddow J. E., Kloza E. M., Knight G. J., and Smith D. E. (1981). Relationship between maternal weight and serum alpha-fetoprotein concentration during the second trimester. *Clin. Chem.*, **27**, 133–4.

28. Wald N. J., Cuckle H., Boreham J., Terzian E., and Redman C. (1981). The effect of maternal weight on maternal serum alpha-fetoprotein levels. *Br. J. Obstet. Gynaecol.*, **88**, 1094–6.

29. Watt H. C., Wald N. J., Smith D., Kennard A., and Densem J. (1996). Effect of allowing for ethnic group in prenatal screening for Down's syndrome. *Prenat. Diagn.*, **16**, 691–8.

30. Wald N. J., Kennard A., Hackshaw A., and McGuire A. (1997). Antenatal screening for Down's syndrome. *J. Med. Screen.*, **4**, 181–246.

31. Crandall B. F., Lebherz T. B., Schroth P. C., and Matsumoto M. (1983). Alpha-fetoprotein concentration in maternal serum: relation to race and body weight. *Clin. Chem.*, **29**, 531–3.

32. Wald N., Cuckle H., and Stirrat G. (1978). Maternal serum alpha-fetoprotein levels in triplet and quadruplet pregnancy. *Br. J. Obstet. Gynaecol.*, **85**, 124–6.

33. Wald N. J., Cuckle H., Stirrat G. M., and Turnbull A. C. (1978). Maternal serum alpha-fetoprotein and birth weight in twin pregnancies. *Br. J. Obstet. Gynaecol.*, **85**, 582–4.

34. Wald N. J., Barker S., Peto R., Brock D. J. H, and Bonnar J. (1975). Maternal serum alpha-fetoprotein levels in multiple pregnancy. *Br. Med. J.*, **1**, 651–2.

35. O'Brien J. E., Dvorin E., Yaron Y., Ayoub M., Johnson M. P., Hume R. F. Jr., and Evens M. I. (1997). Differential increases in AFP, hCG, and uE3 in twin pregnancies: impact on attempts to quantify Down's syndrome screening calculations. *Am. J. Med. Genet.*, **73**, 109–12.

36. Wald N., Barker S., Cuckle H., Brock D. J. H., and Stirrat G. (1977). Maternal serum alpha-fetoprotein and spontaneous abortion. *Br. J. Obstet. Gynaecol.*, **84**, 357–62.

37. Read A. P., Donnai D., Harris R., and Donnai P. (1980). Comparison of pregnancy outcome after amniocentesis for previous neural tube defect or raised maternal serum alpha-fetoprotein. *Br. J. Obstet. Gynaecol.*, **87**, 372–6.

38. Monk A. M. and Goldie D. J. (1976). The significance of raised maternal serum alpha-feto protein levels. *Br. J. Obstet. Gynaecol.*, **83**, 845–52.

39. Gordon Y. B., Grudzinskas J. G., Kitau M. J., Usherwood M. M., Letchworth A. T., and Chard T. (1978). Fetal wastage as a result of an alpha-fetoprotein screening programme. *Lancet*, **i**, 677–8.

40. Haddow J. E., Kloza E. M., Smith D. E., and Knight G. J.(1983). Data from an alpha-fetoprotein pilot screening program in Maine. *Obstet. Gynecol.*, **62**, 556–60.

41. Robinson L., Grau P., and Crandall B. (1989). Pregnancy outcome after increasing maternal serum alpha-fetoprotein levels. *Obstet. Gynecol.*, **74**, 17–20.

42. Bernstein I. M., Barth R. A., Miller R., and Capeleless E. L. (1992). Elevated maternal serum alpha-fetoprotein: association with placental sonolucencies, fetomaternal hemorrhage, vagi-

nal bleeding, and pregnancy outcome in the absence of fetal abnormalies. *Obstet. Gynecol.*, **79**, 71–4.

43. Maher J. E., Davis R. O., Goldenberg R. L., Boots L. R., and DuBard M. B. (1994). Unexplained elevation in maternal serum alpha-fetoprotein and subsequent fetal loss. *Obstet. Gynecol.*, **83**, 138–41.

44. Hsieh T. T., Hung T. H., Hsu J. J., Shau W. Y., Su C. W., and Hsieh F. J. (1997). Prediction of adverse perinatal outcome by maternal serum screening for Down's syndrome in an Asian population. *Obstet. Gynecol.*, **89**, 937–40.

45. Wald N. J. and Cuckle H. S. (1981). Raised maternal serum alpha-fetoprotein levels in subsequent pregnancies. *Lancet*, **i**, 1103.

46. Spencer K. (1997). Between-pregnancy biological variability of maternal serum alpha-fetoprotein and free beta hCG: implications for Down's syndrome screening in subsequent pregnancies. *Prenat. Diagn.*, **17**, 39–45.

47. Wald N., Cuckle H., Stirrat G. M., Bennett M. J., and Turnbull A. C. (1977). Maternal serum alpha-fetoprotein and low birth-weight. *Lancet*, **ii**, 268–70.

48. Brock D. J. H., Barron L., Jelen P., Watt M., and Scrimgeour J. B. (1977). Maternal serum alpha-fetoprotein measurements as an early indicator of low birthweight. *Lancet*, **ii**, 267–8.

49. Macri J. N., Weiss R. R., Libster B., and Cagan M. A. (1978). Maternal serum alpha-fetoprotein and low birthweight. *Lancet*, **i**, 660.

50. Wald N. J., Cuckle H. S., Boreham J., and Turnbull A. C. (1980). Maternal serum alpha-fetoprotein and birth weight. *Br. J. Obstet. Gynaecol.*, **87**, 860–3.

51. Haddow J. E. and Wald N. J. (ed.). (1981). *Alpha-fetoprotein screening. The current issues. A report of the Third Scarborough Conference.* Foundation of Blood Research, Scarborough, Maine.

52. Pacsa A. S. and Pejtsik B. (1979), ELISA for monitoring serum AFP. *Lancet*, **i**, 443.

53. Seppala M., Karjalainen O., Rapola J., and Lindgren J. (1976). Maternal alpha-fetoprotein and fetal exomphalos. *Lancet*, **i**, 303–31.

54. Clarke P. C., Gordon Y. B., Kitau M. J., Chard T., and McNeal A. D. (1977). Alpha-fetoprotein levels in pregnancies complicated by gastrointestinal abnormalities of the fetus. *Br. J. Obstet. Gynaecol.*, **84**, 285–9.

55. Young L. J. and Crawford J. W. (1977). Omphalocoele and raised alpha-fetoprotein in maternal serum. *Br. J. Obstet. Gynaecol.*, **84**, 578–9.

56. Wald N. J., Cuckle H. S., Barlow R. D., Smith A. D., Stirrat G. M., Turnbull A. C., Bobrow M, Brock D. J. H., and Stein S. M. (1980). Early antenatal diagnosis of exomphalos. *Lancet*, **i**, 1368–9.

57. Seppala M., Aula P., Rapola J., Karjalainen O., Huttunen N. P., and Ruoslahti E. (1976). Congenital nephrotic syndrome: prenatal diagnosis and genetic counselling by estimation of amniotic fluid and maternal serum alpha-fetoprotein. *Lancet*, **ii**, 123–4.

58. Albright S. G., Warner A. A., Seed J. W., and Burton B. K. (1990). Congential nephrosis as a cause of elevated alpha-fetoprotein. *Obstet. Gynecol.*, **76**, 969–71.

59. Heinonen S., Ryynanen M., Kirkinen P., Penttila I., Syrjanen K., Seppala M., and Saarikoski S. (1996). Prenatal screening for congential nephrosis in east Finland: results and impact on the birth prevalence of the disease. *Prenat. Diagn.*, **16**, 207–13.

60. Palomaki G. E., Knight G. J., Haddow J. E., Canick J. A., Wald N. J., and Kennard A. (1993). Cigarette smoking and levels of maternal alpha-fetoprotein, unconjated estriol and hCG: impact on Down's syndrome screening. *Obstet. Gynecol.*, **81**, 675–8.

61. Bartels I., Hoppe-Sievert B., Bockel B., Herold S., and Casear J. (1993). Adjustment formulae for maternal serum alpha-fetoprotein, human chorionic gonadotropin and unconjugated oestriol to maternal weight and smoking. *Prenat. Diagn.*, **13**, 123–30.
62. Walters B. N. J., Lao T., and Smith V. (1985). Alpha-fetoprotein and proteinuric pre-eclampsia. *Br. J. Obstet. Gynaecol.*, **92**, 341–4.
63. Waller D. K., Lustig L. S., Cunningham G. C., Feuchtbaum L. B., and Hook B. (1996). The association between maternal serum alpha-fetoprotein and preterm birth, small for gestational age infant, preeclampsia, and placental complication. *Obstet. Gynecol.*, **88**, 816–22.
64. Wenstrom K. D., Owen J., Davis R. O., and Brumfield C. G. (1996). Prognostic significance of unexplained elevated amniotic fluid alpha-fetalprotein. *Obstet. Gynecol.*, **87**, 213–16.
65. Palomaki G. E., Knight G. J., Haddow J. E., Canick J. A., Saller D. N., and Panizza D. S. (1992). Prospective intervention trial of a screening protocol to identify trisomy 18 using maternal serum alpha-fetoprotein, uncongugated oestriol, and human chorinic gonadotropin. *Prenat. Diagn.*, **12**, 925–30.
66. Palomaki G. E., Haddow J. E., Knight G. J., Wald N. J., Kennard A., Canick J. A., Saller D. N., Blizer M. G., Dickeman L. H., and Fisher R. (1995). Risk-based prenatal screening for trisomy 18 using alpha-fetoprotein, unconjugated oestriol and human chorionic gonadotropin. *Prenat. Diagn.*, **15**, 713–23.
67. Barkai G., Goldman B., Ries L., Chaki R., Zer T., and Cuckle H. (1993). Expanding multiple marker screening for Down's syndrome to include Edward's syndrome. *Prenat. Diagn.*, **13**, 843–50.
68. Wald N. J., Cuckle H., Boreham J., Stirrat G. M., and Turnbull A. C. (1979). Maternal serum alpha- fetoprotein and diabetes mellitus. *Br. J. Obstet. Gynaecol.*, **86**, 101–5.
69. Milunsky A., Alpert E., Kitzmiller J. L., Younger M. D., and Neff R. K. (1982). Prenatal diagnosis of neural tube defects. The importance of serum alpha-fetoprotein screening in diabetic prenant women. *Am. J. Obstet. Gynecol.*, **142**, 1030–2.
70. Crossley J. A., Berry E., Aitken D. A., and Connor J. M. (1996). Insulin-dependent diabetes mellitus and prenatal screening results: current experience from a regional screening programme. *Prenat. Diagn.*, **16**, 1039–42.
71. Brock D. J. H., Baron L., Duncan P., Scrimgeour J. B., and Watt M. (1979). Significance of elevated mid-trimester maternal plasma alpha-fetoprotein values. *Lancet*, **i**, 1281–2.
72. Rasmussen-Loft A. G., Nanchahal K., Cuckle H. S. *et al.* (1990). Amniotic fluid acetylcholinesterase in the antenatal diagnosis of open neural tube defects and abdominal wall defects: a comparison of gel electrophoresis and a monoclonal antibody immunoassay. *Prenat. Diagn.*, **10**, 449–59.
73. Wald N. J., Cuckle H. S., and Nanchahal K. (1989). Amniotic fluid acetylcholinesterase measurement in the prenatal diagnosis of open neural tube defects. Second Report of the Collaborative Acetylcholinesterase Study. *Prenat. Diagn.*, **9**, 813–29.
74. Tabor A., Philip J., Madsen M., Bang J., Obel E. B., and Norgaard-Pederson B. (1986). Randomised controlled trial of genetic amniocentesis in 4606 low-risk women. *Lancet*, **i**, 1287–93.
75. Richards D. S., Seeds J. W., Katz V. L., Lingley L. H., Albright S. G., and Cefalo R. C. (1988). Elevated maternal serum alpha-fetoprotein with normal ultrasound: is amniocentesis always appropriate? A review of 26,069 screened patients. *Obstet. Gynecol.*, **71**, 203–7.
76. Drugan A., Zador I. E., Syner F. N., Sokol R. J., Sacks A. J., and Evans M. I. (1988). A normal ultrasound does not obviate the need for amniocentesis in patients with elevated serum alpha-fetoprotein. *Obstet. Gynecol.*, **72**, 627–30.

4 *Down's syndrome*

Nicholas Wald

INTRODUCTION

Down's syndrome is the commonest cause of severe mental retardation. It is due to an extra copy of chromosome 21 or part of its long arm. The disorder can be diagnosed antenatally by examining the chromosomes in fetal cells from anmiotic fluid or the placenta. The birth prevalence of Down's syndrome is associated with maternal age and various biochemical and ultrasound markers. Screening methods based on maternal age and these markers can be used to identify pregnancies with a high enough risk of Down's syndrome to justify an amniocentesis or chorionic villus sampling so that a diagnostic fetal chromosome analysis can be performed. The parents of affected fetuses can then decide whether to have a termination of pregnancy.

THE DISORDER

Ninety-five per cent of infants with Down's syndrome have three copies of chromosome 21, so each cell has 47 chromosomes.[1] In 4 per cent of cases of Down's syndrome the extra chromosome 21 is attached to another chromosome—so-called translocation.[1] Usually the two long arms of chromosome 21 are fused, and the two short arms lost (Robertsonian translocation) so that there are still 46 chromosomes. The extra chromosome 21 can also be attached to chromosomes 13, 14, 15, or 22 instead of chromosome 21. About 1 per cent of Down's syndrome cases are 'mosaics' in which only a proportion of cells in an individual have trisomy 21.[1] The extra chromosome 21 is of maternal origin in about 88 per cent of cases and paternal in 9 per cent, the remaining 3 per cent arising from post zygotic mitosis.[2] About 75 per cent of the maternal cases are due to non-dysjunction at the first meiotic division.[2]

Birth prevalence

The natural birth prevalence of Down's syndrome increases with maternal age (see Fig. 4.1). Under the age of 25 the birth prevalence of Down's syndrome is about 1 in 1500, increasing to about 1 in 1000 at age 30, and 1 in 100 at age 40. Data from the National Down Syndrome Cytogenetic Register show that in 1997 the expected birth

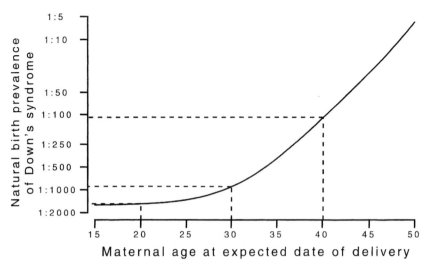

Fig. 4.1 Natural birth prevalence of Down's syndrome according to maternal age, based on Cuckle *et al.* (1987).[3]

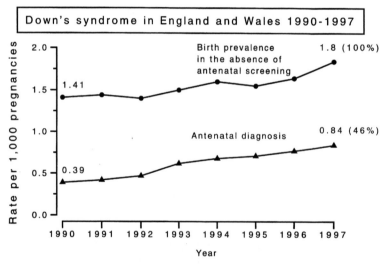

Fig. 4.2 Natural birth prevalence of Down's syndrome in England and Wales 1990–7 and those detected by antenatal screening and diagnosis, based on the National Down Syndrome Cytogenetic Register (personal communication, E. Alberman, D. Mutton, and J. Morris).

prevalence in England and Wales would have been 1.8 per 1000 in the absence of antenatal screening and selective abortion (Fig. 4.2), an increase from a rate of about 1.3 per 1000 10–15 years previously. This increase was due to women having their babies at an older age. The Register also showed that the proportion of affected pregnancies diagnosed antenatally increased as well—to 46% in 1997 (see Fig. 4.2).

Natural history

In about 1 in 150 pregnancies the fetus has Down's syndrome but over three-quarters of these end in a miscarriage.[2] The incidence of miscarriage is about 43 per cent for

Down's syndrome fetuses alive at 10 weeks of gestation, and 23 per cent for those alive at 16 weeks.[4]

About 55 per cent of liveborn infants with Down's syndrome have structural congenital abnormalities. The most common of these are abnormalities of the heart, which affect an estimated 46 per cent of children born with Down's syndrome.[5] The next most common group of abnormalities are those of the intestinal tract, notably duodenal atresia. Table 4.1 shows the proportions of liveborn infants with Down's syndrome affected by congenital heart defects in general, by atrio-ventricular canal defects (the specific heart defect most strongly linked to Down's syndrome), and by duodenal atresia. Duodenal atresia occurs in about 0.018 per cent of all births and is about 300 times more frequent in Down's syndrome (see Table 4.1). Down's syndrome is also associated with urinary tract malformations, limb defects, and congenital cataract.

The extent of mental retardation in Down's syndrome individuals tends to be substantial. In one study the range of IQs at age 21 was 8–67, with a mean of 42, very much lower than the distribution of IQs in the general population (mean 100, SD 15). At age 21 the mean mental age was found to be about five, with a range of 1–8 years.[9]

Other medical problems associated with Down's syndrome include leukaemia, thyroid disorders, epilepsy, and Alzheimer's disease. The risk of developing these

Table 4.1 Approximate likelihood ratio of three congenital abnormalities in Down's syndrome livebirths. Taken from Noble (1998)[6]

Abnormality	Prevalence in Down's syndrome livebirths (%)†	Prevalence in all births (%)	Approximate likelihood ratio
Congenital heart defect	46	0.8‡	60
Atrio-ventricular canal defect	17	0.04‡	420
Duodenal atresia	6	0.018*	300

† From Hayes et al. (1997).[5]
‡ From Heinonen et al. (1977).[7]
* From Leck et al. (1968).[8]

Table 4.2 Approximate likelihood ratio of four major medical problems associated with Down's syndrome.† Taken from Noble (1998)[6]

Medical problem	Prevalence in individuals with Down's syndrome (%)	Prevalence in general population	Approximate likelihood ratio
Leukaemia	1.7‡	0.04*	43
Primary congenital hypothyroidism	0.7**	0.026***	27
Epilepsy	9#	0.8#	11
Alzheimer's disease (up to age 70)	77~	2~~	39

† From Cuckle and Wald (1990).[10]
‡ From Zipursky et al. (1997).[11]
* From Mutton et al. (1997).[12]
** From Stewart (1994).[13]
*** From Fort et al. (1984).[14]
# From Paul (1997).[15]
~ From Visser et al. (1997).[16]
~~ From Holland and Oliver (1995).[17]

disorders is shown in Table 4.2. Individuals with Down's syndrome may develop a type of leukaemia (acute megakaryoblastic leukaemia) in the first few years of life that is almost never seen in individuals without Down's syndrome. In spite of the very high relative risk (43), only about 1–2 per cent of individuals with Down's syndrome develop leukaemia. The absolute risk of hypothyroidism is also low (0.7 per cent), but the risks of epilepsy and Alzheimer's are high, about 9 per cent and 77 per cent respectively.

Life expectancy of individuals with Down's syndrome increased from about 12 to 50 years between 1947 and 1988, mainly due to treatment of infections and congenital heart disease.[18,19]

A summary of some of the key points relating to the natural history of Down's syndrome is given in Table 4.3.

Recurrence risks

Women who have had a pregnancy with Down's syndrome have an increased chance of having a second affected child. In the absence of a translocation (i.e. in non-inherited Down's syndrome) the recurrence risk represents an *added* 0.34 per cent risk at term or 0.42 per cent at mid trimester (see Fig. 4.3). To calculate a woman's risk of having an affected pregnancy this excess risk should be added to her age-specific risk. In cases where parents have a balanced translocation the risk of an affected pregnancy can vary widely, reaching 100 per cent in surviving fetuses if either parent has a 21–21 Robertsonian translocation.

SCREENING TESTS

The relationship between maternal age and the risk of having a pregnancy with Down's syndrome was reported by Penrose in 1933.[20] Twenty-six years later the presence of an extra chromosome 21 was shown to be a diagnostic feature of Down's syndrome.[21] In 1966 the chromosome analysis of human amniotic fluid cells was achieved,[22] and two years later the first antenatal diagnosis of Down's syndrome was made.[23] Screening was then introduced on the basis of selecting women of advanced maternal age for a diagnostic amniocentesis so that those with affected fetuses could be offered termination of pregnancy. An age cut-off of

Table 4.3 Down's syndrome: a summary of the extent of the disability. Taken from Noble (1998)[6]

- 23% of fetuses with Down's syndrome diagnosed *in utero* at 16 weeks would be lost spontaneously if termination of pregnancy were not performed
- 50% of livebirths with Down's syndrome have one or more additional serious congenital abnormalities (other than intellectual handicap)
- 46% have congenital heart defects
- 96% without and 80% with heart defects survive the first year
- 20% die before age 5; after age 5 survival to adulthood is likely
- at age 21 mean IQ is 42 (range 8–67) and mental age is 5 years (range 1–8 years)
- about 2% develop leukaemia
- at least 10% develop epilepsy
- 11% develop Alzheimer's disease by age 50 and 77% by age 70 (mean age of onset 56)
- 44% of liveborns survive to age 60
- life expectancy is 50–55

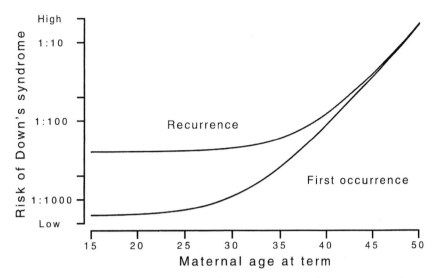

Fig. 4.3 Risk of Down's syndrome at term according to maternal age: first occurrence and recurrence. Taken from Cuckle and Wald (1990).[10]

between 35 and 37 was generally used, and an amniocentesis performed at about 16 weeks of pregnancy. Maternal age screening performed in this way identified about 30 per cent of pregnancies with Down's syndrome by offering an amniocentesis to the oldest 5 per cent of women.

In 1984 Merkatz and his colleagues reported an association between pregnancies with aneuploidies (including Down's syndrome) and low serum alphafetoprotein (AFP) levels.[24] This led to a study of a bank of stored antenatal serum samples that were linked to pregnancies in which Down's syndrome was diagnosed. The study showed that between 14 and 22 weeks of pregnancy the median AFP value in Down's syndrome pregnancies was about 25 per cent lower than for unaffected pregnancies.[25] The relationship was independent of maternal age, and because the study was performed before the introduction of serum screening the results related to Down's syndrome births, thereby avoiding any bias that might occur if women with positive screening results who had an affected pregnancy destined to miscarry were included.

In 1987, levels of maternal serum human chorionic gonadotrophin (hCG) were shown to be, on average, higher in Down's syndrome pregnancies than in unaffected pregnancies.[26] At about the same time levels of unconjugated oestriol (uE_3) were found to be about 25 per cent lower in affected pregnancies.[27,28] In 1988 a new method of screening was reported in which the three biochemical markers (AFP, uE_3, and hCG) were used, together with maternal age, in a single antenatal screening test for Down's syndrome. This became known as the 'triple test'. Performed between 15 and 22 weeks of pregnancy, it detects about 60 per cent of Down's syndrome pregnancies while maintaining a false-positive rate of 5 per cent.[29] The report of this method presented the concept and methodology of 'risk screening' in which the risk estimate itself is used as the screening variable. In this approach the results of the components of a screening test are used to estimate the risk that the fetus has Down's syndrome and the result of the test is considered to be positive when the risk estimate it yields exceeds a certain cut-off level. If gestational age is determined using an ultrasound scan examination the detection rate is nearly 70 per cent for the same 5 per cent false-positive rate.[30] Later it was shown that the free subunits of hCG (α- and β-hCG) had value in screening.[31]

In 1996 the addition of inhibin-A to the triple test was shown to increase the detection rate to 76 per cent for a 5 per cent false-positive rate and the new test was called the quadruple or 'quad' test.[32,33]

In the early 1990s first trimester maternal serum markers of Down's syndrome were assessed, including pregnancy associated plasma protein A (PAPP-A)[34,35] and free β-hCG.[36] Between 8 and 14 weeks, these two serum markers, used together with maternal age, detected 62 per cent of Down's syndrome pregnancies for a 5 per cent false-positive rate.[37]

Ultrasound was also shown to be useful in the detection of Down's syndrome in the first trimester. Between about 10 and 13 weeks of gestation, a widened space at the back of the fetal neck between the spine and the skin, referred to as increased nuchal translucency, was shown to be associated with Down's syndrome.[38–40]

In 1997 the methodology behind the triple test was used to combine maternal age, nuchal translucency, PAPP-A, and free β-hCG into a single first trimester screening test for Down's syndrome.[41] This was called the combined test, and has an estimated detection rate of 80% (later revised to 85%) for a 5% false-positive rate.

In 1999, 11 years after the publication of the triple test, the first trimester combined test and the second trimester quadruple test were integrated into a single test. This was called the integrated test. It has a high detection rate (85 per cent) for a substantially reduced false-positive rate (0.9 per cent) compared with previous screening methods.[42]

In summary, the last 16 years have seen the development of screening based on multiple tests during the second trimester, the first trimester, and both these trimesters together. These three screening strategies will now be considered in turn.

Screening at 14–22 weeks of pregnancy

Six serum markers have been found to be useful in Down's syndrome screening between 14 and 22 weeks of pregnancy, namely AFP, uE₃, total hCG, free β-hCG, free α-hCG, and inhibin-A.[43–96] Table 4.4 summarizes the median levels of these markers in Down's syndrome pregnancies in multiples of the normal median (MoM) based on

Table 4.4   Principal second trimester markers of Down's syndrome. Taken from Wald *et al.* (1997)[97]

Marker	No. of studies	No. of Down's syndrome pregnancies	Median MoM in Down's syndrome pregnancies	95% CI
AFP	38	1328	0.75	0.72–0.78
uE₃	21	733	0.72	0.68–0.75
hCG	28	907	2.06	1.95–2.17
free α-hCG	7	239	1.43	1.12–1.82
free β-hCG	12	562	2.2	2.07–2.33
inhibin-A	6	375	1.92	1.75–2.15

the published studies reviewed by Wald *et al.*[97] Table 4.5 similarly summarizes other second trimester biochemical markers of Down's syndrome. Table 4.6 shows the distribution parameters (medians, standard deviations, correlation coefficients) for AFP, uE_3, hCG and its subunits free $\alpha-$ and free β-hCG, and inhibin-A, based on the

Table 4.5 Other second trimester biochemical markers of Down's syndrome. Taken from Wald *et al.* (1997)[97]

Marker	No. of studies	No. of Down's syndrome pregnancies	Median MoM in Down's syndrome pregnancies	95% CI
SP1	7	379	1.47	1.23–1.76
α-inhibin	4	64	1.63	1.01–2.62
URNAP*	2	76	1.65	1.57–1.74

* Urea resistant neutrophil alkaline phosphatase.

Table 4.6 Distribution parameters (medians, standard deviations and correlation coefficients expressed in multiples of the median for unaffected pregnancies) for the principal second trimester screening markers for Down's syndrome. Taken from Wald *et al.* (1994)[86] (without adjustment for weight) with additional data on inhibin-A from Wald *et al.* (1996)[32] and (1997)[33]

Serum marker(s)	Gestational age estimated by dates[1]		Gestational age estimated by scan[2]	
	Down's syndrome ($n = 77$)	Unaffected ($n = 385$)	Down's syndrome ($n = 77$)	Unaffected ($n = 385$)
Median (antilog of mean $\log_{10}$ MoM)				
AFP	0.72	1.00	0.72	1.00
uE_3	0.72	1.00	0.72	1.00
hCG	2.01	1.00	2.01	1.00
free α-hCG	1.31	1.00	1.31	1.00
free β-hCG	2.22	1.00	2.22	1.00
inhibin-A	1.79	1.00	1.79	1.00
Standard deviation ($\log_{10}$ MoM)				
AFP	0.2015	0.1986	0.1932	0.1902
uE_3	0.1478	0.1391	0.1243	0.1138
hCG	0.2665	0.2401	0.2601	0.2330
free α-hCG	0.1772	0.1520	0.1730	0.1471
free β-hCG	0.3067	0.2508	0.3040	0.2475
inhibin-A	0.2023	0.2188	0.2023	0.2188
Correlation coefficient ($\log_{10}$ MoM)				
AFP, uE_3	0.3359	0.2853	0.2048	0.1291
AFP, hCG	0.1681	0.0327	0.2472	0.1119
AFP, free α-hCG	0.0824	0.1401	0.0575	0.1147
AFP, free β-hCG	0.1499	0.0125	0.2278	0.1006
AFP, inhibin-A	0.1416	0.1150	0.1498	0.1221
uE_3, hCG	−0.3565	−0.1423	−0.3073	−0.0244
uE_3, free α-hCG	0.0948	0.2273	0.0532	0.2070
uE_3, free β-hCG	−0.4486	−0.1770	−0.3974	−0.0303
uE_3, inhibin-A	−0.0722	0.0236	−0.0619	0.0530
hCG, free α-hCG	0.4599	0.3235	0.5051	0.3740
hCG, free β-hCG	0.8898	0.8838	0.8734	0.8592
hCG, inhibin-A	0.2929	0.2357	0.2664	0.2081
free α-hCG, free β-hCG	0.2162	0.1539	0.2572	0.2100
free α-hCG, inhibin-A	0.2819	0.1613	0.2922	0.1705
free β-hCG, inhibin-A	0.3836	0.2777	0.3556	0.2457

[1] Time from first day of last menstrual period.
[2] Using crown rump length or biparietal diameter.
'Dates' and 'scan' are defined in this way throughout the chapter.

Oxford–Barts dataset, the only dataset that has details of all the current markers of interest, including inhibin-A, with estimates according to whether gestational age was determined by dates (time from a woman's last menstrual period) or an ultrasound scan examination (using additional Bart's data with scan measurements).

Screening performance

Table 4.7 shows the screening performance for all combinations of the six serum markers (after correction of the marker level for maternal weight, see below). The detection rates are shown for a 5 per cent false-positive rate, together with the odds of being affected given a positive result (OAPR). The main combinations of markers used in practice are shown in bold type in the table. The most effective combination of markers, while retaining AFP for its value in screening for open neural tube defects, is the quadruple test based on inhibin-A and the triple markers AFP, uE₃, and hCG. This yields a 76 per cent detection rate and an OAPR of 1:50 if gestational age is based on an ultrasound scan examination.

Table 4.7 Screening performance for all combinations of serum markers† (All results have been corrected for maternal weight.) Commonly used marker combinations are indicated in bold. Source: Screening performance estimated using statistical parameters in Wald *et al.* (1994),[86] (1996),[32] (1997)[33]

Marker(s)	Gestational age estimated by dates		Gestational age estimated by scan	
	Detection rate (%) for a 5% false-positive rate	OAPR*	Detection rate (%) for a 5% false-positive rate	OAPR*
Maternal age alone:				
≥36 years	30	1:130	30	1:130
Maternal age with one marker:				
AFP	36	1:110	37	1:105
uE₃	41	1:95	49	1:80
hCG	49	1:80	51	1:75
free α-hCG	38	1:100	39	1:100
free β-hCG	49	1:80	51	1:75
inhibin-A	44	1:90	44	1:90
Maternal age with two markers:				
AFP, uE₃	45	1:85	54	1:70
AFP, hCG	**54**	**1:70**	**59**	**1:65**
AFP, free α-hCG	45	1:85	47	1:80
AFP, free β-hCG	**54**	**1:70**	**58**	**1:65**
AFP, inhibin-A	53	1:75	54	1:70
uE₃, hCG	56	1:70	64	1:60
uE₃, free α-hCG	53	1:70	60	1:65
uE₃, free β-hCG	57	1:70	64	1:60
uE₃, inhibin-A	57	1:70	63	1:60
hCG, free α-hCG	51	1:75	53	1:75
hCG, inhibin-A	58	1:70	59	1:65
free α-hCG, free β-hCG	55	1:70	55	1:70
free α-hCG, inhibin-A	51	1:75	51	1:75
free β-hCG, inhibin-A	58	1:65	59	1:65

Table 4.7 Continued

Marker(s)	Gestational age estimated by dates		Gestational age estimated by scan	
	Detection rate (%) for a 5% false-positive rate	OAPR*	Detection rate (%) for a 5% false-positive rate	OAPR*
Maternal age with three markers:				
AFP, uE₃, hCG	**59**	**1:65**	**69**	**1:55**
AFP, uE₃, free α-hCG	56	1:70	64	1:60
AFP, uE₃, free β-hCG	**60**	**1:65**	**68**	**1:55**
AFP, uE₃, inhibin-A	60	1:65	67	1:57
AFP, hCG, free α-hCG	57	1:65	60	1:65
AFP, hCG, inhibin-A	64	1:60	68	1:55
AFP, free α-hCG, inhibin-A	58	1:65	60	1:65
AFP, free β-hCG, inhibin-A	64	1:60	67	1:55
AFP, free α-hCG, free β-hCG	60	1:65	62	1:60
uE₃, hCG, free α-hCG	60	1:65	67	1:60
uE₃, hCG, inhibin-A	64	1:60	71	1:55
uE₃, free α-hCG, inhibin-A	63	1:60	69	1:55
uE₃, free β-hCG, inhibin-A	64	1:60	70	1:55
uE₃, free α-hCG, free β-hCG	62	1:60	69	1:55
inhibin-A, hCG, free α-hCG	59	1:65	60	1:65
free α-hCG, free β-hCG, inhibin-A	61	1:65	62	1:60
Maternal age with four markers:				
AFP, uE₃, hCG, inhibin-A	**67**	**1:55**	**76**	**1:50**
AFP, uE₃, free α-hCG, inhibin-A	66	1:60	73	1:55
AFP, uE₃, free β-hCG, inhibin-A	**67**	**1:55**	**75**	**1:50**
AFP, uE₃, hCG, free α-hCG	63	1:60	72	1:55
AFP, uE₃, free α-hCG, free β-hCG	65	1:60	73	1:55
AFP, inhibin-A, hCG, free α-hCG	65	1:60	69	1:55
AFP, free α-hCG, free β-hCG, inhibin-A	67	1:60	69	1:55
uE₃, inhibin-A, free α-hCG, hCG	66	1:60	73	1:55
uE₃, free α-hCG, free β-hCG, inhibin-A	68	1:58	73	1:55

† Excluding combinations that include both hCG and free β-hCG.
* OAPR = odds of being affected given a positive result; rounded to nearest 5 (based on a natural birth prevalence of 1.3 per 1,000).

Figure 4.4 shows the detection rate for a 5 per cent false-positive rate using maternal age alone, and maternal age with various combinations of the serum markers.

Figure 4.5 shows the distribution of risk estimates in affected and unaffected pregnancies using the quadruple test with gestational age estimated using an ultrasound scan examination. The detection rate corresponding to a 5 per cent false -positive rate is shown.

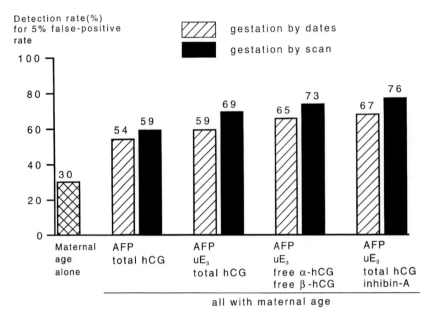

Fig. 4.4   Detection rate for a 5 per cent false-positive rate according to maternal age alone and maternal age with various combinations of serum markers in the second trimester. Taken from Wald *et al.* (1997).[97]

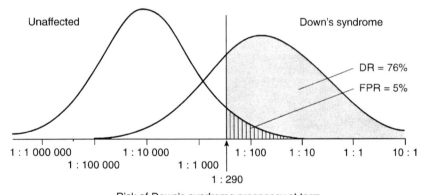

Fig. 4.5   Second trimester distribution of risk estimates of Down's syndrome in affected and unaffected pregnancies using alphafetoprotein (AFP), unconjugated oestriol (uE₃), total human chorionic gonadotrophin (hCG), and inhibin-A with maternal age.

The value of an ultrasound scan to estimate gestational age

An ultrasound scan examination to estimate gestational age is valuable in screening for Down's syndrome and should be done before the serum test is interpreted. The two acceptable ultrasound measurements for estimating gestational age in Down's syndrome screening are a biparietal diameter or a crown rump length, neither of which are systematically increased or decreased in fetuses with Down's syndrome.[98] By improving the precision of estimating gestational age the standard deviation of the serum markers is reduced. The effect is greatest for uE₃ (see Fig. 4.6), the concentration of which changes most with gestational age, and smallest for inhibin-A, the marker that changes least during the period of pregnancy when screening is performed.

Tables 4.8 and 4.9 compare the screening performance using dates and a scan to estimate gestational age; Table 4.8 compares false-positive rates for specified detection rates and Table 4.9 compares detection rates for specified false-positive rates. With a scan estimate of gestational age the false-positive rates in the triple and quadruple tests can be reduced by about a half without loss of detection.

Factors that can influence serum marker levels

Maternal weight

On average, for a 20 kg increase in maternal weight, serum AFP decreases by about 17 per cent, uE₃ decreases by about 7 per cent, and hCG decreases by about 16 per cent.[97] Methods to adjust for maternal weight have been described by Watt *et al.*[99] and Neveux *et al.*[100] Such an adjustment can increase detection by about one percentage point for a given false-positive rate.

Insulin-dependent diabetes

Table 4.10 shows median serum marker levels in pregnant women with and without insulin-dependent diabetes mellitus, based on a review of the literature.[97] After maternal weight adjustment, AFP is about 10 per cent lower in women with insulin-dependent diabetes mellitus, uE₃ is 7 per cent lower, free α-hCG 11 per cent lower, and inhibin-A 9 per cent lower. These differences are statistically significant. There are no statistically significant differences for total hCG and free β-hCG. Adjustment for

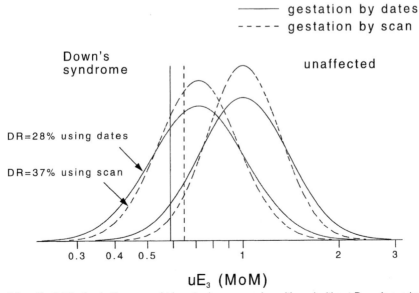

Fig. 4.6 uE₃ distribution in the second trimester in pregnancies with and without Down's syndrome according to method of estimating gestational age. The vertical lines set a 5% false positive rate; dotted line for scan, continuous line for dates.

Table 4.8 Estimates of false-positive rates according to specified detection rates for various combinations of serum markers (all in conjunction with maternal age) and the use of dates or scan to estimate gestational age (all results corrected for maternal weight). Source: Screening performance estimated using statistical parameters in Wald *et al.* (1994),[86] (1996),[32] (1997)[33]

	False-positive rate (%)							
	AFP and total hCG†		AFP, uE₃, hCG†		AFP, uE₃, free α- and free β-hCG		AFP, uE₃, total hCG† and inhibin-A	
Detection rate (%)	Dates	Scan	Dates	Scan	Dates	Scan	Dates	Scan
20	0.3	0.2	0.2	<0.1	0.1	<0.1	<0.1	<0.1
30	0.9	0.7	0.6	0.3	0.3	0.1	0.3	0.1
40	2.0	1.5	1.3	0.7	0.8	0.3	0.7	0.3
50	3.8	3.0	2.8	1.4	1.8	0.8	1.6	0.7
60	6.8	5.4	5.3	2.7	3.5	1.8	3.1	1.6
70	11.7	9.4	9.7	5.2	6.8	4.0	5.9	3.2
80	20.0	16.5	17.6	10.2	13.5	8.9	11.3	6.6

† Results are similar if free β-hCG is used instead of total hCG.

Table 4.9 Estimates of detection rates according to specified false-positive rates for various combinations of serum markers (all in conjunction with maternal age) and the use of dates or scan to estimate gestational age (all results corrected for maternal weight). Source: Screening performance estimated using parameters in Wald *et al.* (1994),[86] (1996),[32] (1997)[33]

	Detection rate (%)							
	AFP and total hCG†		AFP, uE₃, hCG†		AFP, uE₃, free α- and free β-hCG		AFP, uE₃, total hCG† and inhibin-A	
False-positive rate (%)	Dates	Scan	Dates	Scan	Dates	Scan	Dates	Scan
1	31	35	36	46	43	53	44	54
2	40	44	45	55	52	61	54	64
3	46	50	51	62	58	66	60	69
4	51	55	56	66	62	70	64	73
5	54	59	59	69	65	73	67	76
6	58	62	62	72	68	75	70	79
7	60	65	65	74	70	77	73	81
8	63	67	67	76	72	79	75	83
9	65	69	69	78	74	80	77	84
10	67	71	71	80	76	81	78	85

† Results are similar if free β-hCG is used instead of total hCG.

insulin-dependent diabetes mellitus is carried out by dividing the observed MoM value for a woman with diabetes by the corresponding median MoM value in diabetic women without Down's syndrome pregnancies. The risk based on such an adjusted MoM value is termed a 'pseudo risk', because it is not the true one, the calculation of which would require data on the distribution of the markers among insulin-dependent diabetic women with Down's syndrome pregnancies. The pseudo risk adjustment allows women to be classified as either screen positive or screen negative in a way that will keep the false-positive rate in diabetic women approximately the same as in non-diabetic women.

Table 4.10 Median serum marker levels in pregnant women with insulin-dependent diabetes mellitus relative to women without diabetes. Adapted from Table 3.12 in Wald *et al.* (1997)[97]

| Serum marker | Number of women | | | | Median marker level in diabetic women relative to women without diabetes | |
| | Non-diabetic | | Diabetic | | | |
	Weight corrected	Not weight corrected	Weight corrected	Not weight corrected	Weight corrected	Not weight corrected
AFP	40 663	15 617	898	836	0.90	0.84
uE$_3$	25 232	252	202	126	0.93	0.92
total hCG	40 663	15 617	473	360	0.96	0.92
free α-hCG	251	251	126	126	0.89	0.86
free β-hCG	251	251	126	126	1.01	0.96
Inhibin-A	250	250	126	126	0.91	0.88

Twin pregnancies

Table 4.11 shows, in a similar way to the previous table, a summary of the published literature on marker levels in unaffected twin pregnancies compared with unaffected singleton pregnancies. Serum markers in women with twin pregnancies are about twice those found in singleton pregnancies, though for some markers the estimate is slightly above 2 and for others it is somewhat less (see Table 4.11). As with diabetic women, a pseudo risk is calculated by dividing the observed MoM value in a twin pregnancy by the median MoM value in twin pregnancies without Down's syndrome. This is not a true risk, but again it will have the effect of keeping the false-positive rate in twin pregnancies approximately the same as in singleton pregnancies.

Ethnic origin

Table 4.12 summarizes the literature on Down's syndrome markers in black women compared with white women, and Table 4.13 shows the marker levels in South Asian women compared with white women. AFP, total hCG, free β-hCG, and inhibin-A levels show significant differences between black and white women. Marker levels in South Asian women, after adjustment for maternal weight, are not particularly high or low. In calculating risk for black or South Asian women, the observed MoMs can be adjusted using the method of Watt *et al.*[99]

Table 4.11 Median second trimester serum marker levels in unaffected twin pregnancies relative to singleton pregnancies. Adapted from Table 3.13 in Wald *et al.* (1997)[97]

| Serum marker | Number of women | | Median marker level in twins relative to singletons |
	Singleton pregnancy	Twin pregnancy	
AFP	58 572	1892	2.23
uE$_3$	38 360	739	1.65
hCG	42 730	1211	2.01
Free α-hCG	600	199	1.66
Free β-hCG	7261	619	2.08
Inhibin-A	600	199	1.99

Table 4.12   Median second trimester serum marker levels in black women relative to white women. Adapted from Table 3.14 in Wald *et al.* (1997)[97]

| Serum marker | Number of women | | | | Median marker level in black women relative to white women | |
| | White | | Black | | | |
	Weight corrected	Not weight corrected	Weight corrected	Not weight corrected	Weight corrected	Not weight corrected
AFP	159 958	55 984	45 157	7488	1.15*	1.17*
uE₃	14 230	51 803	4584	13 078	1.00	0.99
hCG	16 735	99 450	4894	28 022	1.18*	1.12*
Free α-hCG	922	922	449	449	0.92	0.92
Free β-hCG	922	922	449	449	1.12*	1.09*
Inhibin-A	922	922	449	449	0.92*	0.89*

* Indicates that the ratio was statistically significant.

Table 4.13   Median second trimester serum marker levels in South Asian women relative to white women. Adapted from Table 3.15 in Wald *et al.* (1997)[97]

| Serum marker | Number of women | | | | Median marker level in South Asian women relative to white women | |
| | White | | South Asian | | | |
	Weight corrected	Not weight corrected	Weight corrected	Not weight corrected	Weight corrected	Not weight corrected
AFP	13 693	36 304	4472	4947	0.94	1.02
uE₃	9459	9459	4391	4391	1.07*	1.11
hCG	9459	9459	4391	4391	1.06*	1.12
Free α-hCG	922	922	135	135	1.03	1.11
Free β-hCG	922	922	135	135	0.91	0.99
Inhibin-A	922	922	135	135	1.01	1.09

* Indicates that the ratio was statistically significant.

Smoking

The serum marker levels tend to be different in women who smoke from those in women who do not. Table 4.14 summarizes the literature on marker levels and smoking. Inhibin-A levels in smokers are, on average, about 40 per cent higher than in non-smokers and hCG levels are, on average, about 20% lower. The effect on the other markers is small. Adjusting serum marker levels for smoking status has a very small effect on screening performance; at a given false-positive rate the detection rate increases by less than 1 per cent. The birth prevalence of Down's syndrome in women who smoke appears to be lower than in non-smoking women.[101] The magnitude of this effect is still uncertain. For this reason, and because the effect of adjusting for smoking is small, such an adjustment is not generally made in screening.

Parity

Total hCG tends to decline with increasing parity—on average, by about 3 per cent for each previous birth.[102–105] The reason for this is unknown and the effect is too small to warrant adjustment for parity in Down's syndrome screening.

Table 4.14 Median serum marker levels in smoking and non-smoking pregnant women. Adapted from Table 3.16 in Wald et al. (1997)97 and unpublished observations on inhibin-A

Serum marker	Number of women		Median marker level in smokers relative to non-smokers
	Non-smokers	Smokers	
AFP	>22 789	>6378	1.03
uE$_3$	22 789	6378	0.96
hCG	22 789	6378	0.82
Free β-hCG†			0.94
Inhibin-A	2517	472	1.41

†The numbers of non-smokers and smokers were unspecified—there were 1000 in total.

Assisted reproduction (ovulation induction and in vitro *fertilisation)*

In vitro fertilisation (IVF) is associated with a high false-positive rate relative to the expected rate for women of the same age. The expected rate is itself high (15 per cent) because women having IVF in general tend to be older.[106] hCG levels tend to be higher and uE$_3$ levels somewhat lower in women having IVF. It is reasonable to assume that the effect is due to ovulation induction rather than to IVF *per se*. In view of this it is sensible to adjust the MoM values of women undergoing assisted reproduction in general so that the false-positive rate among such women is approximately the same as among other women.

Routine repeat testing

Routine repeat testing (asking women to come back for a repeat test) adds little to the performance of Down's syndrome screening.[107,108] Given the costs of repeat testing, and the additional anxiety while waiting for a second test result, it is probably not worthwhile introducing repeat testing *policies* in Down's syndrome screening. However, if a second sample has been obtained and tested, this should be taken into account in risk estimation.

Validation of risk using serum markers

Multiple marker screening is based on the methodology outlined in Chapter 2. The method has been validated empirically[109,110] by grouping screened pregnancies according to the predicted (estimated) risk of having an affected pregnancy and comparing the mean predicted risk in each category with the observed prevalence of affected pregnancies in the same category. There was close agreement between the predicted term risk and the prevalence at birth both for the triple test and the quadruple test (see Fig. 4.7). For example, with the quadruple test based on free α- and free β -hCG, with AFP and uE$_3$ measurement, the mean predicted risk in the highest risk group was 1 in 3.3 and the observed prevalence was 1 in 2.6; in the lowest risk group these were 1 in 3000 and 1 in 2300 respectively.

Other potential screening tests
Urinary beta core hCG

Several studies have shown that urinary beta core hCG, a breakdown product of hCG, is raised in Down's syndrome pregnancies compared with unaffected pregnancies.[111–116] In the review by Wald *et al.*[97] the pooled estimate of the median concentration was 3.7 MoM, though more recent information suggests that the effect is much smaller than this.[117]

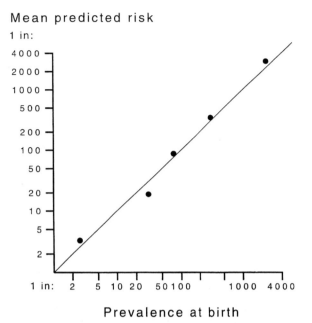

Mean predicted risk

Fig. 4.7   Validation of risk estimates using the quadruple test based on free α-hCG, free β-hCG, AFP, and uE₃. The five groups represented by the full circles were defined according to the quintiles of predicted risk of Down's syndrome in affected pregnancies.

Fetal cells in maternal blood

Several types of nucleated fetal cells which can reveal an extra copy of chromosome 21 can be recovered from maternal blood, such as trophoblastic cells, granulocytes, lymphocytes, and immature red cells. There are about one to two fetal cells for every 10 million maternal cells, although the proportion may be higher in pregnancies with aneuploid fetuses. Various methods have been described for concentrating fetal cells and then determining whether these have trisomy 21. The methods may be useful in screening but none as yet is sufficiently simple, inexpensive, and reliable to be a candidate for routine population screening, and good estimates of screening performance are lacking.[118-120]

Ultrasound markers at 14–22 weeks of pregnancy

These are described in Chapter 18. Several structural abnormalities such as cardiac defects, and other markers such as nuchal fold thickness and femur length, are associated with Down's syndrome. As yet, no algorithm has been produced that combines these markers with a biochemical test suitable for routine screening. A summary of estimates of performance of the various markers is shown in Table 4.15. These summary estimates are based on the simple summation of affected and unaffected pregnancies from studies cited, and because the quality of ultrasound has improved over recent years the studies used to derive these estimates are based on data collected after 1987. There are widely different estimates for detection and false-positive rates across the different studies. The summary estimates, therefore, need to be interpreted cautiously.

Table 4.15 Summary estimates of screening performance of second trimester ultrasound screening markers of Down's syndrome. Derived from Tables 6.A1–6.A8 in Wald *et al.* (1997)[97]

Ultrasound marker	No. of studies	Detection rate (%)	False-positive rate (%)
Nuchal fold thickness ≥6 mm	16	38	1.3
Femur length (comparing observed with expected)	10	34	5.9
Femur length (ratio of BPD to femur length)	4	22	5.9
Humerus length (comparing observed with expected)	6	37	5.3
Femur length and humerus length combined (comparing observed with expected)	3	36	3.7
Pyelectasis	4	19	2.4
Hyperechogenic bowel	3	11	0.7

The main structural abnormality that can be used in screening for Down's syndrome is the presence of heart defects, particularly atrio-ventricular canal defects or ventricular septal defects. About 40–50 per cent of births with Down's syndrome have a heart defect compared with between 0.5 and 1 per cent of births without Down's syndrome so detecting them *in utero* cannot have a performance better than this. The maximum detection rate achievable with a single second trimester ultrasound marker is an estimated 38 per cent using nuchal fold thickness, or about 45 per cent using heart defects, both substantially less than the detection rate achievable with serum screening. Use of these ultrasound markers alone as a primary screening method for Down's syndrome is therefore ruled out, as is their use as a secondary screening test performed on women with positive serum screening results. They could be used in combination with serum markers in primary screening but a suitable algorithm has not yet been specified.

Serum and ultrasound screening at 10–13 weeks of pregnancy
Serum markers
Table 4.16 summarizes the main first trimester serum markers. Two stand out as being discriminatory, PAPP-A and free β-hCG. Table 4.17 shows the Down's syndrome screening performance of these serum markers at 8–14 weeks of gestation based on

Table 4.16 First trimester serum markers of Down's syndrome. Taken from Wald *et al.* (1997)[97]

Marker	No. of studies	No. of Down's syndrome pregnancies	Median MoM in Down's syndrome pregnancies	95% CI
PAPP-A	12	297	0.38	0.33–0.43
free β-hCG	12	308	1.83	1.65–2.03
AFP	16	335	0.78	0.73–0.84
uE$_3$	8	210	0.71	0.59–0.86
hCG	14	352	1.29	1.16–1.44
free α-hCG	6	162	1.00	0.85–1.17

MoM = Multiples of the normal median.

Table 4.17   Down's syndrome screening performance of PAPP-A and free β-hCG at 8–14 weeks of gestation. Source: Wald *et al.* (1995)[120]

Maternal age with:	Detection rate (%) for a 5% false-positive rate
PAPP-A	52
free β-hCG	38
free β-hCG + PAPP-A	62

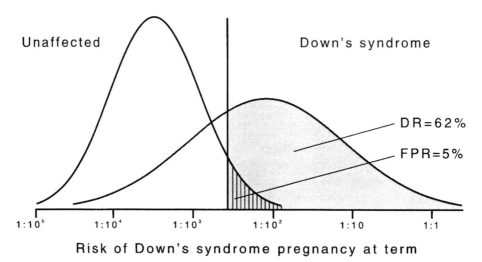

Fig. 4.8 The distribution of risk estimates in affected and unaffected Down's syndrome pregnancies using maternal age with PAPP-A and free β-hCG at 10–13 weeks of pregnancy.

British experience.[121] With free β-hCG, PAPP-A and maternal age, the detection rate for a 5 per cent false-positive rate is 62 per cent. This is illustrated in Fig. 4.8. Similar findings have been reported from the United States.[122]

Nuchal translucency measurement

Nuchal translucency (the width of the space between the skin and cervical spine) is typically about 1 mm at 11 weeks of pregnancy. It increases with gestational age and so it is appropriate to express measurements in multiples of the median for a given gestational age. Figure 4.9 shows the increase with gestational age and Fig. 4.10 shows the distribution of risk in unaffected and Down's syndrome pregnancies using nuchal translucency measurement with maternal age.

The first trimester combined test

Figure 4.11 shows the performance of screening using the first trimester serum markers PAPP-A and free β-hCG combined with the ultrasound marker nuchal translucency and maternal age. The original estimated detection rate for a 5 per cent false-positive rate was 80 per cent.[41] This was later revised to 85%[42] in the light of the publication of updated distribution parameters of nuchal translucency.

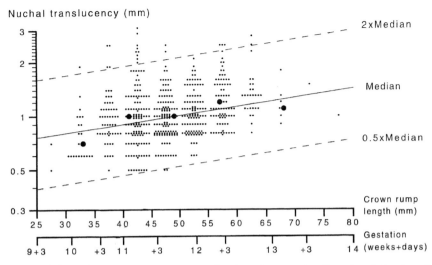

Fig 4.9 Nuchal translucency measurement according to crown rump length and gestational age in pregnancies without Down's syndrome (*n* = 561), from Schuchter *et al.* (1998).[122] Full circles show medians within 10 mm CRL groups.

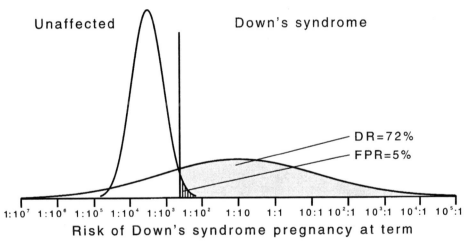

Fig. 4.10 Distributions of estimates of risk of Down's syndrome in affected and unaffected pregnancies using maternal age with nuchal translucency at 10–13 weeks of pregnancy.

Serum and ultrasound screening in the first *and* second trimester: the integrated test

The first trimester serum marker pregnancy associated plasma protein A (PAPP-A) and the ultrasound marker nuchal translucency measurement can be used with maternal age and second trimester serum markers AFP, uE$_3$, hCG, and inhibin-A to form a single integrated test.[42]

The integrated test has an 85 per cent detection rate for a false-positive rate of 0.9 per cent. To achieve the same detection rate, current screening tests would have much higher false-positive rates (see Table 4.18). The integrated test is similarly cost effective

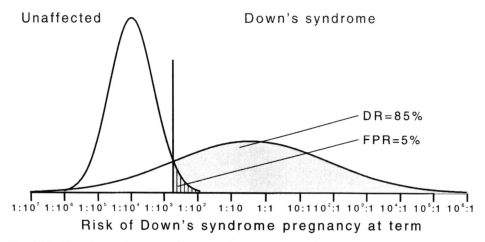

Fig. 4.11 First trimester Down's syndrome screening using the combined test: distributions of estimates of risk of Down's syndrome in affected and unaffected pregnancies using nuchal translucency, PAPP-A, and free β-hCG with maternal age.

to current methods of screening when compared at an 85 per cent detection rate; the extra costs of adding screening markers are largely offset by the savings from the greatly reduced number of amniocenteses or chorionic villus sampling procedures. If the integrated test used in this way were to replace the second trimester triple test as the triple test is currently widely used with a 5 per cent false-positive rate, the detection rate would be greater (85 per cent versus 69 per cent) and the number of amniocenteses and fetal losses from the procedure would be reduced by four-fifths. Table 4.18 also shows the performance of variants of the integrated test. Figure 4.12 compares the positive rates of the different screening tests when used to achieve an 85 per cent detection rate.

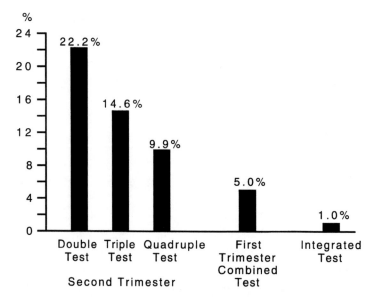

Fig. 4.12 Positive rates of the different screening tests when used to achieve an 85 per cent detection rate.[42]

Table 4.18 Screening to achieve an 85 per cent detection rate for different methods showing the false-positive rate, odds of having an affected pregnancy given a positive result, and number of diagnostic procedure-related fetal losses per Down's syndrome pregnancy diagnosed

Method of screening (all include maternal age)	Risk cut-off level	False-positive rate (%)	Odds of being affected given a positive result	Procedure-related fetal losses per Down's syndrome pregnancy diagnosed*†
First and second trimester				
Integrated test:				
PAPP-A, NT + Quadruple	1 in 120	0.9	1:9	0.08
Integrated test variants				
PAPP-A, NT + Triple	1 in 190	1.5	1:13	0.12
PAPP-A + Quadruple	1 in 410	5.2	1:47	0.42
PAPP-A + Triple	1 in 560	7.7	1:70	0.63
First trimester				
Combined test	1 in 540	4.9	1:45	0.61
Second trimester				
Quadruple test	1 in 630	9.8	1:88	0.79
Triple test	1 in 830	14.5	1:131	1.18
Double test	1 in 1040	22.1	1:200	1.80

NT = nuchal translucency measurement.
* Birth prevalence taken to be 1. 6 per 1000 and uptake of amniocentesis 100 per cent; if birth prevalence were 1.3 per 1000 multiply values in the last three columns by 1.6/1.3.
† Calculated as odds of being unaffected given a positive result × 0.9 per cent.
Source: Wald *et al* (1999).[42]

Table 4.19 compares detection and false-positive rates using the double, triple, quadruple, and integrated tests according to maternal age group. With the integrated test the false-positive rate remains relatively low at all ages.

The integrated test avoids having to select between different tests at different stages of pregnancy. Its use followed by diagnostic karyotyping offers the safest and most effective antenatal screening strategy for Down's syndrome yet described. It is now being assessed in practice at selected centres by formal demonstration projects.

Diagnostic tests

Women in whom the results of a screening test for Down's syndrome are positive are offered a diagnostic amniocentesis or chorionic villus sampling, in order to obtain a sample of cells of the same genetic origin as the fetus. Whether Down's syndrome is present is normally determined by karyotyping either these cells or cells cultured from them (generally the latter, which is the more reliable method). DNA methods such as fluorescence *in situ* hybridization and the polymerase chain reaction (PCR) are also being used to detect Down's syndrome in the fetus. All these diagnostic procedures are

Table 4.19   Detection rates (DR) and false-positive rates (FPR) according to maternal age and method of screening (all tests include maternal age with gestational age estimated using ultrasound)†

Age (years)	Double test		Triple test		Quadruple test		Full integrated test	
	DR (%)	FPR (%)	DR (%)	FPR (%)	DR (%)	FPR (%)	DR (%)	FPR (%)
15–19	35	2.2	50	2.4	63	3.0	78	0.5
20–24	38	2.7	52	2.7	63	3.1	78	0.5
25–29	43	3.7	56	3.4	67	3.9	80	0.7
30–34	57	7.4	66	6.2	75	6.5	84	1.1
15–34	46	4.0	58	3.7	69	4.1	81	0.7
35–39	79	20	82	15	87	15	89	2.6
40+	96	48	96	38	97	33	96	7.5
35+	86	24	88	19	91	17	92	3.3
All	61	5.6	69	4.9	77	5.2	85	0.9

† Women are screen positive if the risk exceeds 1 in 250 for the double and triple tests, 1 in 300 for the quadruple test, and 1 in 120 for the integrated test.

also applicable to other chromosomal disorders. They are discussed at greater length in Chapter 19 (Amniocentesis and chorionic villus sampling).

THE ORGANIZATION OF SCREENING SERVICES

A major challenge in the delivery of Down's syndrome screening services is the need to set up an adequate organizational structure. The state of California is unusual in having achieved this, and as a result provides one of the best screening services in the world. In the absence of an appropriate organizational framework, screening is likely to be introduced piecemeal, leading to gaps in the service through lack of equity in service provision. The precise organizational structure is likely to vary from community to community, but in general, maternity units need to be organized into screening groups of about 20 000 or more deliveries a year. In Britain this would represent about 30 screening groups.

In the structure proposed, each unit would have a clear screening policy agreed centrally and would work in harmony with other screening groups. A screening co-ordinator would be responsible for reporting results to women booking at the maternity unit and coordinating the local screening service. A designated local director of screening, of consultant status, would guide and support the work of the coordinator. The screening coordinators and local directors would form a larger network which would be attentive to advances in screening and their controlled introduction into practice. The policy would need to specify the screening test and the role of ultrasound, and to establish quality control criteria, maximum intervals between the performance and reporting of test results, and the quality of patient information and counselling. Several screening groups would form part of regional groupings that would produce an annual report on the service including an audit of outcome, the uptake of screening, and an assessment as to whether screening performance met expectations on the basis of the age distribution of the women screened. The organizational needs of the screening service are important, and are usually the aspect of screening that is most neglected.

Computer assisted test interpretation

Computer assisted test interpretation is a necessary aspect of screening for Down's syndrome because of the complexity of combining different markers in deriving a woman's risk of having a pregnancy with Down's syndrome. Such computerized interpretations have the advantage of standardizing reporting and ensuring accuracy and quality, provided the software is sound and has been validated. The software also permits the development of a database in which local results can be accumulated and normal medians derived for the calculation of MoM values. The software can vary in levels of sophistication—the best can provide adjustments for all the necessary covariables (for example, ethnic group, and maternal weight), allow for regression to the mean in the interpretation of repeat tests, and provide a wide range of facilities for monitoring the screening programme.

CONCLUSIONS

Figure 4.13 summarizes in the form of a flow diagram the performance of Down's syndrome screening using (1) the second trimester quadruple test, (2) the first trimester combined test, and (3) the first and second trimester integrated test.

Whichever of the three strategies is employed, screening for Down's syndrome is now highly effective. Surveys in Britain and North America[124,125] have shown that serum

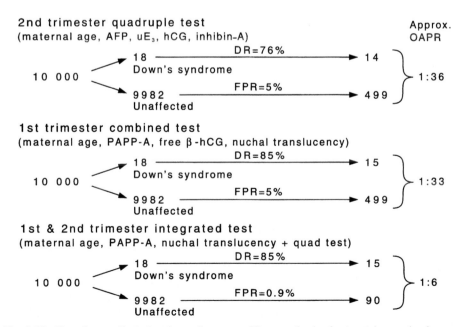

Fig. 4.13 Flow diagram illustrating the performance of three methods of antenatal screening for Down's syndrome (based on a natural birth prevalence of Down's syndrome of 1.8 per 1000, typical of current rates in England and Wales).

screening has been widely introduced over the last 10 years, usually employing the double or triple tests.

Choice is an essential element in screening. Generally about 70 per cent of women take up the offer of screening, and about 70 per cent of those with positive screening results decide to have a diagnostic amniocentesis or chorionic villus sampling procedure. Over 90 per cent with positive diagnostic results opt for a termination of pregnancy. Because among women with positive results those with the highest risk estimates tend to have a diagnostic procedure, and these are the ones most likely to have an affected pregnancy, the expected maximum detection is greater than the simple product of the screening and amniocentesis uptake rates (0.7 × 0.7 or 0.49), but it is still much less than 100 per cent. A reasonable expectation from Down's syndrome screening programme using modern tests is that about 50 per cent of affected pregnancies will be identified and result in a therapeutic abortion.

ACKNOWLEDGEMENTS

I am grateful to Joan Noble, Anne Kennard, Allan Hackshaw, and Hilary Watt for their assistance and collaboration in the work described in this chapter.

REFERENCES

1. Mutton D. E., Alberman E., and Hook E. B., (1996). Cytogenetic and epidemiological findings in Down's syndrome, England and Wales 1989 to 1993. *J. Med.Genet.*, **33**, 387–94.
2. Sherman S. L., Petersen M. B., Freeman S. B. *et al.* (1994). Non-dysjunction of chromosome 21 in maternal meiosis I: evidence for a maternal age-dependent mechanism involving reduced recombination. *Hum. Mol. Genet.* **3**, 1529–35.
3. Cuckle H. S., Wald N. J., and Thompson S. G.. (1987). Estimating a woman's risk of having a pregnancy associated with Down's syndrome using her age and serum alphafetoprotein level. *Br. J. Obstet. Gynaecol.*, **94**, 387–402.
4. Morris J. K., Wald N. J., and Watt H. C. (1999). Fetal loss in Down's syndrome pregnancies. *Prenat. Diagn.*, **19**, 142–5.
5. Hayes C., Johnson Z., Thornton L., *et al.* (1997). Ten-year survival of Down syndrome births. *Int. J. Epidemiol.*, **26**, 822–9.
6. Noble J. (1998). The natural history of Down's syndrome. *J. Med. Screen.*, **5**, 172–7.
7. Heinonen O. P., Slone D., Shapiro S. (1977). *Birth defects and drugs in pregnancy*. Publishing Sciences Group, Littleton, MA.
8. Leck I., Record R. G., McKeown T., and Edwards J. H. (1968). The incidence of malformations in Birmingham, England, 1950–1959. *Teratology*, **1**, 263–80.
9. Carr J. (1988). Six weeks to twenty-one years old: a longitudinal study of children with Down's syndrome and their families. *J. Child Psychol. Psychiatr.*, **29**, 407–31.
10. Cuckle H. S., and Wald N. J. (1990). Screening for Down's syndrome. In: *Prenatal Diagnosis and Prognosis.*, (ed. R. J. Lilford) pp. 657–92. Butterworths, London.
11. Zipursky A., Brown E., Christensen H., Sutherland R., and Doyle J. (1997). Leukaemia and/or myeloproliferative syndrome in neonates with Down syndrome. *Semin. Perinatol.*, **21**, 97–101.

12. Mutton D., Bunch K., Draper G., and Alberman E. (1997). Children's cancer and Down's syndrome. *J. Med. Genet.*, **34**, 65S.
13. Stewart B. (1994). The prevalence of unrecognised thyroid dysfunction in school age children with Down's syndrome in Oxfordshire—diagnostic aspects and approaches to screening and treatment. *Medical issues in Down's syndrome* (conference proceedings, Royal Society of Medicine, June 1994), pp. 43–50. Down's syndrome Association, London.
14. Fort P., Lifshitz F., Bellisario R., Davis J., Lanes R., Pugliese M., Richman R., Post E. M., and David R. (1984). Abnormalities of thyroid function in infants with Down's syndrome. *J. Pediatr.*, **104**, 545–9.
15. Paul A. (1997). Epilepsy or sterotypy? Diagnostic issues in learning disabilities. *Seizure*, **6**, 111–20.
16. Visser F. E., Aldenkamp A. P., van Huffelen A. C., Kuilman M., Overweg J., and van Wijk J. (1997). Prospective study of the prevalence of Alzheimer-type dementia in institutionalised individuals with Down's syndrome. *Am. J. Mental Retard.*, **101**, 400–12.
17. Holland A. J., and Oliver C. (1995). Down's syndrome and the links with Alzheimer's disease. *J. Neurol. Neurosurg. Psychiatry*, **59**, 111–4.
18. Penrose L. S., and Smith G. F. (1966). *Down's anomaly*. Churchill, London.
19. Office of Population Censuses and Surveys (OPCS) (1991). *Mortality statistics (general)*. HMSO, London.
20. Penrose L. S. (1933). The relative effects of paternal and maternal age in mongolism. *J. Genet.*, **27**, 219.
21. Lejeune J., Gautier M., and Turpin R. (1959). Etude des chromosomes somatiques de neuf enfants mongoliens. *C. R. Acad. Sci., Paris*, **248**, 1721–2.
22. Steele M. W., and Breg W. R. (1966). Chromosome analysis of human amniotic-fluid cells. *Lancet*, **ii**, 383–5.
23. Valenti C., Schutta E. J., and Kehaty T. (1968). Prenatal diagnosis of Down's syndrome. *Lancet*, **ii,** 220.
24. Merkatz I. R., Nitowsky H. M., Macri J. N., and Johnson W. E. (1984). An association between low maternal serum alpha-fetoprotein and fetal chromosomal abnormalities. *Am. J. Obstet. Gynecol.*, **148**, 886–94.
25. Cuckle H. S., Wald N. J., and Lindenbaum R. H. (1984). Maternal serum alpha-fetoprotein measurement. A screening test for Down syndrome. *Lancet*, **i**, 926–9.
26. Bogart M., Pandian M. R., and Jones O. W. (1987). Abnormal maternal serum chorionic gonadotropin levels in pregnancies with fetal chromosome abnormalities. *Prenat. Diagn.*, **7**, 623–30.
27. Canick J., Knight G. J., Palomaki G. E., Haddow J. E., Cuckle H. S., and Wald N. J. (1988). Low second trimester maternal serum unconjugated oestriol in pregnancies with Down's syndrome. *Br. J. Obstet.Gynaecol.*, **95**, 330–3.
28. Wald N. J., Cuckle H. S., Densem J. W., Nanchahal K., Canick J. A., Haddow J. E., Knight J. E., and Palomaki G. E. (1988). Maternal serum unconjugated oestriol as an antenatal screening test for Down's syndrome. *Br. J. Obstet.Gynaecol.*, **95**, 334–41.
29. Wald N. J., Cuckle H. S., Densem J. W., Nanchahal K., Royston P., Chard T., Haddow J. E., Knight G. J., Palomaki G. E., and Canick J. A. (1988). Maternal serum screening for Down's syndrome in early pregnancy. *Br. Med. J.*, **297**, 883–8.
30. Wald N. J., Cuckle H. S., Densem J. W., Kennard A., and Smith D. (1992). Maternal serum

screening for Down's syndrome: the effect of routine ultrasound scan determination of gestational age and adjustment for maternal weight. *Br. J. Obstet. Gynecol.*, **99**, 144–9.

31. Ryall R. G., Staples A. J., Robertson E. F., and Pollard A. C. (1992). Improved performance in a prenatal screening programme for Down's syndrome incorporating serum-free hCG subunit analyses. *Prenat. Diagn.*, **12**, 251–61.

32. Wald N. J., Densem J. W., George L., Muttukrishna S., and Knight P. G. (1996). Prenatal screening for Down's syndrome using Inhibin-A as a serum marker. *Prenat. Diagn.*, **16**, 143–53.

33. Wald N. J., Densem J. W., George L., Muttukrishna S., Knight P. G., Watt H., Hackshaw A., and Morris J. (1997). Inhibin-A in Down's syndrome pregnancies: revised estimate of standard deviation. *Prenat. Diagn.*, **17**, 285–90.

34. Brambati B., Lanzani A., and Tului L. (1991). Ultrasound and biochemical assessment of first trimester pregnancy. In *The embryo: normal and abnormal development and growth.* (ed. M. Chapman, G. Grudzinskas, and T. Chard), pp. 181–94. Springer, Berlin.

35. Wald N., Stone R., Cuckle H. S., Grudzinskas J. G., Barkai G., Brambati B., Teisner B., and Fuhrmann W. (1992). First trimester concentrations of pregnancy associated plasma protein A and placental protein 14 in Down's syndrome. *Br. Med. J.*, **305**, 28.

36. Macri J., Kasturi R. V., Krantz B. S., Cook E. J., Moore N. D., Young J. A., Romero D., and Larsen J. W. (1990). Maternal serum Down syndrome screening: Free B-protein is a more effective marker than human chorionic gonadotropin. *Am. J. Obstet. Gynecol.*, **163**, 1248–53.

37. Wald N. J., George L., Smith D., Densem J. W., and Petterson K. (1996). On behalf of the International Prenatal Screening Research Group. Serum screening for Down's syndrome between 8 and 14 weeks of pregnancy. *Br. J. Obstet. Gynaecol.*, **103**, 407–12.

38. Szabo J., and Gellen J., (1990). Nuchal fluid accumulation in trisomy 21 detected by vaginosonography in first trimester. *Lancet*, **336**, 1133.

39. Nicolaides K. H., Azar G., Byrne D., Mansur C., and Marks K. (1992). Fetal nuchal translucency: ultrasound screening for chromosomal defects in the first trimester of pregnancy. *Br. Med. J.*, **304**, 867–9.

40. Pandya P. P., Snijders R. J. M., Johnson S. P., de Loudes Brizot M., and Nicolaides K. H. (1995). Screening for fetal trisomies by maternal age and fetal nuchal translucency thickness at 10 to 14 weeks of gestation. *Br. J. Obstet. Gynaecol.*, **102**, 957–62.

41. Wald N. J., and Hackshaw A. K. (1997). Combining ultrasound and biochemistry in first-trimester screening for Down's syndrome. *Prenat. Diagn.*, **17**, 821–9.

42. Wald N. J., Watt H. C., and Hackshaw A. K. (1999). Integrated screening for Down's syndrome based on tests performed during the first and second trimesters. *N. Engl. J. Med.*, **341**, 461–7.

43. Cowchock F. S., and Ruch D. A. (1984). Low maternal serum AFP and Down syndrome. *Lancet*, **i**, 161–2.

44. Fuhrmann W., Wendt P., and Weitzel H. K. (1984). Maternal serum-AFP as screening test for Down syndrome. *Lancet*, **ii**, 413.

45. Guibaud S., Bonnet-Capela M., Germain D., Dumont M., Thoulon J. M., and Berland M. (1984). Prenatal screening for Down's syndrome. *Lancet*, **ii**, 1359–60.

46. Seller M. J. (1984). Prenatal screening for Down syndrome. *Lancet*, **i**, 1359.

47. Tabor A., Norgaard-Pedersen B., and Jacobsen J. C. (1984). Low maternal serum AFP and Down syndrome. *Lancet*, **ii**, 161.

48. Hershey D. W., Crandall B. F., and Schroth P. S. (1985). Maternal serum alpha-fetoprotein screening of fetal trisomies. *Am. J. Obstet. Gynecol.*, **153**, 224–5.

49. Murday V., and Slack J. (1985). Screening for Down's syndrome in the North East Thames Region. *Br. Med. J.*, **291**, 1315–8.

50. Spencer K., and Carpenter P. (1985). Screening for Down's syndrome using serum alpha fetoprotein: a retrospective study indicating caution. *Br. Med. J.*, **290**, 1940–3.

51. Voitlander T., and Vogel F. (1985). Low alpha-fetoprotein and serum albumin levels in *Morbus* Down may point to a common regulatory mechanism. *Human Genetics*, **71**, 276–7.

52. Doran T. A., Cadesky K., Wong P. Y., Mastrogiacomo C., and Capello T. (1986). Maternal serum alpha-fetoprotein and fetal autosomal trisomies. *Am. J. Obstet. Gynecol.*, **154**, 277–81.

53. Ashwood E. R., Cheng E., and Luthy D. (1987). Maternal serum alpha-fetoprotein and fetal trisomy-21 in women 35 years and older: implications for alpha-fetoprotein screening programs. *Am. J. Med. Genetics*, **26**, 531–9.

54. Tabor A., Larsen S. O., Nielsen J., Nielsen J., Philip J., Pilgaard B., Videbech P., and Norgaard-Pedersen B. (1987). Screening for Down's syndrome using an iso-risk curve based on maternal age and serum alpha-fetoprotein level. *Br. J. Obstet. Gynaecol.*, **94**, 636–42.

55. Dix U., Gams M., Grubisic A., Dericks-Tan J., and Langenbeck U. (1988). Maternal serum alpha-fetoprotein in pregnancies with trisomy 18. *Z. Geburtsh. Perinat.*, **192**, 231–3.

56. Bogart M., Golbus M., Sorg N., and Jones O. W. (1989). Human chorionic gonadotropin levels in pregnancies with aneuploid fetuses. *Prenat. Diagn.*, **9**, 379–84.

57. Del Junco D., Greenberg F., Darnule A., Contant C., Weyland B., Schmidt D., Faucett A., Rose E., and Alpert E. (1989). Statistical analysis of maternal age, maternal serum alpha fetoprotein, B human chorionic gonadotropin, and unconjugated estriol for Down syndrome screening in midtrimester. *Am. J. Hum. Genet.*, **45**, a257.

58. Fisher R. A., Suppnick C. K., Peabody C. T., Zapp A. R., Helwick Loomis D. O., and Schehr A. B. (1989). Maternal serum chorionic gonadotrophin, unconjugated estriol and alpha-fetoprotein in Down syndrome pregnancies. *Am. J. Hum. Genet.*, **45**, a259 (and personal communication).

59. Osathanondh R., Canick J. A., Abell K. B., Stevens L. D., Palomaki G. E., Knight G. J., and Haddow J. E. (1989). Second trimester screening for trisomy 21. *Lancet*, **ii**, 52.

60. Petrocik E., Wassman R., and Kelly J. (1989). Prenatal screening for Down syndrome using maternal serum human chorionic gonadotropin levels. *Am. J. Obstet. Gynecol.*, **161**, 1168–73.

61. Bartels I., Thiele M., and Bogart M. (1990). Maternal serum HCG and SP1 in pregnancies with fetal aneuploidy. *Am. J. Med. Genet.*, **37**, 261–4.

62. Heyl P. S., Miller W., and Canick J. A. (1990). Maternal serum screening for aneuploid pregnancy by alpha-fetoprotein, hCG, and unconjugated estriol. *Obstet. Gynecol.*, **76**, 1025–31.

63. Jacobs S., and, Giles W. (1990). Down's syndrome and low maternal serum alpha-fetoprotein. *Aust. N. Z. J. Obstet. Gynaecol.*, **30**, 335.

64. Macri J. N., Kasturi R. V., Krantz D. A., Cook E. J., Sunderji S. G., and Larsen J. W. (1990). Maternal serum Down syndrome screening: Unconjugated estriol is not useful. *Am. J. Obstet. Gynecol.*, **162**, 672–3.

65. Muller F., and Boue A. (1990). A single chorionic gonadotropin assay for maternal serum screening for Down's syndrome. *Prenat. Diagn.*, **10**, 389–98.

66. Norgaard-Pedersen B., Larsen S. O., Arends J., Svenstrup B., and Tabor A. (1990). Maternal serum markers in screening for Down syndrome. *Clin. Genet.*, **37**, 35–43.

67. Suchy S. F., and Yeager M. T. (1990). Down syndrome screening in women under 35 with maternal serum hCG. *Obstet. Gynecol.*, **76**, 20–4.

68. Bogart M. H., Jones O. W., Felder R. A., Best R. G., Bradley L., Butts W., Crandall B., MacMahon W., Wians F. H., and Loeh P. V. (1991). Prospective evaluation of maternal serum human chorionic gonadotrophin levels in 3428 pregnancies. *Am. J. Obstet. Gynecol.*, **165**, 663–6.

69. Crossley J. A., Aitken D. A., and Connor J. M. (1991). Free ß hCG and prenatal screening for chromosome abnormalities. *J. Med. Genet.*, **28**, 570.

70. Crossley J. A., Aitken D. A., and Connor J. M. (1991). Prenatal screening chorionic gonadotrophin, alpha-fetoprotein, and age. *Prenat. Diagn.*, **11**, 83–101.

71. Kellner L. H., Weiss R. R., Neuer M., and Bock J. L. (1991). Maternal serum screening using alpha-fetoprotein, beta-human chorionic gonadotropin and unconjugated estriol (AFA+) in the second trimester. *Am. J. Obstet. Gynecol.*, **164**, A636.

72. Lewis M., Faed M. J. W., and Howie P. W. (1991). Screening for Down's syndrome based on individual risk. *Br. Med. J.*, **303**, 551–3.

73. MacDonald M. L., Wagner R. M., and Slotnick R. N. (1991). Sensitivity and specificity of screening for Down syndrome with alpha-fetoprotein, hCG, unconjugated estriol, and maternal age. *Obstet. Gynecol.*, **77**, 63–8.

74. Mancini G., Perone M., Dall'Amico D., Bollati C., Albano F., Mazzone R., Russo M., and Carbonara A. (1991). Screening for fetal Down's syndrome with maternal serum markers—an experience in Italy. *Prenat. Diagn.*, **11**, 245–52.

75. Miller C. H., O'Brien T. J., Chatelain S., Butler B. B., and Quirk J. G. (1991). Alteration in age-specific risks for chromosomal trisomy by maternal serum alpha-fetoprotein and human chorionic gonadotropin screening. *Prenat. Diagn.*, **11**, 153–8.

76. Spencer K. (1991). Evaluation of an assay of the free ß-subunit of choriogonadotropin and its potential value in screening for Down's syndrome. *Clin. Chem.*, **37**, 809–14.

77. Zeitune M., Aitken D. A., Crossley J. A., Yates J. R. W., Cooke A., and Ferguson-Smith M. A. (1991). Estimating the risk of a fetal autosomal trisomy at mid-trimester using maternal serum alphafetoprotien and age: a retrospective study of 142 pregnancies. *Prenat. Diagn.*, **11**, 847–57.

78. Herrou M., Leporrier N., and Leymarie P. (1992). Screening for fetal Down syndrome with maternal serum hCG and oestriol: A prospective study. *Prenat. Diagn.*, **12**, 887–92.

79. Mancini G., Perona M., Dall'Amico C., Bollati C., Fulvia A., and Carbonara A. (1992). hCG, AFP, and uE$_3$ patterns in the 14–20th weeks of Down's syndrome pregnancies. *Prenat. Diagn.*, **12**, 619–24.

80. Spencer K., Coombes E. J., Mallard A. S., and Milford Ward A. (1992). Free beta human chorionic gonadotrophin in Down's syndrome screening: a multicentre study of its role compared with other biochemical markers. *Ann. Clin. Biochem.*, **29**, 506–18.

81. Spencer K., and Macri J. N. (1992). Early detection of Down's syndrome using free beta human chorionic gonadotrophin. *Ann. Clin. Biochem.*, **29**, 349–50.

82. Crossley J. A., Aitken D. A., and Connor J. M. (1993). Second trimester unconjugated

oestriol levels in maternal serum from chromosomally abnormal pregnancies using an optimised assay. *Prenat. Diagn.*, **13**, 271–80.

83. Spencer K. (1993). Free α-subunit of human chorionic gonadotrophin in Down syndrome. *Am. J. Obstet. Gynecol.*, **168**, 1.

84. Stone S., Henely R., Reynolds T., and John R. (1993). A comparison of total and free ß-hCG assays in Down syndrome screening. *Prenat. Diagn.*, **13**, 535–7.

85. Norgaard-Pedersen B., Alfthan H., Arends J., Hogdall C., Larsen S. O., Petterson K., and Stenman, S. (1994). A new simple and rapid dual assay for AFP and the free ß-subunit of hCG in screening for Down's syndrome. *Clin. Genet.*, **45**, 1–4.

86. Wald N. J., Densem J. W., Smith D., and Klee G. G. (1994). Four marker serum screening for Down's syndrome. *Prenat. Diagn.*, **14**, 707–16.

87. Forest J. C., Masse J., Rousseau F., *et al.* (1995). Screening for Downs syndrome during the first and second trimesters: Impact of risk estimation parameters. *Clin. Biochem.*, **28**, 443–9.

88. Kellner L. H., Weiss R. R., Weiner Z., *et al.* (1995). The advantages of using triple-marker screening for chromosomal abnormalities. *Am. J. Obstet. Gynecol.*, **172**, 831–6.

89. Wenstrom K. D., Desai R., Owen J., DuBard M. B., and Boots L. (1995). Comparison of multiple marker screening with amniocentesis for the detection of fetal aneuploidy in women ≥35 years old. *Am. J. Obstet. Gynecol.*, **173**, 1287–92.

90. Aitken D. A., Wallace E. M., Crossley J. A., Swanston I. A., van Parenen Y., van Maarle M., Groome N. P., Macri J. N., and Connor J. M. (1996). Dimeric inhibin-A as a marker for Down's syndrome in early pregnancy. *N. Engl. J. Med.*, **334**, 1231–6.

91. Cuckle H. S., Holding S., Jones R., Groome N. P., and Wallace E. M. (1996). Combining inhibin A with existing second-trimester markers in maternal serum screening for Down's syndrome. *Prenat. Diagn.*, **16**, 1095–100.

92. Lambert-Messerlian G. M., Canick J. A., Palomaki G. E., and Schneyer A. L. (1996). Second trimester levels of maternal serum inhibin-A., total inhibin, α inhibin precursor and activin in Down's syndrome pregnancies. *J. Med. Screen.*, **3**, 58–62.

93. Spencer K., Wallace E. M., and Ritoe S. (1996). Second trimester dimeric inhibin-A in Down's syndrome screening. *Prenat. Diagn.*, **16**, 1101–10.

94. Wallace E., Swanston I., Grant V., McNeilly A., Ashby J. P., Blundell G., Colder A. A., and Groome N. P. (1996). Second trimester screening for Down's syndrome using serum dimeric inhibin-A. *Clin. Endocrinol.*, **44**, 17–21.

95. Wenstrom K. D., Owen J., and Boots L. (1997). Second trimester maternal serum CA-125 versus estriol in the multiple-marker screening test for Down syndrome. *Obstet. Gynecol.*, **89**, 359–63. (Data on AFP, uE₃, and total hCG are in reference [55].)

96. Wald N. J., Watt H. C., Haddow J. E., and Knight G. J. (1998). Screening for Down's syndrome at 14 weeks of pregnancy. *Prenat. Diagn.*, **18**, 291–3.

97. Wald N. J., Kennard A., Hackshaw A., and McGuire A. (1997). Antenatal screening for Down's syndrome. *J. Med. Screen.*, **4**, 181–246.

98. Wald N. J., Smith D., Kennard A., Palomaki G. E., Salonen R., Holzgreve W., Pejtsik B., Coombes E. J., Mancini G., MacRae A. R., Wyatt P., and Roberson J. (1993). Biparietal diameter and crown-rump length in fetuses with Down's syndrome: implications for antenatal serum screening for Down's syndrome. *Br. J. Obstet. Gynaecol.*, **100**, 430–5.

99. Watt H. C., Wald N. J., Smith D., Kennard A., and Densem J. (1996). Effect of allowing for ethnic group in prenatal screening for Down's syndrome. *Prenat. Diagn.*, **16**, 691–8.

100. Neveux L. M., Palomaki G. E., Larrivee D. A., Knight G. J., and Haddow J. E. (1996). Refinements in managing maternal weight adjustment for interpreting prenatal screening results. *Prenat. Diagn.*, **16**, 1115–19.

101. Cuckle H. S., Alberman E., Wald N. J., Royston P., and Knight G. (1990). Maternal smoking habits and Down's syndrome. *Prenat. Diagn.*, **10**, 561–7.

102. Haddow J. E., Palomaki G. E., and Knight G. J. (1995). Effect of parity on huma chorionic gonadotropin levels and Down's syndrome screening. *J. Med. Screen.*, **2**, 28–30.

103. Zimmermann R., Streicher A., Huch R., and Huch A. (1995). Effect of gravidity and parity on the parameters used in serum screening for trisomy 21. *Prenat. Diagn.*, **15**, 781–2.

104. Wald N. J., and Watt H. C. (1996). Serum markers for Down's syndrome in relation to number of previous births and maternal age. *Prenat. Diagn.*, **16**, 699–703.

105. Barkai G., Goldman B., Ries L., Chaki R., and Cuckle H. S. (1996). Effect of gravidity on maternal serum markers for Down's syndrome. *Prenat. Diagn.*, **16**, 319–22.

106. Wald N. J., White N., Morris J. K., Huttly W., and Canick J. A. (1999). Serum markers for Down's syndrome in women who have had in vitro fertilization: implications for antenatal screening. *Br. J. Obstet. Gynaecol.*, **106**, 1304–6.

107. Hackshaw A. K., Densem J., and Wald N. J. (1995). Repeat maternal serum testing for Down's screening using multiple markers with special reference to free alpha and free beta hCG. *Prenat. Diagn.*, **14**, 1125–30.

108. Hackshaw A., Densem J., and Wald N. (1998). Erratum. *Prenat. Diagn.*, **18**, 525–6.

109. Wald N. J., Hackshaw A. K., Huttly W., and Kennard A. (1996). Empirical validation of risk screening for Down's syndrome. *J. Med. Screen.*, **3**, 185–7.

110. Canick J. A., and Rish S. (1998). The accuracy of assigned risks in maternal serum screening. *Prenat. Diagn.*, **18**, 413–15.

111. Cuckle H. S., Iles R. K., Sehmi I. K., Oakley R. E., Davies S., and Ind T. (1995). Urinary multiple marker screening for Down's syndrome. *Prenat. Diagn.*, **15**, 745–51.

112. Canick J. A., Kellner L. H., Saller D. N., Palomaki G. E., Walker R. P., and Osathanondh R. (1995). Second trimester levels of maternal urinary gonadotropin peptide in Down syndrome pregnancy. *Prenat. Diagn.*, **15**, 739–44.

113. Canick J. A., Kellner L. H., Saller D. N., Palomaki G. E., Tumber M. B., Messerlian G. L., Walker R. P., and Osathanondh R. (1996). A second level evaluation of maternal urinary gonadotropin peptide as a marker for second trimester Down syndrome screening. *3rd Joint Clinical Genetics Meeting, March of Dimes/ACMG*, Syllabus, Abstract 156, 1996.

114. Isozaki T., Palomaki G. E., Bahado-Singh R. O., and Cole L. A. (1997). Screening for Down syndrome pregnancy using β-core fragment: Prospective study. *Prenat. Diagn.*, **17**, 407–13.

115. Spencer K., Aitken D. A., Macri J. N., and Buchanan P. D. (1996). Urine free beta hCG and beta core in pregnancies affected by Down's syndrome. *Prenat. Diagn.*, **16**, 605–13.

116. Hayashi M., and Kozu H. (1995). Maternal urinary beta-core fragment of hCG/creatinine ratios and fetal chromosomal abnormalities in the second trimester of pregnancy. *Prenat. Diagn.*, **15**, 11–16.

117. Cuckle H. S., Canick J. A., Kellner L. H. (1999). Collaborative study of maternal urine

beta-core human chorionic gonadotrophin screening for Down syndrome. *Prenat. Diagn.*, **10**, 911–7.

118. Simpson J. L., and Elias S. (1994). Isolating fetal cells in maternal circulation for prenatal diagnosis. *Prenat. Diagn.*, **14**, 1229–42.

119. Valerio D., Aiello R., Altien V., Malato A. P., Fortunato A., and Canazio A. (1996). Culture of fetal erythroid progenitor cells from maternal blood for non-invasive prenatal genetic diagnosis. *Prenat. Diagn.*, **16**, 1073–82.

120. Ferguson-Smith M. A., Zheng Y. L., and Carter N. P. (1994). Simultaneous immuno-phenotyping and FISH on fetal cells from maternal blood. *Ann. N. Y. Acad. Sci.*, **731**, 73–9.

121. Wald N. J., Kennard A., and Hackshaw A. K. (1995). First trimester serum screening for Down's syndrome. *Prenat. Diagn.*, **15**, 1227–40.

122. Haddow J. E., Palomaki G. E., Knight G. J., Williams J., Miller W. A., and Johnson A. (1998). Screening of maternal serum for fetal Down's syndrome in the first trimester. *N. Engl. J. Med.*, **388**, 955–61.

123. Schuchter K., Wald N. J., Hackshaw A. K., Hafner E., and Liebhardt E. (1998). The distribution of nuchal translucency at 10–13 weeks of pregnancy. *Prenat. Diagn.*, **18**, 281–6.

124. Wald N. J., Huttly W. J., and Hennessy C. F. (1999). Down's syndrome screening in the UK in 1998. *Lancet*, **354**, 1264.

125. Palomaki G. E., Knight G. J., McCarthy M. T., *et al.* (1992). Maternal serum screening for fetal Down syndrome in the United States: a 1992 survey. *Am. J. Obstet. Gynecol.*, **169**, 1558–62.

5   *X-linked disorders*

Sarah Bundey

INTRODUCTION

X-linked disorders are those caused by a mutation in a gene situated on the X chromosome. As a man possesses only one X chromosome, an abnormal gene on it will not be paired with a normal allele; the man is said to be hemizygous for that particular gene. A woman possesses two X chromosomes; if both members of a pair of X-linked genes are identical then she is said to be homozygous. If the members of her gene pair are dissimilar (for example, one might be the normal or 'wild-type' gene and the other be the gene causing Duchenne muscular dystrophy) the woman is said to be a heterozygote, or a carrier, for muscular dystrophy. Female carriers for most X-linked disorders rarely have symptoms. However, in some X-linked disorders, like the Fragile-X syndrome, a significant proportion of female carriers are symptomatic.

The family patterns found in X-linked recessive disorders are as follows: the daughters of an affected man will always be carriers, his sons will always be healthy, half the daughters of a carrier woman will be carriers and half her sons will be affected (Fig. 5.1). Obligatory heterozygotes are those women who are recognized as heterozygotes from the pedigree; they are the daughters of affected men, or women who have one affected son and at least one other affected male relative. Non-obligatory heterozygotes are recognized by other methods, such as by tests of retinal function, or by molecular investigations.

Many X-linked disorders can arise *de novo* as a result of new genetic mutations. In Duchenne muscular dystrophy (DMD), for example, where affected males die before reproducing (so that a third of the mutant genes in circulation are lost with each generation) the disease would disappear were the lost genes not replaced by new mutations. About one-third of boys with DMD are affected by a new mutation occurring in oogenesis, and about two-thirds have carrier mothers. In contrast, X-linked retinitis pigmentosa (XLRP) has little effect on reproduction, and all mothers of affected males are carriers.

A mutation of an X-linked gene may occur in oogenesis or spermatogenesis or during early embryonic development. If it occurs in oogenesis, and the ovum is fertilized by a Y-bearing sperm, an affected male will be born; if the ovum is fertilized by an X-bearing sperm a carrier daughter will be born. If, on the other hand, mutation occurs

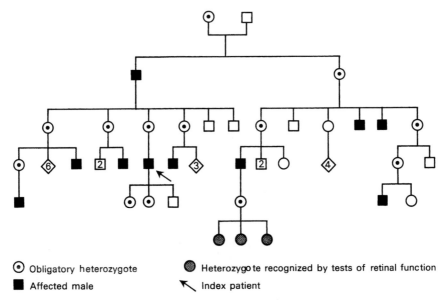

Fig. 5.1 Pedigree of X-linked retinitis pigmentosa.

in spermatogenesis, a carrier girl will be born, for sons do not normally receive their father's X chromosome. Thus, if mutation of an X-linked gene only occurred in oogenesis, an affected male could either have inherited the gene from a carrier mother or have received a new mutation from her. However, if mutation only occurred in spermatogenesis, an affected male would never be born as a result of a new mutation but would always have inherited the abnormal gene from a carrier mother. The relative frequency of mutation in males compared with females is important, since the ability to prevent an X-linked disorder depends firstly upon the ratio of carrier mothers to boys with new mutations, and secondly, upon the extent to which the carrier mothers can be recognized.

Haldane[1] showed that the proportion of new mutants among males with an X-linked disorder equals

$$(1 - f)\,\mu/(\,2\mu + v)$$

where μ equals the mutation rate in female gametes per generation, v equals the mutation rate in male gametes per generation, and f equals the effective fertility (i.e. the mean number of children born to patients divided by the mean number born to their unaffected peers). In X-linked disorders like Duchenne muscular dystrophy where affected males fail to reproduce, this formula shortens to

$$\mu/(\,2\mu + v).$$

If mutation occurs only in males ($\mu = 0$) no boys will be new mutants; if mutation occurs only in females ($v = 0$) then half the affected boys will be new mutants and half will have inherited the abnormal gene from their mothers; if mutation occurs equally in the two sexes ($\mu = v$) then the proportion of new mutants among affected males will be one-third, and two-thirds of mothers will be carriers.

With X-linked disorders which are not fatal, like Becker muscular dystrophy and haemophilia, the proportion of carrier mothers will be greater than two-thirds even if the mutation rates are equal. The exact proportion in a stable equilibrium varies with the fertility of affected males, so that the incidence of carrier females (H) equals

$$2\mu + H/2 + (\text{incidence of affected males} \times f).$$

This formula can be used to calculate the incidence of female carriers for the more benign X-linked disorders of Becker muscular dystrophy and X-linked retinitis pigmentosa, but it cannot apply to the complicated situation that occurs in the Fragile-X syndrome, where women can carry a 'premutation'.

Mutations that occur in early embryonic development will cause mosaicism of somatic tissues, or gonadal tissues, or, most commonly, both.[2] Gonadal mosaicism, with or without somatic mosaicism, can give rise to an unexpected second affected sib in a family where the first case had been thought to be due to a new mutation.[3]

From the point of view of preventing X-linked disease, the recognition of female carriers and the provision of genetic counselling is crucial. Early experience from the West Midlands Muscular Dystrophy Register, before antenatal diagnosis was available, showed that a moderate to high genetic risk for Duchenne muscular dystrophy led to women refraining from becoming pregnant, and therefore to a fall in familial cases of Duchenne muscular dystrophy. When antenatal diagnosis for DMD became available, there was no further alteration in the birth prevalence of preventable cases; however, women were enabled to have healthy children.

Three X-linked disorders for which screening may merit consideration are considered in this chapter—Duchenne muscular dystrophy, the Fragile-X syndrome, and X-linked retinitis pigmentosa. Two other X-linked conditions, haemophilia and glucose 6-phosphate dehydrogenase deficiency, are considered in Chapter 11.

Strategies for screening

As only females can have sons with an X-linked disorder, screening of women in the antenatal clinic for carrier status could be a useful procedure for predicting affected males, supposing that carrier tests suitable for population testing were available. However, unlike screening for Down's syndrome, any risk identified in a woman's pregnancy will apply to each and every pregnancy of hers, not just the current one.

The most useful screening test is to ask a pregnant woman if there is a family history of a severe problem in a child, such as muscular dystrophy, or severe mental retardation; it is also worthwhile to ask about health problems in her parents. About half of women who are carriers of Duchenne muscular dystrophy will have had an affected male relative; about half of women who carry the full mutation for the Fragile-X syndrome will have a retarded male relative, as will a small proportion of women who carry a premutation for the Fragile-X syndrome; and for X-linked retinitis pigmentosa, about three-quarters of carrier women will have a family history of a male with progressive visual loss. X-linked retinitis pigmentosa and Becker muscular dystrophy differ from Duchenne muscular dystrophy and the Fragile-X syndrome because they are milder conditions, and affected males reproduce. It is worth remembering that all daughters of males affected by X-linked disorders will be carriers; hence the importance of asking pregnant women about health problems in their fathers.

After asking about family history in the antenatal clinic, tests for carrier status can be considered, and these will be discussed in the following sections.

It should be remembered that identifying female carriers leads to the detection of only one-quarter of that number of affected fetuses because each carrier has only a 1 in 4 risk of having an affected son in any one pregnancy. The identification of carriers therefore needs to be followed by diagnostic tests on their fetuses. These tests usually make use of cells obtained by amniocentesis or chorionic villus sampling (Chapter 19).

An alternative strategy to antenatal screening is to screen all newborn males and then offer genetic counselling to the families of those shown to be affected.

DUCHENNE MUSCULAR DYSTROPHY (DMD)

The disease

This is a progressive muscular dystrophy characterized by proximal muscle weakness and big calves. Symptoms (in particular, difficulty in walking, a waddling gait, failure to run normally, and difficulty in climbing stairs or in rising from the ground without support) are usually observed at around 18 months to two years, and almost always by the age of three. The mean age of diagnosis is around two years. Affected boys are usually wheelchair-dependent by the age of 10–12 years, and death from pneumonia and respiratory insufficiency supersedes in the late teens or early twenties. No treatment is currently available, although implantation of a gene construct into muscle is a hope for the future. Parents consider DMD to be a serious disease and do not plan further children if genetic risks are high, unless antenatal diagnosis is available.

The disease is caused by deletions or point mutations in the dystrophin gene, a large gene of over 2400 kb situated on the short arm of the X chromosome, at Xp21. Rearrangements and point mutations in this gene can also cause the milder form of Xp21 muscular dystrophy, namely Becker muscular dystrophy. In this condition, onset is usually between 6 and 18 years, progression is slower, and walking is preserved until 25 to 30 years after onset. It is about one-quarter as common as Duchenne muscular dystrophy.[4]

Diagnostic tests in patients

Deletions of the dystrophin gene are found in about 65 per cent of patients with DMD and in about 80 per cent of patients with Becker muscular dystrophy. The deletions are various, and may be detected by a multiplex polymerase chain reaction (PCR) in which several groups of exons are studied simultaneously for deletions. If a deletion is found, this is diagnostic of Xp21 muscular dystrophy, but it is unreliable to predict clinical outcome from the size or the position of a deletion.

If a deletion is not found, the next diagnostic test is to perform immunostaining on a muscle biopsy. In Xp21 muscular dystrophy there is loss or reduction in dystrophin, which is situated at the periphery of muscle fibres. If dystrophin is absent, this indicates the severe disease of DMD. If dystrophin is partially present, this indicates the milder condition of Becker muscular dystrophy. If dystrophin is found to be normal quantitatively and qualitatively, then this indicates an autosomal recessive type of muscular dystrophy involving a mutation in one of the other proteins that form a complex with dystrophin in the muscle fibres.

A pathological point mutation in the dystrophin gene in a male may be recognized by using two tests: automated gene sequencing using dye labelled primers, together with the protein truncation tests, to determine whether a particular point mutation actually results in reduced production of dystrophin.[5]

Family studies

DMD and Becker muscular dystrophy are inherited as straightforward X-linked disorders. Mutation appears to be equally common in ova and sperm. Index boys may have arisen because of a new X-linked mutation occurring in their mother's ovum, or they may be affected because their mother is a carrier. *A priori*, the relative risks of these two situations are 1:2, although with individual families it is usually possible to be more precise than this, through pedigree analysis or through carrier tests on females.

Prevalence

Duchenne muscular dystrophy used to have a prevalence in boys of school age of 2.8 in 10 000 but this has decreased to 2 in 10 000 due to genetic counselling.[4,6-9] Of course, there has been no change in the numbers of affected boys who have no family history of disease, but there has been a fall in the numbers of familial cases. The 2.8 per 10 000 birth frequency among males before genetic counselling was partitioned into about 0.91/10 000 for boys affected as a result of a new mutation, 0.91/10 000 for an affected boy with a carrier mother and no previous case in the family, and 0.98/10 000 for familial cases. It is this last group that has become much less with genetic counselling. The population frequency of women who are carriers for a lethal X-linked disorder like DMD will be 4/3 times the frequency of affected males, namely about 3.7/10 000.

Currently, the most common cause for a second affected boy to be born into a family is when the diagnosis of DMD in his older brother is delayed.[8] This observation has led to the suggestion of neonatal screening for DMD.

Recognition of carrier females
Procedure in women with affected male relatives

A woman is an obligatory carrier for an X-linked disease if she has an affected son and another affected male relative. If there is only one case in the family, she has, *a priori*, a 2 in 3 chance of being a carrier if she is the patient's mother, and a 1 in 3 chance if she is the sister.

Recognition of her status becomes clear if the type of genetic mutation in the affected patient is known, and the same mutation is looked for in the female relative. If the affected boy has a deletion within his dystrophin gene, then automated sequencing of the appropriate exon of the female's dystrophin gene will detect whether she has the same deletion. If the affected boy has a point mutation, this can be looked for in a female relative, again by using an automated gene sequencer targeted at the appropriate part of the gene. If, however, the affected boy has died and there is no sample of DNA from him, then different strategies will have to be used. Firstly, the woman's carrier state should be assessed by comparing the mean of three measurements of her creatine kinase with the distribution in controls and known carriers (in order to discover in which individual the mutation occurred). Secondly, linked markers should be used in the family to try to identify which X chromosome carries the mutation; such linked markers will not define when the mutation occurred, hence the use of creatine kinase tests. However, hopefully such a situation will rarely, if ever, arise, as paediatricians and geneticists now know how essential it is to take blood from affected boys for extraction and analysis of their DNA.

Antenatal screening of women who have no affected male relative

If it were possible to detect all carrier mothers, and if those so identified chose to have antenatal diagnosis of an affected male fetus followed by selective termination of pregnancy, then it would be possible to prevent a third of cases of DMD (that is, about 0.9/10 000) in addition to the third where there is a carrier woman with an affected relative. (The remaining third consists of boys born as a result of new mutations.)

However, antenatal screening for all pathological mutations in the dystrophin gene is not practicable. It is such a large gene that probably every woman has at least one variant within it, consisting of a single base pair change. Over 99 per cent of these variants would not be pathological. However, deletions involving more than one base pair would almost certainly have a pathological effect. Some of these deletions could be recognized by pulsed field gel electrophoresis of appropriately digested DNA, but more comprehensively by the use of an automated gene sequencer. Before using the gene sequencer, the woman's DNA would have to be divided into specific exons of the dystrophin gene, using appropriate probes and PCR. Both procedures are lengthy and would at present be impractible for population screening, although this might be feasible if they became more readily automated. The finding of such a deletion in the dystrophin gene of a woman would indicate that she had a risk of 1 in 2 of having a son affected by Duchenne muscular dystrophy. As about 65 per cent of DMD cases have a deletion, the prevalence of female carriers detected in the general population would be about 65 per cent of 3.7/10 000, which equals about 2.4/10 000.

Diagnostic tests in the fetus

The first test that is indicated in the fetus of a known carrier is sex determination. If the fetus is male, the choice of further tests depends on whether the mother has a deletion. If so, a deletion screen on the fetus will suffice. If not, to have been identified as a carrier the mother must have had an affected relative; and if the precise mutation responsible for this relative's DMD has been documented, the molecular tests for this particular mutation are applied to the fetus. If information about the relative's mutation is not available, it may still be possible to carry out useful studies with linked polymorphic markers, with the hope of identifying which of the mother's two X chromosomes carries the high risk for the Duchenne mutation, and whether this is the X chromosome inherited by the fetus. Using this technique, the detection rate is about 95 per cent and the false positive rate about 4 per cent.

Strategy for antenatal screening

Figure 5.2 presents a scheme for screening 100 000 pregnant women. The expectation is that without intervention these women will have 50 000 sons, of whom 14 will have DMD (based on a birth frequency of 2.8 in 10 000). About 36 women will have a family history of DMD, half of whom will be carriers. Such women hopefully will be known to the Regional Clinical Genetics Service, through its register of DMD

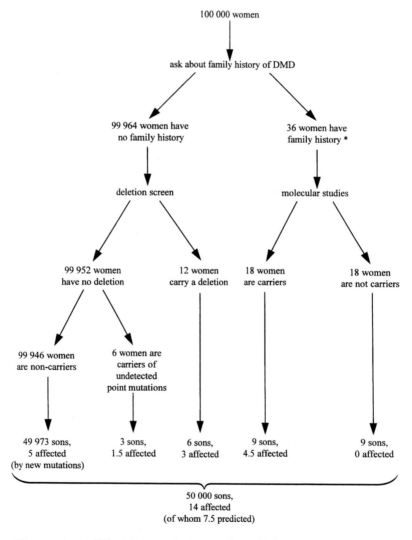

* These women should already be known to a Regional Genetics Unit.

Fig. 5.2   Algorithm of antenatal screening for Duchenne muscular dystrophy.

families. However, if some of these 18 female carriers are not already known, then they should be identified through asking about a family history in the antenatal clinic. There will be another 18 female carriers, of whom 12 could be detected through a deletion screen.

However, screening for deletions by automated sequencing would cost £200 per test, i.e. nearly £20 million for screening 100 000 women. This figure includes salaries for laboratory workers, but not the salaries of nurses or counsellors to explain the tests beforehand and support the 12 women found to be deletion carriers. Most of these 12 women, and other carriers who might be detected among their families, might benefit from advice and support for the future. However, the fetuses in only three of the 12 current pregnancies would be likely to be affected males, so that the cost per affected pregnancy detected would be over £6 million. Even if this cost was to fall by 90 per cent, it would probably still be regarded as prohibitive.

This leaves questioning pregnant women about family history and carrying out molecular studies when this is positive as the only realistic method of screening for DMD. Figure 5.3 is a flow chart illustrating antenatal screening of this kind in a population of a million pregnant women.

Neonatal screening

Such screening makes use of the fact that creatine kinase levels in an asymptomatic boy can predict Duchenne muscular dystrophy. Creatine kinase levels may be very high in the neonatal period,[10,11] but these fall within 8–10 weeks and the diagnosis of Duchenne muscular dystrophy in a boy at risk may be confidently made if the creatine kinase level is over 2000 iu/litre after eight weeks of life. The disease may equally confidently be excluded in a boy at risk if the creatine kinase level at this time is below 200 iu/litre. Probably no infants in the presymptomatic stage of DMD will have levels below 2000 iu/litre but occasional normal infants will have levels between 200 and 2000 iu/litre, and so will children having some other neuromuscular conditions, such as spinal muscular atrophy. It is not yet known whether the presymptomatic state of Becker muscular dystrophy is accompanied by high creatine kinase levels in infancy.

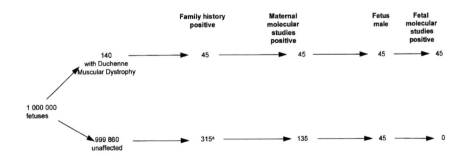

a 180 non-carriers; 90 carriers with daughters; 45 carriers with unaffected sons.

Fig. 5.3   Flow chart for antenatal screening for Duchenne muscular dystrophy.

In one neonatal screening programme on infants with no family history of DMD,[12] blood is taken by a heel prick at 6–7 days of life, and tested for creatine kinase level if the parents agree. Levels of over 2000 iu/litre are found in about 38/100 000 boys. These 38 are retested later, and persistent elevation is found in 23 of them. These 23 are studied to see if a deletion of the dystrophin gene is present, and immunostaining for dystrophin is carried out on a muscle biopsy. This staining can be expected to be diagnostic of DMD in 20 boys. The other three would have other forms of muscular dystrophy.

Among the 20 boys with DMD, 10 would be likely to have carrier mothers as opposed to new mutations. Reproductive patterns suggest that these 10 carriers would only bear five further children between them, of whom a quarter would be expected to have DMD. The most that neonatal screening could achieve is therefore to prevent the birth of 1.25 subsequent cases for every 100 000 neonates screened, which seems too poor a return to justify such screening.

It should be noted that while testing of families after the first affected case of DMD can lead to the prevention of all or nearly all familial cases, there can be no effect on the incidence of cases born as a result of new mutations. This is in contrast to the situation with the next X-linked disorder, the Fragile-X syndrome.

FRAGILE-X SYNDROME

The disease

This is an X-linked mental retardation syndrome which affects both sexes. Affected males tend to be moderately retarded with a range of IQ of 35–70. Affected females are mildly retarded. There are accompanying physical features, more obvious in males than in females, which consist of large heads, hands and feet, large post-pubertal testes, protruding ears, and stocky build.[13] Diagnosis should be considered in any child with unexplained mental retardation, autism, hyperactivity or learning disorder, and cases may be missed because some children with IQs between 50 and 70 are never referred for a medical opinion, but only assessed by educational psychologists. It is not a progressive disorder and life span does not appear to be reduced. Adult males will rarely be able to lead independent lives and will need sheltered accommodation, if not residential care. The lifetime cost of a Fragile-X male will be greater than that for Down's syndrome because of the longer lifespan, and will probably amount to about £¼ million (unpublished data).

Underlying cause

The syndrome takes its name from the finding of 'fragility' of the X chromosome in the band Xq27.3. Using specific culturing techniques, the 'fragile-site' may be visualized in chromosome preparations. However, only a proportion of cells, 4–40 per cent, of an affected male will exhibit the fragile site. In a female, the fragile site is present on a small proportion of one of her X chromosomes. The cytogenetic techniques are sensitive to culture conditions, and the results are somewhat unreliable. Indeed, molecular studies have demonstrated that over half the children once diagnosed as having the Fragile-X syndrome on cytogenetic grounds did not in fact have the Fragile-X mutation.[13] Molecular diagnosis has now superseded chromosomal diagnosis.

In 1991, three groups of workers[14-16] demonstrated that the mutation present in almost all Fragile-X males was an expanded run of CGG (cytosine–guanine–guanine) repeats in the DNA at Xq27.3. This expansion is at the upstream end (exon 1) of what was subsequently identified as the causative gene, now known as the *FRAX-A* gene (or *FMR1* gene) to distinguish it from other causes of fragility in that region. Everyone has a length of CGG repeats in exon 1 of the *FRAX-A* gene; the normal range is 6 to 52 repeats; the range 52–200 is said to be in the premutation range; and the range of 200 or over is accompanied by moderate mental retardation in all males, and by mild retardation in about half the females. An expanded run of more than 200 CGG repeats is associated with methylation, both in the length of repeats itself and 200 base pairs upstream from this in a CpG island which is part of the promotor involved in regulating the gene. This methylation causes 'switching off' of the *FRAX-A* gene. As a result of the 'switching off', or methylation, no FRAX-A protein is produced.[17] The protein produced by the *FRAX-A* gene is known as the FMR protein. The other interesting point about this variable expansion of CGG repeats is that above the size of 50 repeats, there is instability in female meiosis, so that the repeat length tends to increase between mother and offspring. In this way, a woman who is a carrier of a premutation may have a daughter or son with the full mutation or a larger premutation than she has. The chance of a premutation increasing in size to a full mutation depends upon the initial size (see later). In males, studies of sperm have shown only the presence of normal or premutations; full mutations from Fragile-X men are virtually never found in their sperm. These unusual molecular characteristics explain the patterns of inheritance observed in the Fragile-X syndrome.

Family patterns

Because the repeat length of CGGs changes between generations, once they number more than 50, unusual X-linked patterns of inheritance are found. All affected males have a carrier mother, and a carrier grandparent. This may be the maternal grandfather (who is said to be a normal transmitting male because he is clinically unaffected) or the maternal grandmother, a premutation carrier. The daughters of normal transmitting males are all carriers, but never affected, for an expansion of CGG repeats into the affected range of more than 200 only occurs during female meiosis. A woman who is a premutation carrier may have affected sons, unaffected sons who carry an expanded repeat, unaffected sons who do not carry an expanded repeat, affected daughters who are carriers, unaffected daughters who are carriers, and unaffected daughters who are not carriers. The proportions will vary according to the size of the premutation, but for women with over 100 repeats, the proportions of these types of offspring are 0.2, 0.05, 0.25, 0.12, 0.12, 0.25. In summary, retarded children are only born to carrier women, leading Pembrey *et al.*[18] to suggest a 'change' occurring during female meiosis. This change has now been demonstrated to be an expansion of the run of CGG repeats, and there is some evidence that this expands further during the mitosis that follows fertilization of an affected ovum.[19]

About one-sixth of affected males have another affected male relative when they are first ascertained, and only a minority of females who carry a full mutation or a premutation will already have had the experience of a mentally retarded Fragile-X child in their families.

Prevalence

Because the Fragile-X syndrome has different effects in the two sexes, its prevalence among retarded children has to be considered for each sex separately. The prevalence of the syndrome among boys with non-specific severe or moderate mental retardation is about 1 in 15; the proportion of affected girls among those who are mildly retarded is lower than this, about 1 in 20.[13,20,21]

Looking at the population of all school-age children, the Fragile-X syndrome affects about 2.5 in 10 000 males. One report suggests that the proportion of females who are mildly retarded because of the Fragile-X syndrome is similar,[13] but one would expect this to be half as great (p. 125). In addition, a further number of females will carry the full mutation but be clinically unaffected. As the syndrome does not affect longevity, the population prevalence equals the birth prevalence. In New South Wales, where there has been an extensive programme of ascertaining families and offering genetic counselling and antenatal diagnosis, the birth frequency has already fallen to 1 in 10 000 (G. Turner, personal communication 1995).

In Turner's experience, 90 per cent of carrier women with an affected relative choose to have antenatal diagnosis. Moreover, energetic 'cascade' testing of families ascertained through all affected males in a population will lead to the ascertainment of most females who carry a full mutation (G. Turner, personal communication 1995).

In a following section, antenatal screening for carrier women will be considered. It is therefore important to assess now the population frequencies for full and premutations and their implications. Turner et al.[22] observed that of 200 mothers of Fragile-X boys, two-thirds had premutations and one-third had full mutations. This group, and others,[19,23,24] reported that the risks of male offspring being affected were greatest with the longest premutations, and ranged from 1 in 16 with under 60 repeats to 1 in 2 with 120 or more.

However, the above data come from families in which there has been at least one Fragile-X male. Population data are now available from Rousseau et al.[25] who tested 10 624 samples from females tested at a haematology laboratory, and found that 41 carried 55–101 CGG repeats. (Full mutation carriers were not detected by their techniques.) This is a very high frequency of premutation carriers, about 4 in 1000, and suggests that the large majority, about 96 per cent, do not have affected male offspring.

Theoretical modelling on the distribution of premutation alleles in the population, and on the number of generations it takes for a premutation of 50 to reach a full mutation, has been carried out by Morton and Macpherson[26] and Kolehmainen.[27] It is predicted that about 60 per cent of premutations lie in the 50–59 size range, and about 80 per cent lie in the 50–70 size range. Overall, premutations are eleven to twelve times commoner than full mutations. The premutations of size 130 repeats and over, which on Turner's data appear to confer on each son a 1 in 2 risk of being affected, only account for about 6 per cent of all premutations. Kolehmainen[27] also calculated that on average it takes 13 generations for a premutation to reach a full mutation, which would fit with genealogical studies from northern Sweden, where present-day Fragile-X patients can be traced back to a few ancestors.[28]

The figures in Table 5.1 are derived from the data of Turner et al.[22] and Rousseau et al.[25] From the point of view of screening a population of women because of their

Table 5.1 Approximate prevalence per 1000 births for three X-linked disorders

Disorder	Birth prevalence of affected males before genetic counselling	Birth prevalence of carrier females with 1 in 2 risk for a son to be affected	Birth prevalence of premutation carriers who have a less than 1 in 2 risk for a son to be affected	Birth prevalence after cascade family testing*	Birth prevalence after antenatal screening*	Birth prevalence after cascade family testing + neonatal screening (with tests on family when positive)*
Duchenne muscular dystrophy	0.28	0.38		0.19	0.13	0.17
Fragile-X syndrome	0.25	0.17 with full mutation, plus 0.33 with premutation, equals 0.5	4.0 minus 0.33 equals 3.67	0.125	no cases	0.1
X-linked retinitis pigmentosa	0.08	0.16		0.02**	not possible	not possible

* Assuming all female carriers will choose selective terminations of affected pregnancies.

** However, antenatal diagnosis is rarely wanted or possible.

genetic risks, it is probably best to take a cut-off point for significant premutations that is no lower than 70 repeats, which would select for the top 20 per cent of pre-mutation carriers.

Antenatal screening

The aim here is to detect women at risk of having a child who carries the full Fragile-X mutation and its associated risk of mental retardation (100 per cent for males, 50 per cent for females). Such women will have either a premutation or a full mutation. A minority of these women will have a family history of a retarded male relative.

For screening purposes in women with no family history of the Fragile-X syndrome, the PCR test is the best, being quick, relatively inexpensive and with the advantage that it can be carried out on a buccal smear. This test amplifies the region of the CGG repeat and an expansion can be measured against control expansions run alongside on the same gel. This method will detect all premutations and small full mutations, but will fail to detect large full mutations, which occur in about 8/100 000 women who have no family history of the Fragile-X syndrome. The PCR test misses these muta-tions, partly due to difficulties in amplification of a large expansion, and partly because a large expansion often causes somatic mosaicism in tissues leading to a faint smear on a gel which is not easy to recognize. In addition, some women (perhaps 20 per cent) will appear only to have one band on PCR because they have exactly the same length of expansion on each of their two X chromosomes.[29] Some examples of PCR tests on women are shown in Fig. 5.4. It can be seen that the right-hand woman, who is a carrier of a full mutation, has the same profile as a woman with identical numbers of repeats on each of her two X chromosomes (the third of the 'normal women'). Therefore women who appear only to have one band on the PCR test and others suspected of carrying a full mutation need to be re-investigated using Southern blotting on DNA extracted from a blood sample. As the PCR result will be available within 24–48 hours, it should logistically be possible to arrange a blood sample for a week later. Southern blotting analysis will take about two weeks. It is usually per-formed using two test methods: in one the extracted DNA is digested with restriction enzymes *Eco*R1 and *Eag*1 and then hybridized with probe *StB*12.3, and in the other the enzyme is *Pst*1 and the probe is *Oxo*.55.

Testing in batches

PCR testing would be more manageable for screening if specimens were tested in batches.[25] Only if a batch showed an expansion would the individual samples within it need to be investigated to identify which carried a premutation. Unlike individual testing, this method would not detect the women with large full mutations who appear to have only normal bands on PCR because their expanded CGG repeats do not show up clearly. The offspring of these women include about one-fifth of the individuals with Fragile-X syndrome who have a negative family history. Each of the women has a 1 in 4 risk of carrying an affected son and a 1 in 8 risk of carrying an affected daughter (Fig. 5.5).

Diagnostic tests for affected fetuses

One test consists of Southern blotting of DNA obtained from chorionic villus sampling. This test can determine with 100 per cent reliability whether the fetus is a

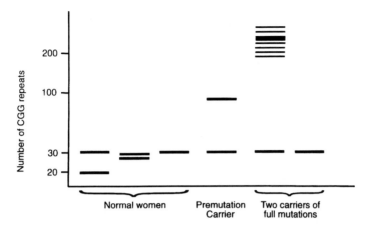

Fig. 5.4 Examples of Fragile-X PCR reactions in six women.

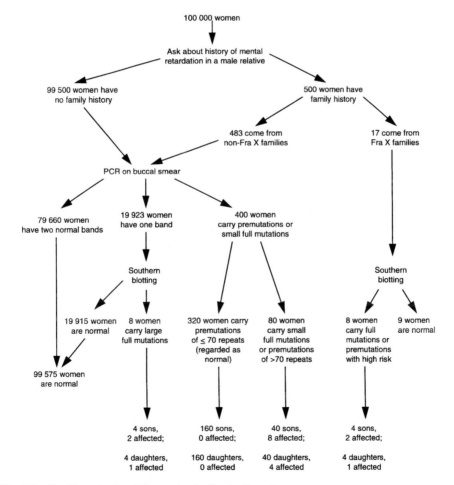

Fig. 5.5 Algorithm of antenatal screening for Fragile-X syndrome.

full mutation or just a premutation who would be clinically normal. Although methylation studies are usually performed to discover if the *FRAX-A* gene is methylated (i.e. is not transcribed), these at present are unreliable on chorionic villi.[30] Methylation studies on amniocentesis cultures are more reliable, but one would still have to explain to a woman that there would be uncertainty about the clinical status of a full mutation-carrying daughter. She would have a 1 in 2 chance of being mildly mentally retarded and a 1 in 2 chance of being mentally fit. In males in whom a large premutation has been diagnosed on a chorionic villus sample, methylation studies on amniocentesis cultures should be carried out to exclude premutation/full mutation mosaicism, since this can cause retardation. A further test appropriate for male fetuses only is to carry out immunological studies, as described in the section on neonatal screening below.

Strategy for antenatal screening

Figure 5.5 shows a strategy for antenatal screening. It also indicates what the results might be if this strategy were applied in 100 000 pregnant women, including 12 whose sons would have the Fragile-X syndrome. In the present state of knowledge, many of these figures can only be speculative.

The first screening test is to ask about severe or moderate mental retardation in a male relative when taking the family history. About 500 of the 100 000 women might report having such a relative.[31] The retardation would be due to the Fragile-X syndrome in the relatives of about 17 of these 500 women (one-thirtieth of the total or one-fifteenth where the male relative's retardation was non-specific). Provided that retarded males were routinely tested for Fragile-X, enquiry to the Regional Clinical Genetics Service should enable these 17 women to be identified. When tested by Southern blotting, about eight of these 17 women might prove to be carriers, and their offspring might include two affected sons.

The 99 983 women not found to have Fragile-X families would be tested by the PCR. This might identify premutations and small full mutations in 400 (0.4 per cent). Only one band might be detected in a total of 19 923, eight with large full mutations and 19 915 with two identical normal bands. The latter figure is 20 per cent of the total without premutations or mutations (99 500 + 483 − 8 − 400) tested by the PCR. Southern blot testing of the 19 923 would identify the mutation carriers among them.

Among the 400 mothers with premutations and small mutations, about 320 would have 70 repeats or less. It has been suggested that about 1 per cent of all affected boys are born to mothers with up to 60 repeats;[32] and it will be assumed here that the percentage whose mothers have 61–70 repeats is not much greater. If so, 100 000 infants might well include no affected boys whose mothers had 70 repeats or less. It is therefore suggested that the PCR test should only be regarded as positive in women in whom it reveals more than 70 repeats.

Figure 5.6 is a flow chart illustrating antenatal screening of this kind for Fragile-X. The strategy described could lead to antenatal diagnosis of all affected fetuses except for those whose mothers carry premutations of 70 repeats or less. The laboratory costs of screening would include £15 for each PCR and £30 for each Southern blotting, so that it would cost nearly £20 million to screen one million women (£160 000 per affected male detected), excluding salaries of nurses and genetic counsellors.

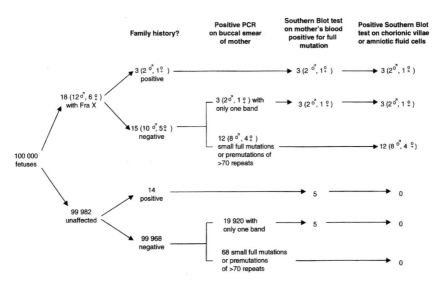

Fig. 5.6 Flow chart for antenatal screening for Fragile-X syndrome.

The strategies for screening and their cost have been admirably discussed by Palomaki.[32] However, since his paper it has become apparent that the population frequency of Fragile-X males is not 1 in 1250 males as originally thought, but about 1 in 4000, and that the frequency of premutation carriers is as high as 4 in 1000. Moreover, experience from New South Wales (G. Turner, personal communication 1995) has shown that full ascertainment of currently affected cases, and energetic counselling of families, can reduce the frequency to 1 in 10 000. Thus population screening is not so obviously beneficial as it appeared in 1994.

A further point is that such screening strategies presuppose that pregnant women will wish to abort a male fetus with moderate mental retardation and will not be too distressed by the uncertainty over the clinical state of a female fetus carrying the full mutation. However, this presupposition may well be unfounded, and doctors would be well advised to refrain from antenatal screening for Fragile-X until there is evidence that the majority of women in the general population want such a test.

Detection of affected males

If screening is not carried out, there should be strong encouragement to test all boys with developmental delay for the Fragile-X syndrome, in order to identify the mothers, who will all be carriers, and to offer them and their relatives appropriate genetic counselling, thus providing the option of selective termination of subsequent affected fetuses.

A reliable test can be used to diagnose affected males, using one to two drops of blood in which the lymphocytes are treated with monoclonal antibodies against the Fragile-X protein (the FMR protein). Controls, and premutation carriers, and all females express the Fragile-X protein. Retarded males have no Fragile-X protein, do not react with the antibody and can readily be distinguished from controls.[33] This test could probably be used, for example, to test large numbers of mentally retarded males, or for neonatal screening; but this is not yet generally accepted, and experience needs to be gained. The test does not identify carrier females who will have some Fragile-X protein produced by their healthy X chromosome. As with early detection of Duchenne muscular dystrophy, there is no advantage to a boy in being identified as having the Fragile-X syndrome before developmental delay has become apparent.

X-LINKED RETINITIS PIGMENTOSA

This disorder has a birth prevalence of at least 1 in 12 000 males.[34] Symptoms of night blindness develop during the first decade and reduction of visual acuity is apparent by the age of 20, a patient becoming blind between 20 and 40 years. Diagnosis is made by finding the characteristic pigmentation in the fundi, together with markedly impaired retinal function tests. Since there are many autosomal types of retinitis pigmentosa, the diagnosis of the X-linked form also requires the presence of an affected male relative or a carrier female relative. Various treatments have been tried but none has been successful.

Recognition of female carriers

In the experience of the Genetic Eye Clinic in Birmingham, every mother of a patient with X-linked retinitis pigmentosa is a carrier. Other females in the family will have their risk halved for each step in relationship between them and the mother. The risks will be reduced by the presence of only healthy sons. Families tend to contain many affected male relatives, and extensive pedigrees, like the one partially represented in Fig. 5.1, occur. X-linked retinitis pigmentosa provides a contrast to Duchenne muscular dystrophy and the Fragile-X syndrome because of its relatively late onset, with diagnosis usually occurring in the teens, and because affected males reproduce. Because of its relatively late onset, it is usually not possible to provide genetic counselling to families before the births of brothers of the first case in a family. However, it should be possible to offer genetic counselling before the births of nephews and grandsons. Only a minority of women consider X-linked retinitis pigmentosa sufficiently severe to warrant limitation of families, but all carriers should be provided with the genetic information so that they can make decisions that are appropriate for them.

Clinical tests for carriers

Carrier females generally have no symptoms, although some have difficulty in seeing at night, and about 5 per cent start to lose their visual acuity after the age of 50.[35] The most frequent sign of the carrier state in a female at risk is the appearance of the peripheral retina, with patches of depigmentation and patches of increased pigmentation. However, in a study from Birmingham, four out of 17 obligatory heterozygotes aged under 20 had normal fundi, and so did one out of 11 older heterozygotes. A negative fundal examination should therefore be followed by tests which assess the peripheral function of the retina: the measurement of the visual fields; the measurement of the eye's ability to see objects as the light decreases (dark adaptation); the difference in the standing ocular potential measured in light and dark (electro-oculography); and the amplitudes and latencies of the retinal a- and b-waves in light and dark (electroretinography).[36] The measurements of the visual fields and dark adaptation depend upon cooperation. In young girls, or in uncooperative women of any age, assessment of the carrier state has to depend upon the examination of the fundi and the objective tests of electro-oculography and electroretinography, which are age-dependent. The results from two series, one assembled by Bird[35] and the other by Bundey and Crews (unpublished), are presented in Table 5.2. The data from Bird have been reduced, to include only those women who are obligatory heterozygotes and to exclude those women whose abnormal retinal function tests were responsible for their isolated affected male relative being classified as having X-linked retinitis pigmentosa.

Table 5.2 shows how tests were not always abnormal under the age of 20. At all ages, the most common abnormal finding was the characteristic patchiness of the peripheral retina; however, the fundi of one woman aged 31 were quite normal, although she did have abnormalities on tests of retinal function. Two obligatory heterozygotes, aged 22 and 46, had abnormal fundi, but no abnormality of retinal function tests. Overall, at least one abnormality was present in all 21 obligatory heterozygotes aged 20 or over.

Molecular analysis in the detection of carriers

Linkage studies reveal the presence of three well-separated X-linked loci;[37] unfortunately clinical features do not distinguish the genes at these loci. If a family is sufficiently large for linkage studies to indicate which of the X-linked loci are responsible (which is true in approximately one-fifth of familial cases), then linked markers may be used as an adjunct in carrier testing and as a method of detecting an affected male fetus. Such linkage studies, however, will carry a few per cent risk of error. One of the genes for X-linked retinitis pigmentosa has recently been identified.[38] This is the gene hitherto called *RP3*, which accounts for about 70 per cent of all X-linked retinitis pigmentosa. Through further studies of this gene, and through mutation analysis, it will be possible to offer more accurate genetic counselling to families of patients, with accurate identification of female carriers, and accurate diagnosis of affected male fetuses. However, the mutations so far described in this gene are various, and technically difficult to document, so that mutation analysis is not suitable for screening women in whom there is no family history of retinitis pigmentosa.

Table 5.2 **Abnormalities in tests of retinal function in women who are obligatory carriers for X-linked retinitis pigmentosa**

Age of woman	Fundi	Visual fields	Dark adaptation	ERG[a]	EOG[b]	In at least one test	In either EOG or ERG
Under 20	19/23	9/17	3/13	4/15	7/18	19/23	8/18
20–39	7/8	4/8	4/8	3/6	3/8	8/8	4/8
40 and over	17/17	15/17	9/11	9/11	7/11	17/17	11/13

[a] Electro-retinography.
[b] Electro-oculography.

Outcome of screening

It should be possible to identify three-quarters of carriers by asking each pregnant woman whether any male in her family has become blind under the age of 40, obtaining clinical details of any such relatives, and testing the retinal function of women whose relatives are found to have had X-linked retinitis pigmentosa (Fig. 5.7). However, except in families large enough for linkage analysis, the only investigation that can be carried out in the fetuses of carriers is to identify the males, only half of whom will be affected.

GENERAL POINTS ON SCREENING FOR X-LINKED DISORDERS

The effectiveness of screening in reducing the birth frequency of an X-linked disorder depends upon what proportion of cases are due to new mutations, to what extent female carriers can be recognized, and on the views of those female carriers regarding selective termination of affected pregnancies. In Duchenne muscular dystrophy, for example, one-third of boys are affected by new mutations, and therefore however good carrier tests are, the birth frequency of the disease can only be reduced to the mutation rate in oogenesis. In the Fragile-X syndrome and X-linked retinitis pigmentosa, all mothers of affected cases are carriers. The recognition of affected male cases and genetic tests within families should enable a large proportion of female carriers for X-linked retinitis pigmentosa to be identified, although not always before they have started their families. The main uncertainty with the fragile-X syndrome arises because of the high frequencies of premutation carriers in the general population and the lack of good data on the level of risks belonging to these carriers, together with the fact that most premutation carriers will not have an affected male relative. The effectiveness of different methods of screening for carriers is summarized in Tables 5.1 and 5.3.

Population screening will also have a small effect on gene frequencies, because in most families an aborted affected male fetus will be replaced by either a healthy son, or by a daughter who could be a carrier. Overall, the incidence of carriers would increase by about one-sixth per generation. In practice, such an increase in carrier

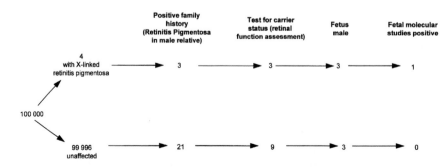

Fig. 5.7 Flow chart for antenatal screening for X-linked retinitis pigmentosa.

Table 5.3 Summary of antenatal screening strategies for carriers of X-linked conditions

Condition	Proportion of carriers		False-positive rate of first test for carriers	Proportion of affected male fetuses which were predicted*
	Positive on first test (family history)*	Positive on second test (molecular studies)*		
Duchenne muscular dystrophy	18/36 (50%)	30/36 (83%)	0.02%	7.5/14 (54%)
Fragile-X syndrome	8/96† (8%)	96/96† (100%)	0.49%	12.3/12.5 (98%)
X-linked retinitis pigmentosa	12/18 (75%)	16/16 (99%)‡	0.012%	3/4 (75%)

* Based on 100 000 pregnancies.
† Carriers of full mutations or premutations of > 70 repeats.
‡ Figure anticipated when genes identified .

frequency would not matter, so long as carrier detection, genetic counselling, and antenatal diagnosis remained available.

Neonatal screening for Duchenne muscular dystrophy and for males with the Fragile-X syndrome is worthy of consideration. Such neonatal screening programmes could not lead to a cure of either disease, but could assist in management by early intervention for their physical or mental disabilities. The main aim of neonatal screening is, however, to provide prompt genetic counselling to the boys' families.

Costs of screening

These are heavy, particularly in terms of salaries of laboratory workers and genetic counsellors, as illustrated by the costs per detected cases of DMD and Fragile-X syndrome (about £6 million and £600 000 respectively) in the screening programmes shown in Figs. 5.2 and 5.5. To these financial considerations should be added the cost of anxiety of those being tested, and the distress of those women found to be carriers when there has been no earlier affected case in their families.

Summary

Taking a good family history from pregnant women is a simple and cost-effective method of screening for all three of the above X-linked disorders, with detection rates of about 32 per cent for Duchenne muscular dystrophy (Fig. 5.3), 16 per cent for Fragile-X syndrome (Fig. 5.6), and 75 per cent for X-linked retinitis pigmentosa (Fig. 5.7). Coupled with energetic genetic counselling, this type of screening can substantially reduce the birth prevalence of familial cases, because generally parents at high risk choose to take avoiding actions.[7–9,20]

Screening by molecular analysis in pregnancies where the family history is negative is not yet technically possible for retinitis pigmentosa and is too expensive to consider for Duchenne muscular dystrophy. It is in principle feasible to offer screening based on a PCR test for Fragile-X to pregnant women whose family history is negative, but various issues with a bearing on whether such screening would be appropriate have still to be resolved.

REFERENCES

1. Haldane, J. B. S. (1935). The rate of spontaneous mutation of a human gene. *Journal of Genetics*, **31**, 317–26.
2. Edwards, J. H. (1989). Familiarity, recessivity and germ-line mosaicism. *Annals of Human Genetics*, **53**, 33–47.
3. Van Essen, A. J., Abbs, S., Baiget, M. *et al.* (1992). Parental origin and germline mosaicism of deletions and duplications of the dystrophin gene: a European study. *Human Genetics*, **88**, 249–57.
4. Bushby, K. M. D., Thambyayah, M., and Gardner-Medwin, D. (1991). The prevalence and incidence of Becker muscular dystrophy. *Lancet*, **337**, 1022–4.
5. Gardner, R. J., Bobrow, M., and Roberts, R. G. (1995). The identification of point mutations in Duchenne muscular dystrophy patients by using reverse-transcription PCR and the protein truncation test. *American Journal of Human Genetics*, **57**, 311–20.
6. Gardner-Medwin, D. (1970). Mutation rate in Duchenne type of muscular dystrophy. *Journal of Medical Genetics*, **7**, 334–7.
7. Gardner-Medwin, D., and Sharples, P. (1989). Some studies of the Duchenne and autosomal recessive types of muscular dystrophy. *Brain Development*, **11**, 91–7.
8. Norman, A. M., Rogers, C., Sibert, J. R., and Harper, P.S. (1989). Duchenne muscular dystrophy in Wales: a 15-year study 1971–1986. *Journal of Medical Genetics*, **26**, 560–4.
9. Bundey, S., and Boughton, E. (1989). Are abortions more or less frequent once prenatal diagnosis is available? *Journal of Medical Genetics*, **26**, 794–5.
10. Gilboa, N., and Swanson, J.R. (1976). Serum creatine phosphokinase in normal newborns. *Archives of Disease in Childhood*, **51**, 283–5.
11. Drummond, L. M. (1979). Creatine phosphokinase levels in the newborn and their use in screening for Duchenne muscular dystrophy. *Archives of Disease in Childhood*, **54**, 362–6.
12. Bradley, D. M., Parsons, E. P., and Clarke, A. (1993). Experience with screening newborns for Duchenne muscular dystrophy in Wales. *British Medical Journal*, **306**, 357–60.
13. Morton, J. E., Bundey, S., Webb, T. P., MacDonald, F., Rindl, P. M., and Bullock, S. (1997). Fragile-X syndrome is less common than previously estimated. *Journal of Medical Genetics*, **34**, 1–5.
14. Oberle, I., Rousseau, F., Heitz, D. *et al.* (1991). Instability of a 550-base pair DNA segment and abnormal methylation in Fragile-X syndrome. *Science*, **252**, 1097–102.
15. Yu, S., Pritchard, M., Kremer, E. *et al.* (1991). Fragile-X genotype characterized by an unstable region of DNA. *Science*, **252**, 1179–81.
16. Verkerk, A. J., Pieretti M., Sutcliffe, J. S. *et al.* (1991). Identification of a gene (FMR-1) containing a CGG repeat coincident with a break point cluster region exhibiting length variation in Fragile-X syndrome. *Cell*, **65**, 905–14.
17. Pieretti, M., Zhang, F., Fu, Y. H. *et al.* (1991). Absence of expression of the FMR-1 gene in Fragile-X syndrome. *Cell*, **66**, 817–22.
18. Pembrey, M. E., Winter, R. M., and Davies, K. E. (1985). A premutation that generates a defect at crossing over explains the inheritance of fragile-X mental retardation. *American Journal of Medical Genetics*, **21**, 709–17.
19. Ashley, A. E., and Sherman, S. L. (1995). Population dynamics of a meiotic/mitotic expansion model for the Fragile-X syndrome. *American Journal of Human Genetics*, **57**, 1414–25.

20. Turner, G., Robinson, H., Laing, S. *et al.* (1992). Population screening for fragile X. *Lancet*, **339**, 1210–13.
21. Slaney, S. F., Wilkie, A. O., Hirst, M. C. *et al.* (1995). DNA testing for fragile-X syndrome in schools for learning difficulties. *Journal of Medical Genetics*, **72**, 33–7.
22. Turner, A. M., Robinson, H., Wake, S., Laing, S. J., Leigh, D., and Turner, G. (1994). Counselling risk figures for fragile-X carrier females of varying band size for use in predicting the likelihood of retardation in their offspring. *American Journal of Medical Genetics*, **51**, 458–62.
23. Fu, Y. H., Kuhl, D. P. A., Pizzutti, A. *et al.* (1991). Variation of the CGG repeat at the fragile-X site results in genetic instability: resolution of the Sherman paradox. *Cell*, **67**, 1047–58.
24. Heitz, D., Devys, D., Imbert, G., Kretz, C., and Mandel, J-L. (1992). Inheritance of the fragile-X syndrome: size of the fragile-X premutation is a major determinant of the transition to full mutation. *Journal of Medical Genetics*, **29**, 794–801.
25. Rousseau, F., Rouillard, P., Morel, M-L., Khandjian, E. W., and Morgan, K. (1995). Prevalence of carriers of premutation—size alleles of the FMR1 gene—and implications for population genetics of the fragile-X syndrome. *American Journal of Human Genetics*, **57**, 1006–18.
26. Morton, N. E., and Macpherson, J. N. (1992). Population genetics of the fragile-X syndrome: multiallelic model for the FMR1 locus. *Proceedings of the National Academy of Sciences USA*, **89**, 4215–17.
27. Kolehmainen, K. (1994). Population genetics of fragile X: a multiple allele model with variable risk of CGG repeat expansion. *American Journal of Medical Genetics*, **51**, 428–35.
28. Holmgren, G., Blomquist, H. K., Drugge, U., and Gustavson, K-H. (1988). Fragile-X families in a northern Swedish county—a genealogical study demonstrating apparent paternal transmission from the 18th century. *American Journal of Medical Genetics*, **30**, 673–9.
29. Brown, W. T., Houck, G. E., Jeziorowska, A. *et al.* (1993). Rapid fragile-X carrier screening and prenatal diagnosis using a non-radioactive PCR test. *Journal of the American Medical Association*, **270**, 1569–75.
30. Castellví-Bel, S., Milà, M., Solar, A., *et al.* (1995). Prenatal diagnosis of fragile-X syndrome: (CGG)$_n$ expansion and methylation of chorionic villus samples. *Prenatal Diagnosis*, **15**, 801–7.
31. Herbst, D. S., and Miller, J. R. (1980). Non-specific X-linked mental retardation. II: the frequency in British Columbia. *American Journal of Medical Genetics*, **7**, 461–9.
32. Palomaki, G. E. (1994). Population based prenatal screening for the fragile-X syndrome. *Journal of Medical Screening*, **1**, 65–72.
33. Willemsen, R., Mohkamsing, S., De Vries B. *et al.* (1995). Rapid antibody test for fragile-X syndrome. *Lancet*, **345**, 1147–8.
34. Bundey, S., and Crews, S. J. (1984). A study of retinitis pigmentosa in the City of Birmingham. I Prevalence. II Clinical and genetic heterogeneity. *Journal of Medical Genetics*, **21**, 417–28.
35. Bird, A. C. (1975). X-linked retinitis pigmentosa. *British Journal of Ophthalmology*, **59**, 177–99.
36. Stavrou, P., Good, P. A., Broadhurst, E. J., Bundey, S., Fielder, A. R., and Crews, S. J.

(1996). ERG and EOG abnormalities in carriers of X-linked retinitis pigmentosa. *Eye*, **10**, 581–9.

37. Ott, J., Bhattacharya, S., Chen, J. D. *et al.* (1989). Localising multiple X-linked retinitis pigmentosa loci using extended multi-locus homogeneity tests. *Proceedings of the National Academy of Sciences USA*, **87**, 701–4.

38. Meindl, A., Dry, K., Herrmann, K. *et al.* (1995). A gene (RPGR) with homology to the RCC1 quanine nucleotide exchange factor is mutated in X-linked retinitis pigmentosa (RP3). *Nature Genetics*, **13**, 35–42.

6 *Tay–Sachs disease*

Feige Kaplan and Charles R. Scriver

INTRODUCTION

Tay–Sachs disease (TSD)*[1] provides an illustration of a fatal metabolic genetic disease which is generally rare but for which it is realistic to screen because cases occur primarily within a well-defined subpopulation on which biochemical testing can be focussed. Within the last 30 years, the discovery of the enzymatic basis of the disease, namely deficiency of the enzyme hexosaminidase A (Hex A), has made possible both enzymatic diagnosis of TSD and heterozygote identification. In the last decade, the cloning of the *HEXA* gene and the identification of more than 80 associated TSD-causing mutations has permitted molecular diagnosis in many instances.

THE DISORDER

Clinical aspects

The clinical picture of TSD was described in 1881 by Warren Tay,[1] a British ophthalmologist, and later (in 1887 and 1896) by Bernard Sachs,[2,3] an American neurologist. They each described independently an infantile disorder characterized by cerebral degeneration, blindness, and loss of motor function. Symptoms appeared at four to six months, progressed thereafter and led to death in the third or fourth year of life. For a detailed description of the clinical phenotype and associated pathophysiology the reader is referred to a recent review.[4] There is no effective therapy for patients affected with TSD, nor are there prospects for adequate therapeutic intervention in the near future.

---

[1] Abbreviations and Nomenclature: TSD, Tay–Sachs disease; Hex, hexosaminidase; Hex A, hexosaminidase A enzyme, an αβ heterodimeric polypeptide; Hex B, hexosaminidase B enzyme, a ββ homodimer; *HEXA*, gene for α subunit of Hex A; *HEXB*, gene for the β subunit of Hex A and Hex B; G_{M2}, the predominant ganglioside in TSD brain and natural substrate of Hex A; 4MUG, 4-methylumbelliferyl, *N*-acetyl glucosaminide, synthetic substrate of Hex enzymes; 4MUGS, 4-methyl-umbelliferyl, *N*-acetyl glucosaminide-sulfate, Hex A-specific synthetic substrate; carrier couple, both partners are heterozygous for a disease-causing *HEXA* mutation.

Metabolic and enzymic features

The metabolic abnormality in TSD was shown by Klenk (1939, 1942)[5,6] to affect a previously uncharacterized class of lipids called gangliosides, located principally in the central nervous system. Svennerholm (1962)[7] identified G_{M2} ganglioside (a branched tetrasaccharide), as the predominant ganglioside of TSD brain. In TSD, G_{M2} accumulates throughout the body; the accumulation in the central nervous system is responsible for the progressive fatal disease.

Enzymatic hydrolysis of G_{M2} and its derivatives requires the interaction of three different gene products: (1) Hex A[8,9], a heterodimer composed of one α- subunit (which hydrolyses both neutral and charged substrates, including G_{M2}) and one β subunit; (2) Hex B, a $\beta\beta$ dimer (which hydrolyses only electrically neutral substrates such as the asialo derivative of G_{M2} ganglioside); and (3) a non-enzymatic activator protein which is coded for by the G_{M2A} gene, binds to G_{M2} ganglioside monomers,[10,11] and presents them to the α subunit active site of Hex A.

Hex A and Hex B are hexosaminidase isozymes. Hex A, the anionic form of Hex, is deficient in tissues and fluids obtained from TSD patients. Hex B, the more cationic species, is normal or elevated in these patients, but is deficient in a similar autosomal recessive disorder, Sandhoff disease. Hex A is more thermolabile than Hex B, and the standard test for TSD makes use of this difference: the activity of Hex in breaking down a synthetic substrate, 4 methylumbelliferyl-N-acetyl-glucosaminide (4MUG), is measured in two samples of serum, one previously heated and the other not, and Hex A activity is estimated by subtracting the heated from the unheated value.

Deficiency of activator protein is associated with a clinical presentation similar to that observed in TSD and Sandhoff disease.[12–,13,14] Affected patients have normal activities of both Hex A and B when assayed *in vitro* with synthetic substrate. However, the *in vivo* hydrolysis of G_{M2} ganglioside is compromised. G_{M2} activator activity can be tested in fibroblast extracts, by measurement of the ability of purified Hex A to stimulate G_{M2} ganglioside hydrolysis *in vitro*[15] and also by immunochemical assay of G_{M2} activator protein by ELISA.[16]

Several variants of Hex A, Hex B, and the activator protein occur, although all are rare.

Variants of Hex A

Certain *HEXA* alleles produce a normally processed Hex A protein which has defective catalytic activity toward G_{M2} ganglioside substrate and 'normal' activity toward the artificial substrate, 4MUG.[17] B1 phenotypes, which result from these alleles, were first recognized as TSD cases with either normal or carrier-like serum Hex A activity.[15,18–25] In at least one such case, heterozygous-like Hex A activity in amniocytes in a patient led to an incorrect fetal diagnosis and birth of a clinically affected infant.[26]

Variants of Hex B

A number of *HEXB* alleles produce a thermolabile Hex B enzyme. In some instances they are associated with a G_{M2} gangliosidosis (i.e. a variant form of Sandhoff disease[27–29]); in others they appear to be benign.[30,31] In Israel, 0.6 per cent of screened 'carriers' have thermolabile Hex B.[32] Individuals who carry a heat-labile *HEXB* allele will have *apparently* elevated Hex A activity.

The AB variant

This is produced by G_{M2A} mutations. It is the most difficult variant to diagnose and requires specific ways to prove that the activator protein is deficient.[4] The trait is suspected when G_{M2} gangliosidosis exists in the presence of 'normal' Hex activity when assayed with each of two synthetic substrates, 4MUG and 4MUGS.

Other related conditions

Some degree of hexosaminidase deficiency (Hex A alone or Hex A and B) has been observed in neurological phenotypes without a predominantly cerebral pathology, such as cerebellar ataxia,[33,34] motor-neurone disorder[35] and amyotrophic lateral sclerosis.[36,37] Partial or complete Hex A deficiency has also been described in adults with no neurological deficits.[38–40] Some apparently healthy adults[40] with complete or partial Hex A deficiency (as assessed by serum or leucocyte 4MUG-cleaving activity[41]) are believed to be compound heterozygotes for a classical TSD gene and an allele encoding a form of Hex A which does not hydrolyse 4MUG but which permits G_{M2} ganglioside cleavage.[42] Many of these individuals eventually develop neurological symptoms associated with adult-onset forms of G_{M2} gangliosidosis;[35–37,43,44] others, when evaluated quite late in life, are completely devoid of clinical symptoms.[38,39]

Birth prevalence

The birth prevalence of TSD varies in different ethnic groups. The carrier frequency for TSD in Ashkenazi Jewish populations (i.e. Jews of Central and Eastern European ancestry) is about 1/30. This is the *observed* frequency from screening programmes. It is consistent with the rate estimated from birth rates of affected cases in the population at presumed Hardy–Weinberg equilibrium. The birth prevalence (1/3600) in Ashkenazi Jews is 100 times higher than that in non-Ashkenazi Jewish populations (1/360 000). The birth prevalence of TSD is also increased in French Canadians in Eastern Quebec,[45] and among Franco-Americans in New England,[46] probably reflecting a founder effect[47] and migration. An increased prevalence of TSD has also been reported in Moroccan Jews living in Israel.[48–50]

Genetic basis

The gene for the α subunit of Hex A (*HEXA*) maps to chromosome 15q23–24,[51,52] the gene for the β subunit of Hex A and for Hex B (*HEXB*) to chromosome 5q13,[53] and the *GM2A* gene to chromosome 15q32–33.[54,55] All three genes have been cloned and sequenced.[56–58] The Hex A α and β subunit propeptide gene products have 65 per cent homology[59] and the exon–intron boundaries are identical for 13 of the 14 exons.[60] One hundred *HEXA*, 25 *HEXB*, and *4GMZA* alleles have been identified to date.[4]

A relational database recording allelic variation at the *HEXA* gene locus (disease-producing and polymorphic) is accessed on the Worldwide Web at http://data.mch.mcgill.ca/hexadb and presently records one hundred mutations along with additional information [*HEXAdb*] Seventy-eight are listed as causing a G_{M2} gangliosidosis with a known clinical phenotype, three as benign, seven as producing neutral polymorphisms. Among twelve alleles for which no associated clinical phenotype has been described, six are predicted to be disease causing.[61]

The first TSD causing mutation identified is the most common allele in French

Canadians originating in eastern Quebec. It is a deletion mutation including the entire first exon and flanking sequences resulting in the loss of 7.6 kb of genomic DNA.[62] This mutation has yet to be found on an Ashkenazi Jewish or any other TSD chromosome![47] With the exception of the 7.6 kb deletion, all *HEXA* mutations identified thus far involve either nucleotide substitutions, or small insertions/deletions.

Three alleles account for 92–98 per cent of *HEXA* mutations in Ashkenazi Jews:[63–66] (1) a TATC insertion in exon 11[67] which occurs in 70–90 per cent of Ashkenazi TSD carriers; (2) a G→C transition at the splice junction in intron 12[68–70] in 10–25 per cent of carriers; and (3) a G805A allele associated with adult-onset forms of TSD[71–73] in 3 per cent of carriers. The exon-11 TATC mutation also occurs among non-Jewish European-derived populations (8 per cent of non-Jewish heterozygotes[74]), and should be ruled out regardless of the origin of the patient. An IVS 9+1 mutation (G→A) is the most frequent allele (10 per cent of non-Jewish heterozygotes) among non-Jews of northern European origin.[75] Among French Canadians, knowledge of demographic and geographic origins of the family is a useful guide; the most frequent mutation here, the 7.6 kb deletion, has a centrer of diffusion south of the St Lawrence River in the Gaspé region of the province of Quebec.[47,76] A less frequent mutation (IVS 7+1 G→A) has been found thus far exclusively among families originating in a genetic isolate north of the St Lawrence River in the Lac St Jean region of Quebec.[77] The 4bp insertion in exon 11 is uncommon in French Canadians. Three mutations cluster in Moroccan Jews; ʌf304/305, R170Q, and IVS 5–2 A→G[47,48] (R Navon, personal communication).

Rare variant TSD phenotypes, some with adult onset,[41–44,78] represent about 3 per cent of cases in Jews and 2 per cent in non-Jews. They are often due to the G805A mutation.[71–73]

There are also benign Hex A deficiency alleles (pseudodeficiency alleles), which produce positive findings in tests for Hex A deficiency without leading to any clinical disorder. It appears that these alleles encode a form of Hex A which does not hydrolyse 4MUG but which permits G_{M2} ganglioside cleavage.[42] In the Ashkenazi Jewish population the frequency of benign Hex A deficiency alleles is ~1/1200.[79] In the Moroccan Jewish community, though data are insufficient to estimate gene frequencies precisely, pseudoalleles appear to be rare (R. Navon, personal communication). In non-Jewish populations, by contrast, two different pseudo-deficiency alleles can account for over one-third of enzyme-defined—'carriers'.[80,81] An early observation that the 'TSD' carrier frequency among non-Jews was 1/167 by population screening,[82] rather than the predicted value (1/300) based on birth prevalence, is now explained by the frequency of pseudodeficiency alleles in this population.

Carriers (heterozygotes) of TSD and Sandhoff disease are asymptomatic. TSD heterozygotes are detectable because they usually have Hex A levels less than about 55 per cent of total Hex activity; in affected individuals (homozygotes) Hex A is almost completely absent. In many instances, carriers can also be detected by DNA analysis.

SCREENING

Primary screening test

The initial screening test for Tay–Sachs disease is so simple that it is often not regarded as a screening test at all. It is to ask an individual whether he or she is Jewish or has a Jewish parent (or in Quebec and New England, a French Canadian). In addition, one can determine whether a woman has had a previously affected pregnancy. One can determine further whether Jews are of Ashkenazi origin (eastern European descent) or of Moroccan ancestry, but often this is not done, e.g. in Israel.

Second screening test

The second screening test is the measurement of heat-labile Hex A activity (Hex A test), from which carrier status can be inferred. The major technical problem affecting the measurement of Hex A activity with non-specific synthetic substrates is the presence of non-Hex A isozymes. Hex isozymes differ in a number of their properties, and TSD carriers can be identified by heat-independent electrophoretic and pH-stability differences and by use of non-serum (tears, cells) samples; but the most useful characteristic for distinguishing between Hex A and non-Hex A forms is the difference in thermolability. Under precise conditions (temperature, pH, ionic strength, and protein concentration), Hex A inactivation by heat is complete and Hex B is unaffected. (For a review of effects of reaction variables in Hex assay see Kaback *et al.*[83]).

The Hex A test is initially carried out in serum in men and non-pregnant women, and in leucocytes in pregnant women. The test also identifies Sandhoff carriers (Hex B deficient). As carried out in serum, it is by general agreement the preferred standard. It involves the following steps.[84,85]

1. Exposure of one of a set of duplicate samples to an exact temperature for a precise interval (e.g. 5 min at 60°C for serum or 2 h at 52°C for leucocytes). These conditions must result in no loss of Hex activity from the serum (or leucocytes) of individuals affected with the classical form of TSD.

2. Incubation of heated and unheated samples with 4MUG substrate at 37°C followed by quantitation of released 4MU in a fluorimeter and conversion of results into enzymatic units (e.g. nanomoles substrate hydrolyzsed per hour per ml for serum or per hour per mg of protein for leucocytes).

The heated sample produces the Hex B value for *tissue* extracts. For *serum*, the heat-stable Hex activity is the sum of Hex B plus the intermediate forms I_1 and I_2.[86] For both serum and tissue extracts, Hex A is the difference between the values for heated and unheated samples.

Calibration of the conditions for assay is best done using serum from a homozygous affected (Hex A nul) TSD patient.

The index of Hex A activity used by most laboratories is the percentage of Hex activity accounted for by Hex A ('% Hex A'). No threshold % Hex A value has been prescribed for distinguishing between positive and negative Hex A test results. Instead, the threshold is set at each laboratory after examining the distribution of levels obtained there in homozygous normal individuals and heterozygotes. A group of randomly chosen non-Jewish individuals is usually selected to serve as normal control subjects since such a sample is expected to contain not more than 1 in 167 whose serum enzyme activity is in the heterozygote range. A more difficult problem has been to obtain a sufficient number of samples from 'obligate' heterozygotes (i.e. parents of an affected TSD child) to define the 'carrier' range of values. However, it is now possible for individuals certain to be 'carriers', independent of their serum Hex A and B enzyme values (or whatever other reference), to be confirmed by DNA analysis and detection of a HEXA mutation known to cause TSD.

Time of screening

Screening can be carried out in pregnancy or before pregnancy. If a woman has previously had an affected pregnancy and has not changed her partner, there is no need to perform the secondary test on either of the couple; the woman can proceed directly to antenatal diagnosis.

Screening in pregnancy

The second screening (Hex A) test is usually undertaken in pregnancy if both partners are Jewish or each has a Jewish parent. Some programmes offer the Hex A test to couples in which *either* partner is Jewish.

The Hex A test is performed on *serum* collected from the *father* (since pregnancy can cause false-positives). If the father is found to be positive, a leucocyte Hex A test is performed on the father since this is more discriminatory (see Table 6.1). This is not done as a matter of routine since the test is more complicated and expensive. If the father's leucocyte Hex A test is positive, a leucocyte Hex A test is done on the mother. If this is positive (so both parents are judged to be carriers), antenatal diagnosis is carried out using amniocentesis or CVS.

Pre-marital couple screening

This approach has been adopted by the ultra-orthodox Jewish community, using a programme called 'Dor Yeshorim'.[61,88] The programme tests young people and records on a register whether each person is a carrier. When a marriage is being considered, a search of the register is made to see if the potential couple are both carriers. If they are, the idea of marriage can be abandoned. If neither or only one is a carrier, the marriage can be encouraged—the screen is negative. This approach is a variant of the process of couple screening as described for cystic fibrosis.[89]

Community-based screening

In community screening programmes, members of the Jewish community are invited to come forward to have their Tay–Sachs disease carrier status determined. The initiative is largely from the individuals being screened, and instances of both poor and effective take-up have been reported.[90–94]

Detection rates and false-positive rates

Since the initial screening test is whether a couple is Jewish (or belongs to another high-risk group), non-Jewish TSD carrier couples will not normally be identified. In

Table 6.1   Two-standard-deviation ranges of Hex A activity in normals and carriers for serum and leukocytes

	Serum* (nmol/ml per hour)	Leukocytes** (% Hex A)
Normals	316–620	63–79
Carriers	142–420	46–62

* From Kaback *et al.*[83]
** From Saifer and Perle.[87]

communities where Jews represent about 1 per cent of the population (for example, Britain) this means that about half of carrier couples (and affected pregnancies) will occur in non-Jews and be missed. In countries such as the USA where Jews represent about 2 per cent of the community, about one-third of cases of Tay–Sachs disease will be missed. The calculation is as follows: in a million pregnancies in Britain, for example, there will be 10 000 Jews and 990 000 non-Jews. With a birth prevalence of 1/3600 in Jews, there will be three cases expected. Among the remaining 990 000 pregnancies, with a birth prevalence of 1/360 000, there will be a further three affected pregnancies; hence the detection rate of 50 per cent (3/6).

The false-positive rate of the initial screening enquiry (Are you or either of your parents Jewish?) will, in effect, be the prevalence of Jews in the community (about 1 per cent in Britain and 2–3 per cent in the USA) because the disease is so rare.

In the secondary screening test (measurement of Hex A), it is usual to set the threshold high enough for the detection rate to be almost 100 per cent, on the ground that missing carriers has graver consequences than submitting some non-carriers to further testing (the outcome if they are classified as positive). In Israel, the threshold is commonly set at 57 per cent Hex A; i.e., subjects in whom less than 57 per cent of Hex activity is attributed to Hex A are investigated further (L. Peleg and E. Akstein, personal communication). With this threshold, virtually no cases are missed but the false-positive rate is 13 per cent.

Instead of a threshold being defined in terms of % Hex A alone, heat-labile (Hex A) and heat-stable (Hex B) activity may be treated as separate variables. For example, the bivariate distributions of Hex A and Hex B activity were established for heterozygotes and normal homozygotes in the Montreal programme. These distributions were then used to calculate the equation for the 0.01 probability line for heterozygosity (i.e. the line beyond which 99 per cent of heterozygotes would fall if the Hex A value of each was plotted against its Hex B value on a scatter diagram, implying a detection rate of 99 per cent if this line is used as a threshold; see Fig. 6.1).[95] Discrimination between heterozygotes and normal homozygotes is more accurate with this approach than with a threshold based on % Hex A. However, there is still overlap between the two distributions, so that supplementary tests are again needed in persons classified as screen-positive.

Heterozygotes for benign Hex A deficiency alleles are one group in whom the 4MUG-based secondary screening test yields false-positive findings. These alleles can account for over one-third of positive results in non-Jewish populations,[80,81] which heightens the need for supplementary tests in persons with 4MUG-positive tests in these populations.

Supplementary tests for carriers

When the 4MUG-based Hex A test in serum is positive, there are three alternative supplementary tests that may be used: a 4-MUG-based Hex A test on leucocytes; a further serum test using 4-methyl, *N*-acetyl glucosaminide-sulphate (4MUGS) instead of 4MUG; and a DNA analysis.

4MUG-based Hex A test on leucocytes

The Hex A test is normally carried out on serum because this is much less labour-intensive than a leucocyte Hex A test; but the latter test is widely used to distinguish

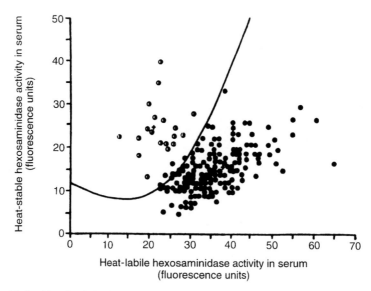

Fig. 6.1 Method for discrimination of genotypes by measure of two non-independent quantitative phenotypes: serum heat-labile and heat-stable hexosaminidase activities. Individuals represented by points above and to left of the hyperbola have greater than 0.01 probability of TSD carrier status. Half-shaded circles, obligate Ashkenazim heterozygotes; full circles, normal Gentile homozygotes. (From Gold *et al.*[95])

between carriers and normals in whom the serum Hex A test is positive, since the distributions of leucocyte Hex A in heterozygotes and homozygous normals do not overlap as the serum Hex A distributions do (Table 6.1). Also, leucocytes are used instead of serum when testing for Hex A in pregnant women. This is because during pregnancy the serum contains a placental species of Hex with thermolability properties similar to those of Hex B,[96–98] so that % Hex A is reduced and the woman would be classified as a carrier if the serum were tested. The isozyme content of leucocytes does not change in pregnancy, and is not affected by oral contraceptives.[99]

In leucocytes as well as in serum, the 4MUG-based test is positive for carriers of benign Hex A deficiency as well as of TSD; but this is not a serious contraindication to leucocyte testing in programmes directed at Jews, in whom benign Hex A deficiency alleles are rare.

4MUGS-based Hex A test

Whereas 4MUG measures total Hex activity (A and B), its sulphated derivative 4MUGS is specific for Hex A (including the variant of this which benign Hex A deficiency alleles produce). Compared with 4MUG, 4MUGS therefore has the advantages of (1) not giving false-positive results for the benign Hex A deficiency alleles or for the *HEXB* alleles which produce thermolabile Hex B enzymes (p. 140), and (2) not giving false-negative results for the B1 *HEXA* alleles (p. 140) which produce enzymes that act on 4MUG but not on G_{M2} ganglioside.[100–103] Despite these advantages, 4MUGS is used only in supplementary testing; it has not replaced 4MUG as the substrate in the test offered to all members of high-risk ethnic groups, because its higher cost is prohibitive and because most available preparations of 4MUGS are not sufficiently free of 4MUG.

DNA analysis

Various DNA-based tests for *HEXA* mutations have been described. The conditions for PCR amplification of each *HEXA* exon (including flanking sequences) have been published.[104] Inclusion of the flanking intronic regions in the amplification products permits detection of mutations which affect splicing as well as those which alter the coding sequences. Four analytical procedures have proven useful for mutation detection: heteroduplex analysis, restriction enzyme digestion, allele-specific hybridization, and allele-specific amplification (reviewed by Hechtman and Kaplan[105]).

Mutation analysis can be offered to all carrier couples identified by a screening test, but it is not appropriate to screen for carriers by DNA analysis because of the extensive *HEXA* allelic heterogeneity. DNA testing for three *HEXA* mutations will identify 92–98 per cent of *HEXA* alleles in Ashkenazi Jews[63–66] (p. 142). In non-Jewish Americans of European descent, DNA testing for five mutations will identify up to 60 per cent of *HEXA* alleles.[74]

Quality control (The International TSD Heterozygote Screening Programme)

At the time of the first International Conference on Tay–Sachs Disease Screening and Prevention (1977), over 45 centres were operating programmes to identify TSD heterozygotes. Whereas all subscribed to a shared set of operating principles (TSD occurs predominantly in defined populations or communities; the heterozygous state can be determined by an accurate and inexpensive laboratory method; prenatal diagnosis of TSD in early pregnancy is possible, and allows for selective abortion of affected fetuses, and permits birth of unaffected infants[106]), it was apparent that a programme to maintain quality control was important. Accordingly, an international centre for TSD Testing, Quality Control, and Data Collection was established in the mid-1970s, with the support of the National Association for Tay–Sachs Disease and Allied Disorders, a non-profit lay organization in the US and Canada.[107] The TSD Quality Control programme now carries out annual blinded proficiency testing with serum and leucocyte samples. Virtually all laboratories throughout the world involved in TSD testing participate voluntarily. The few laboratories that could not 'pass' have since given up testing. The list of proficient laboratories is widely known and accessible.[74]

DIAGNOSIS

If both parents of a fetus are carriers, antenatal testing can determine if the fetus is homozygous affected. This requires Hex A and Hex B measurement in cultured fetal amniocytes or chorionic villus samples. In general, there are more technical problems associated with CVS samples and amniocentesis is preferred. The usual test performed is determination of Hex A activity in the amniocytes. DNA mutation analysis can also be performed on the amniocyte although this requires knowledge of the parental mutation in order to know which mutations to look for. If both parents are Ashkenazi Jews, it is appropriate to test for the three alleles that are common in the Ashkenazi community (TATC insertion in exon 11, G→C at the splice junction of intron 12, and G805A). DNA testing rarely produces diagnostic errors.

For practical purposes the detection rate is 100 per cent and the false-positive rate is 0 per cent.

There are a number of supplementary procedures that may also be used antenatally or later in the diagnosis of homozygosity for TSD.

1. Direct assessment of deficient-Hex A activity is feasible with radiochemically labelled G_{M2} ganglioside. The latter is prepared by extraction from post mortem brain tissue[108] followed by enzymatic or chemical labelling of the *N*-acetygalactosamine,[109,110] sialic acid,[111] or sphingosine[112] component of G_{M2} ganglioside. Although the expense of substrate preparation and the limited sources of G_{M2} ganglioside make its use in routine enzymatic measurement prohibitive, assays measuring G_{M2} ganglioside hydrolysis have been developed for specialized diagnostic purposes.

2. Cell-free cleavage of the 3H [gal-NAc] GM2 ganglioside has been used to distinguish between the early and late-onset TSD variants.[113] The assay employs purified human kidney activator protein and distinguishes between the fibroblasts of cases of infantile, juvenile, and adult-onset TSD, and of benign Hex A deficiency, by their levels of residual enzymatic activity.

3. A procedure involving ^{3}H [sphingosine] G_{M2} ganglioside loading of cultured fibroblasts and intracellular cleavage by intact cells is not as sensitive to small differences in residual enzyme activity as the cell-free assays, but it distinguishes late-onset TSD from the form in which the Hex A deficient adult is healthy.[114]

4. Proof (for counselling purposes) that the cause of Hex A deficiency is mutation at the *HEXA* locus rests ultimately in DNA analysis. In the absence of proof, Sandhoff (*HEXB*), and AB (*GM2A*) mutations must be considered.

SCREENING PROGRAMMES IN PRACTICE

Antenatal screening

The main method of screening is antenatal screening, the first aim of which is to identify Jewish couples. In the USA and Canada, this has proven to be highly effective. Given that about 2 per cent of the population is Jewish and that TSD is 100 times as common in Jews as in non-Jews, one would expect that, in the absence of screening, the ratio between the numbers of births with Tay–Sachs disease among Jewish couples and non-Jewish couples would be 2:1 (p. 145). During the 1980s and early 1990s the ratio has been 1:3,[74] which implies a detection rate among Jews of 83 per cent.

Screening high-school pupils

The Montreal programme has existed since 1972[115] and a 20-year analysis of process and outcome variables has been completed.[90] The programme operates in the context of health care in Canada;[116] it is centred in high schools, and it has three separate components: one for education, another for screening, and a third for counselling after the results of the screening test are distributed. The programme, which focusses on senior high-school students, in regions of the city where the majority of Ashkenazi Jews live and attend school, was initiated and maintained by the community itself after pilot studies, and approval by the School Boards and community leaders and spokespersons. The programme is supported largely by funds from the Health Ministry through the Quebec Network of Genetic Medicine[117] but also by community funding; it continues to operate for and in the community it serves.

Four process and outcome variables have been measured:[90] (1) the proportion of the high-school cohort reached by the educational programme; (2) the uptake rate for the screening test; (3) the origin of carrier couples seeking the prenatal diagnosis option; (4) the change in birth prevalence of TSD over the past two decades. Some of our findings are compared with worldwide experience in Table 6.2.

The educational programme has reached 89 per cent of the high-school cohort. Participation in the screening phase, in the first decade, involved only the students' own consent (valid under Quebec law at the time); in the second decade, signed consent by both parent and student was added. The overall uptake rate of screening was 67 per cent. By 1992, 14 844 Ashkenazi Jewish students had been screened and 521 TSD carriers identified (carrier frequency 1 in 28); carriers were identified by the serum hexosaminidase assay (4MUG substrate).

Virtually all carriers identified in the screening phase took up the options of reproductive counselling *and* prenatal diagnosis if they found themselves to be a partner in a carrier couple. This shows that carriers have not been deterred by their genotype in their choice of partner, that they do not forget their test result, and that if one has a partner who was not tested in the school programme, he or she is tested later. Nor were carrier couples deterred from conceiving; in the two decades covered by our analysis, ten carrier couples in which one or both partners had been identified as carriers by the high-school programme asked for antenatal diagnosis, as did six couples with a family history of TSD. The ten couples that included carriers identified in the high-school programme had 17 pregnancies, and the six with a positive family history had 15. Four fetuses in each of these two groups of pregnancies were affected, and all eight affected pregnancies were voluntarily terminated.

Table 6.2   Tay–Sachs carrier screening and disease avoidance

A. Community-based screening

Region	Persons tested	Carriers detected (rate)	Carrier couples (via screening)
Worldwide[a]	953 004	36 418 (3.8%)	1056
Montreal high schools[b]	14 844	521 (3.5%)	10

B. Prenatal diagnosis in carrier couples

Region	Pregnancies monitored	Affected fetuses (and terminations)	Unaffected live births
Worldwide[a]	1298	201 (201)	1054
Montreal: from high-school programme)[b]	17	4 (4)	13

[a] From Kaback *et al.*[74]
[b] From Mitchell *et al.*;[90] 20-year outcome analysis of program where high-school students were screened (part A); their uptake of antenatal diagnosis later in life (part B) approaches 100 per cent of those identified as carrier couples by screening/testing.

At the present time in Montreal, all couples using antenatal diagnosis for Tay–Sachs disease have discovered their status through the high-school screening programme. The idea that Tay–Sachs disease *can* be avoided has permeated the community which is now well aware of the potential benefits in participation in the aforementioned programme. This and the introduction of testing in high-risk groups in Quebec has been associated with a 90 per cent fall in the number of cases of Tay–Sachs disease born in Quebec, reflecting both a general decline in birth rate and the effect of carrier screening.[90] The rare case today is born outside the region where the screening programme operates, and always to an unscreened, usually non-Jewish, couple.

The Dor Yeshorim programme

In the ultraorthodox Jewish community, marriages are arranged through a *shadchen* (matchmaker). In the Dor Yeshorim programme, before matrimonial introductions take place and often when the young people concerned are still attending school, blood spots are collected from them and tested for heterozygosity for various autosomal recessive disorders, including Tay–Sachs disease, cystic fibrosis and Canavan disease, a severe demyelinating disease that develops in infancy due to a deficiency of the enzyme aspartoacylase. The results are recorded in New York in a confidential central register, linked to index numbers which the individuals keep. If an introduction with a view to marriage is being considered, the index numbers of the prospective couple are sent by the parents to the registry. If both members of the proposed marriage are carriers of the same disease, a report to this effect is passed to the parents.

This programme thus meets the needs of a community in which pre-natal diagnosis and abortion is forbidden; anonymity regarding carrier status is preserved; stigma is avoided; the common goal, avoidance of a lethal disease, is accomplished. The Dor Yeshorim programme was first developed by the ultra-orthodox community in New York and has since been adopted in Israel and Montreal. No TSD child has been born to screened newlywed couples in Israel since the programme was instituted there in 1986.[118]

CONCLUSION

Figure 6.2 gives an overview of screening for TSD in pregnancy in a population like that of the United States and Canada where about 2 per cent of people are Jewish. Although it would normally be difficult to justify mounting a programme of biochemical testing to prevent a disease that only occurs in about 1/100 000 pregnancies, this is made feasible by the fact that the number tested in this way can be reduced to 2 per cent of the population by putting one question , namely 'Are you and your partner Jewish or of Jewish parentage?'—to all pregnant women. Together with the screening of future parents, this programme is estimated to be preventing about five-sixths of the cases that would otherwise occur in Jews, and therefore rather more than half of all cases in the United States and Canada. By helping carriers to bear normal children instead of affected ones, such screening enhances family and community life.

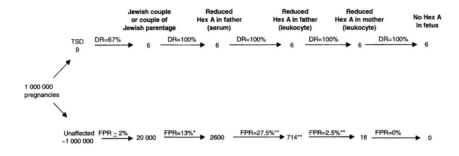

* L Peleg & E Akstein, personal communication

** Estimated on the assumption that one-thirtieth of the partners of carrier fathers will be carriers; 24 x 30 = 720 carrier fathers, and six of these 720 will have offspring with TSD, so that 714 will not. False-positive rates given for Hex A (leukocyte) tests for mothers and fathers are derived from the estimated numbers of false-positive results in these and the fathers' Hex A (serum) tests. DR = detection rate; FPR = false-positive rate.

Fig. 6.2 Flow diagram for antenatal screening for TSD in a community where 2% of people are Jews.

ACKNOWLEDGEMENTS

The authors wish to thank Peter Hechtman, our colleague in Tay–Sachs disease research, and Lynne Prevost for assistance in the preparation of the text.

REFERENCES

1. Tay, W. (1881). Symmetrical changes in the region of the yellow spot in each eye of an infant. *Trans. Opthal. Soc.*, **1**, 55–7.

2. Sachs, B. (1887). On arrested cerebral development, with special reference to its cortical pathology. *J. Nerv. Ment. Dis.*, **12**, 541–53.

3. Sachs, B. (1892). Family form of idiocy, generally fatal, associated with early blindness (Amaurotic Family Idiocy). *J. Nerv. Ment. Dis.*, **21**, 475–81.

4. Gravel, R. A., Clarke, J. T. R., Kaback, M. M., Mahuran, D., Sandhoff, K., and Suzuki, K. (1995). The GM2 Gangliosidoses. In *The metabolic basis of inherited disease* (ed. C.R. Scriver, A.L. Beaudet, W.S. Sly, and D. Valle), pp. 2839–82. McGraw-Hill, New York.

5. Klenk, E. (1939). Beiträge zur Chemie der Lipoidsen, Niemann-Picksche Krankheit und Amaurotische Idiotie. *H-S Z. Physiol. Chem.*, **262**, 128–43.

6. Klenk, E. (1942). Gangliosides, a new group of sugar-containing brain lipids. *H-S Z. Physiol. Chem.*, **273**, 76–86.

7. Svennerholm, L. (1962). The chemical structure of normal human brain and Tay–Sachs gangliosidies. *Biochem. Biophys. Res. Commun.*, **9**, 436–41.

8. Lalley, P. A., Rattazzi, M. C., and Shows, T. B. (1974). Human β-D-N-acetylhexosaminidases A and B: Expression and linkage relationships in somatic cells hybrids. *Proc. Natl. Acad. Sci. U.S.A.*, **71**, 1569–73.

9. Kytzia, H.-J. and Sandhoff, K. (1985). Evidence for two different active sites on human β-hexosaminidase A: Interaction of G_{M2} activator protein with β-hexosaminidase A. *J. Biol. Chem.*, **260**, 7568–72.

10. Conzelmann, E., Burg, J., Stephan, G., and Sandhoff, K. (1982). Complexing glycolipids

and their transfer between membranes by the activator protein for degradation of lysosomal ganglioside G_{M2}. *Eur. J. Biochem.*, **123**, 455–64.

11. Hechtman, P., Isaacs, C., and Smith-Jones, L. (1985). Substrate binding properties of the human liver hexosaminidase A activator protein. *Can. J. Biochem. Cell Biol.*, **63**, 830–8.

12. Conzelmann, E., and Sandhoff, K. (1978). AB variant of infantile G_{M2} gangliosidosis: Deficiency of a factor necessary for stimulation of hexosaminidase A-catalyzed degradation of ganglioside G_{M2} and glycolipid G_{A2}. *Proc. Natl. Acad. Sci. U.S.A.*, **75**, 3979–83.

13. Hirabayashi, Y., Li, Y.-T., and Li, S.-C. (1983). The protein activator specific for the enzymic hydrolysis of G_{M2} ganglioside in normal human brain and brains of three types of G_{M2} gangliosidosis. *J. Neurochem.*, **40**, 168–75.

14. Hechtman, P., Gordon, B. A., and Ng Ying Kin, N. M. K. (1982). Deficiency of the hexosaminidase A activator protein in a case of G_{M2} gangliosidosis; Variant AB. *Pediatr. Res.*, **16**, 217–22.

15. Kytzia, H. J., Hinrichs, U., Maire, I., Suzuki, K., and Sandhoff, K. (1983). Variant of G_{M2} gangliosidosis with hexosaminidase A having a severely changed substrate specificity. *EMBO J.*, **2**, 1201–5.

16. Banerjee, A., Burg, J., Conzelmann, E.,Carroll, M., and Sandhoff, K. (1984). Enzyme-linked immunosorbent assay for the ganglioside GM2 activator protein. Screening of normal human tissues and body fluids, of tissues of GM2 gangliosidosis, and for its subcellular localization. *Hoppe-Zeyler's Z. Physiol. Chem.*, **365**, 347–56.

17. Sonderfeld-Fresko, S., and Proia, R. L. (1989). Analysis of the glycosylation and phosphorylation of the lysozymal enzyme, beta-hexosaminidase B, by site-directed mutagenesis. *J. Biol. Chem.*, **264**, 7692–7.

18. Goldman, J. E., Yamanaka, T., Rapin, I., Adachi, M., and Suzuki, K. (1980). The AB variant of G_{M2} gangliosidosis: Clinical, biochemical and pathological studies of two patients. *Acta Neuropathol. (Berl.)*, **52**, 189–202.

19. Li, Y.-T., Hirabayashi, Y., and Li, S.-C. (1983). Differentiation of two variants of type AB G_{M2} gangliosidosis using chromogenic substrates. *Am. J. Hum. Genet.*, **35**, 520–2.

20. Inui, K., Grebner, E. E., Jackson, L. G., and Wenger, D. A. (1983). Juvenile G_{M2} gangliosidosis (AmB) variant: Inablility to activate hexosaminidase A by activator protein. *Am. J. Hum. Genet.*, **35**, 551–64.

21. Conzelmann, E., Nekrkorn, H., and Kytzia, H.-J. (1985). Prenatal diagnosis of G_{M2} gangliosidosis with high residual hexosaminidase A activity (variant B1, pseudo AB). *Pediatr. Res.*, **19**, 1220–4.

22. Charrow, J., Inui, K., and Wenger, D. A. (1985). Late onset G_{M2} gangliosidosis: An α-locus genetic compound with near normal hexosaminidase activity. *Clin. Genet.*, **27**, 78–84.

23. Bayleran, J., Hechtman, P., Kolodny, E., and Kaback, M. (1987). Tay–Sachs disease with hexosaminidase A: Characterization of the defective enzyme in two patients. *Am. J. Hum. Genet.*, **41**, 532–48.

24. Gordon, B. A., Gordon, K. E., Hinton, G. G., Cadera, W., Feleki, V., Bayleran, J., and Hechtman, P. (1988). Tay–Sachs disease: B1 variant. *Pediatr. Neurol.* **4**, 54–7.

25. Tanaka, A., Ohno, K., Sandhoff, K., Maire, I., Kolodny, E. H., Brown, A., and Suzuki, K. (1990). G_{M2}-gangliosidosis B1 variant: analysis of beta-hexosaminidase alpha gene abnormalities in seven patients. *Am. J. Hum. Genet.*, **46**, 329–39.

26. Kolodny, E. H., Raghavan, S. S., Lyerla, T. A., Proia, R. L., Neufeld, E. F., and Grebner,

E. E. (1983). Misdiagnosis in a fetus with an unstable hexosaminidase A catalytically inactive toward G_{M2} ganglioside. *Am. J. Hum. Genet.*, **35**, 47A.

27. Momoi, T., Suco, M., Tanaka, K., and Nakas, Y. (1978). Tay–Sachs disease with altered β-hexosaminidase B; a new variant? *Pediatr. Res.*, **12**, 77–81.

28. Lowden, J. A. (1979). Evidence for a hybrid hexosaminidase isoenzyme in heterozygotes for Sandhoff disease. *Am. J. Hum. Genet.*, **31**, 281–9.

29. Lane, A. B., and Jenkins, T. (1978). Two variant hexosaminidase β-chain alleles segregating in a South African family. *Clin. Chim. Acta*, **87**, 219–28.

30. Hechtman, P. and Rowlands, A. (1979). Apparent hexosaminidase B deficiency in two healthy members of a pedigree. *Am. J. Hum. Genet.*, **31**, 428–38.

31. Navon, R., Nutman, J., Kopel, R., Gaber, L., Gadoth, N., Goldman, B., and Nitzan, M. (1981). Hereditary heat-labile hexosaminidase B: Its implication for recognizing Tay–Sachs genotypes. *Am. J. Hum. Genet.*, **33**, 907–15.

32. Peleg L., and Goldman B. (1994). Detection of Tay–Sachs disease carriers among individuals with thermolabile hexosaminidase B. *Eur. J. Clin. Chem. Biochem.*, **32**, 65–9.

33. Willner, J. P., Grabowski, G. A., Gordon, R. E., Bender, A. N., and Desnick, R. J. (1981). Chronic G_{M2} gangliosidosis masquerading as atypical Friedreich ataxia: Clinical, morphological, and biochemical studies of nine cases. *Neurology*, **31**, 787–98.

34. Rapin, I., Suzuki, K., and Valsamis, M. P. (1976). Adult (chronic) G_{M2} gangliosidosis. *Arch. Neurol.*, **33**, 120–9.

35. Johnson, W. G., Wigger, H. J., Karp, H. R., Glaubiger, L. M., and Rowland, L. P. (1981). Juvenile spinal muscular atrophy: A new hexosaminidase deficiency phenotype. *Ann. Neurol.*, **11**, 11–16.

36. Yaffe, M. G., Kaback, M., Goldberg, M., Miles, G., Itabashi, H., McIntyre, H., and Mohandas, T. (1979). An amyotrophic lateral sclerosis-like syndrome with hexosaminidase A deficiency: A new type of G_{M2} gangliosidosis (abstract). *Neurology*, **29**, 611. (Abstract)

37. Argov, Z., and Navon, R. (1984). Clinical and genetic variations in the syndrome of adult G_{M2} gangliosidosis resulting from hexosaminidase A deficiency. *Ann. Neurol.*, **16**, 14–20.

38. Vigdoff, J., Buist, N. R., and O'Brien, J. S. (1973). Absence of β-N-acetyl-D-hexosaminidase A activity in a healthy woman. *Am. J. Hum. Genet.*, **25**, 372–81.

39. Grebner, E. E., Mansfield, A. A., Raghavan, S. S., Kolodny, E. H., d'Azzo, A., Neufeld, E. F., and Jackson, L. G. (1986). Two abnormalities of hexosaminidase A in clinically normal individuals. *Am. J. Hum. Genet.*, **38**, 505–15.

40. Navon, R., Padeh, B., and Adam, A. (1973). Apparent deficiency of hexosaminidase A in healthy members of a family with Tay-Sachs disease. *Am. J. Hum. Genet.*, **25**, 287–93.

41. Navon, R., Geiger, B., Ben Yoseph, Y., and Rattazzi, M. C. (1976). Low Levels of β Hexosaminidase A in healthy individuals with apparent deficiency of this enzyme. *Am. J. Hum. Genet.*, **28**, 339–49.

42. Tallman, J. F., Brady, R. O., Navon, R., and Padeh, B. (1974). Ganglioside catabolism in hexosaminidase A-deficient adults. *Nature*, **252**, 254–5.

43. Navon, R., Brand, N., and Sandbank, U. (1980). Adult (G_{M2}) gangliosidosis: neurologic and biochemical findings in an apparently new type. *Neurology*, **30**, 449–50.

44. Navon, R., Argov, Z., Brand, N., and Sandbank, U. (1981). Adult G_{M2} gangliosidosis in association with Tay–Sachs disease: a new phenotype. *Neurology*, **31**, 1397–401.

45. Andermann, E., Scriver, C. R., Wolfe, L. S., Dansky, L., and Andermann, F. (1977). Genetic variants of Tay–Sachs disease: Tay–Sachs disease in French Canadians, juvenile

Tay Sachs disease in Lebanese Canadians and a Tay Sachs screening program in the French Canadian population. *Prog. Clin. Biol. Res.*, **18**, 161–88.

46. Triggs-Raine, B., Richard, M., Wasel, N., Premce, E. M., and Natowicz, M. R. (1995). Mutational analysis of Tay–Sachs disease: Studies on Tay–Sachs carriers of French Canadian background living in New England. *Am. J. Hum. Genet.*, **56**, 870–9.

47. De Braekeleer, M., Hechtman, P., Andermann, E., and Kaplan, F. (1992). The French Canadian Tay–Sachs disease deletion mutation: Identification of probable founders. *Hum. Genet.*, **89**, 83–7.

48. Drucker, L., Proia, R., and Navon, R. (1992). Identification and rapid detection of three Tay–Sachs mutations in the Moroccan Jewish population. *Am. J. Hum. Genet.*, **51**, 371–7.

49. Kaufman, M., Grinshpun-Cohen, J., Karpati, M., Peleg, L., Goldman, B., Akstein, E., Adam, A., Navon R. (1997). Tay-Sachs disease and *HEXA* mutations among Moroccan Jews. *Hum. Mutat.*, **10**, 295–300.

50. Navon, R., and Proia, R. L. (1991). Tay–Sachs disease in Moroccan Jews: Deletion of a phenylalanine in the α-subunit of ß-hexosaminidase. *Am. J. Hum. Genet.*, **48**, 412–19.

51. Chern, C.J., Kennett, R., Engel, E., Mellman, W. J., and Croce, C. M. (1977). Assignment of the structural genes for the α-subunit of hexosaminidase A, mannose phosphate isomerase and pyruvate kinase to the region of 22-qter of human chromosome 15. *Som. Cell Genet.*, **3**, 553–60.

52. Takeda, K., Nakai, H., Hagiwara, H., Tada, K., Shows, T. B., Byers, M. G., and Myerowitz, R. (1990). Fine assignment of beta-hexosaminidase A alpha-subunit on 15q23-q24 by high resolution *in situ* hybridization. *Tohoku. J. Exp. Med.*, **160**, 203–11.

53. Dana, S. L., and Wasmuth, J. J. (1982). Selective linkage disruption in human–Chinese hamster cell hybrids: deletion mapping on the leu S, Hex B, emt B, and chr genes on chromosome 5. *Mol. Cell. Biol.*, **2**, 1220–8.

54. Burg, J., Conzelmann, E., Sandhoff, K., Solomon, E., and Swallow, D. M. (1985). Mapping of the gene coding for the human G_{M2} activator protein to chromosome 5. *Ann. Hum. Genet.*, **49**, 41–5.

55. Swallow, D. M.,Islam, I., Fox, M. F., Povey, S., Klima, H., Schepers, U., and Sandhoff, K. (1993). Regional localization of the gene coding for the G_{M2} activator protein (*GM2A*) to chromosome 15q32-33 and confirmation of the assignment of *GM2AP* to chromosome 3. *Ann. Hum. Genet.*, **57**, 187–93.

56. Myerowitz, R., and Proia, R. L. (1984). cDNA clone for the α-chain of human β-hexosaminidase: deficiency of α chain mRNA in Ashkenazi Tay-Sachs fibroblasts. *Proc. Natl. Acad. Sci.*, **81**, 5394–8.

57. O'Dowd, B. F., Quan, F., Willard, H. F., Lambonwah, A.-M., Korneluk, R. G., Lowden, J. A., Gravel, R. A., and Mahuran, D. J. (1985). Isolation of cDNA clones coding for the β subunit of human β-hexosaminidase. *Proc. Natl. Acad. Sci.*, **82**, 1184–8.

58. Klima, H., Tanaka, A., Schnabel, D., Nakano, T., Schröder, M., Suzuki, K., and Sandhoff, K. (1991). Characterization of full-length cDNAs and the gene coding for the human G_{M2} activator protein. *FEBS. Lett.*, **289**, 260–4.

59. Myerowitz, R., Piekarz, R., Neufeld, E. F., Shows, T., and Suzuki, K. (1985). Human β-hexosaminidase α chain: coding sequence and homology with the β chain. *Proc. Natl. Acad. Sci.*, **82**, 7830–4.

60. Proia, R. L., and Soravia, E. (1987). Organization of the gene encoding the human beta-hexosaminidase alpha-chain. *J. Biol. Chem.*, **262**, 5677–81.
61. Kaplan, F., (1998). Tay-Sachs disease carrier screening: A model for prevention of genetic disease. *Genetic Testing*, **2**, 271–91.
62. Myerowitz, R., and Hogikyan, N. D. (1987). A deletion involving Alu sequences in the beta-hexosaminidase alpha-chain gene of French Canadians with Tay–Sachs disease. *J. Biol. Chem.*, **262**, 15396–9.
63. Triggs-Raine, B., Feigenbaum, A. S., Natowicz, M., Skomorowski, M., Schuster, S. M., Clarke, J. T. R., and Mahuran, D. J. (1990). Screening for carrier of Tay–Sachs disease among Ashkenazi Jews. A comparison of DNA-based and enzyme-based tests. *N. Engl. J. Med.*, **323**, 6–12.
64. Paw, B. H., Tieu, P. T., Kaback, M. M., Lim, J., and Neufeld, E. F. (1990). Frequency of three HEXA mutant alleles among Jewish and non-Jewish carriers identified in a Tay–Sachs screening program. *Am. J. Hum. Genet.*, **47**, 698–705.
65. Landels, E. C., Ellis, II. H., Fensom, A. H., Green, P. M., and Bobrow, M. (1991). Frequency of the Tay–Sachs Disease splice and insertion mutations in the U.K. Ashkenazi Jewish population. *J. Med. Genet.*, **28**, 177–80.
66. Fernandes, M. J. G., Kaplan, F., Clow, C., Hechtman, P., and Scriver, C. R. (1992). Specificity and sensitivity of hexosaminidase assays and DNA analysis for the detection of Tay–Sachs carriers among Ashkenazi Jews. *Genet.Epidem.*, **9**, 169–75.
67. Myerowitz, R., and Costigan, F. C. (1988). The major defect in Ashkenazi Jews with Tay–Sachs disease is an insertion in the gene for the alpha-chain of beta-hexosaminidase. *J. Biol. Chem.*, **263**, 18587–9.
68. Myerowitz, R. (1988). A splice junction mutation in some Ashkenazi Jews with Tay– Sachs disease: Evidence against a single defect within this ethnic group. *Proc. Natl. Acad. Sci.*, **85**:, 3955–9.
69. Arpaia, E., Dumbrille Ross, A., Maler, T., Neote, K., Tropak, M., Troxel, C., Stirling, J. L., Pitts, J. S., Bapat, B., Lamhonwah, A. M., *et al.* (1988). Identification of an altered splice site in Ashkenazi Tay–Sachs disease. *Nature*, **333**, 85–6.
70. Ohno, K., and Suzuki, K. (1988). Multiple abnormal beta-hexosaminidase alpha chain mRNAs in a compound-heterozygous Ashkenazi Jewish patient with Tay–Sachs disease. *J. Biol. Chem.*, **263**, 18563–7.
71. Paw, B. H., Kaback, M. M., and Neufeld, E. F. (1989). Molecular basis of adult-onset and chronic G_{M2} gangliosidoses in patients of Ashkenazi Jewish origin: substitution of serine for glycine at position 269 of the alpha-subunit of beta-hexosaminidase. *Proc. Natl. Acad. Sci.*, **86**, 2413–17.
72. Navon, R., Kolodny, E. H., Mitsumoto, H., Thomas, G. H., and Proia, R. L. (1990). Ashkenazi-Jewish and non-Jewish adult G_{M2} gangliosidosis patients share a common genetic defect. *Am. J. Hum. Genet.*, **46**, 817–21.
73. Navon, R., and Proia, R. L. (1989). The mutations in Ashkenazi Jews with adult G_{M2} gangliosidosis, the adult form of Tay–Sachs disease. *Science*, **243**, 1471–4.
74. Kaback, M. M., Lim-Steele, J., Dabholkar, D., Brown, D., Levy, N., and Zeiger K. (for the International TSD Data Collection Network). (1993). Tay–Sachs disease-carrier screening, prenatal diagnosis, and the molecular era. *J. Am. Med. Assoc.*, **270**, 2307–15.
75. Akerman, B. R., Zielenski, J., Triggs-Raine, B. L., Prence, E. M., Natowicz, M. R., Lim-Steele, J. S. T., Kaback, M. M., Mules, E. H., Thomas, G. H., Clarke, J. T. R., and Gravel,

R. A. (1992). A mutation common in non-Jewish Tay–Sachs disease: Frequency and RNA studies. *Hum. Mut.*, **1**, 303–9.

76. Hechtman, P., Kaplan, F., Bayleran, J., Boulay, B., Andermann, E., de Braekeleer, M., Melancon, S., Lambert, M., Potier, M., Gagne, R., Kolodny, E., Clow, C., Capua, A., Prevost, C., and Scriver, C. R. (1990). More than one mutant allele causes infantile Tay–Sachs disease in French-Canadians. *Am. J. Hum. Genet.*, **47**, 815–22.

77. Hechtman, P., Boulay, B., de Braekeleer, M., Andermann, E., Melançon, S., Larochelle, J., Prevost, C., and Kaplan, F. (1992). The intron 7 donor splice site transition: A second Tay–Sachs disease mutation in French Canada. *Hum. Genet.*, **90**, 402–6.

78. Navon, R., Argov, Z., and Frisch, A. (1986). Hexosaminidase A deficiency in adults. *Am. J. Hum. Genet.*, **24**, 179–96.

79. Greenberg, D. A. and Kaback, M. M. (1982). Estimation of the frequency of hexosaminidase A variant alleles in the American Jewish population. *Am. J. Hum. Genet.*, **34**, 444–51.

80. Triggs-Raine, B. L., Mules, E. H., Kaback, M. M., Lim-Steele, J. S. T., Dowling, C. E., Akerman, B. R., Natowicz, M. R., Grebner, E. E., Navon, R., Welch, J. P., Greenberg, C. R., Thomas, G. H., and Gravel, R. H. (1992). A pseudodeficiency allele common in non-Jewish Tay–Sachs carriers: Implications for carrier screening. *Am. J. Hum. Genet.*, **51**, 793–801.

81. Cao, Z., Natowicz, M. R., Kaback, M. M., Lim-Steele, J. S., Prence, E. M., Brown D., Chabot, T., and Triggs-Raine B. L. (1993). A second mutation associated with apparent beta-hexosaminidase A pseudodeficiency: Identification and frequency estimation. *Am. J. Hum. Genet.*, **53**, 1198–1205.

82. Kaback, M. M., Hirsh, P., Roy, C., Greenwald, S., and Kirk, M. (1978). Gene frequencies for Tay–Sachs (TSD) and Sandhoff's disease (SD) in Jewish and non-Jewish populations. *Pediatr. Res.*, **12**, 530A.

83. Kaback, M. M., Bailin, G., Hirsch, P., and Roy, C. (1977). Automated thermal fractionation of serum hexosaminidase: Effects of alteration in reaction variables and implications for Tay–Sachs disease heterozygote screening. In *Tay–Sachs disease: screening and prevention* (ed. M. M. Kaback), pp. 197–212. Alan R.Liss Inc., New York.

84. Delvin, E., Scriver, C. R., Pottier, A., Clow, C., and Goldman, H. (1972). Maladie de Tay–Sachs: Dépistage et diagnostic prénatal. *L'Union Médicale du Canada* , **101**, 683–688.

85. Lowden, J. A., Skomorowski, M. A., Henderson, F., and Kaback, M. (1973). Automated assay of hexosaminidases in serum. *Clin. Chem.*, **19**, 1345–9.

86 Price, R. G. and Dance, N. (1972). The demonstration of multiple heat stable forms of N-Acetyl-β-glucosaminidase in normal human serum. *Biochim. Biophys. Acta*, **271**, 145–153.

87. Saifer, A., and Perle, G. (1977). Hexosaminidase A analysis of various biological fluids by Ph inactivation for the identification of Tay–Sachs disease genotypes. In *Tay–Sachs disease: screening and prevention* (ed. M. M. Kaback), pp. 227–38. Alan R. Liss, Inc., New York.

88. Merz, B. (1987). Matchmaking scheme solves Tay–Sachs problems. *J. Am. Med. Assoc.*, **258**, 2636–9.

89. Wald, N. J. (1991). Couple screening for cystic fibrosis. *Lancet*, **338**, 1318–1319.

90. Mitchell, J. J., Capua, A., Clow, C., and Scriver, C. R. (1996). Twenty-year outcome of genetic screening programs for Tay–Sachs and ß-thalassemia diseases in high schools. *Am. J. Hum. Genet.*, **59**, 793–8.

91. Steele, M. W. (1980). Lessons from the American Tay–Sachs programme. *1980. Lancet*, **ii**, 914.

92. Lowden, J. A. and Davidson, J. (1977). Tay–Sachs screening and prevention: the Canadian experience. In *Tay–Sachs disease: screening and prevention* (ed. M. M. Kaback), pp. 37–46. Alan R. Liss Inc., New York.

93. Padeh, B., Schachar, S., Modan M., and Goldman, B. (1978). Screening and prevention of Tay–Sachs disease in Israel. *Monogr. Hum. Genet.*, **9**, 170–5.

94. Evans, P. R. (1977). Tay–Sachs screening in Britain. In *Tay–Sachs disease: screening and prevention* (ed. M. M. Kaback), pp. 55–9. Alan R. Liss Inc., New York.

95. Gold, R. J. M., Maag, U. R., Neal, J. L., and Scriver, C. R. (1974). The use of biochemical data in screening for mutant alleles and in genetic counselling. *Ann. Hum. Genet.*, **37**, 315–26.

96. Potier, M., Boire, G., Dallaire, L., and Melancon, S. B. (1977). N-Acetyl-β-hexosaminidase isoenzymes of amniotic fluid and maternal serum. Their relevance to prenatal diagnosis of the G_{M2} gangliosidoses. *Clin. Chim. Acta*, **76**, 309–15.

97. Lowden, J. A. (1979). Serum β-hexosaminidases in pregnancy. *Clin. Chim. Acta*, **93**, 409–17.

98. Stirling, J. L. (1972). Separation and characterization of N-acetyl-β-glucosaminidases A and P from maternal serum. *Biochim. Biophys. Acta*, **271**, 154–73.

99. Desnick, R. J., Truex, J. H., and Goldberg, J. D. (1977). A fully automated method for identification of Tay–Sachs disease carriers by tear β-hexosaminidase assay. *Prog. Clin. Biol. Res.*, **18**, 245–65.

100. Fuchs, W., Navon, R., Kaback, M. M., and Kresse, H. (1983). Tay–Sachs disease: one step assay of β-N-acetylhexosaminidase in serum with sulfated chromogenic substrates. *Clin. Chim. Acta*, **133**, 253–61.

101. Bayleran, J., Hechtman, P., and Saray, W. (1984). Synthesis of 4-methyl-umbellifery-β-D-N-acetylglucosamine-6-sulfate and its use in classification of G_{M2} gangliosidosis genotypes. *Clin. Chim. Acta*, **143**, 73–89.

102. Inui, K., and Wenger, D. A. (1984). Usefulness of 4-methylumbelliferyl-6-sulfo-2-acetamido-2-deoxy-β-D- glucopyrnoside for the diagnosis of G_{M2} gangliosidosis in leucocytes. *Clin. Genet.*, **26**, 318–21.

103. Ben-Yoseph, Y., Reid, J. E., Shapiro, B., and Nadler, H. J. (1985). Diagnosis and carrier detection of Tay–Sachs disease: Direct determination of Hex A using 4-methyl-umbelliferyl derivatives of N-acetylglucosamine-6-sulfate and N-acetylgalactos-amine-6-sulfate. *Am. J. Hum. Genet.*, **37**, 733–48.

104. Triggs-Raine, B. L., Akerman, B. R., Clarke, J. T. R., and Gravel, R. A. (1991). Sequence of DNA flanking the exons of the HEXA gene, and identification of mutations in Tay–Sachs disease. *Am. J. Hum. Genet.*, **49**, 1041–54.

105. Hechtman P., and Kaplan F. (1993). Tay–Sachs disease screening and diagnosis: Evolving technologies. *DNA Cell Biol.*, **12**, 651–65.

106. Kaback, M. M., Nathan, T. J., and Greenwald, S. (1977). Tay–Sachs disease: Heterozygote screening and prenatal diagnosis—U.S. experience and world perspective. In *Tay–Sachs disease: screening and prevention* (ed. M. M. Kaback), pp. 13–36. Alan R. Liss Inc., New York.

107. Kaback, M. M., Shapiro, L. J., Hirsch, P., and Roy, C. (1977). Tay–Sachs disease heterozygote detection: A quality control study. In *Tay Sachs disease: screening and prevention* (ed. M. M. Kaback)., pp. 267–80. Alan R. Liss Inc., New York.

108. Wolfe, L. S. (1972). Methods for separation and determination of gangliosides. In *Research methods in neurochemistry* (ed. N. Marks and R. Rodnight), pp. 233–48. Plenum, New York.

109. Suzuki, Y., and Suzuki, K. (1972). Specific radioactive labeling of terminal N-acetylgalactosamine of glycosphingolipids by the galactose oxidase-sodium borohydride method. *J. Lipid Res.*, **13**, 687–90.

110. Novak, A., Lowden, A., Gravel, Y. L., and Wolfe, L. S. (1979). Preparation of radio-labelled G_{M2} and G_{A2} gangliosides. *J. Lipid Res.*, **20**, 678–80.

111. Kolodny, E. H., Brady, R. O., Quirk, J. M., and Kanfer, J. N. (1970). Preparation of radioactive Tay–Sachs ganglioside labelled in the sialic acid moiety. *J. Lipid Res.*, **11**, 144–9.

112. Schwarzmann, G. (1978). A simple and novel method for tritium labeling of gangliosides and other sphingolipids. *Biochim. Biophys. Acta*, **529**, 106–14.

113. Conzelmann, E., Kytzia, H.-J., Navon, R., and Sandhoff, K. (1983). Ganglioside G_{M2} N-acetyl-β-D-galactosamine activity in cultured fibroblasts of late-infantile and adult G_{M2} gangliosidosis patients and of healthy probands with low hexosaminidase level. *Am. J. Hum. Genet.*, **35**, 900–13.

114. Raghavan, S. S., Krusell, A., Krusell, J., Lyerla, T. A., and Kolodny, E. H. (1985). G_{M2}-Ganglioside metabolism in hexosaminidase A deficiency states: Determination in situ using labeled G_{M2} ganglioside added to fibroblast cultures. *Am. J. Hum. Genet.*, **37**, 1071–82.

115. Beck, E., Blaichman, S., Scriver, C. R., and Clow, C. L. (1974). Advocacy and compliance in genetic screening. Behaviour of physicians and clients in a voluntary program of testing for the Tay–Sachs gene. *New Engl. J. Med.*, **291**, 1166–70.

116. Evans, R. G. (1992). 'We'll take care of it for you.' Health care in the Canadian community. *Daedalus*, **117**, (4), 155–89.

117. Scriver, C. R., Laberge C., Clow, C. L., and Fraser, F. C. (1978). Genetics and medicine: An evolving relationship. *Science*, **200**, 946–52.

118. Broide, E., Zeigler, M., Eckstein, J., and Bach, G. (1993). Screening for carriers of Tay–Sachs disease in the ultraorthodox Ashkenazi Jewish community in Israel. *Am. J. Med. Genet.*, **47**, 213–15.

7 Infections

Catherine S. Peckham and Marie-Louise Newell

INTRODUCTION

Although the vast majority of infections in pregnancy have no effect on the developing fetus, some can lead to severe damage and disability. These are listed in Table 7.1. Overall, infections in pregnancy are thought to be responsible for less than 1 per cent of severe anatomical malformations,[1] but the proportion of early-onset visual and auditory impairment and cerebral palsy that they cause is greater than this. Except for rubella, they affect mainly already formed organs. Most produce no symptoms in the mother by which they can be identified. This makes serological screening of great importance.

Infections of the fetus are acquired as a result of systemic blood-borne maternal infection crossing the placenta, or from ascending infection from the lower genital tract. Transplacental infection may occur with or without infection of the placenta, and placental infection does not necessarily imply fetal infection. Infections of the newborn may also be acquired from contact with contaminated vaginal secretions or blood during delivery. Infections of the fetus and newborn may result from a primary maternal infection, reactivation of a latent maternal infection, or from exposure to infectious agents that constitute part of the lower genital tract flora. The main outcomes of fetal infection include fetal loss, stillbirth, preterm delivery, low birthweight, congenital abnormalities, symptoms or signs of disease at birth, and late development or manifestation of damage, which may not be apparent until months or years after birth. Some infectious agents continue to replicate in the infant for months or years after birth (e.g. CMV, rubella, HSV, toxoplasma, syphilis) and cause continued tissue destruction.

The impact of a specific infection on the fetus or newborn may depend on the timing of infection during pregnancy. Rubella, for example, is of concern if it occurs during the first trimester when the risk of fetal damage is high, whereas damage from cytomegalovirus may occur following exposure to infection in all trimesters of pregnancy. With toxoplasmosis the risk of fetal infection increases with duration of pregnancy, but the proportion of infected infants with fetal damage declines. In contrast, other infectious agents such as herpes simplex virus or chlamydia are usually

Table 7.1 Maternal infections that can affect the fetus or newborn infant

Viruses:	Rubella
	Cytomegalovirus (CMV)
	Hepatitis B (HBV)
	Hepatitis C (HCV)
	Herpes simplex
	Varicella zoster
	Human immunodeficiency virus 1 and 2 (HIV-1, HIV-2)
	Human T-cell leukaemia virus type 1 (HTLV-1)
	Parvovirus B19
Bacteria:	*Treponema pallidum*
	Listeria monocytogenes
	Neisseria gonorrhoeae
	Group B streptococcus
	Chlamydia trachomatis
Protozoa:	*Toxoplasma gondii*

acquired by the neonate at the time of delivery as a result of exposure to the organism after the rupture of the membranes.

The justification of screening for specific infections in pregnancy is to prevent or reduce the adverse consequences of these infections for the fetus or newborn, through treatment or termination of the pregnancy. At the present time in the UK, antenatal screening is recommended for syphilis, hepatitis B, HIV infection, and rubella. The aim in screening for syphilis, hepatitis B, and HIV infection is to identify infected women in pregnancy so that treatment can be initiated and fetal/neonatal infection and damage avoided. Screening for rubella does not aim to reduce fetal abnormalities in the current pregnancy, but to establish whether a woman is susceptible to infection, thereby identifying those women who require post-partum vaccination to protect a subsequent pregnancy.

There is an ongoing public and professional debate as to the relative merits of extending antenatal screening to include other infections such as toxoplasmosis, cytomegalovirus, herpes simplex, chlamydia, and streptococcal B infection. The development and wider availability of laboratory tests together with advances in prenatal diagnosis, such as fetal blood sampling and improved ultrasound techniques, have increased the scope and pressure for possible interventions to reduce the consequences of congenital and perinatal infections. There is no simple universal screening procedure to cover all these infections and different screening schedules are required for each specific infection.

Decisions about the value of introducing a screening programme must be based on detailed information relating to the infection, and benefits and risks must be carefully balanced. Specific information required in reaching a decision to screen includes the prevalence of infection in the pregnant population, rates of mother-to-child transmission, the reliability of the screening and subsequent diagnostic tests, assessment of disease burden in both symptomatic and asymptomatic congenitally infected infants, and the effectiveness, acceptability, and possible risks of intervention or treatment. In this chapter we discuss infections that may have an adverse effect on the fetus or newborn and for which screening has been considered, including those where there are already screening programmes in place, those where there is ongoing debate as to whether programmes should be introduced, and those where there is still insufficient evidence to recommend screening. For as many infections as possible, we include estimates of the proportion of children damaged by the infection when there is no screening, and of the reduction in this proportion which screening makes possible. Even when based on limited data (as some of our estimates are), approximate estimates are better than none and are helpful when considering the possibility of screening.

RUBELLA

Rubella is a mild disease with few complications, but when acquired in early pregnancy it may cause serious fetal damage. Fetal infection results from a primary infection in pregnancy and reinfection has only been described in a few case-reports.[2] The widespread rubella immunization of school girls and susceptible women in the UK since 1970, the introduction of measles, mumps, rubella (MMR) vaccine in 1988, and the 1994 mass campaign to immunize all school children aged 5–16 years with measles/rubella vaccine have significantly reduced the circulation of rubella virus in the community. As a result the incidence of congenital rubella has also fallen, reaching an all time low in 1995, when only one case was reported in the UK. However, the figure for 1996 was higher (12 cases), demonstrating that continued surveillance is essential.[3]

Congenital rubella

It is estimated that about 80 per cent of infants exposed to rubella in the first three months of pregnancy will have rubella-associated defects, and the risk of damage then declines to about 10–20 per cent by 16 weeks.[4] After this stage of pregnancy fetal damage is rare.[5,6] Major clinical manifestations of congenital rubella include congenital heart disease, cataracts, sensorineural hearing loss, microphthalmos, microcephaly, cerebral palsy, and mental retardation. Some congenital rubella abnormalities such as cataracts or congenital heart defects are obvious at birth, but others such as hearing impairment may not become apparent, or even develop, for months or years. Exposure to rubella in early pregnancy is likely to result in fetal infection with multiple defects whereas damage following exposure to infection in the third or fourth month usually results in a single defect, sensorineural hearing loss. This is the most frequent rubella defect and before the introduction of rubella vaccine accounted for nearly 20 per cent of moderate/severe congenital deafness in children.[7]

A definitive diagnosis of congenital rubella can be established by virus isolation or by serological findings, including IgG antibody persisting without a significant decline beyond six to nine months of age (when passively acquired maternal antibody can usually no longer be detected). The presence of rubella-specific IgM, which may persist until three to six months of age, is also indicative of infection.

Frequency

The frequency of congenital rubella can be estimated either from notifications of affected children or from the reported incidence of rubella in pregnant women and the risk to the offspring of infected women. During 1991–6, 31 affected children (about seven per million born) were notified to the congenital rubella surveillance programme in the UK.[3] This figure is likely to be an under-estimate, since only severely affected infants are likely to be diagnosed, and since affected fetuses from terminated pregnancies are not included. In England and Wales, 43 terminations for maternal rubella disease (29) or contact (14) were reported in 1991–5.

According to a study of the incidence of rubella in pregnant women in England and Wales,[8] 2.0 per cent of women in their first pregnancies and 1.2 per cent of women in their second or later pregnancies in 1994–5 were susceptible to rubella infection, and the infection rate among susceptible pregnant women in 1990–5 was about 3/1000 in first pregnancies and 1/1000 in later ones. From the evidence that the prevalence of defects due to rubella in the offspring falls from 80 per cent after maternal infection during the first trimester to almost zero after infection more than four months after conception (p. 161), one would expect about 30 per cent of the offspring of women infected during pregnancy to be affected. If so, and if the above susceptibility and infection rates in pregnancy were correct, the prevalence of affected fetuses in the general population would be about 18 (i.e. $0.3 \times 0.003 \times 20\,000$) per million first pregnancies and 4 (i.e. $0.3 \times 0.001 \times 12\,000$) per million later ones. Data on maternal susceptibility by ethnic group and on the origins of mothers of affected children show that the children of immigrants to Britain are at much higher risk.[8]

Intervention

A woman's decision whether to have her pregnancy terminated will be influenced by the risk and severity of defects. Because risk and severity decline rapidly during the second trimester, termination is not generally advised in pregnancies in which infection arises after 16 weeks.

Current screening programme in the United Kingdom

The aim of the antenatal screening programme is not to identify women who acquire rubella infection in pregnancy, but to identify those who are susceptible so that they can be offered rubella vaccination after the pregnancy. It therefore has no implications for the management of the current pregnancy, but aims to protect subsequent pregnancies. Women with rubella IgG antibody levels below 15 iu are normally reported as rubella susceptible and immunization is recommended in the postnatal period. A 'susceptible' result from a screening test may simply reflect low levels of antibody and this is likely to account for the majority of cases where women with evidence of previous immunity, due to infection or vaccination, are reported to be susceptible.

Screening policy

Once established, all screening programmes need to be kept under review and if necessary modified to ensure that they are achieving their objectives. Even if the UK practice of screening pregnant women and later vaccinating those who are not immune reduced the prevalence of non-immunity in women in their second or later pregnancies to zero, it would be unlikely to prevent more than about three cases of congenital rubella per million births. This estimate is obtained by dividing the estimated prevalence of the rubella syndrome in first-born infants (18/million) by three (since susceptible women are only one third as likely to be infected in their second or later pregnancies as in their first—see p.162) and halving the resulting figure of 6/1 000 000 (since only about half of all infants are not first-born).

Screening all pregnant women for susceptibility therefore does little to prevent congenital rubella, in contrast to the policy of general infant and childhood vaccination also adopted in the UK. Susceptibility testing can however be used in samples to monitor the success of this policy in rendering the population immune, and may also have a place in the care of women from groups known to be at high risk of having affected children—e.g. those who immigrated to the UK at adult ages and have no history of rubella vaccination.[8]

It is important to appreciate that an 'immune' result in the rubella screening test does not preclude recent or current infection. Women who report contact with rubella or present with symptoms suggestive of rubella infection in the first 16 weeks of pregnancy should be offered diagnostic tests and appropriate counselling, irrespective of vaccination history or screening results.

SYPHILIS

Syphilis is a serious and preventable disease. The place of screening in its management is discussed at length in a review from the UK Public Health Laboratory Service.[9]

In adults the primary lesion of syphilis appears at the initial site of the infection with *Treponema pallidum* about three weeks after exposure, followed by a more generalized illness involving skin rashes and condylomata after 6–12 weeks (secondary syphilis). If untreated, this stage is self-limited and the patient usually progresses to a latent stage of infection during which the only evidence of syphilis is positive serology. During the early latent phase (within two years of onset) organisms can be seeded intermittently into the blood stream.

Congenital syphilis

Treponema pallidum can be transmitted from an infected woman to her fetus, particularly when her infection is untreated and in the primary, secondary, or early latent stage.[10] Transmission usually occurs after the 18th week of pregnancy. Untreated syphilis in pregnancy may result in significant perinatal mortality and morbidity, the risk depending on the stage of infection in the mother and levels of spirochetes in the blood stream.[11]

If a mother has a primary or secondary infection in pregnancy it is unlikely that she will deliver a normal term infant. During the first two years of untreated latent maternal infection an estimated 20 per cent of infants will die *in utero* or in the neonatal period, 20 per cent will be premature but otherwise normal, 40 per cent will be infected and damaged, and 20 per cent will be uninfected.[12] After the second year of maternal infection the probability of fetal infection diminishes, and transmission is rare after the fourth year.

Congenital syphilis has traditionally been divided into two stages. When clinical features of the disease are apparent in the first two years of life, and a direct result of active infection and inflammation, the disease is designated as early congenital syphilis. After two years it is termed late congenital syphilis, and presents with mal-formations and stigmata that represent the scars induced by initial lesions of early syphilis or reactions to persisting or ongoing inflammation. The most common neonatal presentation includes hepatomegaly, jaundice, and osteochondritis; lymph-adenopathy, pneumonia, and myocarditis are less common clinical manifestations. Clinical features do not become apparent until 2–12 weeks of age. The most common clinical manifestation of late congenital syphilis is interstitial keratitis, occurring in about 40 per cent of affected children, usually between six and 14 years. Bone and joint lesions, and disease leading to deafness and neurological involvement, may result in a minority of children.

Diagnosis of congenital syphilis is difficult, even when infection is suspected, because many infected infants are asymptomatic at birth and the presence of mater-nal antibody makes infants' serology difficult to interpret. Definitive proof with the identification of *T. pallidum* is rare since the organism cannot be cultured and few infants have skin lesions to produce a specimen for dark-field microscopy.[13] As a result good reporting criteria for congenital syphilis are difficult to formulate. The CDC definition of congenital syphilis includes infants with clinical evidence of active infec-tion, asymptomatic infants, and stillbirths.[14] All infants at risk require a full clinical evaluation at birth and follow-up until non-treponemal and treponemal tests are negative and maternal antibody has disappeared.

Frequency

Information on the number of women identified and treated during pregnancy and on the incidence of congenital syphilis in the UK has recently become available from a survey in which all paediatricians and genito-urinary physicians in the United Kingdom were asked to report cases seen in a three-year period, during which there were 2.2 million births.[15] Based on the results, the review from the UK Public Health Laboratory Service concluded that the prevalence of maternal infection might lie between 90 and 120 per million.[9]

Four per cent of the maternal cases reported had primary or secondary syphilis and 20 per cent were in the early latent phase of infection.[15] From these figures and the proportions of children of untreated women with syphilis at different stages who die in fetal or neonatal life or are damaged by the infection (see above), it can be estimated that if there was no screening the total incidence of congenital syphilis in the UK would be 20 per million (four in infants of mothers with primary or secondary syphilis, 12 (i.e. 20 × 60 per cent) with mothers in the early latent phase, and occa-sional cases with mothers in the late latent phase). Under the current screening programme, the recent three-year UK survey identified four presumptive and four possible cases of congenital syphilis per million births.[15] The programme may there-fore prevent 60–80 per cent of cases (12–16 cases per million births).

As these figures illustrate, congenital syphilis has become a relatively rare condition in developed countries, and most doctors in the UK will never have seen a case.[13] However, over the past two decades, increases in the incidence of acquired and con-genital syphilis have been reported from both developed and developing countries. In the USA the rate of congenital syphilis among infants increased from 43 per million in 1982 to 947 per million in 1992. This closely reflected the increase in primary and secondary syphilis in women of child-bearing age[16] which was related to social deprivation, drug use, exchange of sex for drugs, and failure to receive antenatal care. This highlights the importance of monitoring trends in the UK.

Intervention

In order to prevent congenital syphilis, pregnant women are tested serologically and those who are seropositive are treated with penicillin, which is effective. When these measures are taken in early pregnancy they prevent most cases of congenital syphilis, since the disease is not usually transmitted to the fetus before the 19th week of gestation.[17] Detection in late pregnancy is less effective, but may prevent some of the sequelae. Infants with suspected congenital syphilis should be examined clinically during their first months of life, and they should be treated if maternal treatment was suboptimal or if there is a suspicion of active infection in the child.

Screening tests

Screening and confirmatory tests for syphilis are both varied and complex. Serological screening is performed on blood samples collected at the first antenatal visit, by standard tests such as the Venereal Disease Reference Laboratory (VDRL) test or the flocculation test.[18,19] Since these are non-specific tests and detect non-treponemal antibodies, all positive or dubious results require confirmation by a specific treponemal test such as the *T. pallidum* immobilization test (TPI) or the fluorescent treponemal antibody absorption (FTA) test. Other treponemal infections such as yaws, bejel, and pinta are serologically indistinguishable. The proportion of uninfected women who test positive has been estimated to be 0.2 per cent when a non-treponemal test alone is used and 0.1 per cent when secondary screening by a treponemal test is included.[9]

Screening policy

In a detailed economic analysis using Swedish data, Stray-Pedersen[12] concluded that a programme of screening and treatment of women for syphilis was cost-effective despite the rarity of syphilis. Even when the incidence of maternal syphilis was as low as 50 per million pregnancies, the benefit outweighed the cost of the syphilis screening programme. Antenatal screening was also supported on economic grounds by Williams[20] and Bowell *et al.*[21] in the UK, and by Garland and Kelly[22] in Australia.

The marginal cost of antenatal screening for syphilis in the UK is £0.88 per pregnancy screened.[9] If, in the absence of screening, syphilis would cause death or disability in 20 per million fetuses or infants in the UK, as estimated above, it follows that the cost of screening per prospective case of congenital syphilis would be £44 000 (i.e. 0.88 × 1000 000/20). The recent review from the UK Public Health Laboratory Service concludes that this expenditure is justified, given that screening also benefits women who would otherwise develop tertiary syphilis and that the incidence of syphilis may increase in the future, as it did during the 1990s in some developed and developing countries and in one British city (Bristol).[9,23] The situation needs to be kept under review, with adequate surveillance systems to monitor trends of syphilis in pregnant women and children.[23]

HUMAN IMMUNODEFICIENCY VIRUS

The human immunodeficiency virus (HIV) is a retrovirus, which has as its main target cell the helper/inducer T-lymphocytes. The destruction of these lymphocytes results in immunosuppression and increased susceptibility to common infections and AIDS. There are at least two types of HIV of which HIV-1 is the most prevalent and pathogenic. HIV-2 is uncommon in Western countries and less transmissible, and in this section we refer to HIV-1.

HIV infection is transmitted in three ways: sexually, through contaminated blood and vertically from mother to child. Vertical transmission is the major mode of acquisition of infection for children and currently accounts for about 85 per cent of cases of paediatric AIDS. It can occur before or during birth or through breastfeeding. In Europe, the estimated rate of mother-to-child transmission in the absence of breast-feeding is 15–20 per cent.[25–27]

Mothers with evidence of immunodeficiency or high viral load are two to three times more likely to transmit the virus than those whose immune status is relatively intact. Breastfeeding approximately doubles the rate of transmission.[28] An elective caesarean section reduces the risk of transmission by 50–80 per cent, irrespective of maternal virus load.[29]

HIV infection in infancy

The initial clinical presentation of HIV infection in infants is often non-specific and may involve a wide spectrum of manifestations, such as generalized lymphadenopathy, hepatomegaly and/or splenomegaly, persistent parotitis, diarrhoea, and fever. Other more serious manifestations include persistent oral candida, lymphoid interstitial pneumonitis, lymphoma, and serious bacterial and other opportunistic infections. Acquired Immune Deficiency Syndrome (AIDS) denotes a group of serious HIV-related manifestations indicative of severe immune deficiency. One-quarter of infected children develop AIDS or die in the first year of life. After this age, disease progression is slower and by five years of age, an estimated 40 per cent of infected children will have developed AIDS and 25 per cent will have died.[30] The long-term picture is unknown, but it is likely that all infected children will develop AIDS and few, if any, will survive into adulthood. The prognosis after the diagnosis of AIDS is variable and may depend not only on treatment but also on the age of AIDS onset and the presenting symptoms/signs.

The diagnosis of HIV infection in infants is complicated by the presence of passively acquired maternal antibody, which may persist for up to 18 months. An earlier diagnosis can be made by virus culture, polymerase chain reaction (PCR), the detection of p24-antigen or IgA. Culture of HIV is the definitive method of diagnosis but it is slow, expensive, and limited to specialized laboratories. An ELISA for detection of p24-antigen is the most commonly used antigen test. Its sensitivity has been improved by incorporating acid or heat dissociation of antibody–antigen complexes. The polymerase chain reaction (PCR) is a method of amplification of DNA sequences in a cell-free system. It is of particular value in infants born to HIV seropositive mothers, where serological diagnosis is not helpful in determining infection status. PCR sensitivity in the first few days of life is about 40 per cent and increases rapidly to about 100 per cent by one month of age.[31]

Frequency

The prevalence of maternal HIV infection varies widely even within the UK. In anonymous seroprevalence surveillance surveys based on neonatal blood samples, infection rates among women delivering livebirths in 1996–7 ranged between 0.02 per cent and 0.49 per cent in districts of London, and between zero and 0.08 per cent in districts of England outside London. The highest rates found were in inner London. For all districts combined, the rates were 19.9/10 000 births in London, 1.6/10 000 in the rest of England and Wales and 2.3/10 000 in Scotland.[32] If the vertical transmission rate is 15–20 per cent in artifically fed infants and is doubled by breastfeeding (see p. 166), the infection would probably be transmitted to at least a quarter of the infected women's children, i.e. to 5.0/10 000 children born in London in 1996–7, 0.4/10 000 in the rest of England and Wales, and 0.6/10 000 in Scotland.

In London most infections are associated with births to women from high prevalence countries, whereas in Edinburgh, Dundee, and Dublin injecting drug use is a more important source.

Intervention

The administration of antiretroviral therapy with zidovudine during pregnancy, labour, and early infancy significantly reduces the rate of transmission. In an American-French trial, the rate of vertical transmission was 7.6 per cent in the treated group and 22.6 per cent in the placebo group.[33,34] Zidovudine was well tolerated in pregnancy and in the newborn, and although anaemia was more common in the treated newborns, it resolved when treatment was discontinued. In the USA, zidovudine treatment is recommended for all pregnant women identified with HIV infection.[35] The transmission rate following treatment is now less than 5 per cent. However, questions remain about the optimum time of initiation of therapy during pregnancy, and possible long-term sequelae in the infants, the large majority of whom will not be infected anyway. Further trials with shorter regimens have shown a lower but still substantial reduction in risk.

In populations where safe and affordable alternatives are available, HIV infected women should be encouraged not to breastfeed.[36] The suggestion from observational studies that a caesarean section delivery may reduce the rate of mother-to-child transmission[26] has been confirmed by the results from an international randomized trial of mode of delivery[29].

Antenatal screening to identify infected women is recommended principally so that they can be offered advice and treatment such as the above to reduce the risk of transmission of infection to their infant and its serious consequences. There are also benefits for the HIV infected mother herself and for those infants who acquire infection. Table 7.2 summarizes the benefits of identifying HIV infection in pregnancy.

Table 7.2   The benefits of identifying HIV infection in pregnancy

Reducing mother-to-child transmission:	Avoidance of breastfeeding
	Anti-retroviral therapy
	Elective caesarian delivery
Improved management of the infected child:	Early diagnosis
	Pneumocystis carinii pneumonia prophylaxis
	Anti-retroviral therapy
Management of the infection in the mother:	Appropriate prophylaxis
	Anti-retroviral treatment
	Prevention of sexual transmission

Screening tests

Current serological tests for HIV-specific IgG antibody are of high specificity and sensitivity. Sera found to be reactive for anti-HIV on screening should be retested with the same ELISA and the results confirmed by another ELISA system or Western Blot. For diagnostic purposes it is prudent to obtain a repeat sample from the woman to confirm infection.

The majority of infected women seroconvert within six to eight weeks after infection, although in some cases antibody may not appear until three months later. Thus a negative antibody test is reliable only if the woman has not been exposed to the virus in the previous three months. A false-negative test result may occur if the woman is tested in the window period between infection and seroconversion. A screening brief in the *Journal of Medical Screening* suggests that ELISA testing for maternal HIV-specific antibody identifies 99 per cent of women who have been infected for over 3 weeks. With repeat testing in women whose initial test is positive, the proportion of all uninfected women who remain test-positive is 0.1 per cent if the initial sample is used for the repeat test and close to zero if a second sample is used.[37]

Screening policy

The cost-effectiveness of screening for HIV in pregnancy, as of other programmes, depends on the local prevalence and the proportion of infected women diagnosed for the first time as a result of antenatal screening.[38] The uptake of screening by those most at risk is another factor. In the UK, evaluation of existing antenatal screening programmes through active case reporting systems and anonymous testing of antenatal or neonatal samples has highlighted that the uptake of screening is poor although there has been some improvement recently. In 1997 in London, 32 per cent of infected women were identified as such before the end of pregnancy. Three-fifths of these were known about before the pregnancy.[32]

Until 1999, the UK Department of Health recommended that antenatal testing for HIV be provided in populations with a high prevalence of HIV infection, and that elsewhere testing should be available to those who request it and those identified in routine clinical practice as being at risk.[39] A prevalence of 50 maternal infections per 100 000 pregnancies was independently suggested as the level above which routine screening should be provided.[37]

In 1999, the UK Department's policy changed to one of offering and recommending an HIV test to *all* pregnant women in England as an integral part of their antenatal care.[40,41] According to the anonymous seroprevalence survey data,[32] this would involve testing 5.6 times as many women as would be included if testing were only carried out in areas where more than 50/100 000 pregnant women were HIV-positive. It would identify HIV infection in 41/100 000 instead of 30/100 000 pregnant women in the country as a whole. The numbers of infant lives saved would be about one fifth as great (i.e. 8/100 000 and 6/100 000 respectively), since about a quarter of children of HIV-positive mothers are infected and die in the absence of intervention, and an estimated four fifths of these deaths can be prevented by zidovudine treatment. The preventive effects might be somewhat greater, since infected mothers can also be offered caesarian delivery and advice not to breast-feed. It follows that in England as a whole, with about 700 000 births annually, at least 56 children per year would be saved by universal testing, as against 42 with testing in high-risk areas only. The simplicity and equity of universal testing and the improved level of public protection it confers justify its extra cost.

HEPATITIS B VIRUS

Hepatitis B virus (HBV) is a small enveloped DNA virus and an important cause of morbidity and mortality worldwide. After the acute infection a proportion of individuals develop persistent infection, which can be identified through the detection of hepatitis B surface antigen (HBsAg). A second antigen, HBeAg, is also detected in some chronic carriers, and is associated with high infectivity. Most chronic carriers are symptomless.

Transmission of infection from HBsAg carrier mothers to their infants is one of the most important factors contributing to the high prevalence of HBV in many parts of the world. Hence prevention of the development of carrier status is of importance. Carrier status in childhood not only produces a reservoir of infection which facilitates intrafamilial and community transmission but perpetuates the cycle of perinatal transmission. In southeast Asia and sub-Saharan Africa where the prevalence of HBV infection is high, most infections are acquired in childhood. The high prevalence in the Far East is maintained by vertical transmission from mother to baby during the perinatal period,[42] although in Africa infection is usually acquired horizontally from other routes.[43]

Perinatal hepatitis B infection

The usual route of vertical transmission during the perinatal period is contact with infected vaginal secretions or maternal blood to which the infant is exposed at the time of birth. The virus does not cross the placenta and the few intrauterine infections that occur are probably due to leakage of maternal blood into the fetal circulation. Risk of mother-to-child transmission of HBV is related to the infectivity of maternal blood and the degree of exposure at birth.[44] Infectivity is related to the presence of high titres of HBsAg in the mother's circulation and to the presence of hepatitis B e antigen (HBeAg), which correlates with a high level of HBV DNA. The prevalence of HBeAg varies in different populations and is particularly high in southeast Asia.

Nearly 90 per cent of infants born to mothers who are HBeAg positive become infected. Among mothers with HBsAg who are HBeAg-negative, the risk of transmission is about 10 per cent in those with HBe antibody (the majority) and 40 per cent in those lacking HBe antibody.[45]

Infants infected with HBV at birth are generally not mature enough to mount an adequate immune response. As a result, most are asymptomatic and more than 90 per cent become chronic carriers. The risk of persistent carriage being established following infection after birth declines with age, e.g. to about 25 per cent after infection at five years and 10 per cent after infection at 15 years according to surveys in both developed and developing countries.[46]

Among all the infants (infected and uninfected) born to carrier mothers, 81.7 per cent (95 per cent CI 77.7, 85.7) of those whose mothers are HBeAg-positive and 9.5 per cent (95 per cent CI 5.7, 13.2) of those whose mothers are HBeAg-negative become chronic carriers according to all the available studies combined.[47]

HBV carrier children are at risk of developing chronic active hepatitis, liver cirrhosis, and primary hepatocellular carcinoma.[48] They also constitute a reservoir of virus for infection of others.

Frequency

The prevalence of chronic carrier mothers varies greatly between countries and between populations within a country. In countries in southeast Asia and Africa, where prevalence is high, 70–80 per cent of adults have evidence of past HBV infection and 8–20 per cent of pregnant women are chronic symptomless carriers of HBV and at risk of transmitting infection to their newborn infant. In intermediate prevalence countries, such as Japan, Eastern Europe, Russia, and the Mediterranean countries, 20–30 per cent of women have evidence of past infection, and 2–7 per cent are carriers.

In northern Europe and North America where the prevalence is low, fewer than 10 per cent of adults have experienced HBV infection and less than 1 per cent of pregnant women are chronic carriers of the virus.[49] In The Netherlands, where pregnant women are screened routinely for hepatitis B antigens, 4.4/1000 carry HBsAg, and one-tenth of these carriers are also HBeAg-positive.[50] National data for the UK are not available. One per cent of pregnant women screened in Inner London, 1.8/1000 in Glasgow, and 0.5/1000 in Cambridge were found in recent studies to carry HBsAg.[51] Twenty per cent of HBsAg carriers in the largest study in the UK were HBeAg-positive.[52] These figures suggest that in the UK as a whole, HBsAg may be carried by between 1 and 2/1000 pregnant women—0.8–1.6 HBeAg-negative carriers and 0.2–0.4 HBeAg-positive per 1000.

In low-prevalence countries, most infections are acquired through sexual contact or injecting drug use, and perinatal infection is uncommon. Among injecting drug users, 40–60 per cent have evidence of HBV infection, and 3–9 per cent are carriers. Immigrants in low-prevalence countries have similar carrier rates to women in their countries of origin.

Given that 10 per cent of neonates with HBeAg-negative carrier mothers and 82 per cent of those with HBeAg-positive mothers become chronic carriers, it can be estimated that the carrier status arises as a result of infection at birth in between 0.2 and 0.5/1000 infants in the UK, i.e. between $[(0.10 \times 0.8) + (0.82 \times 0.2)]$ and $[(0.10 \times 1.6) + (0.82 \times 0.4)]$. Between 30 per cent and 50 per cent of carriers infected at birth develop chronic liver disease.

Intervention

The development of carrier status can be prevented in 85–95 per cent of infants of carrier mothers by giving hepatitis B immunoglobulin immediately after birth, before antigenaemia has developed, together with a three-dose schedule of acellular vaccine starting at birth.[53] Antenatal screening for maternal carrier status is necessary if these measures are to be applied.

Screening and diagnostic tests

There are a variety of screening tests available for the detection of HBsAg, the most popular being ELISAs, which have a high sensitivity. Commercial ELISA kits are available for the detection of HBeAg and antibody, HBsAg and antibody, HB core antibodies, and IgM. Pregnant women are first screened for HBsAg, and if positive tested for HBe antigen and antibody to determine infectivity and for anti-core IgM antibody to differentiate recent acute infection from the carrier state. Experience in The Netherlands suggests that with repeat testing of samples that test positive, screening for HBsAg identifies at least 98 per cent of infected women, and is only positive in 0.002 per cent of uninfected women according to the results of retesting at delivery.[50]

Screening policy

The cost-effectiveness of antenatal screening and intervention depends on the prevalence of HBV infection in the population.[54] In areas of high prevalence, and this often includes inner cities in countries with a low prevalence, the most effective approach to prevention is universal testing. In areas of low endemicity one possible approach is two-step screening, first identifying people thought to be at high risk on account of country of origin, place of residence, and particular high-risk life styles (e.g. injecting drug use) and then testing these people serologically. Questions that will satisfactorily deal with the first step without causing offence and without missing too many cases are difficult to identify, and the effectiveness of this approach has therefore been questioned.[55,56] In one low-prevalence area of the UK (East Anglia) it was estimated that one-step antenatal screening would result in 11.7 fewer childhood carriers per 100 000 children than two-step screening. This would prevent an estimated 2.9 deaths/100 000 from occurring 40–50 years later, at a cost of £2437 per year of life saved, which suggested that the introduction of universal screening in the UK would be beneficial.[57]

In the UK the Department of Health instructed in 1998 that antenatal screening based on measuring HBsAg be carried out as a one-step procedure in all pregnant women,[58] as had been independently recommended.[59] This approach has been adopted in many European countries and has been shown to be cost-effective in The Netherlands.[50,60-62] In the USA routine antenatal screening and immunization of children at risk, which is now current policy,[63] was shown to be cost-effective at a prevalence of 0.06 per cent when both direct and indirect costs were taken into account.[64]

Over the country as a whole, if between 0.2 and 0.5/1000 infants would acquire carrier status at birth in the absence of prophylaxis and if immunization at birth can reduce the risk by 90 per cent, as suggested above, one-step antenatal screening could prevent carrier status in between 18 and 45/100 000 neonates, or between 100 and 300 per year. It is more effective to introduce antenatal HBV screening than to screen all neonates or to introduce HBV into routine vaccination schedules during childhood, since recent seroprevalence data show that most HBV infection in British children results from vertical transmission.[65]

CYTOMEGALOVIRUS

Cytomegalovirus (CMV) is a DNA virus and a member of the herpes family of viruses which also includes herpes simplex, Epstein–Barr, and varicella-zoster virus. Like other viruses in the herpes family, once primary infection has occurred the virus establishes itself in the host in a latent form and may periodically reactivate. Both primary and recurrent infection are associated with viral shedding in body fluids, including urine, saliva, semen, cervical secretions, and breast milk. In healthy individuals, symptoms of CMV infection are usually mild or inapparent and it rarely causes serious illness. However, infection can be life-threatening in immunocompromised individuals and premature infants, and when acquired in pregnancy can cause fetal damage.

In addition to intrauterine infection, infants born to seropositive mothers may acquire infection during delivery, or in early life as a result of breastfeeding or prolonged close contact with an infected individual. In the UK about 20 per cent of children become infected by 12 months,[66] but infection acquired after birth is rarely associated with adverse outcome, except in the very premature infant. In non-industrialized countries most women of childbearing age are seropositive, having acquired infection in early life, whilst in industrialized countries, such as the UK, about 50 per cent of women are susceptible to CMV infection. There is considerable age-specific variation in sero-prevalence according to ethnic group.[67] About one in every 100 women found to be susceptible in early pregnancy will acquire a primary infection during pregnancy and about 40 per cent of infected women are likely to transmit the infection to their fetus.[68]

Congenital CMV infection

Both primary and recurrent maternal infection during pregnancy can result in fetal infection, but the risk of damage following a maternal recurrent infection appears to be extremely low, although defects compatible with congenital CMV infection have been reported.[68,69] In the UK about two-thirds of congenital infections result from primary maternal infection. Between 5 per cent and 10 per cent of infants who are infected congenitally by mothers with a primary infection are symptomatic at birth. Clinical manifestations include hepatomegaly, splenomegaly, thrombocytopenia, prolonged neonatal jaundice, pneumonitis, growth retardation, microcephaly, and occasionally cerebral calcification. Most infants with signs of infection at birth suffer long-term complications which are often multiple and may include cerebral palsy, mental retardation, optic atrophy, and sensorineural deafness.[70,71] In contrast most infants who are asymptomatic at birth develop normally, although a small proportion, about 5–10 per cent, will have long-term neurological sequelae, sensorineural hearing loss being the most frequent problem.[67,72,73] It follows that long-term sequelae occur in about 6 per cent of all infants whose mothers experience primary CMV infections during pregnancy, i.e. in about 15 per cent of the subset of these infants who themselves become infected (Fig. 14.1).

Sensorineural hearing loss is the most common single defect attributable to congenital CMV. It has been estimated that 12 per cent of bilateral congenital sensorineural hearing loss is due to CMV[74] and this has replaced congenital rubella as the most common viral cause of congenital deafness. Furthermore, an estimated 7 per cent of cerebral palsy is due to congenital CMV. Unlike rubella, which only harms the fetus when exposure occurs in early pregnancy, CMV can lead to fetal damage following primary maternal infection at any time in pregnancy.

Frequency

The birth prevalence of congenital CMV infection varies between populations from 0.2 to 2.2 per cent of livebirths.[75] From the above findings that 50 per cent of pregnant women are susceptible to CMV infection, that 1 per cent of susceptible pregnant women acquire a primary infection, that vertical transmission occurs in 40 per cent of these infections, and that two-thirds of cases of congenital CMV infection are acquired from mothers with primary infections, it can be estimated that in the UK 3/1000 fetuses (i.e. $0.5 \times 0.01 \times 0.4 \times 1.5$) are infected.[67] The proportion of infants born who can be expected to suffer long-term sequelae of infections is about 3/10 000 (Fig. 7.1).

Intervention

There is no effective treatment for either maternal or fetal CMV infection. Antenatal screening has been suggested to enable termination to be offered if infection is found, and neonatal screening to identify children at risk of neurological problems, particularly sensorineural hearing loss, so that special care and education can be arranged.

Antenatal screening

Antenatal screening for primary maternal infection would require an initial test for seropositivity, after which all seronegative women would need repeated serological testing throughout pregnancy, since most maternal infections are asymptomatic. Among women who were initially seropositive, it would be possible to distinguish those who had only become so within the last few months by testing for CMV-specific IgM; but this would not identify exclusively those infected after conception, since IgM may persist for three to six months after primary infection or even longer. Testing for fetal infection by amniocentesis and attempted isolation of CMV from amniotic fluid has also been proposed[76] but isolation of virus in the amniotic fluid is not proof of fetal infection or damage, and negative results do not exclude fetal infection. In view of the limitations of these procedures and the low risk of fetal damage following CMV infection (Fig. 7.1), the case for screening with a view to offering termination of pregnancy is weak.

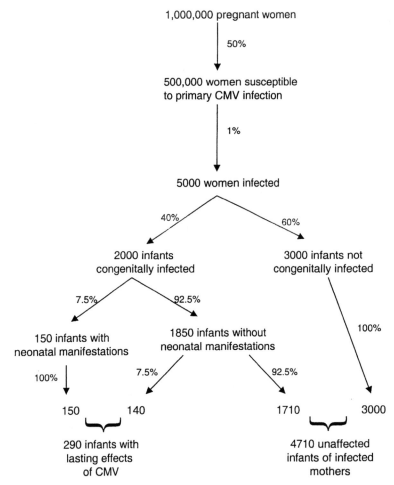

Fig. 7.1   Estimated impact of primary CMV in pregnancy.

Neonatal screening

In neonates, congenital infection is indicated by the presence of CMV in a throat swab or urine sample obtained in the first two or three weeks of life. Virus isolation beyond this period does not distinguish congenital from acquired infection, which commonly occurs in the early months of life and is not associated with complications. As fewer than 10 per cent of asymptomatic infants identified as congenitally infected would subsequently develop a CMV-related problem and there is at present no treatment to offer, there is little benefit from neonatal screening. Also, neonatal screening could be harmful, causing unnecessary distress for parents, most of whose children will be healthy. In the absence of screening, most affected infants who later needed special care or education would still be identified in early childhood by routine screening for problems such as hearing impairment. Neonatal as well as antenatal screening for CMV is therefore unjustified.

TOXOPLASMOSIS

Toxoplasmosis is caused by the protozoan parasite *Toxoplasma gondii* and although its life cycle has been well described the precise mode of transmission to humans is not well understood. Infection can be acquired through the consumption of undercooked meat containing toxoplasma tissue cysts, especially lamb and pork, and the ingestion of oocysts from the faeces of infected kittens, either directly or from contaminated garden soil and poorly washed garden produce. The relative importance of each of these routes is not known. In most healthy women newly acquired infection is not recognized clinically but it can result in fetal infection with potentially serious consequences for the newborn infant. It is generally held that fetal infection is associated with acute toxoplasmosis infection in the mother, and not with chronic infection. Based on this precept serological screening programmes have been adopted in some countries.

Congenital toxoplasmosis

The overall risk of transmission to the fetus based on studies carried out in Europe and North America in the 1960s is about 40 per cent.[77] This ranges from about 15 per cent after maternal infection in the first trimester to about 30 per cent and 60 per cent following exposure in the second and third trimesters respectively.[78] In contrast, the likelihood of an infected fetus being damaged is much higher when infection occurs in early pregnancy than when it occurs later.[79] Manifestations range from the 'classic triad' of retino-choroiditis, cerebral calcification, and hydrocephalus, to non-specific signs such as low birthweight, hepatosplenomegaly, jaundice, thrombocytopenia, and convulsions. In a minority of infected infants, about 5–10 per cent, severe manifestations present at birth or during infancy, and long-term sequelae, including neurological impairment, epilepsy, and impaired vision due to retinochoroiditis occur in most children of this subgroup who survive.[80] However, most infants with congenital toxoplasmosis (90–95 per cent) are asymptomatic at birth or have non-specific signs such as intrauterine growth retardation, hepatomegaly, splenomegaly, purpura, and jaundice. Some of this subgroup subsequently develop sequelae, of which retinochoroiditis is the most commonly recognized and may not appear until adulthood. Small studies suggest that the prevalence of visual impairment in congenitally infected young adults who had no specific signs at birth is about 25 per cent, but there have been no large-scale prospective studies and no reliable estimates are available.[81]

Frequency

The prevalence of infection varies markedly from country to country and between groups within a country. In the UK, less than 20 per cent of pregnant women have serological evidence of prior toxoplasma infection and over 80 per cent remain susceptible to infection. The seropositivity rate among pregnant women relates to their country of birth: women born in the UK, regardless of their ethnic origin, have a significantly lower seroprevalence than those born in southern Europe or Africa.[82] There is some evidence from Sweden and the UK that seroprevalence has fallen over the past

20 years.[83] Such reductions may reflect improvements in food hygiene, increased use of frozen meat, or the introduction of successful health education programmes.

The best estimate of the incidence of toxoplasmosis in pregnancy in the UK is around 2 per 1000.[84] From this figure, and from the above-quoted estimates that the fetus is infected in 40 per cent of pregnancies in which primary infection occurs and that 5–10 per cent of fetal infections have severe effects which present in infancy and lead to lasting damage, one would expect these effects to be present in 40–80 per million infants born. If a quarter of the remaining 90–95 per cent of fetal infections led to visual impairment, this would be expected to develop in a further 180–190 per million infants (Fig. 7.2). However, active paediatric ascertainment of cases in 1989–90[81] together with analysis of laboratory reports revealed a maximum of only about 30 diagnosed cases of congenital toxoplasmosis per million births. The disparity between the expected and observed figures shows the need for further studies on the incidence and natural history of gestational toxoplasmosis in the UK.

Interventions

If maternal infection is diagnosed, the use of the antibiotic spiramycin to reduce the risk of fetal infection is widely recommended, and is commonly continued until term if fetal infection is not detected. The case for this practice is based on comparison with historical controls, and its efficacy has never been evaluated in a randomized controlled trial.[85] If fetal infection is diagnosed, three-week courses of spiromycin are alternated with combination therapy of sulphadiazine, pirethamine, and folinic acid. These drugs are not given in early pregnancy because of their toxicity and possible teratogenic effects. All four drugs are generally given for one year from birth to infants who are known to have been infected, on the assumption that this treatment will limit tissue damage.

Screening and diagnostic tests

Where antenatal screening for toxoplasmosis is practised, its purpose is to identify maternal infections arising after conception so that fetal infection can be prevented or treated. The first antenatal blood sample is therefore tested for toxoplasma-specific IgG and IgM antibodies. Those with no antibodies can then be retested to detect seroconversions later in pregnancy. Those in whom the initial screening test for IgM is positive (which may indicate that a post-conceptional infection has already occurred) need further blood sampling to confirm the finding.

Numerous methods are available for the detection of toxoplasma-specific IgG and IgM, but there is a wide variation in the reported performance of the assays. The accepted reference test is the Sabin Feldman dye test, which measures both IgG and IgM antibodies, but as it requires live, viable parasites, it is rarely performed outside a reference laboratory. Tests based on the detection of IgM in sera may be difficult to interpret because IgM may persist, although in decreasing concentrations, for several months or even years after infection, so that a sensitive test today may detect it even if the woman was infected before conceiving. Tests based on IgA and the measurement of IgG avidity are now becoming available and may clarify whether the infection was likely to have occurred during the pregnancy.[86]

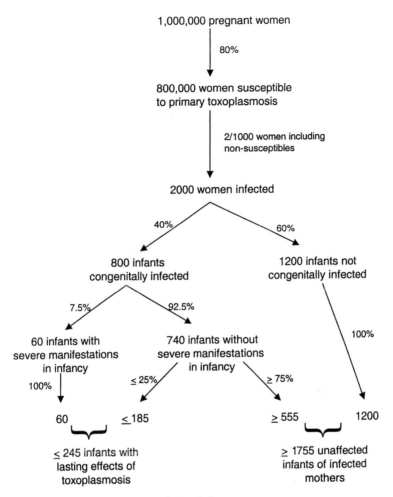

Fig. 7.2 Estimated impact of primary toxoplasmosis in pregnancy.

These new serological tests are likely to play an important role in any future screening programme.

No maternal screening test will identify fetal infection, but women in whom infection has been confirmed can be offered amniocentesis or cordocentesis to establish whether fetal infection has occurred, and thereby avoid termination of an uninfected fetus. However, these investigations carry a risk of associated pregnancy loss. Fetal diagnosis is confirmed by recovering the parasite from fetal blood or amniotic fluid. Where available, a polymerase chain reaction test (PCR) on amniotic fluid is the preferred method for rapid diagnosis of infection.

In the newborn the diagnosis of congenital infection may be problematic even when signs of congenital toxoplasmosis are present. Diagnosis depends on the identification of toxoplasma-specific IgM in neonatal blood samples or the demonstration of persistent IgG antibodies. Toxoplasma IgM assays are relatively insensitive, and a negative result does not exclude infection. IgG antibody must be measured sequentially for at least the first year of life in order to demonstrate changes in IgG titre that differentiate between antibodies acquired passively from the mother and true fetal infection.

Screening policy

Antenatal screening programmes have been set up in some European countries, notably Austria and France, and over recent years there has been increased pressure in the UK to follow a similar course. However, there is insufficient evidence at the present time to recommend routine screening for toxoplasmosis in the UK.[81,87-89] Reports from some European countries with higher seroprevalence rates than the UK also conclude that screening is not justified.[90] Testing for seroconversion requires repeat samples from all women who are seronegative at booking. In the UK this would necessitate the retesting of more than 80 per cent of women throughout pregnancy so that treatment could be initiated as soon as possible after the onset of maternal infection. Screening algorithms range from monthly to three-monthly retesting of susceptible women, but they lack a clear scientific rationale due to the absence of information about the effect of delaying treatment during pregnancy. As already indicated, reliable information is also lacking as to the efficacy of spiramycin in preventing vertical transmission, and as to the prevalence and nature of long-term damage (especially in children with no major neonatal symptoms) following congenital toxoplasmosis; and IgM assays are sometimes misleading. A survey of 28 countries in Europe found that only seven currently recommend systematic screening and no country has a programme whose impact on congenital toxoplasmosis can be assessed.[91] There is therefore too little information at present to determine whether antenatal screening with treatment of women with proven recent infection would be cost-effective in the UK or elsewhere in Europe. Some authorities consider that primary health education would be more important and cost-effective than serological screening to detect infection after it has occurred.

HERPES SIMPLEX VIRUS

Herpes simplex virus (HSV) belongs to the family of human herpes viruses, DNA viruses with the ability to establish latency and reactivate throughout life. There are two strains of HSV, HSV-1 and HSV-2. HSV-1 is usually acquired in early life, whereas HSV-2 is seldom found until after puberty and is associated with onset of sexual activity. However, virus type alone is not necessarily a good indicator of source of infection. In adults, primary genital herpes is generally caused by HSV-2, although HSV-1 is increasing as a cause of first episode genital disease. HSV infection is widespread and 80-100 per cent of many adult populations will have antibodies. HSV-2 seropositivity is rare before adolescence and then rises with increasing age; the annual rate of seroconversion in USA studies is about 2 per cent. The prevalence of HSV-2 shows geographic, socio-economic, and racial variation, and is related to number of sexual partners. In STD populations 20 per cent to over 60 per cent are seropositive.

Congenital and perinatal infection

There have been isolated case reports of maternal infection in early pregnancy associated with fetal abnormality, but evidence that transplacental transmission of HSV causes abnormality is inconclusive,[92,93] and the major problem which maternal HSV infection poses for the fetus and infant is vertical transmission either during passage through the birth canal or from ascending infection after rupture of the membranes. Recurrent maternal genital HSV infection poses a low risk of transmission and most cases of neonatal infection result from a primary and often asymptomatic infection acquired in late pregnancy.[94–98]

Neonatal HSV infection is a potentially serious disease associated with high mortality and morbidity, even with antiviral therapy.[99] Neonatal infection may present with isolated skin lesions, localized neurological disease, or disseminated disease involving multiple organs. Disseminated infection is associated with a high mortality, and neurological development is impaired in 50 per cent of children who survive after disseminated infection or encephalitis. Neonates presenting with localized infection have a much better prognosis.[100]

About 70 per cent of neonatal HSV infections in the USA, 50 per cent in the UK, and 30 per cent in Japan are caused by HSV-2 infection. The reason for the higher incidence of HSV-2 as the cause of this condition in the USA is not clear.

Frequency

The estimated rate of neonatal herpes in the USA is about 20–50/100 000 deliveries per year.[99] In contrast neonatal herpes is rare in the UK. During a five and a half year period of active national surveillance (1986–91) through the British Paediatric Association Surveillance Unit[24] 76 cases of neonatal infection (between 7 and 19 cases each year) were notified in the UK and Eire. Two-thirds of cases presented with disseminated infection or herpes encephalitis and one-third with localized infection. The incidence was 1.65 per 100 000 livebirths. This is likely to be a minimum estimate of the size of the problem since the diagnosis may have been missed in some neonates because of the non-specific nature of the clinical presentation.[101] A rate of 6.5/100 000 births has been reported from Sweden.[102]

One-quarter of children in the British study died in the neonatal period, and another third died later or had significant long-term sequelae.

Intervention

If there is clinical evidence of primary maternal infection in late pregnancy, it is recommended that the possibility of vertical transmission from the birth canal should be avoided by caesarean section.[103,104] Also, all infants exposed to primary maternal genital infection at delivery should be closely monitored, and be given antiviral therapy if symptoms develop.[99] A trial of antiviral therapy revealed no difference in effectiveness between acyclovir and vidarabine. Their use was associated with a reduction in the proportions of infections resulting in mortality (to 19 per cent) and in lasting morbidity as fewer infections were disseminated.[99,100]

Tests for infection

Virus isolation is the definitive method of diagnosis of HSV infection, but it is limited by the duration of viral shedding. DNA PCR is increasingly being used and may be the gold standard in the future. A swab for virus isolation should be taken from any infant suspected of having neonatal herpes, and where possible from the genital tract of the mother. Virus may be isolated from the neonate from several sites, including skin, mouth, throat, nose, eye, and cerebrospinal fluid. Testing of paired sera for evidence of infection in the infant or its mother may demonstrate seroconversion.

Screening policy

In the USA, the high frequency of neonatal herpes led in the early 1980s to recommendations that pregnant women should be screened by asking them about recurrent genital HSV infection, and that those with such a history should be tested weekly during the third trimester for virus shedding in the cervix. Caesarean section was then recommended if virus shedding was detected in the week of delivery or if lesions were present.[105] However, with the accumulation of evidence that neonatal herpes generally results from primary and often asymptomatic maternal infection in late pregnancy rather than from recurrence, it was realized that screening was likely to have prevented very few cases of neonatal infection at the cost of large numbers of additional caesarean deliveries.[106–108] On the basis of this information and the low risk of neonatal herpes in the absence of genital lesions in the mother, the policy of testing women with a past history of infection has been abandoned.

In the UK, where the prevalence of neonatal HSV infection probably lies between 2 and 10/100 000 births and is therefore much lower than in the USA, there is even less justification for the introduction of routine antenatal screening.[109] Among the 76 cases gathered by active surveillance mentioned above, in only about 25 per cent was there any indication of either a history of maternal genital infection or evidence of primary infection in pregnancy. Even when such information was available, it had usually come to light only after the diagnosis of neonatal herpes was made.[101] It follows that even if the neonatal prevalence was as high as 10/100 000, screening would not be justified, since it would lead to the prevention of fewer than 25 cases per million births at the cost of many unnecessary caesarean sections carried out to prevent vertical transmission.

CHLAMYDIA

Chlamydia is a common, sexually transmitted bacterial pathogen which can be transmitted from mother to infant by direct contact of the fetus with an infected endocervix during delivery. Most maternal infections are asymptomatic. Neonatal infection may result in conjunctivitis, pneumonia, and possibly otitis media, and has been associated with low birthweight.[110,111]

There is conflicting evidence on whether chlamydia is causally related to late spontaneous abortion, stillbirth, prematurity, and early neonatal death. Factors associated with increased risk of maternal chlamydia are also associated with a poorer pregnancy outcome and this needs to be taken into account when assessing the adverse effect of chlamydia infection in pregnancy.[112]

Perinatal infection

Neonatal infection occurs in up to two-thirds of infants exposed to maternal infection during delivery.[113] The major entry to the fetus is through the eye, leading to conjunctivitis. Subsequently the nasopharynx is colonized. Healing usually occurs without complications but nasopharyngeal infection may lead to pneumonia. Chlamydia is one of the most common causes of pneumonia during the first few months of life. Cases usually present with cough and tachypnoea but no fever. Chlamydia pneumonia is often but not always preceded by conjunctivitis.[113,114]

Frequency

The reported prevalence of genital chlamydia varies widely in different populations. In the USA 2.8–9.4 per cent of women screened at selected family planning clinics tested positive,[115] and chlamydia has been isolated from 20–30 per cent of women attending clinics for sexually transmitted diseases. Infection rates are high not only in women with a history of STDs or a partner with previous STD infection but also in young women, women with early onset sexual activity or multiple sexual partners, and women of single marital status.[116] In UK studies, infection was detected in 2–3 per cent of women of reproductive age attending for routine cervical smear tests[117] and in 4–12 per cent of attenders at genito-urinary medicine clinics and clinics for termination of pregnancy.[118]

American experience suggests that conjunctivitis occurs in 20–50 per cent and pneumonia in 10–20 per cent of infants exposed to infection during passage through the birth canal.[114] If the same rates occurred in Britain, and if infection was as prevalent in parturient women as in attenders for routine cervical smears, the prevalence of clinical infection in all infants would be of the order of 1 per cent. Without data on the overall prevalence of infection in parturient women, and on the incidence of clinical disease in exposed infants in Britain, one cannot be more precise.

Infants born by caesarean section are at low risk of acquiring infection unless premature rupture of the membranes has occurred.

Intervention

Chlamydia infections respond well to erythromycin. It follows that most cases of neonatal infection could be prevented by treating carrier mothers before delivery if they could be reliably identified by screening, and that when neonatal infection occurs long-term sequelae are rare if prompt treatment is given. This treatment should include local application of erythromycin therapy to eradicate potential nasopharyngeal colonisation.

Screening and diagnostic tests

There is a lack of inexpensive, widely available, accurate tests for chlamydia infection; and which if any of these tests should be used for antenatal screening remains uncertain, despite recent improvements in the laboratory kits available and the development of non-invasive urine-based kits. During the last decade, chlamydia trachomatis infections have generally been detected by cell culture or by enzyme immunoassays applied to cervical samples. Results have shown wide laboratory variation, and are highly dependent on sampling techniques and the handling of specimens. Culture has been regarded as the gold standard against which non-cultural methods should be compared. However, although false-positive results are not a problem with culture, false-negative findings are. It probably detects fewer than 70 per cent of infections. Conventional non-cultural tests also under-estimate the prevalence of infection. It has been proposed that specimens be regarded as positive if either cell culture or both of two non-culture tests give positive results, and that this combination of procedures be used as an 'expanded gold standard' against which to evaluate the performance of other tests. The recently developed ligase chain reaction assay, which is an *in vitro* nucleic acid amplification technique that exponentially amplifies selected DNA sequences, appears to yield few false-negative or false-positive results when compared with the 'expanded gold standard', and its use in detecting infection from urine samples is encouraging. However, this test is expensive and not widely available, and the optimal strategy for screening and diagnosis remains to be determined.[119]

Screening policy

The ease with which neonatal chlamydia infections can be diagnosed and treated suggests that antenatal screening would only be justified if it could be done more economically than the treatment of neonatal infections. In the USA, a cost–benefit analysis estimated this to be the case when cervical infection rates were above 6 per cent.[114]

Although the USA has been the scene of strong support for screening pregnant women systematically for chlamydia infection, this is not currently practised or contemplated. If it was to be introduced, it would be most appropriate during the third trimester. With earlier screening, more women would be treated unnecessarily (since carriage is intermittent) whilst infection arising during late pregnancy would be missed. Given the costliness of universal screening, selective testing of high-risk groups has been proposed; but even this would be premature without more information. Priority needs to be given to determining the prevalence of infection in neonates, and to comparing the cost-effectiveness of the different screening tests and relating this to the cost of treatment in the newborn, so as to arrive at a rational screening policy.

GROUP B STREPTOCOCCAL INFECTION

Group B streptococcal infection is an important cause of neonatal bacterial sepsis. Healthy women may carry group B streptococci and be a source of peripartum infection of their offspring. There is also some evidence that colonization in pregnancy may be associated with chorioamnionitis, premature rupture of the membranes, and preterm delivery.[120] There has been an ongoing debate, particularly in the USA, about whether or not pregnant women should routinely be tested for colonization of the birth canal by group B streptococci, so that those found to be positive could be prescribed antibiotics to reduce transmission of infection to the infant at birth.

Perinatal infection

Group B streptococcal disease in infants can be divided into early onset disease (<7 days), and late onset disease (7–89 days). The majority of infections, about 80 per cent, constitute early onset disease in which the case fatality rate is about 6 per cent.

Prematurity is a major cause of death in these cases. Two-thirds of early onset disease presents within six hours of birth and the most common manifestations are neonatal sepsis and pneumonia.[121] Immature infants are at high risk, as are babies born after prolonged rupture of the membranes, amniotic colonization, or maternal fever during labour, which increase the duration of exposure and/or the concentration of bacteria.

Late onset disease usually manifests as meningitis. The route of infection is peripartum exposure in about 50 per cent of cases. In the remainder infection is acquired from nosocomial or community contacts.

Frequency

There is considerable geographical variation in colonization rates. In the USA about 15–40 per cent of pregnant women are asymptomatic carriers of group B streptococci. The vertical transmission rate based on positive culture is between 40 and 73 per cent, and 1–2 per cent of culture-positive infants (3 per 1000 infants born) develop disease.[120] Based on active case surveillance in the USA an estimated 7600 cases of disease and 310 deaths due to infection (a case fatality ratio of 4 per cent) occurred in infants of 90 days or younger in 1990.

In western Europe, invasive group B streptococcal infection is less common in neonates (generally less than 1/1000 births and only 0.3/1000 in a nationwide British study), possibly because of lower rates of vaginal carriage (<10 per cent) and of premature delivery.[122]

Intervention

Most maternal and neonatal infections with group B streptococci respond to antibiotics such as penicillin. In a randomized trial of intrapartum ampicillin in carrier women with premature onset of labour or rupture of membranes[123] colonization was observed in 51 per cent of control neonates and in 9 per cent whose mothers had been treated, suggesting that the antibiotic reduced the vertical transmission rate by more than 80 per cent; and 6 per cent of control neonates but none born after treatment were affected by bacteraemia. According to another randomized trial, vaginal lavage with chlorhexidine during labour may reduce the risk of clinical disease in the children of carrier mothers.[124]

Screening and diagnostic tests

Culture of swabs from the genital tract is the standard method of identifying carrier women. Rapid diagnostic tests which use latex agglutination or ELISA technology to identify group-specific polysaccharide antigen have also been developed. These rapid tests have lower detection rates and higher false-positive rates than occur with cultures, but they have the advantage that results may be available in less than an hour.

Screening policy

In the USA, the high prevalence of the carrier state and the economic burden that this imposed led the American Academy of Pediatrics to recommend in 1992 that all pregnant women should be screened for group B streptococci at 26–28 weeks of gestation, and that those with positive results in whom risk factors for vertical transmission were also present should be treated. Subsequently the American College of Obstetricians and Gynecologists recommended against routine antenatal screening except in populations where the prevalence of infection was extremely high, proposing instead that women with risk factors such as onset of labour before 37 weeks, rupture of the membranes more than 18 hours before the beginning of labour, or maternal fever during labour should have swabs taken from the genital tract and tested, so that women with positive results could receive intrapartum antibiotics such as ampicillin.[120,125]

The main reason for arguing against routine antenatal screening followed by antibiotic treatment of all infected women is that clinical disease as a result of infection only occurs in about 1 per cent of their infants. This policy is therefore expensive in relation to the number who benefit, and may do more harm than good by leading both to adverse reactions to the antibiotic used and to the development of antibiotic-resistant organisms. If clinical infection subsequently develops, effective antibiotic treatment may then be difficult.

Given that the proportion of all British neonates reported to be affected by clinical disease due to group B streptococci (0.3/1000) is only a tenth of the USA figure, the case against introducing universal maternal screening is even stronger in the UK. Here too, a more economic approach would be to restrict testing for carrier status to women in whom clinical indications such as premature onset of labour are present, using rapid diagnostic tests to enable those found to be carriers to begin chemotherapy as soon as possible. The future may lie with the use of vaccines against the group B streptococcus, which are currently under development.

CONCLUSION

In this chapter, we have focused on the prevention of neonatal disease rather than on the prevention of maternal cases. We summarize our observations and conclusions in Table 7.3. It gives estimates of the proportions of British infants affected in the absence of screening, and the impact that screening would have on these proportions. We conclude that antenatal screening for HIV, the hepatitis B virus, and possibly *Treponema pallidum*, are justified in part or all of the UK. Testing pregnant women for rubella susceptibility is difficult to justify except in some ethnic minorities. There are no convincing reasons for screening all pregnant women by laboratory tests for infection with cytomegalovirus, *Toxoplasma gondii*, herpes simplex virus, *Chlamydia trachomatis*, or group B streptococci, although tests for some of these agents (e.g. herpes simplex virus and *C. trachomatis*) may be appropriate in high-risk groups.

The prevalence of the infections considered varies from country to country and between populations within a country, and as a result policies also may justifiably vary. For example, the prevalence of hepatitis B carrier mothers is much higher in some countries than in others. Even within Europe, much higher rates occur in the more southern countries than in Scandinavia and the UK. In view of this, a common European approach to hepatitis B screening in pregnancy is not appropriate. Within the UK, universal antenatal testing for hepatitis B antigens seems to be indicated; but there is a strong case for confining the screening of all pregnant women for HIV infection to selected areas.

Toxoplasmosis is another infection for which antenatal screening is not equally

Table 7.3 Summary of effectiveness of methods of antenatal or neonatal screening for infections if applied in the United Kingdom

	Rubella	Syphilis	HIV infection	Hepatitis B	Cytomegalovirus infection	Toxoplasmosis	Herpes simplex	Chlamydia trachomatis infection	Group B streptococcal infection
Aim of screening	Prevention of maternal infection	Prevention or early treatment of fetal infection	Prevention or early treatment of fetal infection	Early treatment of neonatal infection	Prevention of birth of affected fetuses / Early detection of affected children	Prevention of early treatment of fetal infection	Prevention of intra-partum infection of child	Prevention of intra-partum infection of child	Prevention of intra-partum infection of child
Method of screening	Blood test for maternal antibody	Blood test for maternal antibodies	Blood test for maternal antibodies	Blood test for maternal antigen	Blood test for maternal antibodies / Virus isolation from child	Blood test for maternal antibodies	Virus isolation from maternal swab	Virus isolation from maternal swab	Culture or test for antigen in maternal swab
Suggested management of screen-positive	Postnatal immunization	Chemotherapy	Chemotherapy: no breast feeding; elective caesarian section	Immunoglobulin plus vaccination	Termination of pregnancy / Surveillance for sensory or motor disabilities	Chemotherapy	Caesarean section	Chemotherapy	Chemotherapy
Percentage of cases of disease in fetus or child that are preventable by above policy[a]	≤ 25%	70%	≥ 80%	90%	_c / 0%	_c,e	≤ 25%	_f	> 80%

Table 7.3 Continued

	Rubella	Syphilis	HIV infection	Hepatitis B	Cytomegalovirus infection	Toxoplasmosis	Herpes simplex	Chlamydia trachomatis infection	Group B streptococcal infection
Estimated number of cases of disease per million births:-									
(a) occurring in the absence of screening	12	20	100	140[b]	300	≤ 245	< 100	10 000	300
(b) preventable with screening	3	14	> 80	126	–	–	< 25	–	> 240
Case for screening	Weak	More information needed	Strong	Strong	Weak[d]	Weak[e]	Weak	More information needed[f,g]	Weak[g,h]

[a] Assumed to be 90 per cent for diseases for which treatment is effective but quantitative data not found.
[b] Assuming that 40 per cent of those infected will develop chronic liver disease.
[c] Varies with frequency with which seronegative women are retested.
[d] Positive test results leading to offer of termination would occur in 12–25 unaffected fetuses for every one with disease.
[e] Lack of reliable data on efficacy of treatment.
[f] Lack of reliable data on accuracy of screening.
[g] Neonates with clinical infection can be treated effectively.
[h] High false-positive rate (> 98 per cent); treatment can have maternal side-effects.

appropriate everywhere. In France, this infection is more prevalent than in England. As a result, only about 20 per cent of pregnant French women but 80 per cent of English are susceptible to infection, and the susceptible French women are at higher risk than the susceptible English ones of becoming infected during pregnancy. Repeat testing of all susceptible women throughout pregnancy is therefore both less costly and more productive in France than it would be in England.

Knowledge of the prevalence of the different infections is thus essential if rational decisions on screening policy are to be made.

In this chapter we have only considered those infections for which screening has been proposed. There are other infections that have the potential to damage the fetus or newborn infant, such as varicella zoster infection. These infections are uncommon in pregnancy, as most women of childbearing age are immune and those infected usually present with clinical manifestations or a history of contact. However, the list of conditions for which screening is being suggested continues to grow as diagnostic tools become more readily available and cheaper. Recent examples include hepatitis C and HTLV-1 infection.

REFERENCES

1. Leck, I. (1994). Structural birth defects. In *The Epidemiology of Childhood Diseases*, (ed. I.B. Pless), pp. 66–117. Oxford University Press, New York.
2. Miller, E. (1990). Rubella reinfection. *Archives of Disease in Childhood*, **65**, 820–1.
3. Tookey, P. A., and Peckham, C. S. (1999). Surveillance of congenital rubella in Great Britain, 1971–96. *British Medical Journal*, **318**, 769–70.
4. Miller, E. (1991). Rubella in the United Kingdom. *Epidemiology and Infection*, **107**, 31–42.
5. Miller, E., Craddock-Watson, J. E., and Pollock, T. M. (1982). Consequences of confirmed maternal rubella at successive stages of pregnancy. *Lancet*, **2**, 781–4.
6. Grilner, L., Forsgren, M., Barr, B., Bottiger, M., Danielsson, L., and de Verdier, C. (1983). Outcome of rubella during pregnancy with special reference to the 17th–24th weeks of gestation. *Scandinavian Journal of Infectious Diseases*, **15**, 321–5.
7. Peckham, C. S., Martin, J. A. M., Marshall, W. C., and Dudgeon, J. A. (1979). Congenital rubella deafness: a preventable disease. *Lancet*, **i**, 258–61.
8. Miller, E., Waight, P., Gay, N., Ramsay, M., Vurdien, J., *et al.* (1997). The epidemiology of rubella in England and Wales before and after the 1994 measles and rubella vaccination campaign; fourth joint report from the PHLS and the National Congenital Rubella Surveillance Programme. *Communicable Diseases Report*, **7**, 26–32.
9. STD Section, HIV and STD Division, PHLS Communicable Disease Surveillance Centre, with the PHLS Syphilis Working Group (1998). *Report to the National Screening Committee. Antenatal syphilis screening in the UK—a systematic review and national options appraisal with recommendations*. Public Health Laboratory Service, London.
10. Fiumara, N. (1952). The incidence of prenatal syphilis at the Boston City Hospital. *New England Journal of Medicine*, **247**, 48–52.
11. Wendel, G. D. (1988). Gestational and congenital syphilis. *Clinics in Perinatology*, **15**, 287–303.
12. Stray-Pedersen, B. (1983). Economic evaluation of maternal screening to prevent congenital syphilis. *Sexually Transmitted Diseases*, **10**, 167–72.

13. Ewing, C. I., Roberts, C., Davidson, D. C., and Arya, O. P. (1985). Early congenital syphilis still occurs. *Archives of Disease in Childhood*, **60**, 1128–33.

14. Centers for Disease Control (1992). *Congenital syphilis case investigation and reporting form instructions.* Centers for Disease Control.

15. Hurtig, A.-K., Nicoll, A., Carne, C., Lissauer, T., Connor, N., Webster, J.P., and Ratcliffe, L. (1998). Syphilis in pregnant women and their children in the United Kingdom: results from national clinician reporting surveys 1994–7. *British Medical Journal*, **317**, 1617–19.

16. Rolfs, R. T., and Nakshima, A. K. (1990). Epidemiology of primary and secondary syphilis in the United States, 1981 through 1989. *Journal of the American Medical Association*, **264**, 1432–7.

17. Ingall, D., Sanchez, P.J., and Musher, D.M. (1995). Syphilis. In *Infections Diseases of the Fetus and Newborn Infant* (ed. J.S. Remington and J.D. Klein), 4th edn, pp. 524–64. Saunders, Philadelphia.

18. Larsen, S. A., Hunter, E. F., and Kraus, S. J. (1990). *A manual of tests for syphilis.* American Public Health Association, Washington, DC.

19. Young, H. (1992). Syphilis: new diagnostic directions. *International Journal of STD and AIDS*, **3**, 391–413.

20. Williams, K. (1985). Screening for syphilis in pregnancy: an assessment of the costs and benefits. *Community Medicine*, **7**, 37–42.

21. Bowell, P., Mayne, K., Puckett, A., Entwistle, C., and Selkon, J. (1989). Serological screening tests for syphilis in pregnancy: results of a five year study (1983–7) in the Oxford Region. *Journal of Clinical Pathology*, **42**, 1281–4.

22. Garland, S. M., and Kelly, V. N. (1989). Is antenatal screening for syphilis worth while? *Medical Journal of Australia*, **151**, 368–72.

23. Welch, J. (1998). Antenatal screening for syphilis—still important in preventing disease. *British Medical Journal*, **317**, 1605–6.

24. Nicoll, A., and Moisley, C. (1994). Antenatal screening for syphilis. *British Medical Journal*, **308**, 1253–4.

25. Kind, C., Brandle, B., Wyler, C-A., Calame, A., Rudin, C., Schaad, U. B., Schupback, J., Senn, H-P., Perrin, L., and Matter, L. (Swiss Neonatal HIV Study Group) (1992). Epidemiology of vertically transmitted HIV-1 infection in Switzerland: results of a nationwide prospective study. *European Journal of Pediatrics*, **151**, 442–8.

26. European Collaborative Study (1994). Caesarean section and risk of vertical transmission of HIV-1 infection. *Lancet*, **343**, 1464–7.

27. Mayaux, M-J., Blanche, S., Rouzioux, C., Le Chenadec, J., Chambrin, V., Firtion, G., Allemon, M-C., Vilmer, E., Vigneron, N. C., Tricoire, J., Guillot, F., and Courpotin, C. (French Pediatric HIV Infection Study Group) (1995). Maternal factors associated with perinatal HIV-1 transmission: The French Cohort Study: 7 years of follow-up observation. *Journal of Acquired Immune Deficiency Syndromes and Human Retrovirology*, **8**, 188–94.

28. Newell, M.L., and Peckham, C.S. (1993). Risk factors for vertical transmission of HIV-1 and early markers of infection in children. *Aids*, **7**, S591–7.

29. European Mode of Delivery Collaboration (1999). Elective caesarian section versus vaginal delivery in preventing HIV-1 transmission: a randomised clinical trial. *Lancet*, **353**, 1035–9.

30. European Collaborative Study (1994). Natural history of vertically acquired human immunodeficiency virus-1 infection. *Pediatrics*, **94**, 815–19.

31. Dunn, D. T., Brandt, C. D., Krivine, A., Cassol, S. A., Roques, P., Borkowsky, W., *et al.* (1995). The sensitivity of HIV-1 DNA polymerase chain reaction in the neonatal period and the relative contributions of intra-uterine and intra-partum transmission. *AIDS*, **9**, F7-F11.

32. PHLS AIDS and STD Centre, Scottish Centre for Infection and Environmental Health, Institute of Child Health, London and Oxford Haemophilia Centre (1999). AIDS and HIV infection in the United Kingdom: monthly report. *Communicable Disease Report*, **9**, 45–8.

33. Connor, E. M., Sperling, R. S., Gelber, R., Kiselev, P., Scott, G., O'Sullivan, M. J., *et al.* (1994). Reduction of maternal–infant transmission of human immunodeficiency virus type 1 with zidovudine treatment. *New England Journal of Medicine*, **331**, 1173–80.

34. Sperling, R.S., Shapiro, D.E., Coombs, R.W., Todd, J.A., Herman, S.A., McSherry, G.D., *et al.* (1996). Maternal viral load, zidovudine treatment, and the risk of transmission of human immunodeficiency virus type I from mother to infant. *New England Journal of Medicine*, **335**, 1621–9.

35. Centers for Disease Control and Prevention (1994). Recommendations for the use of zidovudine to reduce perinatal transmission of human immunodeficiency virus. *Morbidity and Mortality Weekly Report*, **43 RR-11**, 1–20.

36. World Health Organization (1992). Consensus statement from the WHO/UNICEF: Consultation on HIV transmission and breast-feeding. *Weekly Epidemiological Record*, **67**, 177–9.

37. Anon. (1997). Screening brief: AIDS from maternally transmitted HIV infection. *Journal of Medical Screening*, **4**, 177.

38. Dunn, D. T., Nicoll, A., Holland, F. J., and Davison, C. F. (1995). How much paediatric HIV infection could be prevented by antenatal HIV testing? *Journal of Medical Screening*, **2**, 35–40.

39. Department of Health (1992). *Guidelines for offering voluntary named HIV antibody testing to women receiving antenatal care.* DoH, London.

40. NHS Executive (1999). Reducing mother to baby transmission of HIV. *Health Service Circular* 1999/183.

41. Nicoll, A., and Peckham, C. (1999). Reducing vertical transmission of HIV in the UK. *British Medical Journal*, **319**, 1211–12.

42. Stevens, C. E., Beasley, R. P., Tsui, J., and Lee, W. L. (1975). Vertical tranmission of hepatitis B antigen in Taiwan. *New England Journal of Medicine*, **292**, 771–4.

43. Davis, L. G., Weber, D. J., and Lemon, S. M. (1989). Horizontal transmission of Hepatitis B virus. *Lancet*, **i**, 889–93.

44. Burk, R. D., Hwang, L., Ho, G. Y. F., Shafritz, D. A., and Beasley, R. P. (1994). Outcome of perinatal hepatitis B virus exposure is dependent on maternal virus load. *Journal of Infectious Diseases*, **170**, 1418–23.

45. Stevens, C. E., Neurath, R. E., Beasley, R. P., and Szmuness, W. (1979). HBe Ag and anti-HBe detection by radioimmunoassay: correlation with vertical transmission of hepatitis B virus in Taiwan. *Journal of Medical Virology*, **3**, 237–41.

46. Edmunds, W.J., Medley, G.F., Nokes, D., Hall, A.J., and Whittle, H.C. (1993). The influence of age on the development of the hepatitis B carrier state. *Proceedings of the Royal Society of London B*, **253**, 197–201.

47. Jordan, R., and Law, M. (1997). An appraisal of the efficacy and cost-effectiveness of antenatal screening for hepatitis B. *Journal of Medical Screening*, **4**, 117–27.

48. Beasley, R. P. (1982). Hepatitis B virus as the etiologic agent in hepatocellular carcinoma: Epidemiologic considerations. *Hepatology*, **2**, 21S-26S.
49. Krugman, S. (1988). Hepatitis B virus and the neonate. *Annals of the New York Academy of Sciences*, **549**, 129–34.
50. Grosheide, P. M., Wladimiroff, J. W., Heijtink, R. A., Mazel, J. A., Christiaens, G.C., Nuijten, A. S., and Schalm, S. W. (Dutch Study Group On Prevention of Neonatal Hepatitis) (1995). Proposal for routine antenatal screening at 14 weeks for hepatitis B surface antigen. *British Medical Journal*, **311**, 1197–9.
51. McMenamin, J. (1996). Hepatitis B in the UK: who is at risk, who succumbs? Role of screening. In *Prevention of Hepatitis B in the Newborn, Children and Adolescents*, (ed. A. Zuckerman), pp. 1–8. The Royal College of Physicians, London
52. Harrison, T.J., Bal, V., Wheeler, E.J., Meacock, T.J., Harrison, J.F., and Zuckerman, A.J. (1985). Hepatitis B virus DNA and e antigen in serum from blood donors in the United Kingdom positive for hepititis B surface antigen. *British Medical Journal*, **290**, 663–4.
53. Sangfelt, P., Reichard, O., Lidman, K., von Sydow, M., and Forsgren, M. (1995). Prevention of hepatitis B by immunization of the newborn infant—a long term follow-up study in Stockholm, Sweden. *Scandinavian Journal of Infectious Diseases*, **27**, 3–7.
54. Arevalo, J. A., and Washington, A. E. (1988). Cost-effectiveness of prenatal screening and immunization for hepatitis B virus. *Journal of the American Medical Association*, **259**, 365–9.
55. Cruz, A. C., Frentzen, B. H., and Behnke, M. (1987). Hepatitis B: A case for prenatal screening of all patients. *American Journal of Obstetrics and Gynecology*, **156**, 1180–3.
56. Chrystie, I., Sumner, D., Palmer, S., Kenney, A., and Banatvala, J. (1992). Screening of pregnant women for evidence of current hepatitis B infection: selective or universal? *Health Trends*, **24**, 13–15.
57. Dwyer, M.J., and McIntyre, P.G. (1996). Antenatal screening for hepatitis B surface antigen: an appraisal of its value in a low prevalence area. *Epidemiology and Infection*, **117**, 121–31.
58. NHS Executive (1998). Screening of pregnant women for hepatitis B and immunisation of babies at risk. *Health Service Circular* 1998/127.
59. Anon. (1998). Screening brief: hepatoma and chronic liver disease from maternally transmitted hepatitis B infection. *Journal of Medical Screening*, **5**, 54.
60. Grosheide, P. M., Klokman-Houweling, J. M., Conyn-van Spaendonck, M. A. E., and the National Hepatitis B Steering Committee (1995). Programme for preventing perinatal hepatitis B infection through screening of pregnant women and immunization of infants of infected mothers in the Netherlands, 1989–92. *British Medical Journal*, **311**, 1200–2.
61. Schalm, S. W., Mazel, A., de Gast, G. C., Heytink, R. A., Botman, M. J., Banffer, J. R. J., *et al.* (1989). Prevention of hepatitis B infection in newborns through mass screening and delayed vaccination of all infants of mothers with hepatitis B surface antigen. *Pediatrics*, **83**, 1041–7.
62. Stroffolini, T., Pasquini, P., and Mele, A. (Collaborating Group Against Hepatitis B in Italy) (1989). A nationwide vaccination programme in Italy against hepatitis B virus infection in infants of hepatitis B surface antigen carrier mothers. *Vaccine*, **7**, 152–4.
63. Advisory Committee Immunization Practices (1991). Hepatitis B virus: a comprehensive strategy for eliminating transmission in the United States through universal childhood vaccination. *Morbidity and Mortality Weekly Report*, **40**, RR–13, 1–25.

64. Kane, M. A., Hadler, S. C., Margolis, H. S., and Maynard, J. E. (1988). Routine prenatal screening for hepatitis B surface antigen. *Journal of the American Medical Association*, **259**, 408–9.

65. Hesketh, L.M., Rowlatt, J.D., Gay, N.J., Morgan-Capner, P., and Miller, E. (1997). Childhood infection with hepatitis A and B viruses in England and Wales. *Communicable Disease Review*, 7, R60-R63.

66. Peckham, C. S., Johnson, C., Ades, A., Pearl, K., and Chin, K. S. (1987). The early acquisition of cytomegalovirus infection. *Archives of Disease in Childhood*, **62**, 780–5.

67. Peckham, C. S. (1991). Cytomegalovirus infection: congenital and neonatal disease. *Scandinavian Journal of Infectious Disease*, **78**, Suppl., 82–7.

68. Stagno, S., Pass, R. F., and Dworsky, M. E. (1982). Congenital cytomegalovirus infection: the relative importance of primary and recurrent maternal infection. *New England Journal of Medicine*, **306**, 945–9.

69. Rutter, D., Griffiths, P. D., and Trompeter, R. S. (1985). Cytomegalic inclusion disease after recurrent maternal infection. *Lancet*, **ii**, 1182.

70. Pass, R. F., Stagno, S., Myers, G. J., and Alford, C. A. (1980). Outcome of symptomatic congenital cytomegalovirus infection: results of long-term longitudinal follow-up. *Journal of Pediatrics*, **66**, 758–62.

71. Ramsey, M. E. B., Miller, E., and Peckham, C. S. (1991). Outcome of confirmed symptomatic congenital cytomegalovirus infection. *Archives of Disease in Childhood*, **66**, 1068–9.

72. Ahlfors, K., Ivarsson, S., Johnsson, T., and Svanberg, L. (1979). A prospective study on congenital and acquired cytomegalovirus infections in infants. *Scandinavian Journal of Infectious Diseases*, **11**, 177–8.

73. Saigal, S., Lunyk, O., Larke, R. P. B., and Chernesky, M. A. (1982). The outcome in children with congenital cytomegalovirus infection. *American Journal of Diseases of Children*, **136**, 896–905.

74. Peckham, C. S., Stark, O., Dudgeon, J. A., Martin, J. A. M., and Hawkins, G. (1987). Congenital cytomegalovirus infection: a cause of sensorineural hearing loss. *Archives of Disease in Childhood*, **62**, 1233–7.

75. Stagno, S., Pass, R. F., Dworsky, M. E., and Alford, C. A. (1983). Congenital and perinatal cytomegalovirus infections. *Seminars in Perinatology*, **7**, 31–42.

76. Grose, C., Meehan, T., and Weiner, C. (1992). Prenatal diagnosis of congenital cytomegalovirus infection by virus isolation after amniocentesis. *Pediatric Infectious Disease Journal*, **11**, 605–7.

77. Desmonts, G., and Couvreur, J. (1974). Toxoplasmosis in pregnancy and its transmission to the foetus. *Bulletin of the New York Academy of Medicine*, **50**, 146–59.

78. Remington, J. S., McLeod, R., and Desmonts, G. (1995). Toxoplasmosis. In *Infectious Diseases of the Fetus and Newborn Infant*. (ed. J. S. Remington and J. O. Klein), pp. 140–267. Saunders, Philadelphia.

79. Mombro, M., Perathoner, C., Leone, A., Nicocia, M., Rugenini, A. M., Zotti, C., *et al.* (1995). Congenital toxoplasmosis: 10-year follow up. *European Journal of Pediatrics*, **154**, 635–9.

80. Roizen, N., Swisher, C. N., Stein, M. A., Hopkins, J., Boyer, K. M., Holfels, E., *et al.* (1995). Neurologic and developmental outcome in treated congenital toxoplasmosis. *Pediatrics*, **95**, 11–20.

81. Hall, S. M. (1992). Congenital toxoplasmosis. *British Medical Journal*, **305**, 291–7.

82. Gilbert, R. E., Tookey, P. A., Cubitt, W. D., Ades, A. E., Masters, J., and Peckham, C. S. (1993). Prevalence of toxoplasma IgG among pregnant women in west London according to country of birth and ethnic group. *British Medical Journal*, **306**, 185.

83. Walker, J., Nokes, D. J., and Jennings, R. (1992). Longitudinal study of toxoplasma sero-prevalence in South Yorkshire. *Epidemiology and Infection*, **108**, 99–106.

84. Ades, A. E. (1992). Methods for estimating the incidence of primary infection in pregnancy: a reappraisal of toxoplasmosis and cytomegalovirus data. *Epidemiology and Infection*, **108**, 367–75.

85. Peckham, C. S., and Logan, S. (1993). Screening for toxoplasmosis during pregnancy. *Archives of Disease in Childhood*, **68**, 3–5.

86. Lappalainen, M., Koskiniemi, M., Hiilesmaa, V., Ammala, P., Teramo, K., Koskela, P., Lebech, M., Raivio, K. O., and Hedman, K. (The Study Group) (1995). Outcome of children after maternal primary toxoplasma infection during pregnancy with emphasis on avidity of specific IgG. *Pediatric Infectious Disease Journal*, **14**, 354–61.

87. Editorial. (1990). Antenatal screening for toxoplasmosis in the UK. *Lancet*, **ii**, 346–8.

88. O'Callaghan, E., Sham, P., Takei, N., Glover, G., and Murray, R. M. (1991). Schizophrenia after prenatal exposure to 1957 A2 influenza epidemic. *Lancet*, **337**, 1248–50.

89. Royal College of Obstetricians and Gynaecologists (1992). *Prenatal Screening for Toxoplasmosis in the UK: Report of a Multidisciplinary Working Group*, p. 14. RCOG, London.

90. Walpole, I. R., Hodgen, N., and Bower, C. (1991). Congenital toxoplasmosis: a large survey in Western Australia. *Medical Journal of Australia*, **154**, 720–4.

91. Raeber, P.A., Biedermann, K., Just, M., and Zuber, P. (1995). Prevention of congenital toxoplasmosis in Europe. *Schweizerische Medizinische Wochenschift Supplementum*, **65**, 96S-102S.

92. South, M. A., Tompkins, W. A. F., Morris, C. R., and Rawls, W. E. (1969). Congenital malformations of the central nervous system associated with genital type 2 herpes virus. *Journal of Pediatrics*, **75**, 13–18.

93. Florman, A. L., Gershon, A. A., Blackett, P. R., and Nahmias, A. J. (1973). Intrauterine infection with herpes simplex virus: resultant congenital malformations. *Journal of the American Medical Association*, **225**, 129–32.

94. Arvin, A., Hensleigh, P., and Prober, C. (1986). Failure of antepartum maternal cultures to predict the infants risk of exposure to herpes simplex virus at delivery. *New England Journal of Medicine*, **315**, 796–800.

95. Prober, C. G., Sullender, W. M., Yasukawa, L. L., Av, D. S., Yeager, A., and Arvin, A. M. (1987). Low risk of herpes simplex virus infections in neonates exposed to the virus at the time of vaginal delivery to mothers with recurrent genital herpes simplex virus infection. *New England Journal of Medicine*, **316**, 240–4.

96. Prober, C., Hensleigh, P., Boucher, F., Yasukawa, L., Au, D., and Arvin, A. (1988). Use of routine viral cultures at delivery to identify neonates exposed to herpes simplex virus. *New England Journal of Medicine*, **318**, 887–91.

97. Boucher, F. D., Yasukawa, L., Bronzan, R. N., Hensleigh, P. A., Arvin, A. M., and Prober, C. G. (1990). A prospective evaluation of primary genital herpes simplex virus type 2 infections acquired during pregnancy. *Pediatric Infectious Disease Journal*, **9**, 499–504.

98. Brown, Z. A., Benedetti, J., Ashley, R., *et al.* (1991). Neonatal herpes simplex virus infection in relation to asymptomatic maternal infection at the time of labor. *New England Journal of Medicine*, **324**, 1247–52.

99. Whitley, R. J., and Arvin, A. M. (1994). Herpes Simplex virus infection. In *Infectious diseases of the fetus and newborn*, (ed J. S. Remington and J. O. Klein), pp. 354–76. Saunders, Philadelphia.

100. Whitley, R., Arvin, A., Prober, C., Corey, L., Burchett, S., Plotkin, S., *et al.* (1991). Predictors of morbidity and mortality in neonates with herpes simplex virus infections. *New England Journal of Medicine*, **324**, 450–4.

101. Tookey, P., and Peckham, C. S. (1996). Neonatal HSV infection in the British Isles. *Paediatric and Perinatal Epidemiology*, **10**, 432–42.

102. Malm, G., Berg, U., and Forsgren, M. (1995). Neonatal herpes simplex: clinical findings and outcome in relation to type of maternal infection. *Acta Paediatrica*, **84**, 256–60.

103. American College of Obstetricians and Gynecologists (1988). Perinatal herpes simplex virus infections. *American College of Obstetricians and Gynecologists Technical Bulletin*, **122**, 1–21.

104. Anon. (1989). Sexually transmitted diseases treatment guidelines. *Morbidity and Mortality Weekly Report*, **38**, 8–16.

105. Committee on Fetus and Newborn (1980). Perinatal herpes simplex virus infection. *Pediatrics*, **66**, 147–8.

106. Binkin, N. J., Koplan, J. P., and Cates, W. (1984). Preventing neonatal herpes: the value of weekly viral cultures in pregnant women with recurrent genital herpes. *Journal of the American Medical Association*, **251**, 2816–21.

107. Libman, M.D., Dascal, A., Kramer, M.S., and Mendelson, J. (1991). Strategies for the prevention of neonatal infection with herpes simplex virus: a decision analysis. *Reviews of Infectious Diseases*, **13**, 1093–104.

108. Prober, C. and Arvin A.M. (1995). Perinatal herpes: current status and obstetric management strategies: the pediatric perspective. *Pediatric Infectious Disease Journal*, **14**, 832–5.

109. Anon. (1988). Virological screening for herpes simplex virus during pregnancy. *Lancet*, **i**, 722–3.

110. Schaefer, C., Harrison, R., Boyce, W. T., and Lewis, M. (1985). Illnesses in infants born to women with *Chlamydia trachomatis* infection. A prospective study. *American Journal of Diseases of Children*, **139**, 127–33.

111. Hammerschlag, M.R., Cummings, C., Roblin, P. M., Williams, T. H., and Delke, J. (1989). Efficacy of neonatal ocular prophylaxis for the prevention of chlamydial and gonococcal conjunctivitis. *New England Journal of Medicine*, **320**, 769–72.

112. Preece, P. M., Anderson, J. M., and Thompson, R. G. (1989). Chlamydia trachomatis infection in infants: a prospective study. *Archives of Disease in Childhood*, **64**, 525–9.

113. Schachter, J., Grossman, M., Sweet, R. L., Holt, J., Jordan, C. X., and Bishop, E. (1986). Prospective study of perinatal transmission of *Chlamydia trachomatis*. *Journal of the American Medical Association*, **255**, 3374–7.

114. Schachter, J., and Grossman, M. (1995). Chlamydia. In *Infectious Disease of the Fetus and Newborn Infant*, (ed. J. S. Remington and J. O. Klein), pp. 657–67. Saunders, Philadelphia.

115. Centers for Disease Control (1997). *Chlamydia trachomatis* genital infections: United States 1995. *Morbidity and Mortality Weekly Report*, **46**, 193–8.

116. Centers for Disease Control. (1985). Policy guidelines for prevention and control: *Chlamydia trachomatis* infections. *Morbidity and Mortality Weekly Report*, **34**, 53S-74S.

117. Grun, L., Tassano-Smith, J., Carder, C., Johnson, A.M., Robinson, R., Murray, E., *et al.* (1997). Comparison of two methods of screening for genital chlamydial infection in women attending in general practice: cross-sectional survey. *British Medical Journal*, **315**, 226–30.

118. Fish, A.N.J., Fairweather, D.V.I., Oriel, J.D., and Ridgway, G.L. (1989). *Chlamydia trachomatis* infection in a gynaecology clinic population: identification of high risk groups and the value of contact tracing. *European Journal of Obstetrics, Gynaecology and Reproductive Biology*, **31**, 67–74.

119. Taylor-Robinson, D. (1996). Tests for infection with *Chlamydia trachomatis*. *International Journal of STD and AIDS*, **7**, 19–25.

120. American Academy of Pediatrics Committee on Infectious Diseases and Committee on Fetus and Newborn (1992). Guidelines for prevention of group B streptococcal (GBS) infection by chemoprophylaxis. *Pediatrics*, **90**, 775–8.

121. Payne, N. R., Burke, B. A., Day, D. L., Christenson, P. D., Thompson, T. R., and Ferrieri, P. (1988). Correlation of clinical and pathologic findings in early onset neonatal Group B streptococcal infection with disease severity and prediction of outcome. *Pediatric Infectious Disease Journal*, **7**, 836–47.

122. Mayon-White, T. R. (1985). The incidence of GBS disease in neonates in different countries. *Antibiotics and Chemotherapy*, **35**, 17–27.

123. Boyer, K. M., and Gotoff, S. P. (1986). Prevention of early-onset neonatal group B streptococcal disease with selective intrapartum chemoprophylaxis. *New England Journal of Medicine*, **314**, 1665–9.

124. Burman, L. G., Christensen, P., Christensen, K., Fryklund, B., Helgesson, A-M., Svenningsen, M. W., and Tullus, K. (Swedish Chlorhexidine Study Group) (1992). Prevention of excess neonatal morbidity associated with group B streptococci by vaginal chlorhexidine disinfection during labour. *Lancet*, **340**, 65–9.

125. Towers, C. V. (1995). Group B streptococcus: the US controversy. *Lancet*, **346**, 197–9.

8 Disorders associated with hyperglycaemia in pregnancy

R. J. Jarrett

INTRODUCTION

The maternal and fetal risks associated with hyperglycaemia are almost invariably described in relation to diagnostic categories—insulin-dependent diabetes mellitus (IDDM), non-insulin-dependent diabetes mellitus (NIDDM), and gestational diabetes mellitus (GDM), the definitions of which are listed below:

1. Insulin-dependent diabetes mellitus (IDDM: type 1 diabetes): A form of diabetes with peak incidence in adolescence. Usually presents with classical symptoms–thirst, polyuria, and weight loss, sometimes with symptoms/signs of ketoacidosis. Several circulating antibodies to body constituents, including the islet cells, may be found. Associated strongly with certain HLA loci and variants.

2. Non-insulin-dependent diabetes mellitus (NIDDM: type 2 diabetes): Uncommon before age 30 years; thereafter increases in incidence with age. Strong genetic component to aetiology. Commonly associated with obesity, particularly abdominal obesity. Often asymptomatic and diagnosed by case finding/screening.

3. Gestational diabetes mellitus (GDM): Usually defined currently as diabetes or glucose intolerance first recognized in pregnancy. The WHO Study Group[1] recommends that the criteria and classification (into Impaired Glucose Tolerance (IGT) and NIDDM, respectively) used in adults generally should also be used for pregnant women. Other bodies recommend a version of the criteria originally proposed in the United States based on a glucose tolerance test and which includes both gestational glucose intolerance and NIDDM within the same category.

Most of the data in the literature relate to IDDM in Europid (of European origin[2]) women, in whom IDDM is the predominant form of diabetes during the reproductive years. However, in many other ethnic groups—South Asians, Hispanic Americans, Native Americans, Polynesians, Micronesians—NIDDM is not only substantially more frequent than in Europid populations, but presents earlier, so that it is the more common form of diabetes in women of reproductive age.[3]

The main question considered in this chapter is whether screening in order to identify new cases of diabetes of any kind in pregnancy is worthwhile. In IDDM the benefits of good blood glucose control during pregnancy seem clear, but the clinical manifestations enable most of the few cases that present in pregnancy to be recognized without screening. This discussion therefore focuses mainly on NIDDM and GDM and concludes that there is insufficient evidence to justify screening.

MATERNAL AND FETAL DISORDERS ASSOCIATED WITH HYPERGLYCAEMIA

Women with unrecognized IDDM are at risk of developing ketoacidosis, whether pregnant or not. As recently as 1950 perinatal mortality rates associated with IDDM exceeded 20 per cent.[4] These rates have declined subsequently and in some centres approach those in the general obstetric population.[4] The decline is attributed to more intensive glycaemic control throughout the pregnancy in addition to improved obstetric and neonatal management.

The frequency of both minor and major congenital abnormalities is increased in offspring of mothers with IDDM and NIDDM.[5,6] Animal studies suggest that hyperglycaemia during embryogenesis, together with other associated metabolic disturbances, is responsible.[5] A Swedish study of 532 women with IDDM[7] observed that both spontaneous abortions and congenital malformations were substantially and significantly more frequent when the glycated haemoglobin level, measured at an average gestational age of nine (range 5–16) weeks, exceeded 10.1 per cent; this value was stated to be eight standard deviations above the mean (5.3 per cent, 95 per cent CI 3.5–7.1) of a non-pregnant control group, but appears to be nearer five. The authors found no other variables to be significantly related to malformation or abortion rates.

Macrosomia is often quoted as a complication of IDDM, NIDDM, and GDM, though it is most commonly associated with maternal obesity without hyperglycaemia.[8,9] Unfortunately, there is no consensus definition of macrosomia and it is sometimes regarded as a birth weight exceeding 4 or 4.5 kg or one exceeding the 95th (or some other) centile in relation to gestational age. The classical fetopathy associated with very poor control in IDDM comprises a birth weight above the 99th centile, increased total body protein, glycogen, and fat, with hypertrophied internal organs due to cellular hyperplasia and hypertrophy.[5] Good glycaemic control diminishes the frequency of macrosomia,[4] however defined,[10] but even in well-controlled IDDM there remains a higher frequency of large for gestational age neonates.[4] Similar comparative data for NIDDM are lacking.

Because of the way in which GDM is defined, prevailing blood glucose levels in untreated GDM range from the upper normal to those found in NIDDM. Until very recently reports of outcomes in GDM did not, or did not adequately, separate GDM which was only glucose intolerance (i.e. hyperglycaemia provoked by an oral glucose load) from that which was really NIDDM (i.e. with hyperglycaemia in the fasting state). Nevertheless, the only consistently reported association of GDM is a higher frequency of macrosomia, though it is not possible to state with conviction whether this is due to the increased frequency of obesity in women with GDM, to hyperglycaemia, or to both. One randomized study has demonstrated a reduction in average birth weight and frequency of macrosomia in the offspring of mothers with GDM who were treated with an intensive insulin regime, but most of the women in this study were Hispanic Americans who, judging by the levels of glycated haemoglobin in early pregnancy, must have included a high proportion of women with NIDDM antedating the pregnancy.[9]

Birth weight exceeding 4.5 kg is associated with a higher rate of shoulder dystocia during labour and this may cause injury to the brachial plexus and/or clavicles of the fetus.[10] However, only 4 per cent or so of women with untreated gestational glucose intolerance deliver infants weighting 4.5 kg or more compared with about 2 per cent of the general obstetric population.[10] Reported caesarean section rates are usually higher in women with GDM, which may be in part due to the higher frequency of macrosomia, but may also be in part due to the effect of the diagnostic label upon the obstetrician. As there is no study where the medical attendants have been blinded to the diagnosis, the reasons remain speculative.

One study, funded by the US National Institutes of Health, the Hyperglycaemia Adverse Pregnancy Outcome (HAPO) Study, will involve 25 000 unselected pregnant women in three continents.[11] A 75g oral glucose tolerance test will be performed at 28 weeks of gestation and only women satisfying the WHO criteria for diabetes will be treated, allowing the analysis of lesser degrees of glucose intolerance in relation to outcome. The study is recognition of the uncertainty regarding screening for gestational diabetes and is an attempt to assess moderate hyperglycaemia in pregnancy in relation to outcome.

POSSIBLE SCREENING

Current practices are extremely diverse with regard to who should be screened, the timing of screening, type of screening test, nature of gold standard test, and blood glucose criteria for diagnosis.[12,13] This diversity is not surprising given the lack of consensus regarding the purpose(s) of screening. Some regard the principal reason as the potential prevention of macrosomia, but given that macrosomia is not a serious problem and that most macrosomic infants are offspring of women who do not have any form of diabetes, this does not justify screening for GDM, as the Canadian Task Force concluded after a thorough review of the literature.[8] The other principal reason suggested for screening is to identify women at high risk of developing NIDDM subsequently.[14] However, there is probably nothing special about the glucose intolerance associated with pregnancy,[15] and non-pregnant women or men of similar age and degrees of glucose intolerance are not at present offered screening although they also are at increased risk of developing NIDDM.[3] (There are no data bearing on possible differences in relative risk.) There is an argument, in part based upon ideas of 'good practice', for case finding, i.e. identifying early in pregnancy those women with pre-existing but undiagnosed NIDDM. Treatment of women so identified would be unlikely to influence the rate of congenital abnormalities, given that embryogenesis is completed by the seventh week of gestation. However, assuming that NIDDM resembles IDDM in this respect,[4] detecting florid hyperglycaemia early in pregnancy might allow a reduction in associated perinatal mortality. The number of cases detected would, however, be small. In the Swedish general population[16] the incidence of NIDDM (not specifically discovered by screening) in women increased with age in the range 15–34 years, incidence rates in successive five-year age groups being 0.9, 1.1, 3.3, and 4.3 per 100 000 per year, respectively. Epidemiological studies find, on average, one unknown for every known person with NIDDM, so screening would be expected to yield a similar incidence rate. In those ethnic groups particularly at risk of NIDDM, one might expect from prevalence data that incidence would be increased by three to six times. Thus, even in women aged more than 30 years in those populations most at risk, about 4000 pregnant women would have to be screened to discover one with undiagnosed NIDDM. Other estimates can be derived from two studies which screened only those pregnant women deemed to be at risk of glucose intolerance/NIDDM. Both used the WHO 'epidemiological' definition of NIDDM (i.e. adequate for population estimates but not for individual, clinical diagnosis), which comprises a plasma glucose level measured two hours after a 75 g oral glucose in excess of 11.1 mmol/l (200 mg/dl).[1] In Leicester[17] 314 of 4561 South Asian and 504 of 7444 Europid women were screened. Eight South Asian and two Europid women were found to have undiagnosed diabetes according to the WHO definition, i.e. 0.18 per cent and 0.03 per cent of the total populations. A study in Belfast[18] was of similar design, but confined to a local population which is predominantly Europid. Screening tests were performed in 953 consecutive singleton pregnancies, representing 7 per cent of the total obstetric population. Seven women were positive, i.e. 0.05 per cent of the total population, similar to the Leicester figures for Europid women.

Although the incidence rates of 18/10 000 (Asian) and 4/10 000 (Europid) are higher than the rates extrapolated from the Swedish data, they may be under-estimates since not all (albeit those most at risk) members of the study population were screened. Nevertheless, these, like the Swedish figures, suggest that the incidence in Europid women is low. The Belfast and Leicester reports gave no data on the severity of the hyperglycaemia in those who screened positive, beyond stating that they met the WHO criteria. In both studies the women with positive tests were older, with average ages of 32–33 years.

Screening tests

If screening for the disorders associated with hyperglycaemia were contemplated, whether in pregnancy or in non-pregnant women or in men, at present the test would be the oral glucose tolerance test (OGTT). This is because other tests, such as fasting or casual blood glucose, glycated haemoglobin and serum fructosamine, while having specificity, lack sensitivity when the WHO two-hour glucose level is used as the gold standard. Furthermore, research in pregnancy has been influenced by the concept of GDM, which if it is to include glucose intolerance *must* utilize the OGTT in order to detect it. The OGTT has many problems, both in administration and interpretation, not least the lack of reproducibility, so that an individual may be labelled as glucose intolerant or even NIDDM on one occasion but not on a second—and vice versa. If physicians and obstetricians were content to screen with the object of finding those women who enter pregnancy with hyperglycaemia (fasting, post-prandial, casual) *not* provoked by a glucose load, then a simple and specific test could be employed. But based upon the estimates above, the yield, even in high-risk populations, would be very low. In any case, the matter is of little practical interest in the absence of evidence of benefit.

CONCLUSION

There is no good evidence that screening for gestational glucose intolerance benefits mothers or their offspring. While women at risk of developing NIDDM in later life may be identified, there is unfortunately no guaranteed preventive action. Screening for glucose intolerance sufficient to attract the diagnostic label NIDDM could be regarded as 'good practice' but has only theoretical value for the index pregnancy; it could not, for instance, affect rates of congenital anomalies. Even in high-risk populations the yield of NIDDM according to the WHO epidemiological criteria is low and of more florid hyperglycaemia would be even lower. The status of screening for NIDDM in pregnant women is similar to that in the general population – controversial and lacking satisfactory screening tests.[19]

REFERENCES

1. WHO (1985). Diabetes mellitus: report of a WHO Study Group. *WHO Technical Reports Series* 727. WHO, Geneva.
2. Freedman B. J. (1984). Caucasian. *Br. Med. J.*, **288**, 696–8.
3. Jarrett R. J. (1989). Epidemiology and public health aspects of non-insulin dependent diabetes mellitus. *Epidemiol. Rev.*, **11**, 151–71.
4. Kühl C., and Møller-Jensen B. (1989). Intensified insulin treatment in diabetic pregnancy. In *Carbohydrate Metabolism in Pregnancy and the Newborn*, (ed. H. W. Sutherland, J. M. Stowers, and D. W. M. Pearson), pp. 161–71. Springer, London.
5. Eriksson U. J. (1995). The pathogenesis of congenital malformations in diabetic pregnancy. *Diabetes Metabolism Rev.*, **11**, 63–82.
6. Bennett P. H., Webner C., and Miller M. (1979). Congenital anomalies and the diabetic and prediabetic pregnancy. In *Pregnancy Metabolism, Diabetes and the Fetus*, CIBA Foundation Symposium 63, (ed. K. Elliot *et al.*), pp. 207–18. Excerpta Medica, Amsterdam.
7. Hanson U., Persson B., and Thunell S. (1990). The relation between HbAlc in early diabetic pregnancy and the occurrence of spontaneous abortion and malformation in Sweden. *Diabetologia*, **33**, 100–4.
8. Canadian Task Force on the Periodic Health Examination (1992). Periodic health examination, 1992 update: 1. Screening for gestational diabetes mellitus. *Can. Med. Assoc. J.*, **147**, 435–43.
9. de Veciana M., Major C. A., Morgan M. A., Asrat T., Toohey J. S., Lien J. M., and Evans A. T. (1995). Postprandial versus preprandial blood glucose monitoring in women with gestational diabetes mellitus requiring insulin therapy. *New Engl. J. Med.*, **333**, 1237–41.
10. Ales K. L., and Santini D. L. (1989). Should all pregnant women be screened for gestational glucose intolerance? *Lancet*, **1**, 1187–91.

11. Dornhurst A., and Frost G. (2000). Jelly-beans, only a colourful distraction from gestational glucose-challenge tests. *Lancet*, **355**, 674.
12. Gabbe S. G., and Landon M. B. (1989). Management of diabetes in pregnancy: survey of materno-fetal specialists in the United States. In *Carbohydrate Metabolism in Pregnancy and the Newborn*, (ed. H. W. Sutherland, J. M. Stowers, and D. W. M. Pearson), pp. 309–17. Springer, London.
13. Nelson Piercy C., and Gale E. A. M. (1994). Do we know how to screen for gestational diabetes? Current practice in one regional health authority. *Diabetic Med.*, **11**, 493–8.
14. Dornhorst A., and Beard R. W. (1993). Gestational diabetes: a challenge for the future. *Diabetic Med.*, **10**, 897–905.
15. Harris M. I. (1988). Gestational diabetes may represent discovery of pre-existing glucose intolerance. *Diabetes Care*, **11**, 402–11.
16. Blohmé G., Nystrom L., Arnqvist H. J., Lither E., Littorin B., Olsson P. O., Scherstén B., Wibell L., and Ostman J. (1992). Male predominance in insulin-dependent (Type 1) diabetes mellitus in young adults: results of a five-year prospective nationwide study in the 15–34 year age group in Sweden. *Diabetologia*, **35**, 56–62.
17. Samanta A., Burden M. L., Burden A. C., and Jones G. R. (1989). Glucose tolerance during pregnancy in Asian women. *Diabet. Res. Clin. Prac.*, **7**, 127–35.
18. Roberts R. N., Moohan J. M., Foo R. L. K., Harley J. M. G., Traub A. I., and Hadden D. R. (1993). Fetal outcome in mothers with IGT in pregnancy. *Diabetic Med.*, **10**, 438–43.
19. Knowler W. C. (1994). Screening for NIDDM: opportunities for detection, treatment, and prevention. *Diabetes Care*, **17**, 445–50.

9 *Disorders associated with high blood pressure*

Michael de Swiet and Ian Leck

INTRODUCTION

In the United Kingdom there are about 730 000 births per year.[1] It has been recommended that a pregnant woman should attend an antenatal clinic on about 10 occasions.[2] It is standard practice to measure the blood pressure at each antenatal visit. Therefore, the blood pressure is probably measured in pregnancy on seven or eight million occasions in the UK each year. Measurement of the blood pressure in pregnancy is in effect screening; indeed, it must be the most frequent screening test applied in pregnancy. The reason for all this screening is that very high blood pressure in pregnancy is associated with various adverse outcomes in mother or child.

HIGH BLOOD PRESSURE DURING PREGNANCY AND ITS COMPLICATIONS

It is generally accepted that high blood pressure is not a disease, but represents the upper part of a continuous distribution of blood pressure values. Although some cases of high blood pressure are due to known causes (e.g. phaeochromocytoma, coarctation of the aorta) these cases represent only a very small proportion of the hypertensive population, much less than 5 per cent. In the rest of the population, high blood pressure is important as a risk factor for various diseases or complications, some cases of which can be prevented by lowering the blood pressure.

In pregnancy, high blood pressure has long been the most widely used marker for the condition often referred to as pre-eclampsia. This condition is a placental disorder of unknown cause. It is recognized by signs that develop in late pregnancy and regress after delivery. These signs include not only high blood pressure but also proteinuria, fluid retention, hyperuricaemia, thrombocytopaenia, abnormal liver enzyme activity, and haemoconcentration; but these features are not usually all found in the same patient. No one of them (not even high blood pressure) is invariably present.[3,4] The adverse outcomes of pregnancy that are associated with the disorder include not only eclampsia but also the HELLP syndrome (severe disseminated intravascular coagulation combined with liver dysfunction and acute haemolysis[5]), abruptio placentae, cerebral haemorrhage, and renal and left ventricular haemorrhage in the mother, and intra-uterine growth restriction, preterm birth, and perinatal death in the child.

Although the term 'pre-eclampsia' has been used broadly of the above disorder,[3,4,6] many authorities use this term more specifically, to denote a combination of an increase in blood pressure during pregnancy with proteinuria and/or oedema (the easiest signs of the disorder to detect in practice).[7-9] Since most epidemiological studies have been based on pre-eclampsia defined in the latter manner, this practice is followed in this chapter.

Even an increase in blood pressure during pregnancy without proteinuria or oedema suggests that the placental disorder is present, and therefore that the other signs may appear later. It is therefore usual to distinguish high blood pressure which develops during pregnancy ('pregnancy-induced hypertension') from high blood pressure originating before the onset of pregnancy ('pregnancy-associated hypertension'). In this chapter, the words 'hypertension' and 'normotension' are in general avoided, since they are not categorically distinct entities; but on grounds of convenience, the terms 'pregnancy-associated hypertension' (PAH) and 'pregnancy-induced hypertension' (PIH) are used as defined above, and the term 'hypertensive disease of pregnancy' (HDP) is used to denote disease of which PAH or PIH is a sign.*

The course of blood pressure during pregnancy
Normal findings

During pregnancy, blood pressure is generally believed to follow the course described by MacGillivray[10] (Fig. 9.1). There is little change in the mean systolic blood pressure which is approximately 105 mmHg throughout pregnancy (sitting). However, diastolic blood pressure falls from 70 mmHg to about 55 mmHg at 20 weeks of gestation, rising to 65 mmHg at term. The standard deviations of these measurements of systolic and diastolic blood pressure are about 10 mmHg.

Pregnancy-associated and pregnancy-induced hypertension (PAH and PIH)

The distribution of blood pressure is continuous in pregnant women, as in the rest of the population, which makes it arbitrary to use any 'cut-off' point to separate hypertension in pregnancy from normotension. This practice also ignores the fact that the whole distribution of blood pressure is shifted upwards with increased age. For example, Miall and Oldham[11] found an increase of 11 mmHg in the mean systolic pressure of non-pregnant women between the ages of 20 and 40 years. Despite these considerations, for management purposes pregnant women are generally defined as hypertensive if their diastolic pressure is 90 mmHg or above at any time during pregnancy.

---

* Some authorities use the terms PAH and PIH in a different way. They describe hypertension detected before 20 weeks of gestation as 'essential' (whether it is truly essential or due to very rare secondary causes such as phaeochromocytoma), since it is believed that, with very few exceptions, hypertension which appears before 20 weeks is not directly due to pregnancy. When hypertension appears *de novo* after 20 weeks it is attributed to pregnancy, and is described in the alternative nomenclature as PIH when associated with proteinuria and as PAH otherwise, because fetal and maternal morbidity are much more common when proteinuria is present than when it is not.

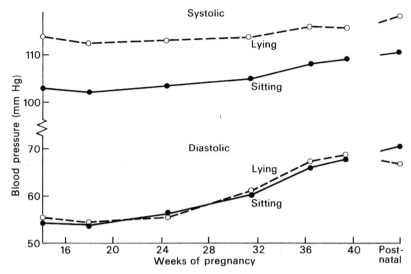

Fig. 9.1 Mean systolic and diastolic blood pressures sitting and lying during pregnancy.[10]

It has long been believed that the prognosis is worse for a pregnancy with PIH than for a pregnancy with PAH in which the blood pressure is equally high. It is also thought that patients who start pregnancy with PAH are more likely to develop PIH than those who are normotensive at the beginning of pregnancy.

Women with diastolic pressures of 90 mmHg or more are generally classified as cases of PAH if the diastolic pressure is found to be at this level by 20 weeks of gestation, and as cases of PIH without PAH if an increase to this level occurs later.[6] Women with PAH are considered to have PIH as well if they develop proteinuria or if their diastolic pressure increases by at least 10 mm[6] or 15 mm[8] after 20 weeks. Some authorities use additional criteria either in defining PAH and PIH or in subdividing these two categories. Examples of these definitions are given in Appendix 1.

Just as the blood pressure levels used in defining PAH and PIH are somewhat arbitrary, so is the rule that a woman should only be considered to have PIH if her blood pressure passes the designated level beyond 20 weeks of gestation. Most clinicians accept that it is possible for patients to have the disease process associated with PIH before 20 weeks of gestation, as judged by the associated clinical features. Indeed the placental pathology probably starts at 12–14 weeks.[12]

If a patient is seen for the first time after 20 weeks of gestation, and has a blood pressure in excess of 90 mmHg, we cannot usually tell whether she has PAH or PIH, although attempts to do so have been made using the history and some laboratory investigations (e.g. measurements of serum uric acid,[13] platelet count, and factor VIII estimation[14]).

The above problems of definition mean that epidemiological investigations involving large numbers of patients assessed only by blood pressure are difficult to interpret, since women cannot all be classified into groups with PAH, PIH, and normal blood pressure.

Table 9.1   Distribution of British singleton pregnancies according to blood pressure category

Category	Definition	Year of survey			
		1958[16]		1970[6]	
		Number	Percentage of classifiable pregnancies*	Number	Percentage of classifiable pregnancies*
Blood pressure not raised	MDP† <90; no proteinuria	10 996	70.2	10 787	71.1
PAH without PIH	MDP ≥90 before 20 weeks; no rise of ≥10 later; no proteinuria	285	1.8	321	2.1
PAH + PIH	MDP ≥90 before 20 weeks; rise of ≥10 later, and/or proteinuria	157	1.0	163	1.1
PIH without PAH	MDP <90 before 20 weeks; MDP ≥90 later, and/or eclampsia	2205	14.1	2659	17.5
Blood pressure raised; not specified whether PAH or PIH	MDP not recorded before 20 weeks; MDP ≥90 later	2023	12.9	1240	8.2
Proteinuria not elsewhere classified	MDP not recorded or <90; proteinuria	398	–	937	–
Other	MDP and whether proteinuria not recorded	930	–	708	–
Total		16 994	100	16 815	100

* Denominator excludes 'proteinuria not elsewhere classified' and 'other' categories.
† MDP = maximum diastolic pressure (mmHg).

The prevalence of high blood pressure during pregnancy

Estimates of the prevalence of high blood pressure vary widely. Data from 41 studies (35 hospital-based and six population-based) in 14 countries were presented at a World Health Organization (WHO) Conference in 1977.[15] Among these studies, the reported prevalence of hypertensive disease of pregnancy varied from 0.1 per cent in the only Ethiopian hospital in the study to 31.4 per cent in one of five hospitals in the United States. Although the differences reported may have been partly genuine, they were probably due largely to variations in the quality of obstetric care (and hence the frequency of measurement), in the criteria used to define hypertensive disease, and in the factors influencing selection for admission to the hospitals which provided statistics.

The population-based studies considered at the 1977 WHO Conference included two nationwide British surveys, one in 1958[16] and one in 1970,[6] in each of which all pregnancies ending in a birth during a single week were studied by a retrospective survey of the case notes. The results of analysing these cohorts by blood pressure and by whether proteinuria was recorded are shown in Table 9.1. For between 8 per cent and 10 per cent of pregnancies in each cohort, there was not enough information to classify them. Diastolic pressures of 90 mmHg or more were reported in about 30 per cent of the remaining pregnancies—3 per cent with PAH (in one-third of which PIH also developed), 14–18 per cent without PAH in which PIH developed, and 8–13 per cent in which there was no record of diastolic pressure before 20 weeks to indicate whether the hypertension was PAH or PIH.

Table 9.2 Distribution of British pregnancies with PIH or hypertension not fully specified, by severity of hypertensive disease

Severity	Definition	Year of survey			
		1958[16]		1970[6]	
		Number	Percentage of classifiable pregnancies*	Number	Percentage of classifiable pregnancies*
Mild	MDP† after 20 weeks 90–99; no proteinuria or eclampsia	2669	17.0	2459	16.2
Moderate	MDP after 20 weeks 100–109; no proteinuria or eclampsia	611	3.9	610	4.0
Severe	MDP after 20 weeks ≥110, and/or proteinuria with MDP ≥90, and/or eclampsia	948	6.1	830	5.5
Total		4228	27.0	3899	25.7

* Denominator excludes 'proteinuria not elsewhere classified' and 'other' categories.
† MDP = maximum diastolic pressure (mmHg).

Since PIH without PAH was five times as common as PAH in the pregnancies for which diastolic pressure before 20 weeks was known, the distribution of cases of high blood pressure by severity was analysed for both cohorts on the assumption that the cases in which pressure before 20 weeks was not known had PIH as opposed to PAH. The results (Table 9.2) suggested that mild PIH occurs in 16–17 per cent of British pregnancies, moderate PIH in 4 per cent, and severe PIH in 5–6 per cent.

None of these three categories correspond to pre-eclampsia (PIH with proteinuria). The 'severe PIH' group included all cases of PIH with proteinuria, but also non-proteinuric cases with diastolic pressure readings of at least 110 mmHg. Pre-eclampsia has been reported in 2.6 per cent of United States pregnancies.[17]

Adverse outcomes of pregnancy related to maternal hypertension
Perinatal mortality

Most clinicians have the impression that perinatal mortality is much higher in PIH than PAH. This impression is based on extreme cases. A young primigravid patient who suddenly develops a blood pressure of 160/105 and heavy proteinuria at 26 weeks of gestation has severe PIH and will be lucky to have a live baby. A patient whose blood-pressure measurement is 160/105 at 12 weeks of gestation has PAH and may show no change in blood pressure during pregnancy, or even a fall in blood pressure, in which case the prognosis for the fetus is only marginally impaired.

It is difficult to determine whether the clinical impression that PIH is more hazardous than PAH for the fetus is correct, mainly because many cases of high blood pressure in pregnancy are not sufficiently specified to be accurately classified as PAH or PIH. The impression that there is a difference in prognosis is not supported by the perinatal mortality experience of the nationwide British cohorts of pregnancies studied in 1958 and 1970 (Table 9.3). There were no significant perinatal mortality differences between all cases of PAH and all cases of PIH without PAH; but each of these two groups included a minority in which perinatal mortality was much higher than in the rest of the group. The high-risk minorities were the cases of PAH who also developed PIH, and the 'severe' cases of PIH without PAH (i.e. those with a diastolic

Table 9.3   Perinatal mortality by blood pressure in British singleton pregnancies

Category	Definition	Year of survey					
		1958[16]			1970[6]		
		Perinatal deaths	All births	Perinatal mortality per 1000	Perinatal deaths	All births	Perinatal mortality per 1000
Blood pressure not raised	MDP* <90; no proteinuria	279	10 996	25	207	10 787	19
PAH	MDP before 20 weeks ≥90						
without PIH	No rise of ≥10 later; no proteinuria	10	285	35 ⎫	5	321	16 ⎫
with PIH	Rise of ≥10 later, and/or proteinuria	10	157	64 ⎭ 45	5	163	31 ⎭ 21
PIH without PAH†	MDP before 20 weeks <90 or ?						
mild	MDP 90–99 later; no proteinuria or eclampsia	75	2669	28 ⎫	48	2459	20 ⎫
moderate	MDP 100–109 later; no proteinuria or eclampsia	27	611	44 ⎬ 41	11	610	18 ⎬ 22
severe	MDP ≥110 later; and/or proteinuria with MDP ≥90, and/or eclampsia	70	948	74 ⎭	28	830	34 ⎭
Proteinuria not elsewhere classified and other	MDP <90 with proteinuria, or not recorded	93	1328	70	56	1645	34

* MDP = maximum diastolic pressure (mmHg).
† Including hypertension not fully specified.

pressure of 110 mmHg or more and/or proteinuria and/or eclampsia). With these exceptions, mortality in 1970 was no higher when PAH or PIH was present than when it was not, although this was not true in 1958 (when the perinatal mortality difference between normotensive and hypertensive pregnancies was much greater than in 1970).

These findings are consistent with the view that with good antenatal care, including early delivery in selected cases, the risks of perinatal death are not materially affected by raised blood pressure (whether PAH or PIH) unless this reaches a level around 160/110 or unless there is proteinuria. The main reason for identifying women with diastolic pressure between 90 and 110 mmHg is to enable maternal and fetal monitoring to be intensified with a view to timely delivery if required by the condition of either mother or fetus. This is more important than treatment of the blood pressure.

More recent studies than the nationwide British surveys provide further support for the view that perinatal mortality is unaffected by modest increases in blood pressure if there is good antenatal care. In these studies, significant increases in perinatal mortality were only observed in cases in which PAH[8,18] or PIH[19] was complicated by proteinuria and/or oedema, or in which diastolic pressures above 110 mmHg or systolic pressures above 160 mmHg were detected.[20] Findings from one of these studies is shown in Table 9.4. A further finding was that in cases of PIH in which the

Table 9.4 Perinatal mortality rate in 13 988 primigravidae in Aberdeen, 1958–71[19]

Maternal condition	No. of mothers	No. of perinatal deaths	Perintal death-rate (per 1000)
Normal blood pressure	10 017	207	20.7
Late hypertension only	3443	65	18.9
Hypertension with proteinuria	528	29	55.0

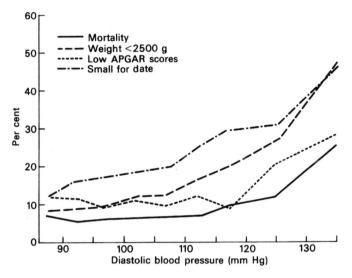

Fig. 9.2 Relationship of diastolic blood pressure to fetal outcome in 4404 women with signs of HDP in Helsinki & Würzburg, 1960–69.[20]

diastolic pressure had increased by 25 mmHg or more, perinatal mortality was almost five times as high as in normotensive women.[21]

The impact that hypertensive disease of pregnancy (HDP) would have on perinatal mortality in the absence of screening and treatment cannot be precisely assessed from the above observations, since these were made when some screening and treatment were already taking place. However, the data in Table 9.3 can be used to assess the impact of HDP on perinatal mortality in Britain in 1958 and 1970, and the effect of changes in management between these dates. In the 1958 cohort the perinatal mortality rate was 41.1/1000 pregnancies with PIH or PAH, 25.4/1000 pregnancies in which blood pressure was not raised, and 30.1/1000 of these groups combined. These figures suggest that HDP may have been responsible for 38 per cent (i.e. (41.1 – 25.4)/41.1) of perinatal deaths associated with high blood pressure, and for 16 per cent (i.e. (30.1 – 25.4)/30.1) of all perinatal deaths.

The corresponding perinatal death rates for the 1970 cohort were 22.1/1000 with PIH or PAH, 19.2/1000 without raised blood pressure, and 20.0/1000 of these groups combined, suggesting that only 13 per cent of perinatal deaths associated with high blood pressure and 4 per cent of all perinatal deaths were attributable to HDP. Interestingly, the latter percentage is close to the proportion of perinatal deaths for which maternal hypertension has been certified as a main cause of death in England and Wales in more recent years (e.g. 5.2 per cent in 1997[22]).

The figures in Table 9.3 indicate that the ratio between the perinatal mortality rates for pregnancies with and without high blood pressure declined from 1.62:1 in 1958 to 1.15:1 in 1970. It seems reasonable to attribute this improvement to advances in the management of HDP, and to suppose (1) that if these advances had not occurred, mortality would have fallen by the same proportion in pregnancies with and without high blood pressure, and (2) that the offspring of affected women would experience the same perinatal mortality as other fetuses and infants if all deaths due to HDP were prevented. If these suppositions are correct, it follows that advances in the management of HDP between 1958 and 1970 were successful in preventing about three-quarters of the HDP-related perinatal deaths that would otherwise have occurred.

The pathology in stillbirths and neonatal deaths attributed to HDP is variable. Among those recorded in England and Wales in 1992, the most commonly certified main fetal conditions were prematurity in 31 per cent, non-infectious respiratory disorders (e.g. respiratory distress syndrome) in 16 per cent, and birth asphyxia in 12 per cent.[23]

Other fetal outcomes

Intrauterine growth restriction, and pre-term birth with its associated problems such as respiratory distress syndrome and intraventricular haemorrhage, are relatively common in the surviving infants of hypertensive mothers as well as in those who die. Pre-term birth in hypertensive pregnancies is sometimes caused by active intervention because of the fear that the infant will otherwise die *in utero*, but nevertheless it remains a complication of hypertension.

The influence of blood pressure on these non-fatal outcomes is even more difficult to quantify than its impact on perinatal mortality, since data on non-fatal outcomes are less 'hard' and fewer analyses of their relationship to blood pressure are available; for example, analyses of this kind are not included in the reports of the 1958 and 1970 cohort studies.

In one study of the relationship of fetal growth restriction to maternal blood pressure,[24] the term 'hypertension' was used of pregnancies in which mean arterial pressure (diastolic pressure + 1/3 pulse pressure) exceeded 104 mmHg more than once during the third trimester, and infants were defined as small for gestational age if they were born at 37 weeks of gestation or later weighing less than 2500 g. In this study, the proportion of liveborn white American infants who were small for gestational age ranged from 2 per cent when maternal blood pressure was normal to 12 per cent in pregnancies with pre-eclampsia (defined as 'hypertension' and a proteinuria test result of ++ or more).

Fetal growth restriction may even be associated with increases in maternal blood pressure which are too small to affect perinatal mortality. Thus, in the data of Tervilä *et al.*[20] the risk of fetal growth restriction started to increase with diastolic pressure at a lower level (about 90 mmHg) than did perinatal mortality (Fig. 9.2), and McCowan *et al.*[8] reported that the offspring of women with PAH but no pre-eclampsia (whose perinatal mortality was not significantly increased) included 11 per cent with a birth-weight below the fifth centile for gestation.

There is also evidence that hypertensive disease in pregnancy is a risk factor for childhood disability. In Dundee, Scotland, diastolic pressures of above 110 mmHg, or above 90 mmHg with proteinuria, were reported for 11 per cent of pregnancies preceding the birth of children with neurodevelopmental disability and for 5 per cent of control pregnancies.[25]

Maternal outcomes

Maternal death

In New York from 1980 to 1984, hypertension was reported to have caused 10 per cent of all maternal deaths. Two causes were reported more often—pulmonary embolism (13 per cent) and complications of ectopic pregnancy (13 per cent).[26] The most recent report on maternal mortality in Britain (covering 1994–6) attributed 15 per cent of direct maternal deaths, or 9.1 deaths per million maternities, to hypertensive disorders of pregnancy, making them the most common cause of maternal mortality except for pulmonary embolism (36 per cent of deaths). Maternal death due to hypertensive disease generally used to be brought about by eclampsia (reported in about half these deaths) and/or by renal failure, placental abruption, left ventricular failure, or cerebral haemorrhage.[1] With modern intensive care the major causes of death from hypertensive disorders of pregnancy are cerebral and pulmonary. Most women with severe hypertension survive when treated by modern methods, but even the survivors may lose their babies (e.g. by placental abruption) or be disabled (e.g. by brain damage).

Eclampsia

The aspects of non-fatal fetal outcomes described above which make it difficult to quantify their relationship to hypertensive disease also apply to non-fatal maternal outcomes, except for eclampsia. This is a manifestation of hypertensive disease by definition—'the occurrence of convulsions unrelated to coincidental neurologic disease in a woman with pre-eclampsia'.[7] Eclampsia may occur in more than 1 per cent of pregnancies in some developing countries[15] but is only reported in about 0.5/1000 in the United States[17] and the United Kingdom[27] and in 0.27/1000 in Sweden (where most women receive early and regular antenatal care).[28] Death occurred in nearly 2 per cent of women with eclampsia in the United Kingdom study (which covered the year 1992) and 7 per cent of the offspring of affected women died between 20 weeks of gestation and one year after birth.[27]

SCREENING TESTS

Blood pressure measurement

The healthy pregnant woman is generally encouraged to attend a medical facility (e.g. hospital antenatal clinic or general practitioner's surgery) on many occasions—e.g. every four weeks from about 12 to 26 weeks, every two weeks from then until 36 weeks, and then weekly until term. One of the main reasons for this practice is to enable her blood pressure to be measured. This is done at booking in order to detect PAH and establish a baseline, and repeatedly thereafter because PIH may develop at any time during the second half of pregnancy. Evidence is lacking as to whether much would be lost if low-risk women were examined less often, so as to reduce costs; but frequent examinations are now so firmly established a practice, that randomized trials of a change of this kind would be difficult to introduce, especially as the outcomes of interest (e.g. eclampsia, or perinatal death due to blood-pressure-related maternal disease) are so rare that very large numbers of pregnancies would need to be included.

Equipment

Even in surveys, blood pressure in pregnancy is usually measured by conventional sphygmomanometry, and this is also the technique which should be used clinically. Because of the risk of observer bias, including digit preference, special sphygmomanometers have been developed (e.g. random zero sphygmomanometer[29] and London School of Hygiene sphygmomanometer[30]) which enable the blood pressure to be recorded without the observer knowing what it is until after the recordings have been made. Such instruments have been used in surveys but are now replaced by automated sphygmomanometers.

Cuff size is also important.[31] Patients who are obese probably do have higher blood pressure than the normal population.[32] But much of the 'hypertension' seen in obese patients relates to their large arms. If a standard cuff is used, the inflation bag may not be long enough or wide enough to transmit the pressure inside the cuff to the brachial artery. This over-estimates the blood pressure. Under-estimation of the blood pressure caused by using too large a cuff is theoretically possible, but probably rare in clinical practice.[33] As a working rule, the sphygmomanometer cuff inflation bag should extend round at least two-thirds of the arm's circumference, and should cover half the length of the upper arm.[34]

Procedure

Blood pressure should be measured in patients sitting or semirecumbent in the left lateral position. There is no consistent agreement as to the magnitude or even the direction of changes in blood pressure between these two positions in pregnancy.[35] However, it is clear that the blood pressure should not be measured in patients lying on their backs, particularly in late pregnancy. In this position the uterus compresses the inferior vena cava and reduces venous return, which results in a decrease in cardiac output and a false reduction of blood pressure.[36]

The diastolic blood pressure is taken to be the pressure at which the Korotkoff sounds are muffled (K_4) or disappear (K_5). In the past K_4 was recommended for the measurement of diastolic blood pressure in pregnancy in the belief that too many patients would have Korotkoff sounds audible to zero pressure to make K_5 practical. Recent work[37] challenges this concept. In a rigorous study using seven pairs of observers in 250 pregnant women, K_5 was always audible and the observers could only agree as to the presence of K_4 in 48 per cent of cases. K_5 is now therefore the preferred end point for diastolic blood pressure measurement in pregnancy.[38] In practice, the consistency of blood pressure measurements made at different times in pregnancy is more important than the absolute level recorded.

Sphygmomanometer readings of blood pressure often differ considerably from the intra-arterial pressure.[39] In the study cited, the 95 per cent confidence limits for K_5 were +28.2 to –6.0 mmHg, taking intra-arterial as the 'true' diastolic blood pressure.[39] Therefore a diastolic blood pressure recorded as 90 mmHg (to the nearest 5 mmHg as is often the case) could be as high as 92.4 + 28.2 = 120.6 mmHg or as low as 87.6 – 6.0 = 81.6 mmHg.

Systolic blood pressure is a better predictor of fetal outcome than diastolic.[20] One reason for this is that the errors in measurement of systolic blood pressure are smaller. It would therefore be more logical to rely on systolic blood pressure measurement than diastolic,[40] but it seems unlikely that the ingrained habits and clinical trial data of many generations will be overturned.

Whatever pressure reading is used, the extreme between-occasion variability of blood pressure means that one cannot assume that any single reading is typical. This limitation could be overcome by non-invasive ambulatory monitoring of blood pressure, when the blood pressure is repeatedly sampled over at least a 24 hour period.[41] In the short term, i.e. when measurements are made within a few weeks of delivery, ambulatory monitoring is a better predictor of fetal and maternal outcomes than is casual measurement.[42] However, at present ambulatory measurement should be considered a research tool.

Performance of screening for perinatal death

In order to determine the performance of screening for any adverse outcome by measuring blood pressure, one would need information about the distribution by blood pressure of (1) pregnancies in which the adverse outcome would occur if there was no effective screening-based treatment programme, and (2) all other pregnancies. In practice, such information may not exist. The adverse outcome for which the most extensive data are available is perinatal mortality; but in the large populations where this has been analysed in relation to maternal blood pressure, clinical management was

Table 9.5   Performance of blood pressure screening as a predictor of perinatal mortality in British pregnancies surveyed in 1958

(a) Positive result = MDP* ≥90 at any time in pregnancy.

	Result of screening test		
	Positive	Negative	Total
Perinatal death	192 (true-positive)	279 (false-negative)	471
No perinatal death	4478 (false-positive)	10 717 (true-negative)	15 195
Total	4670	10 996	15 666

Detection rate = 192/471 = 40.2%.
False-positive rate = 4478/15 195 = 29.5%.
Odds of being affected given a positive result = 192:4478 = 1:23.
* MDP = maximum diastolic pressure in mmHg.

(b) Positive results = MDP* ≥90 before 20 weeks, rising by ≥10 later; MDP ≥110 after 20 weeks; proteinuria with MDP ≥90; eclampsia.

	Result of screening test		
	Positive	Negative	Total
Perinatal death	80 (true-positive)	391 (false-negative)	471
No perinatal death	1025 (false-positive)	14 170 (true-negative)	15 195
Total	1105	14 561	15 666

Detection rate = 80/471 = 17.0%.
False-positive rate = 1025/15 195 = 6.7%.
Odds of being affected given a positive result = 80:1025 = 1:13.
* MDP = maximum diastolic pressure in mmHg.

influenced by blood pressure, and some perinatal deaths that would have occurred if there had been no screening programme may therefore have been prevented.

It was concluded above (p. 208) that blood pressure control had far less effect on perinatal mortality in the first of the two British cohorts analysed in Tables 9.1–9.3 (i.e. the cohort born in 1958) than in the second (born in 1970). Table 9.5 shows estimates of the detection rate and false-positive rate of blood pressure screening as a predictor of perinatal mortality in 1958, calculated on the assumption that no lives were saved by screening at that time. In this case, the detection rate would be the proportion of perinatal deaths associated with HDP, and the false-positive rate would be the proportion of survivors associated with HDP.

Two alternative criteria for the presence of HDP (i.e. definitions of a positive test) are considered in Table 9.5. One of these definitions is a diastolic pressure of 90 mmHg or more at any time in pregnancy, for which the detection rate is 40 per cent, the false-positive rate is 29 per cent, and the odds of being affected given a positive result (OAPR) is 1:23 (Table 9.5(a)). The other definition considered is that used to define PAH with PIH and severe PIH without PAH in Table 9.3, for which the detec-

Table 9.6   Estimated performance of blood pressure screening as a predictor that perinatal mortality would occur if there was no screening, for a population of 10 000 British pregnancies in the late 1990s

(a) Positive result = MDP[a] ⩾ 90 at any time in pregnancy.

	Result of screening test		
	Positive	**Negative**	**Total**
Perinatal death	38[d] (true-positive)	55[c] (false-negative)	93
No perinatal death	2943 (false-positive)	6964 (true-negative)	9907
Total	2981[b]	7019	10 000

Detection rate = 38/93 = 40.9%.
False-positive rate = 2943/9907 = 29.7%.
Odds of being affected given a positive result = 38:2943 = 1:77.
[a] MDP = maximum diastolic pressure in mmHg.
[b] 10 000 × 4670/15 666 (from Table 16.5(a)).
[c] 7019 × 7.9/1000. Perinatal death is assumed to occur in 7.9/1000 normotensive pregnancies.
[d] 2981 × 1.62 × 7.9/1000. Perinatal death is assumed to occur in 1.62 × 7.9/1000 'positive' pregnancies (see text). Remaining figures obtained by addition or subtraction from ones derived above.

(b) Positive results = MDP ⩾ 90 before 20 weeks, rising by ⩾ 10 later; MDP ⩾ 110 after 20 weeks; proteinuria with MDP ⩾ 90; eclampsia.

	Result of screening test		
	Positive	**Negative**	**Total**
Perinatal death	16[g] (true-positive)	77 (false-negative)	93[f]
No perinatal death	689 (false-positive)	9218 (true-negative)	9907
Total	705[e]	9295	10 000

Detection rate = 16/93 = 17.2%.
False-positive rate = 689/9907 = 7.0%.
Odds of being affected given a positive result = 16:689 = 1:43.
[e] 10 000 × 1105/15 666 (from Table 16.5(b)).
[f] from Table 16.6(a).
[g] 705 × 2.85 × 7.9/1000. Perinatal death is assumed to occur in 2.85 × 7.9/1000 'positive' pregnancies (see text). Remaining figures obtained by addition or subtraction from ones derived above.

tion rate is 17 per cent, the false-positive rate is 7 per cent, and the OAPR is 1:13 (Table 9.5(b)). With either definition of a positive test, the detection rate and the OAPR would no doubt be higher if deaths that were clearly not caused by HDP (e.g. those from lethal malformations) were not counted as perinatal deaths; but the data one would need to do this are not available.

OAPR is likely to be much lower now than it was in 1958, since even if blood pressure screening in pregnancy had saved no lives the perinatal mortality in pregnancies with high blood pressure would probably have fallen in response to the changes that have caused the decline in overall perinatal mortality. Tables 9.6(a) and (b) show the results that screening using the lower and higher cut-offs of 'positive' might now achieve, assuming (1) that the perinatal mortality rate from deaths not ascribed to hypertension (7.9/1000[22]) applies to pregnancies in which diastolic pressure remains below 90 mmHg and (2) that in the absence of screening, the perinatal mortality rates in pregnancies that are 'positive' according to the broader and narrower definitions would exceed 7.9/1000 by 62 per cent and 185 per cent respectively. The figures of 62 per cent and 185 per cent are the excesses in perinatal mortality in the pregnancies of the 1958 cohort that were 'positive' according to the broader and narrower definitions (Table 9.3).

Table 9.6(a) suggests that if all women with diastolic pressures of 90 mmHg or more were to be treated for HDP, 40 per cent of *all* women whose fetuses would die if there was no screening of blood pressure would receive treatment, and our analysis of the 1958 and 1970 cohorts (p. 208) suggests that this treatment would prevent perinatal death in at least three-quarters of those fetuses which without screening would die as a result of HDP. However, for every one woman treated for HDP whose fetus would die in the absence of screening, nearly 80 others would also be treated—between one in three and one in four of all pregnancies.

If additional care was to be restricted to women with PIH that was severe or combined with PAH, the number of women receiving this care whose fetuses would survive without it would be reduced to one in 15 of all pregnancies—40 times as many as the number treated in which perinatal death would occur in the absence of additional care; but the latter number would only include 17 per cent of all the fetuses who would die if there was no screening (Table 9.6(b)). Current obstetric practice would regard it as unethical to restrict additional care to women with such severe hypertension, and would demand some form of intervention once the diastolic pressure exceeded 100 mmHg and often at lower pressures.

Screening may be rather more accurate than these estimates suggest. This would be so if, in the absence of screening, perinatal mortality would have fallen less since 1958 in pregnancies with high blood pressure than in other pregnancies. In Table 9.6 it is assumed that perinatal mortality would have fallen by the same proportion in both groups.

Screening for outcomes other than perinatal death

The above assessment of the accuracy of blood pressure screening in identifying pregnancies threatened by perinatal death could not have been made without data on perinatal mortality at different blood pressures. It is not possible to make similar assessments of the accuracy of screening in identifying pregnancies threatened by maternal mortality or non-fatal disease, since we lack the necessary data on the frequency of maternal deaths and non-fatal disorders of mother and offspring at different blood pressures.

So far as maternal mortality is concerned, its frequency (about six direct maternal deaths per 100 000 pregnancies in Britain[1]) is so low in relation to the prevalence of high blood pressure that if blood pressure screening were used to predict it, the odds of being affected given a positive test would be even lower than those we have seen for fetal mortality. Also, the report on Confidential Enquiries into Maternal Deaths in the United Kingdom[1] does not give sufficient details to estimate what level of blood pressure might be critical for maternal mortality. Most clinicians would be concerned for the mother's safety if the blood pressure rose above 110 mmHg diastolic or 170 mmHg systolic; but the rapidity with which blood pressure rises is also very important.

Other procedures

Testing for proteinuria

As already noted, some authorities limit the term 'pre-eclampsia' to maternal hypertension combined with proteinuria of at least 500 mg/l;[9] and the classification of hypertension followed in Tables 9.1–9.3 treats all pregnancies with the combination of proteinuria and a diastolic pressure of 90 mmHg or more as cases of either PAH with PIH or severe PIH. These conventions reflect the fact that when maternal hypertension is accompanied by proteinuria, fetal mortality is undoubtedly higher.[24,43]

Testing for proteinuria is clinically indicated at all antenatal visits irrespective of the blood pressure, since in some cases of pre-eclampsia proteinuria can be detected before high blood pressure or in the presence of elevations in blood pressure which would otherwise be considered trivial. However, it should be borne in mind when testing for proteinuria that the dip-stick method, which is the most widely used test, is very sensitive and difficult to quantify; also there are many causes of proteinuria, such as urinary tract infection, contamination by vaginal discharge, and renal disease, apart from the hypertensive diseases of pregnancy.

Measurement of serum markers

During the 1970s, Redman *et al.*[13] reported a perinatal mortality of 50 per cent in hypertensive pregnancies in which serum uric acid was elevated above 6 mg/100 ml (0.36 mmol/litre) before 32 weeks of gestation. It therefore seems possible that uric acid is more powerful than blood pressure as a predictor of fetal outcome, but this remains to be confirmed. Uric acid measurement will not supplant blood pressure measurement, because there will remain individuals with high blood pressures where the mother and fetus are at risk whatever the level of uric acid. Furthermore, measurement of the blood pressure is cheaper than measurement of uric acid, and the result is available immediately.

It has recently been suggested that activin-A and inhibin-A, two proteins produced by the placenta, may be useful serum markers of pre-eclampsia, since the concentrations of both were higher in 20 women with pre-eclampsia than in 20 controls, with no overlap between these groups.[44] This requires further study in a larger cohort.

Measures to predict PIH

The possibility of predicting which women will develop PIH has been explored in various ways. Several workers[24,45,46] have shown that even among women whose blood pressure in early or mid-pregnancy is below what is generally defined as hypertensive, those with pressures towards the upper end of the normal range are more likely to become hypertensive later. Other variables that have been considered as possible predictors of PIH include: Doppler wave-form patterns of the utero-placental arteries;[47] increase in blood pressure when patients roll over from the left lateral to the supine position[48,49] or when they are infused with angiotensin;[50] angiotensin II binding sites on platelets;[51] levels of serum fibronectin (thought to be a marker of endothelial damage),[52,53] of platelet calcium,[54] and of plasma atrial natriuretic factor;[55] high haemoglobin concentration at booking (considered because patients who develop pre-eclampsia are thought not to expand their circulating blood volume to the same extent as normotensive patients);[56] elevation of the ratio of the diene conjugated isomer of linoleic acid 18:2(9,11) to linoleic acid 18:2 (9,12) (attributed to excess free-radical activity);[57] and reduction of the urinary kallikrein-creatinine ratio.[58] The accuracy as screening procedures of most of these tests is either low[55,59-61] or uncertain, and some are too invasive or demand too many resources to be suitable for general use. Even if a test to predict PIH was shown to be free of these limitations, its use for screening would not currently be justified, since women at risk of PIH have not yet been shown to benefit from being identified and treated while still normotensive.

MANAGEMENT OF HIGH BLOOD PRESSURE IN PREGNANCY

The aim in managing cases of high blood pressure in pregnancy is to prevent death and disability in both mother and offspring. Treatment to protect the mother should probably be considered mandatory at levels of blood pressure in excess of 160/105 mmHg, and the most effective way to protect her is to deliver her fetus. However, antihypertensive therapy may also be necessary to control the blood pressure acutely, or to allow pregnancy to continue for one or two weeks in the hope of delivering a viable fetus. The antihypertensive drugs most frequently used for the acute control of blood pressure[62] include sympatholytic agents (labetalol and methyl-dopa), a vasodilator (hydralazine), and a calcium blocker (nifedipine), each given intravenously (or orally in high dosage in the case of methyl-dopa) in order to ensure their rapid action.

In addition, anticonvulsant therapy is sometimes given in pre-eclampsia, with the aim of preventing eclampsia.[62,63] Among the anticonvulsants used, magnesium sulphate is the drug of choice. In recent clinical trials it was much more effective than diazepam and phenytoin in preventing eclamptic fits, including further fits when eclampsia has already developed[64] and first fits in pre-eclampsia.[65] However, whether the good done by anticonvulsant prophylaxis in pre-eclampsia outweighs the possibility for harm is unclear[66] and merits investigation by a placebo-controlled trial of magnesium sulphate.[67] In the United States, an estimated 5 per cent of all pregnant women receive anticonvulsants,[65] but many clinicians now believe that this is generally unnecessary and that 'the key initial step in stopping progression from pre-eclampsia to eclampsia is effective treatment of the hypertension',[67] bearing in mind that only delivery will finally halt the process.

As well as being used in obstetric hypertensive emergencies, sympatholytic agents (especially methyl-dopa and labetalol), vasodilators (usually combined with sympatholytic agents), and calcium blockers (especially nifedipine) are given at blood pressures where the mother's health is not in immediate danger.[68] There have been few satisfactory trials of the effectiveness of such therapy in reducing perinatal mortality. Two studies of methyl-dopa have shown a small improvement in the fetal survival, when compared with no hypertensive therapy at maternal diastolic blood pressures between 95 and 105 mmHg.[69,70] In addition, Gallery *et al.*[71] and Fidler *et al.*[72] have shown that the beta-adrenergic receptor blocking drug oxprenolol is as effective as methyl-dopa in a similar situation; but beta-adrenergic blocking drugs have not been shown to improve fetal survival compared with placebo. Numerous other small trials of many different types of antihypertensive agents have shown differences in 'softer' fetal outcomes such as birth weight and gestational age at delivery. These trials have been well summarized and subjected to meta-analysis by Collins and Wallenburg.[73]

It was thought that low-dose aspirin might reduce the risk of pre-eclampsia and its complications, since pre-eclampsia is associated with excessive production of the vasoconstrictor and platelet-aggregating agent thromboxane, which is reduced by low-dose aspirin. In large randomized clinical trials in pregnant women thought to be at increased risk of pre-eclampsia, the prevalence of pre-eclampsia (which averaged 7–8 per cent in the placebo-treated women) was 10 per cent lower in women on low-dose aspirin. This was not considered sufficient improvement to justify routine low-dose aspirin for all women at risk of pre-eclampsia.[74,75]

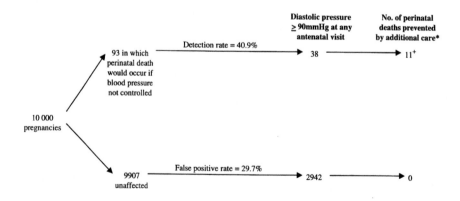

*   'Additional care' = increased frequency of examination, and therapy if indicated - e.g. oral hypotensive drugs if blood pressure ≥ 150/100 mmHg &/or proteinuria; intravenous hypotensive drugs if blood pressure ≥ 160/110 mmHg with proteinuria, followed by oral hypotensive drugs if blood pressure then falls and by early delivery otherwise.

+   Three-quarters of the excess number of deaths predicted to occur without additional care in pregnancies with diastolic pressure ≥ 90 mmHg   (i.e. 0.75 x 2980 x 4.8 /1000; see text).

Fig. 9.3 Performance of screening at each antenatal visit: positive defined by blood pressure alone (≥90 mmHg diastolic). Numbers taken from Table 9.6(a) except where stated.

CONCLUSIONS

As generally defined, high blood pressure in pregnancy has a high prevalence—close to 30 per cent if all pregnancies in which the diastolic pressure is reported ever to have reached 90 mmHg are defined as affected (as was the case in the British cohort studies of 1958[16] and 1970[6] on which the analyses in this chapter largely depend). Adverse outcomes of pregnancy due to HDP are much less common, and it is not possible from the available data to determine the efficacy of screening and treatment in preventing the adverse outcomes. In the absence of blood pressure screening and treatment, perinatal death (the outcome that can be analysed most fully) would occur in 12.7/1000 pregnancies with a diastolic pressure of >90 mmHg recorded at least once (compared with 7.9/1000 other pregnancies) according to the estimates in Table 16.6(a). Screening and treatment can be expected to reduce the excess perinatal mortality in these pregnancies (12.7 – 7.9 = 4.8/1000) by at least three-quarters, given the evidence of a reduction of this magnitude between 1958 and 1970 in the British cohort studies (p. 208). This is summarized in Fig. 9.3, which shows that 11 fetal lives would be saved for every 10 000 women screened using a cut-off of 90 mmHg.

As well as seeming to be effective, screening by blood pressure measurement is an inexpensive test, which requires only a few minutes and can be performed by anyone appropriately trained. Carrying it out at each antenatal visit remains the established practice because blood pressure may rise suddenly at any time in the second half of pregnancy.

One issue that needs further appraisal is whether and when slight or moderate elevation in blood pressure should be treated. Here there may be important financial benefits to be gained from a critical application of screening techniques. Many women

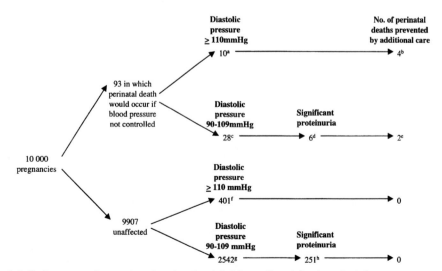

Fig. 9.4 Performance of screening at each antenatal visit: positive defined as diastolic pressure ≥110 mmHg, or ≥90 mmHg with proteinuria. See Appendix 2 for footnotes a-h, which explain how the numbers to which they relate were derived.

with slight elevations in blood pressure are admitted to hospital at considerable cost to themselves and to the health services, and the 30 per cent false-positive rate in Fig. 16.3 is evidence that not all these admissions are necessary.

Figure 9.4 shows (in a similar manner to Fig. 9.3) the estimated impact of a policy of restricting additional care to women whose diastolic pressure reaches 110 mmHg and to those in whom a diastolic pressure of 90–109 mmHg is combined with proteinuria. It is estimated that this 'high cut-off' policy would prevent six perinatal deaths per 10 000 births by treating 6.7 per cent of women (i.e. 10 + 6 + 401 + 251 per 10 000). It would therefore involve treating about 100 women (i.e. 670/6) for each perinatal death prevented. Screening using the lower cut-off (diastolic pressure ≥90 mmHg—see Fig 16.3) would prevent five additional perinatal deaths (i.e. 11 deaths in total), but at a cost of increasing the false-positive rate from below 7 per cent to 30 per cent, i.e. treating nearly a quarter of all pregnant women in addition to those treated under the high-cut-off policy. The marginal benefit of using the lower cut-off would therefore be one perinatal death prevented per 460 (i.e. (3000 – 700)/5) additional women treated.

Research is likely to improve the prediction of adverse outcomes associated with high blood pressure in pregnancy, particularly by further evaluating serum markers such as inhibin-A[44] and other tests such as Doppler ultrasound of the uterine artery.[76]

APPENDIX 1: SOME DEFINITIONS USED IN THE CLASSIFICATION OF HIGH BLOOD PRESSURE IN PREGNANCY

Categories broadly corresponding to PAH as defined in text

1. Essential hypertension: Maximum diastolic pressure before 20 weeks ≥90mmHg.[6]

2. Chronic hypertension: Diastolic pressure before 20 weeks >90 mmHg, or history of having hypertension and being on anti-hypertensive medication before the pregnancy.[8]

3. Chronic hypertension: Known hypertension before pregnancy, or rise in blood pressure to >140/90 mmHg before 20 weeks.[77]

Categories broadly corresponding to PIH as defined in text

1. PIH: Blood pressure before 20 weeks <140/90 mmHg; systolic pressure ≥140 mmHg and/or diastolic pressure ≥90 mmHg later, on at least two occasions four hours or more apart.[9] Some authorities add that the increase in diastolic pressure should be ≥25 mmHg.[21,68]

2. PIH: Blood pressure before 20 weeks <140/90 mmHg; systolic pressure ≥140 mmHg and/or diastolic pressure ≥90 mmHg and/or increase from baseline of ≥30 mmHg systolic pressure and/or ≥15 mmHg diastolic pressure after 20 weeks, on at least two occasions six hours or more apart.[7]

3. Pre-eclampsia: Maximum diastolic pressure before 20 weeks <90 mmHg; ≥90 mmHg later, and/or eclampsia.[6]

Sub-categories of PIH used in nationwide British surveys[6,16]

1. Mild pre-eclampsia: Maximum diastolic pressure after 20 weeks 90–99 mmHg; no proteinuria or eclampsia.

2. Moderate pre-eclampsia: Maximum diastolic pressure after 20 weeks 100–109 mmHg; no proteinuria or eclampsia.

3. Severe pre-eclampsia: Maximum diastolic pressure after 20 weeks $\geqslant 110$ mmHg, or proteinuria with maximum diastolic pressure after 20 weeks 90–109 mmHg, and/or eclampsia.

Other definitions of pre-eclampsia

1. PIH according to first definition above, concurrent with proteinuria $\geqslant 500$ mg/l.[9]

2. PIH according to second definition above, concurrent with proteinuria or oedema or both.[7]

Definitions of PAH with PIH or pre-eclampsia

1. Essential hypertension and pre-eclampsia: Maximum diastolic pressure before 20 weeks of gestation $\geqslant 90$ mmHg; increase of $\geqslant 10$ mmHg later, and/or proteinuria.[6]

2. Chronic hypertension with pre-eclampsia: Diastolic pressure before 20 weeks of gestation $\geqslant 90$ mmHg, or history of having hypertension and being on antihypertensive medication before the pregnancy; blood pressure later at least 140/90 mmHg with an increase of $\geqslant 30$ mmHg in systolic pressure and/or 15 mmHg in diastolic pressure on at least two occasions six hours apart, concurrent with proteinuria $\geqslant 0.3$ g/24 h or $\geqslant +$ on dipstick test on two occasions in the absence of urinary tract infection.[8]

APPENDIX 2: DERIVATION OF VARIOUS NUMBERS IN FIG. 9.4

a. $10 = 16 \times 411/(411 + 257)$. 16 is the number of true positives in Table 9.6(b). 411 and 257 are respectively the estimated numbers per 10 000 pregnancies in which diastolic pressures of $\geqslant 110$ mmHg (with or without proteinuria) and diastolic pressures of 90–109 mmHg combined with proteinuria would be observed. These two estimates were derived from the statistics for the 1958 birth cohort (Table 9.3) by making three assumptions:

> (i) That the pregnancies classified as 'proteinuria not elsewhere classified, and other' (for most of which the diastolic pressure was not known) were distributed between the other categories in the same proportions as the remaining pregnancies (which totalled 15 666). In this case, severe PIH without PAH would have occurred in 605/10 000 pregnancies (i.e. 948/15 666), mild or moderate PIH without PAH in 2094 (i.e. 3280/15 666), and PAH in 282 (i.e. 442/15 666).

(ii) That pregnancies with PAH were distributed by severity in the same proportions as pregnancies with PIH but not PAH. In this case the total number with severe PIH and/or PAH would be 668 (i.e. 605 + [282 × 605/(605 + 2094)]), and the total number with mild or moderate PIH and/or PAH would be 2313 (i.e. 2094 + [282 × 2094/(605 + 2094)]).

(iii) That proteinuria would occur in 10 per cent of pregnancies with PIH and/or PAH which in the absence of proteinuria would be regarded as mild or moderate (i.e. pregnancies with diastolic pressures of 90–109 mmHg). In this case, the 668 pregnancies with severe PIH and/or PAH would include 257 with diastolic pressures of 90–109 mmHg (i.e. one-ninth as many as the 2313 with mild or moderate PIH and/or PAH) and 411 with diastolic pressures of >110 mmHg (i.e. 668 – 257).

b. 4 = 10 – (1.73 × 7.9/1000 × 411). It is assumed that perinatal death would occur in 1.73 × 7.9/1000 pregnancies treated on account of diastolic pressures of ≥110 mmHg. 7.9/1000 is the perinatal mortality to be expected in the absence of HDP (see p. 213). 1.73:1 was the ratio between the perinatal death rate for pregnancies with severe PIH (including PIH + PAH) and the rate for normotensive pregnancies in the 1970 birth cohort (Table 9.3). 411 is the estimated total number of pregnancies with diastolic pressure ≥110 mmHg (see note a).

c. 28 = 38 – 10. 38 is the number of true positives to be expected with a cut-off of 90 mmHg (Table 9.6(a)).

d. 6 = 16 × 257/(411 + 257).*

e. 2 = 6 – (1.73 × 7.9/1000 × 257). 257 is the estimated total number of pregnancies with diastolic pressure of 90–109 mmHg and proteinuria (see note a). 1.73 and 7.9/1000 are as in note b.

f. 401 = 411 – 10.*

g. 2542 = 2313 + 257 – 28.*

h. 251 = 257 – 6.*

REFERENCES

1. Department of Health and Social Security. (1998). *Why Mothers Die: Report on Confidential Enquiries into Maternal Deaths in the United Kingdom 1994–96*. Stationery Office, London.

2. Dewhurst C.J. (1976). *Integrated Obstetrics and Gynaecology for Postgraduates*. Blackwell, Oxford.

3. Roberts J.M. and Redman C.W.G. (1993). Pre-eclampsia: more than pregnancy-induced hypertension. *Lancet*, **341**, 1447–51.

4. Redman C. W. G. and Roberts J. M. (1993). Management of pre-eclampsia. *Lancet*, **341**, 1451–4.

5. Weinstein L. (1982). Syndrome of hemolysis, elevated liver enzymes, and low platelet count: a severe consequence of hypertension in pregnancy. *Am J Obstet Gynecol*, **142**, 159–67.

---

* See note a for sources of figures not shown within the flow chart.

6. Chamberlain C. V. P., Phillipp E., Howlett B., and Masters K. (1978). *British Births, 1970: A Survey under the Joint Auspices of the National Birthday Trust and the Royal College of Obstetricians and Gynaecologists, Vol 2: Obstetric Care.* Heinemann, London.
7. Hughes E. C. (ed.) (1972). *Obstetric–Gynecologic Terminology*, p. 422. Davies, Philadelphia.
8. McCowan L. M. E., Buist R. G., North R. A., and Gamble G. (1996). Perinatal mortality in chronic hypertension. *Br J Obstet Gynaecol*, **10**, 123–9.
9. Davey D. A. and MacGillivray I. (1986). The classification and definition of the hypertensive disorders of pregnancy. *Clin Exp Hypertens*, **B5**, 97–133.
10. MacGillivray I., Rose G. A., and Rowe B. (1969). Blood pressure survey in pregnancy. *Clin Sci*, **37**, 395–407.
11. Miall W. E. and Oldham P. D. (1955). A study of arterial blood pressure and its inheritance in a sample of the general population. *Clin Sci*, **14**, 459–88.
12. Khong T. Y., de Wolf F., Robertson W. B., and Brosens I. (1986). Inadequate maternal vascular response to placentation in pregnancies complicated by pre-eclampsia and by small-for-gestational age infants. *Br J Obstet Gynaecol*, **93**, 1049–59.
13. Redman C. W. G., Beilin L. J., Bonnar J., and Wilkinson R. H. (1976). Plasma-urate measurements in predicting fetal death in hypertensive pregnancy. *Lancet*, **i**, 1370–3.
14. Redman C. W. G., Denson K. W. E., Beilin L. J., Bolton F. G., and Stirrat G. M. (1977). Factor VIII consumption in pre-eclampsia. *Lancet*, **ii**: 1249–52.
15. Davies A. M. (1979). Epidemiology of the hypertensive disorders of pregnancy. *Bull WHO*, **57**, 373–86.
16. Butler N. R. and Bonham D. G. (1963). *Perinatal Mortality (First Report of the British Perinatal Mortality Survey)*. Livingstone, Edinburgh.
17. Saftlas A. F., Olson D. R., Franks A. L., Atrash H. K., and Pokras R. (1990). Epidemiology of pre-eclampsia and eclampsia in the United States. *Am J Obstet Gynecol*, **163**, 460–5.
18. Sibai B. M., Abdella T. N., and Anderson G. D. (1983). Pregnancy outcome in 211 patients with mild chronic hypertension. *Obstet Gynecol*, **61**, 571–6.
19. MacGillivray I. and Campbell D. M. (1980). The effect of hypertension and oedema on birth weight. In *Pregnancy Hypertension*, (ed. J. Bonnar, I. MacGillivray, and E. M. Symonds), pp. 307–11. MTP, Lancaster.
20. Tervilä L., Goecke C., and Timonen S. (1973). Estimation of gestosis of pregnancy (EPH-gestosis). *Acta Obstet Gynec Scand*, **52**, 235–43.
21. Redman C. W. G. and Jefferies M. (1988). Revised definition of pre-eclampsia. *Lancet*, **i** 809–12.
22. Office for National Statistics (1999). *Mortality Statistics: Childhood, Infant and Perinatal.* Series DH3, no. 30 (Review of the Registrar General on deaths in England and Wales, 1997). Stationery Office, London.
23. Office of Population Censuses & Surveys. (1995). *Mortality Statistics Childhood 1992.* Series DH6, no. 6 (Review of the Registrar General on deaths in England and Wales, 1992). Her Majesty's Stationery Office, London.
24. Page E. W. and Christianson R. (1976). Influence of blood pressure changes with and without proteinuria upon outcome of pregnancy. *Am J Obstet Gynecol*, **126**, 821–33.
25. Taylor D. J., Howie P. W., Davidson J., Davidson D., and Drillien C. M. (1985). Do pregnancy complications contribute to neurodevelopmental disability? *Lancet*, **i**, 713–16.

26. Syverson C. J., Chavkin W., Atrash H. K., Rochat R. W., Sharp E. S., and King G. E. (1991). Pregnancy-related mortality in New York City, 1980 to 1984: Causes of death and associated risk factors. *Am J Obstet Gynecol*, **164**, 603–8.

27. Douglas R. A. and Redman C. W. G. (1994). Eclampsia in the United Kingdom. *Br Med J*, **309**, 1395–400.

28. Moller B. and Lindmark G. (1986). Eclampsia in Sweden, 1976–1980. *Acta Obstet Gynecol Scand*, **65**, 307–14.

29. Wright B. M. and Dore C. F. (1970). A random zero sphygmomanometer. *Lancet*, **i**, 337–8.

30. Rose G. A., Holland W. W., and Crowley E. A. (1964). A sphygmomanometer for epidemiologists. *Lancet*, **i**, 296–300.

31. King G. E. (1967). Errors in clinical measurement of blood pressure in obesity. *Clin Sci*, **32**, 223–37.

32. Johnson A. L., Cornoni J. C., Cassel J. C., Tyroler H. A., Heyden S., and Hames C. G. (1975). Influence of race, sex and weight on blood pressure behaviour in young adults. *Am J Cardiol*, **35**, 523–30.

33. Steinfield L., Alexander H., and Cohen M. L. (1974). Updating sphygmomanometry. *Am J Cardiol*, **33**, 107–10.

34. Kirkendall W. M., Burton A. C., Epstein F. H., and Freis E. D. (1967). Report of a subcommittee of the postgraduate education committee, American Heart Association. Recommendations for human blood pressure determination by sphygmomanometers. *Circulation*, **36**, 980–8.

35. de Swiet M. (1991). The Cardiovascular System. In *Clinical Physiology in Obstetrics*, 2nd edn, (ed. F. Hytten and G. Chamberlain), pp.3–38. Blackwell Scientific Publications, Oxford.

36. McLennan C. E. (1943). Antecubital and femoral venous pressure in normal and toxemic pregnancy. *Am J Obstet Gynecol*, **45**, 568–91.

37. Shennan A. H., Gupta M., Halligan A., Taylor D. J., and de Swiet M. (1996). Lack of reproducibility in pregnancy of Korotkoff phase IV as measured by mercury sphygmomanometry. *Lancet*, **347**, 139–42.

38. de Swiet M. and Shennan A. H. (1996). Blood pressure measurement in pregnancy. *Br J Obstet Gynaecol*, **103**, 862–3.

39. Raftery E. B. and Ward A. P. (1968). The indirect method of recording blood pressure. *Cardiovasc Res*, **2**, 210–18.

40. Seligman S. (1987). Which blood pressure? *Br J Obstet Gynaecol*, **94**, 497–8.

41. Margulies M., Zin C., Margulies N. D., and Voto L. S. (1989). Non-invasive ambulatory blood pressure control in normotensive pregnant women. *Am J Hypertens*, **2**, 924–6.

42. Peek M., Shennan A., Halligan A., Lambert P., Taylor D. J., and de Swiet M. (1996). Hypertension in pregnancy: which method of blood pressure measurement is the most predictive of outcome? *Obstet Gynecol*, **88**, 130–3.

43. Ferrazzani S., Caruso A., De-Carolis S., Martino I. V., and Mancuso S. (1990). Proteinuria and outcome of 444 pregnancies complicated by hypertension. *Am J Obstet Gynecol*, **162**, 366–71.

44. Muttukrishna S., Knight P. G., Groome N. P., Redman C. W. G., and Ledger W. L. (1997). Activin A and inhibin A as possible endocrine markers for pre-eclampsia. *Lancet*, **349**, 1285–8.

45. Gallery E. D. M., Hunyor S. N., Ross M., and Gyory A. A. (1977). Predicting the devel-

opment of pregnancy-associated hypertension. The place of standardised blood-pressure management, *Lancet*, **i**, 1273–5.

46. Moutquin J. M., Rainville C., Giroux L., Raynauld P., Amyot G., Bilodeau R., and Pelland R. N. (1985). A prospective study of blood pressure in pregnancy: prediction of pre-eclampsia. *Am J Obstet Gynecol*, **151**, 191–6.
47. Campbell S., Diaz-Recasens J., Griffith D. R. et al. (1983). New Doppler technique for assessing utero placental blood flow. *Lancet*, **i**, 675–7.
48. Gant N. F., Chand S., Worley R. J., Whalley P. J., Crosby U. D., and MacDonald P. C. (1974). A clinical test for predicting the development of active hypertension in pregnancy. *Am J Obstet Gynecol*, **120**, 1–7.
49. Louden K. A. and Broughton Pipkin F. (1991). Prediction of pregnancy-induced hypertensive disorders by angiotensin II sensitivity and supine pressure test. *Br J Obstet Gynaecol*, **98**, 231–3.
50. Gant N. F., Daley G. L., Chand S., Whalley P. J., and MacDonald P. C. (1973). A study of angiotensin II pressor response throughout primigravid pregnancy. *J Clin Invest*, **52**, 2682–9.
51. Baker P. N. , Broughton Pipkin F., and Symonds E. M. (1989). Platelet angiotensin II binding sites in hypertension in pregnancy. *Lancet*, **ii**, 1151.
52. Lockwood C. J. and Peters J. H. (1990). Increased plasma levels of EDI and cellular fibronective precede the clinical signs of pre-eclampsia. *Am J Obstet Gynecol*, **162**, 358–62.
53. Azar R. and Turpin D. (1989). La fibronective plasmatique: marquer de l'hypertension arterielle gravidique? *J Gynaecol Obstet Biol Reprod (Paris)*, **18**, 863–6.
54. Zemei M. B., Zemei P. C., Berry S., Norman G., Kowalczyk C., Sokol R. J., Standley P. R., Walsh M. F., and Sowers J. R. (1990). Altered platelet calcium metabolism as an early predictor of increased peripheral vascular resistance and pre-eclampsia in urban black women. *New Engl J Med*, **323**, 434–8.
55. McCance D. R., McKnight J. A., Traub A. I., Sheridan B., Roberts G., and Atkinson A. B. (1990). Plasma trial natriuretic factor levels during normal pregnancy and pregnancy complicated by diabetes mellitus and hypertension. *J Hum Hypertens*, **4**, 31–5.
56. Murphy J. F., O'Riordan J., Newcombe R. G., and Coles E. C. (1986). Relation of haemoglobin levels in first and second trimesters to outcome of pregnancy. *Lancet*, **i**, 992–4.
57. Eskine K. J., Iversen S. A., and Davies R. (1985). An altered ratio of 18:2 (9,11) to 18:2 (9,12) linoleic acid in plasma phospholipids as a possible predictor of pre-eclampsia. *Lancet*, **i**, 554–5.
58. Millar J., Campbell S., Albano J., Higgins B., and Clark A. (1996). Early prediction of pre-eclampsia by measurement of kallikrein and creatinine on a random urine sample. *Br J Obstet Gynaecol*, **103**, 421–6.
59. Jacobson S. L., Imahof R., Manning N. et al. (1990). The value of Doppler assessment of the utero placental circulation in predicting pre-eclampsia or intrauterine growth retardation. *Am J Obstet Gynecol*, **162**, 110–14.
60. Chesley L. C. and Sibai B. M. (1988). Clinical significance of elevated mean arterial pressure in the second trimester. *Am J Obstet Gynecol*, **159**, 275–9.
61. Dekker G. A., Makovitz J. W., and Wallenburg H. C. S. (1990). Prediction of pregnancy-induced hypertension disorders by angiotensin II sensitivity and supine pressor test. *Br J Obstet Gynaecol*, **97**, 817–21.

62. Chamberlain G. V. P., Lewis P. J., de Swiet M., and Bulpitt C. J. (1978). How obstetricians manage hypertension in pregnancy. *Br Med J*, **i**, 626–9.
63. Slater R. M., Wilcox F. I., Smith W. D., Donnai P., Partick J., Richardson T., Mawer G. E., D'Souza S. W., and Anderton J. M. (1987). Phenytoin infusion in severe pre-eclampsia. *Lancet*, **i**, 1417–20.
64. Eclampsia Trial Collaborative Group (1995). Which anticonvulsant for women with eclampsia? Evidence from the Collaborative Eclampsia Trial. *Lancet*, **345**, 1455–63.
65. Lucas M. J., Levene R. I., and Cunningham F. G. (1995). A comparison of magnesium sulfate with phenytoin for the prevention of eclampsia. *New Engl J Med*, **333**, 201–5.
66. Duley L. and Johanson R. (1994). Magnesium sulphate for pre-eclampsia and eclampsia: the evidence so far. *Br J Obstet Gynaecol*, **101**, 565–7.
67. Neilson J. P. (1995). Magnesium sulphate: the drug of choice in eclampsia. *Br Med J*, **311**, 702–3.
68. Pipkin F. B. (1995). The hypertensive disorders of pregnancy. *Br Med J*, **311**, 609–13.
69. Redman C. W. G., Beilin L. J., Bonnar J., and Ounsted M. K. (1976). Fetal outcome in trial of antihypertensive treatment in pregnancy. *Lancet*, **ii**, 753–6.
70. Leather H. M., Humphreys P., Baker P., and Chadd M. A. (1968). A controlled trial of hypotensive agents in hypertension in pregnancy. *Lancet*, **ii**, 488–90.
71. Gallery E. C. M., Saunders D. M., Hunyor S. N., and Gyory A. Z. (1978). Improvement of fetal growth with treatment of maternal hypertension in pregnancy. *Clin Sci Molec Med*, **55**, 339–61.
72. Fidler J., Smith V., Fayers P., and de Swiet M. (1983). Randomised controlled comparative study of methyl-dopa and oxprenolol for the treatment of hypertension in pregnancy. *Br Med J*, **286**, 1927–30.
73. Collins R. and Wallenburg H. C. S. (1989). Pharmacological prevention and treatment of hypertensive disorder in pregnancy. In *Effective Care in Pregnancy and Childbirth*, Vol. 1, (ed. I. Chalmers, M. Enkin, and M. J. N. C. Keirse), pp. 512–33. Oxford University Press, Oxford.
74. CLASP (Collaborative Low-dose Aspirin Study in Pregnancy) Collaborative Group (1994). CLASP: a randomised trial of low-dose aspirin for the prevention and treatment of pre-eclampsia among 9364 pregnant women. *Lancet*, **343**, 619–29.
75. Caritis S., Sibai B., Hauth J., Lindheimer M. D., Klebanoff M., Thom E., VanDorsten P., Landon M., Paul R., Miodovnik M., Meis P., Thurnau G., and the National Institute of Child Health and Human Development Network of Maternal-Fetal Medicine Units (1998). Low-dose aspirin to prevent preeclampsia in women at high risk. *New Engl J Med*, **338**, 701–5.
76. Chappell L. and Bewley S. (1998). Pre-eclamptic toxaemia: the role of uterine artery Doppler. *Br J Obstet Gynaecol*, **105**, 379–82.
77. Gifford R. W., August P., Chesley L. C. et al. (1990). National high blood pressure education program working group report on high blood pressure in pregnancy. *Am J Obstet Gynecol*, **163**, 1691–712.

10 *Acquired haematological disorders*

Elizabeth A. Letsky and Sir David Weatherall

INTRODUCTION

There are only two groups of acquired haematological disorders which are common enough and of sufficient clinical importance to have led to the development of widespread antenatal or neonatal screening programmes. These are the anaemias of pregnancy and fetomaternal alloimmunization.

The main aim in screening pregnant women for anaemia is to detect and correct iron deficiency so that the prevalence of certain adverse outcomes such as low birthweight is reduced. Iron deficiency is the commonest medical complication of pregnancy. It is responsible for the vast majority of cases of anaemia in pregnancy and can have adverse effects on the mother, fetus, and neonate. The screening test is measurement of the haemoglobin (Hb) level. When carried out at the first antenatal visit, this detects women who are coming into pregnancy already anaemic and enables the cause of the anaemia to be determined. Although most cases are due to iron deficiency of nutritional origin, it is important to identify the various genetic disorders of haemoglobin synthesis described in Chapter 11, and other less common causes of anaemia which affect women of reproductive age. Rescreening the haemoglobin level later in pregnancy will identify those women who have become iron deficient during the course of pregnancy and who are at risk of going into labour and the postpartum period with dangerously low haemoglobin levels.

The main aim in screening for fetomaternal alloimmunization is to prevent haemolytic disease of the fetus and newborn. This problem is considered in Chapter 12. The present chapter includes a discussion of allo-immune thrombocytopenia of the fetus and newborn, in which the alloimmunization involves fetal platelet antigens.

In the past decade or so, it has become convenient to screen for anaemia by carrying out an automated full blood count, which has resulted in unsolicited *de facto* screening using various haematological variables, including platelet count. This leads to the identification of many symptomless women as thrombocytopenic by non-pregnant standards. The question whether any action should be taken in response to this finding is also discussed in this chapter.

The chapter does not deal with selective testing for acquired haematological disorders when the risk of disorders of these kinds is high (e.g. when a routine ultrasound detects fetal hydrops or when drugs with haematological side-effects are used), since testing in these circumstances is not screening but part of clinical care.

IRON DEFICIENCY OF PREGNANCY

The physiological background

There are dramatic changes in the circulating blood during normal pregnancy.[1] It is therefore not possible to assess accurately the haematological status of pregnant women by the criteria used for males and non-pregnant females.

From early pregnancy there is an increased impetus to erythropoiesis, due mainly to a rise in erythropoietin (Epo) production and possibly caused by the actions of other hormones such as placental lactogen. There is a threefold increase in the concentration of Epo in plasma and in urine by the second trimester. Recent studies have also shown a further statistically significant increase in Epo concentration in the presence of anaemia or iron deficiency.[2-5]

In spite of this drive to erythropoiesis the haemoglobin concentration, haematocrit, and red cell count fall as healthy pregnancy progresses because the increase in plasma volume is greater than the rise in red cell mass.[6] The haemoglobin level reaches its nadir at 32–34 weeks when haemodilution is maximal. The rise in plasma volume is approximately 50 per cent while the increase in red cell mass is 18–25 per cent dependent on iron status. The haemoglobin concentration falls to a mean of between 11 and 12 g/dl according to most published series. The WHO recommends that ideally haemoglobin should be maintained at or above 11g/dl and should not be allowed to fall below 10.5g/dl in the second trimester.[7-9]

In pregnancy with adequate iron stores, the Hb concentration is dependent largely on the plasma volume increase, which is controlled independently of iron status and is directly related to the mother's health during pregnancy and labour and to the birth weight of the baby. Women with poorly growing fetuses and poor reproductive performance have a correspondingly poor plasma volume response, and therefore less reduction of the haemoglobin level by haemodilution. This probably explains why an association of high haemoglobin concentration with poor reproductive performance has sometimes been observed,[10,11] although this association has been interpreted elsewhere as evidence that routine iron supplements are unnecessary[12] and may be harmful.[11]

Although the increase in red cell mass represents the major single demand for additional iron during pregnancy, the demands of the fetus also become substantial during the last three months and especially the last four weeks before term. The fetus derives its iron from the maternal serum by active transport across the placenta.[13] A further reduction in maternal iron is occasioned by the blood loss which occurs at delivery, although the haemoglobin returns to pre-pregnancy levels by the end of the first week post partum in iron-replete women with normal blood loss at delivery. Breast feeding results in a further demand for iron, although there is some iron conservation during the months of amenorrhoea. The total requirement of iron during pregnancy and breast feeding is of the order of 700–1400 mg. Overall, the requirement is 4 mg per day but rises from 2 mg per day in the non-pregnant to 6 mg per day in the last few weeks of pregnancy. A normal mixed diet contains an average of about

14 mg of iron each day of which only 1–2 mg (5–10 per cent) is absorbed. Even though absorption from the gut is more efficient in pregnancy the amount of iron that a current Western diet will provide is about 500 mg less than is needed through pregnancy and breast feeding. There is a limited increase in absorption if the mother's reticulo-endothelial iron stores are insufficient to meet this need. Iron depletion and eventually anaemia will follow if her iron intake is not supplemented.

The disorder

Especially for women who become pregnant again not many months after giving birth, it is common to have insufficient reticulo-endothelial iron reserves to cover the high iron requirements of pregnancy, particularly during the last 100–120 days. Iron deficiency is considered to be present when these reserves are totally depleted, and is regarded as having two stages—a first and milder stage in which iron-deficiency erythropoiesis is initiated although the haemoglobin concentration remains normal, and a second and more severe stage in which the haemoglobin concentration is low. Clinical experience shows that even with haemoglobin levels below 11.0g/dl, many apparently healthy women are able to proceed through pregnancy without complications, although investigation indicates that the majority are iron (and folate) deficient. However, both stages of iron deficiency appear to be associated with various non-haematological problems for mother and child.

Maternal problems

In the mother, there is compensation for defects in oxygen-carrying capacity, and overt symptoms of iron deficiency are generally not prominent. However, recent work indicates that impairment of the function of iron-dependent tissue enzymes occurs even in the first stage of iron deficiency, and develops hand-in-hand with the fall in haemoglobin concentration. This may have various consequences. An effect on the brain is suggested by the observation that subjective well-being improves long before haemoglobin level when oral or parenteral iron is given for anaemia.[14] The anecdotal reports of increased blood loss at delivery in anaemic women may indicate that iron deficiency impairs myometrial function by affecting neuromuscular transmission. The reported association between anaemia and preterm birth[15–18] may also be due to various effects of iron deficiency on cellular function.

Fetal problems

Because there is active transport of iron from mother to fetus in the last four weeks of pregnancy, concentrations of ferritin (a marker of iron stores) are substantially higher in the cord blood than in the mother's circulation at term whether she is iron deficient or not; and all cord ferritin levels fall within the normal adult range. However, babies born to iron-deficient mothers have significantly lower cord ferritin levels than other babies. This has an important bearing on iron stores and development of anaemia in the first year of life when iron intake is very poor.[4,19–21]

There is some evidence that the risk of behavioural and learning difficulties is increased by iron deficiency in the child, and therefore indirectly by maternal iron deficiency. Studies have suggested that children with iron deficiency are at increased risk of behavioural abnormalities related to changes in the concentration of chemical indicators in the brain.[22-26] Iron deficiency in the absence of anaemia is associated with poor performance in the Bayley Mental Developmental Index. Moreover, poor performance of 12–18 month-old iron-deficient anaemic infants in mental and motor development can be improved to the level of iron-sufficient infants by treatment with ferrous sulphate.[27]

Even more far-reaching effects of maternal iron deficiency during pregnancy have been suggested. A correlation has recently been shown between maternal iron-deficiency anaemia, high placental weight and an increased ratio of placental to birth weight. This suggests that maternal iron deficiency results in slower fetal than placental growth. High blood pressure in adult life has also been linked to an increased ratio of placental to birth weight, as well as to low birth weight itself. Maternal iron deficiency may therefore increase the risk of adult hypertension, which appears to have its origin in fetal life.[28-30]

Prevalence

In the present state of knowledge it is not possible to estimate the proportion of pregnancies in which outcomes such as pre-term birth, post-partum haemorrhage, and behavioural and learning difficulties and eventual hypertension in the offspring occur as a result of iron deficiency. Even the population prevalence of iron deficiency itself (i.e. the proportion of people whose iron reserves are totally depleted) has not been well documented. The prevalence of anaemia according to the WHO definition (haemoglobin <11.0 g/dl) has been more widely studied and is well over 50 per cent in many developing countries. In industrialized countries, prevalence in the general population is much lower, and most cases are only recognized by laboratory investigation; the classical clinical manifestations of iron deficiency (koilonychia, glossitis, cheilosis, and dysphagia) are seen only rarely. It has been estimated that less than one in 500 men in the USA has iron-deficiency anaemia.[31] However, even in the developed countries anaemia is common in pregnant women who have not received iron supplementation. For example, between 40 per cent and 50 per cent of unsupplemented women in two large surveys had haemoglobin levels below 11 g/dl at term.[32]

It would appear therefore that a high proportion of reproducing women lack storage iron. The reason may be that social changes over the centuries have made it more difficult for women to build up iron stores so that iron balance can be maintained in pregnancy. Iron intake must have fallen with the reduction in meat and fish consumption when human society became based on agriculture instead of hunting and fishing,[33] and dietary changes following industrialization may have had a similar effect.

Prevention

When a pregnant woman's iron stores are depleted, her increased need for iron can be met by provision of supplemental iron through the second and third trimesters of pregnancy. Over the years there have been many studies which have proven without doubt that iron supplements prevent the development of anaemia[34] and that in women on a good diet who are not apparently anaemic at booking, the mean haemoglobin level can be raised by oral iron therapy throughout pregnancy. The difference in favour of those so treated is most marked at term when the need for an adequate haemoglobin level is maximal.

There are almost no risks associated with iron supplementation during pregnancy. It is not possible for this to raise the Hb concentration to supra-normal levels, or to increase the mean corpuscular volume and alter blood flow. There is a potential hazard for women who are homozygous for the gene for haemochromatosis (2–5/1000 of most populations of European origin[35,36]): homozygotes absorb more dietary iron than is normal, which can lead to serious illness due to iron overload, and this process is likely to be accelerated by supplementing their iron intake. However, the clinical disease is only between one-tenth and one-fifth as common in women as in men, which suggests that most female homozygotes are clinically unaffected, particularly in the reproductive years.[37]

There is considerable controversy about whether routine iron supplements for all women during pregnancy are justifiable. Many authors are not able to accept that the physiological requirements for iron in pregnancy are considerably higher than the usual intake of most healthy women with apparently good diets in industrial countries.[11,38] It has been suggested that women should be screened for insufficient iron stores by measuring their serum ferritin, and that those with serum ferritin above 80 μg/l early in pregnancy should not be given supplementary iron.[39,40] On investigation of 669 consecutive women booking for confinement at Queen Charlotte's Hospital, London, with Hb concentration of 11.0 g/dl or above, only 7.6 per cent had serum ferritins above 80 μg/l, and 82.5 per cent had serum ferritins <50 μg/l, including 12 per cent of the total who had totally depleted stores with a ferritin of < 8 μg/l.[41] These findings, together with the increasing evidence that iron depletion affects exercise tolerance, cerebral function, and fetal, neonatal and infant development,[15–27,29] lead us to support the conclusion that it is safer, more practical, and in the long term less expensive in terms of investigation, hospital admission, and treatment, to offer all women iron supplements from 16 weeks of gestation[4,20,34,42] rather than screen for deficient iron stores in the first trimester or wait until overt severe iron-deficiency anaemia develops. Oral supplementation of 60–80 mg elemental iron per day from early pregnancy maintains a haemoglobin level in the normal range in most subjects on a Western diet but does not maintain or restore iron stores. The most recent guidelines for the use of iron supplements to prevent and treat iron deficiency anaemia were issued jointly by the International Nutritional Anemia Consultative Group (INACG), WHO and UNICEF. It is suggested that 60 mg iron plus 400 g folic acid is given daily for six months during pregnancy in communities where the prevalence of anaemia is <40% (e.g. UK), and that where the prevalence is higher these supplements should continue for three months post partum.[43]

Screening and diagnosis
Haemoglobin measurement
Although we recommend giving iron supplementation to all pregnant women rather than to a subset identified by screening, we also support the established practice of screening for anaemia by measuring the haemoglobin concentration at the first ante-natal visit at 10–16 weeks and at around 30 weeks of gestation. This procedure is simple and cheap; and although formal randomized trials have not been carried out to quantify its benefit it is likely to be worthwhile, since it identifies women who may need more than the standard dose of supplementary iron because their iron stores are depleted,

and also detects women who need to be investigated for causes of anaemia other than simple iron deficiency.

Among the disorders other than iron deficiency which cause anaemia, the thalassaemias and sickling disorders are considered in Chapter 7 of this book. They have to be ruled out in any patient of the appropriate racial background. Other causes of anaemia are much less common in Western Europe and North America, although megaloblastic anaemia due to folate deficiency occurs in some racial groups, particularly in the latter half of pregnancy or in the puerperium.[44] In parts of India nutritional vitamin B_{12} deficiency is still extremely common in vegans.[44] In very poor communities, for example Malawi where maize is the staple diet, B_{12} deficiency has been shown with megaloblastic changes in the bone marrow.[45] HIV and its complications contribute to the high incidence of anaemia in an increasing number of populations, particularly in Africa. In many tropical countries chronic malaria and gastrointestinal parasitic infections may lead to severe anaemia early in pregnancy.

Screening for anaemia is generally combined with various other tests for which blood is taken at the first antenatal visit and at around 30 weeks of gestation. A full blood count is performed together with blood grouping and screening for atypical antibodies. In a well nourished population the haemoglobin level should be within the normal female range (12.0–14.0 g/dl) and certainly above 11.0 g/dl. In the first trimester there is no physiological reason why the haemoglobin should not be above 12.0 g/dl, and some obstetric units which do not offer supplements to all women recommend them if the Hb is below 12.0 g/dl at booking.

Tests for iron deficiency

Various tests have been used in the assessment of iron deficiency in pregnancy. We refer first to the tests that we do not recommend for general use for this purpose, giving our reservations. These tests are measurements of mean corpuscular volume (MCV), mean corpuscular haemoglobin content (MCH), mean corpuscular haemoglobin concentration (MCHC), serum iron, total iron binding capacity, transferrin saturation, erythrocyte protoporphyrin, and marrow iron.

MCV, MCH, and MCHC, which are helpful outside pregnancy, are altered during pregnancy due to physiological changes. This makes them poor indicators of iron deficiency which develops during the course of pregnancy. For example, the increased drive to erythropoiesis during pregnancy results in a higher proportion of young large red cells, which appears to mask the effect of iron deficiency on the MCV even when anaemia has become established.[40,46] The MCV, MCH, and MCHC are, however, of help in diagnosis when a woman enters pregnancy with established microcytic hypochromic anaemia due to iron deficiency, or with macrocytic anaemia due to deficiency of folate or vitamin B_{12}. The problems of screening for megaloblastic anaemia in pregnancy are dealt with by Chanarin.[44] Determination of the MCV and MHC is also the screening test for β-thalassaemia (see Chapter 7).

Low serum iron, increase in total iron binding capacity, and a transferrin saturation level of less than one-third, are all signs that less iron than normal is being carried by serum proteins. Although among the earliest indicators of iron-deficient erythropoiesis, they are unreliable. Serum iron fluctuates widely and is affected by recent ingestion of iron and other factors not directly involved with iron metabolism, and total iron binding capacity increases in normal pregnancy.

Erythrocyte zinc protoporphyrin represents unused substrate for haem synthesis, and its level rises when not enough iron is reaching the developing erythrocyte. It too is unreliable as a marker of iron deficiency, since it can also increase in infection, other chronic inflammatory disease, and malignancy.

All the above variables are related more closely to tissue iron status than to iron stores. The most rapid and reliable method of assessing iron stores in pregnancy is by examination of an appropriately stained preparation of a bone marrow sample. However, the need for bone marrow samples for this purpose can be expected to decline as adequate blood tests for iron status (see below) become available.

The most useful blood tests for assessing iron status are those measuring transferrin receptor and ferritin. Ferritin, a high molecular weight glycoprotein which can be measured by immunoradiometric assay, circulates in the blood of healthy adults in a range of 15–300 µg/l. It is stable and not affected by recent ingestion of iron, and in normal circumstances it appears to reflect the iron stores accurately and quantitatively, particularly in the lower range associated with iron deficiency which is so important in pregnancy. It shares with erythrocyte zinc protoporphyrin the drawback of being affected by inflammation and malignancy. It is increased to about three times normal for any given level of storage iron in patients with chronic inflammatory disease, and will often fall in the normal range in individuals with genuine iron-deficient anaemia and co-existing inflammation or neoplasia.

Serum transferrin receptor (TfR) provides a new method for assessing cellular iron status which is reported to be reliable.[31] It is present in all cells as a transmembrane protein which binds transferrin-bound iron and transports it to the cell interior. Nine-tenths of the TfR molecule is located outside the cell. Any reduction in iron supply results in an increase of TfR synthesis. Studies using sensitive immunological techniques have shown that transferrin receptor circulates in small amounts in the plasma of all individuals and that the concentration is proportional to the total body mass of TfR. The only notable exception is in patients with iron-deficiency anaemia in whom the *serum* receptor is elevated some three-fold. This is accompanied by an increase in the density of surface transferrin receptor in iron-deficient cells. There is little or no change in serum receptor concentration during the early stages of storage iron depletion, but as soon as tissue iron deficiency is established the serum TfR concentration increases in direct proportion to the degree of iron deficiency. This change precedes the reduction in MCV and the rise in erythrocyte protoporphyrin and is therefore a valuable measurement for detection of early tissue iron lack. This measurement of iron status is particularly helpful in identifying iron deficiency in pregnancy.[47] It will identify truly iron-deficient women from those who have a low haemoglobin concentration due to haemodilution or those who have low serum ferritin due to storage iron mobilization. It is not in routine use in the UK. Several studies are in progress to assess its value in the management of anaemia in areas of the world where both nutritional iron anaemia and chronic inflammatory disease during pregnancy are common.[48]

In combination, serum ferritin and TfR give a complete picture of iron status—the serum ferritin reflecting iron stores and TfR the tissue iron status.[47]

Conclusions

It is difficult to assess the specific benefits of measuring haemoglobin concentration as a method of screening for iron deficiency and other causes of anaemia. One difficulty is that relatively little is known about the frequency of the non-haematological disorders associated with iron deficiency and the extent to which the associations are causal. Another difficulty is that formal randomized trials to quantify the benefits of measuring haemoglobin in pregnancy have not been carried out, and would be difficult to institute now that the practice is so firmly established. However, we consider that this practice should continue, even if all pregnant women are given routine iron supplements. Its benefits include firstly enabling anaemias that are not prevented by iron supplementation to be identified, and secondly providing a basis for deciding which women should be given more than the routine dose of iron.

THROMBOCYTOPENIA DURING PREGNANCY AND IN THE NEWBORN

There is a sharp distinction to be made between maternal thrombocytopenia during pregnancy and fetal allo-immune thrombocytopenia (FAIT). Maternal thrombocytopenia is sometimes caused by an auto-immune reaction to platelets, in which case the platelet-associated antibody may cross the placenta and cause thrombocytopenia in the fetus and neonate; but fetal thrombocytopenia due to maternal idiopathic thrombocytopenic purpura (the most common diagnosis in clinically recognized cases of maternal auto-immune thrombocytopenia) is not associated with spontaneous fetal haemorrhage.[49] In this respect it differs from FAIT, which occurs when a woman who is negative for the platelet surface antigen HPA[1] has an HPA[1]-positive fetus and produces anti-HPA[1] Ig/G antibody which can cross the placenta and cause fetal thrombocytopenia. FAIT is thus a serious fetal disorder with no maternal consequences,[50] in contrast to idiopathic thrombocytopenia purpura, which is a largely benign maternal disorder with rare fetal morbidity. Both problems have recently been reviewed.[51-53]

Allo-immune fetal thrombocytopenia

The disorder

The platelet surface antigens involved in FAIT have recently been renamed, using the Human Platelet Antigen (HPA) system. Approximately 98 per cent of the population are positive for the platelet antigen HPA[1] (previously Pla[1]) or for one of two allelic variants of it (HPA[1a] and HPA[2]). The maternal immune response is in part genetically determined by genes located in the major histocompatibility complex. HPA[1] negative women with HLA-B8 and HLA-DR3 and DRW52 antigens are at increased risk of allo-immunization if exposed to the HPA[1] antigen.

The second most frequent antigen after HPA[1a] to be implicated in FAIT is HPA[5b]. Data on the immune response against HPA[5b] are limited. Anecdotal reports suggest that FAIT arising from HPA[5b] antibodies has less severe clinical consequences, but an association with intracranial haemorrhage and neurological consequences was reported in one small series.[54]

In contrast to the sparing of first pregnancies, which is a feature of the common red blood cell allo-immune disorders (cf. Rh(D) disease), about 30 per cent of affected cases of FAIT occur in a first pregnancy. These cases in first pregnancies are usually unexpected because platelet and HLA typing are not part of routine antenatal screening. They represent about 9 per cent of all neonatal thrombocytopenias. Subsequent pregnancies are affected in 75 per cent to 90 per cent of cases with similar or increasing severity. Fetal platelet antigens are fully expressed by 18 weeks of gestation, and severe thrombocytopenia has been demonstrated as early as 20 weeks. The specific binding of the platelet antibody to the antigen on the surface of the platelet seriously impairs platelet function (unlike the non-specific IgG antibody in auto-immune thrombocytopenia), and the fetus is at risk of spontaneous haemorrhage *in utero* well before delivery. Ultrasound findings suggestive of intracranial haemorrhage are, however, rare before the third trimester. Intracranial bleeding is the most serious complication of this disease. It occurs in 10–30 per cent of cases and is responsible for a 12–15 per cent mortality rate.[52,55,56]

There is a wide spectrum of clinical presentation. The unexpected first case may be symptomless with thrombocytopenia discovered incidentally (e.g. on examination of cord blood of a child born to a Rh(D) negative woman). There may be petechiae and purpura, and on further investigation evidence of intracranial haemorrhage (e.g. porencephaly due to an old haemorrhage) may be found. In the most severe cases there may be devastating consequences resulting in severe motor and neurological impairment including blindness and mental retardation. The frequency of neurological handicap is difficult to establish because defects may not become apparent until some time after birth, but developmental abnormalities have been reported in up to 25 per cent of cases. Intrauterine death due to massive intracranial haemorrhage has been described either during labour or in the third trimester.

Prevalence

Symptomatic FAIT occurs in about 0.2–1.0 per thousand pregnancies, but it is likely that asymptomatic unrecognized cases occur more frequently. Epidemiological studies are in progress in the UK and in the USA to establish the true frequency. The above figures suggest that the proportion of all fetuses affected by intracranial haemorrhage as a result of symptomatic FAIT lies between 0.02/1000 (i.e. 10 per cent of 0.2/1000) and 0.3/1000 (i.e. 30 per cent of 1/1000). A preliminary study in the UK has recently been published supporting these figures.[57]

Management

The investigation of neonates with unexpected thrombocytopenia, and of intrauterine deaths with intracranial haemorrhage, should involve typing of maternal, fetal/neonatal, and paternal platelet antigens, together with maternal serum testing for antiplatelet antibodies. Couples who have borne an affected child or who appear for other reasons to be at risk of doing so should be referred to a specialist centre before embarking on another pregnancy so that expert and effective counselling and therapy can be planned. The pregnant woman at risk should be referred for assessment at a specialist centre early in pregnancy. If she is HPA[1] antibody-positive and her partner is heterozygous for HPA[1] antigen, the HPA status of the fetus should be determined by DNA analysis of fetal amniotic fluid cells, since HPA[1] negative fetuses do not need fetal blood sampling later in pregnancy. The first-degree female relatives of women whose fetuses are at risk of FAIT should be screened as possible sources of platelets for transfusion, and also to identify those whose own pregnancies may be at risk.

The ideal management of the fetus affected by this potentially devastating condition is controversial and as yet undecided. Trials are ongoing comparing maternal intravenous IgG and pre-delivery fetal platelet transfusions with or without maternal or fetal intravenous IgG.[58] The whole question has been the subject of several reviews.[52,55,56,58-61]

Screening

It was estimated above that between two and 30 fetuses in every 100 000 (equivalent to up to 200 per year in the UK) are affected by intracranial haemorrhage as a result of symptomatic FAIT. If current or future epidemiological studies yield a figure towards or above the upper limit of this range, and if the results of the current trials provide a firm basis for effective prevention or treatment, serious consideration will need to be given to screening all pregnant women for HPA status at the same time as for red cell group. This would need to be followed by HLA testing in HPA[1] negative women, and/or by testing the HPA status of their partners.[57]

Until the case for screening for FAIT by routine HPA testing is settled, it would be worth screening each pregnant woman by asking whether she or a first-degree relative has had a child with FAIT or unexplained brain damage. If the answer was positive, further testing as described above under 'management' would follow.

Maternal thrombocytopenia during pregnancy

All auto-analysers currently used in the routine examination of pregnant women's blood provide a platelet count. Although this has not come about as a result of any decision that platelet counting is a useful population screening test for any disorder, it means that screening of this kind is happening, and that clinicians often receive reports of thrombocytopenia ($<150 \times 10^9$ platelets/litre) in asymptomatic pregnant women. What difference if any should a report of this kind make to the clinical care of an apparently healthy woman? In seeking to answer this question, we shall briefly review the causes of maternal thrombocytopenia and its effects on the fetus, and then consider the implications of this knowledge for clinical management.

Causation

Rarely, maternal thrombocytopenia is the result of under-production of platelets, due to genetic causes, neoplastic infiltration, or toxic depression of megakaryocytes by infection or drugs. However, the vast majority of cases result from an increased rate of platelet consumption. The most important and difficult of these cases in terms of diagnosis and management are those with auto-immune thrombocytopenia. Sometimes this is induced by one of a wide variety of drugs, of which sulphonamides, quinidine, and quinine are among the most frequent offenders. In these cases, the immune reaction is due to antibody being formed against a drug–hapten complex, the platelet being an innocent bystander caught up in the reaction. However, most clinically recognized cases of auto-immune thrombocytopenia are diagnosed as having idiopathic thrombocytopenic purpura (ITP), which is a diagnosis of exclusion.

In an even larger number of cases of maternal thrombocytopenia, as well as there being no identifiable cause there is no purpura or other clinical evidence of an increased risk of bleeding. There is a downward trend in the platelet count during healthy pregnancy.[50] Most investigators agree that low-grade chronic intravascular coagulation within the utero-placental circulation is part of the physiological response of all women to pregnancy. This results in an increased platelet turnover with a larger proportion of young platelets with a greater mean platelet volume and in some cases a significant reduction in number.[62] For example, in one prospective study of 6715 consecutive deliveries,[50] 7.6 per cent of all women had maternal thrombocytopenia immediately pre-partum, and approximately two-thirds of those affected had no history of immune thrombocytopenia or associated conditions such as pre-eclampsia. The platelet count in this group was usually above 80×10^9 per litre but could be as low as 50×10^9 per litre. It is uncertain whether the thrombocytopenia seen in these healthy women is auto-immune, but their platelet counts return to normal shortly after delivery. The risk of bleeding for any given platelet count is less when the proportion of young, large platelets is high, as it is in pregnancy.

Fetal effects

It seems from the above-quoted study of unselected deliveries[50] that the offspring of healthy women with asymptomatic thrombocytopenia have similar cord platelet counts to babies born to non-thrombocytopenic mothers. In both groups there was a frequency of mild neonatal thrombocytopenia of 4 per cent.

In offspring of women with ITP, an analysis of reported cases in the literature[63] suggested an overall incidence of neonatal thrombocytopenia of 52 per cent, with significant morbidity in 12 per cent of births. However, these cases are likely to have been unrepresentative, since symptomatic women and babies are more likely than others to have been reported and some cases of thrombocytopenia with clearly defined causes may have been included.[64] In a much more reliable study based on consecutive pregnancies in women with presumed ITP,[65] the overall incidence of neonatal thrombocytopenia in 162 cases was 11 per cent. In cases in which there was either no history of ITP before pregnancy or a history but no detectable free anti-platelet IgG in the index pregnancy, the risk of severe thrombocytopenia in the fetus at term was found to be negligible.

Management

The above evidence that asymptomatic maternal thrombocytopenia is benign indicates that there is no reason to screen for this condition and no reason to take action on the platelet counts generated in the course of routine blood testing in pregnancy. Low platelet counts not associated with purpura or other evidence of abnormal bleeding are of no consequence. Even when a pregnant woman has symptomatic clinically significant haemorrhage arising from ITP, it seems that there is little risk of fetal or neonatal thrombocytopenia.

Measurement of the platelet count and other haematological variables such as platelet antibody has a place in the investigation of pregnant women (and sometimes in their fetuses) when they have clinical signs of thrombocytopenia or are at increased risk of it, e.g. because of a history either of ITP or of taking drugs that can reduce the platelet count. However, testing for thrombocytopenia in these circumstances is not population screening but part of clinical management. Even its use in this context has not been entirely beneficial, with clinicians reacting to moderately reduced maternal platelet counts by unnecessary interventions such as fetal blood sampling and caesarian section. The current trend in management is to return to a conservative policy of monitoring, supportive therapy, and a mode of delivery determined mainly by obstetric indications and not primarily by either maternal or fetal platelet count.[51,66]

Conclusions

The established routine of screening for maternal thrombocytopenia by measuring the platelet count as part of a full blood count in asymptomatic pregnant women seems to be of no value.

Antenatal screening for platelet antigens and specific allo-antibodies is not an established practice in women with no family history of FAIT. Most severe cases are diagnosed in the neonatal period in the first affected pregnancy. The availability of a whole blood typing assay for HPA[1a,67] and a human monoclonal antibody fragment specific for HPA[1a,68] may facilitate large screening programmes, but the optimal strategy for FAIT screening remains unclear, while the costing, impact on long-term outcome, and the effectiveness of available treatment have not been established.[57]

REFERENCES

1. Letsky E. A. (1998) The haematological system, In *Clinical Physiology in Obstetrics*, 3rd edn, (ed. G. V. P. Chamberlain and F. Broughton-Pipkin). Blackwell Scientific, Oxford.
2. Beguin Y., Lipscei G., Oris R., Thoumsin H., and Fillet G. (1990). Serum immunoreactive erythropoietin during pregnancy and in the early postpartum, *British Journal of Haematology*, **76**, 545–9.
3. Harstad T. W., Mason R. A., and Cox S. M. (1992). Serum erythropoietin quantitation in pregnancy using an enzyme-linked immunoassay, *American Journal of Perinatology*, **9**, 233–5.
4. Milman N., Agger A. O., Nielsen O. J., *et al.* (1994). Iron status markers and serum erythropoietin in 120 mothers and newborn infants. Effect of iron supplementation in normal pregnancy, *Acta Obstetrica et Gynecologica Scandinavica*, **73**, 200–4.
5. Riikonen S., Saijonmaa O., Jarvenpaa A. L., and Fyhrquist F. (1994). Serum concentrations of erythropoietin in healthy and anaemic pregnant women, *Scandinavian Journal of Clinical and Laboratory Investigation*, **54**, 653–7.
6. De Leeuw N. K., Lowenstein L., and Hsieh Y. S. (1966). Iron deficiency and hydremia in normal pregnancy, *Medicine (Baltimore)*, **45**, 291–315.
7. World Health Organization (1972). *Nutritional anaemias*. WHO, Geneva.
8. World Health Organization (1992). *The prevalence of nutritional anaemia in women*. WHO, Geneva.
9. World Health Organization (1993). *Prevention and management of severe anaemia in pregnancy*: report of a Technical Working Group, Geneva, 20–22 May 1991. Geneva, Maternal Health and Safe Motherhood Programme, WHO, Geneva.
10. Murphy J. F., O'Riordan J., Newcombe R. G., Coles E. C., and Pearson J. F. (1986). Relation of haemoglobin levels in first and second trimesters to outcome of pregnancy, *Lancet*, **1**, 992–5.

11. Steer P., Alam M. A., Wadsworth J., and Welch A. (1995). Relation between maternal haemoglobin concentration and birth weight in different ethnic groups, *British Medical Journal*, **310**, 489–91.
12. Editorial (1994). Routine iron supplements in pregnancy are unnecessary, *Drugs and Therapeutics Bulletin*, **32**, 30–1.
13. Hallberg L. (1992). Iron balance in pregnancy and lactation, In *Nutritional Anaemias*, (ed. S. J. Forget and S. Zlotkin), pp. 13–25. Raven, New York.
14. Addy D. P. (1986). Happiness is: iron [editorial], *British Medical Journal*, **292**, 969–70.
15. Allen L. H. (1993). Iron-deficiency anemia increases risk of preterm delivery, *Nutritional Reviews*, **51**, 49–52.
16. Scholl T. O., Hediger M. L., Fischer R. L., and Shearer J. W. (1992). Anemia vs iron deficiency: increased risk of preterm delivery in a prospective study, *American Journal of Clinical Nutrition*, **55**, 985–8.
17. Kaltreider D. F. and Kohl S. (1980). Epidemiology of pre-term delivery, *Clinics in Obstetrics and Gynecology*, **23**, 17–31.
18. Klebanoff M. A., Shiono P. H., Selby J. V., Trachtenberg A. I., and Graubard B. I. (1991). Anemia and spontaneous preterm birth, *American Journal of Obstetrics and Gynecology*, **164**, 59–63.
19. Colomer J., Colomert C., Gutierrez D., *et al.* (1990). Anaemia during pregnancy as a risk factor for infant iron deficiency: Report from the Valencia Infant Anaemia Cohort (VIAC) Study, *Paediatric and Perinatal Epidemiology*, **4**, 196–204.
20. Milman N., Agger A. O., and Nielsen O. J. (1991). Iron supplementation during pregnancy. Effect on iron status markers, serum erythropoietin and human placental lactogen. A placebo controlled study in 207 Danish women, *Danish Medical Bulletin*, **38**, 471–6.
21. Fenton V., Cavill I., and Fisher J. (1977) Iron stores in pregnancy, *British Journal of Haematology*, **37**, 145–9.
22. Aukett M. A., Parks Y. A., Scott P. H., and Wharton B. A. (1986). Treatment with iron increases weight gain and psychomotor development, *Archives of Disease in Childhood*, **61**, 849–57.
23. Lozoff B., Brittenham G. M., and Wolf A. W. (1987). Iron deficiency anemia and iron therapy effect on infant developmental test performance, *Pediatrics*, **79**, 981–95.
24. Walter T., De Andraca I., Chadud P., and Perales C. G. (1989). Iron deficiency anemia: adverse effects on infant psychomotor development, *Pediatircs*, **84**, 7–17.
25. Walter T. (1994). Effect of iron-deficiency anaemia on cognitive skills in infancy and childhood, *Baillieres Clinical Haematology*, **7**, 815–27.
26. Oski F. A. (1985). Iron deficiency–facts and fallacies, *Pediatric Clinics of North America*, **32**, 493–7.
27. Idjradinata P. and Pollitt E. (1993). Reversal of developmental delays in iron-deficient anaemic infants treated with iron, *Lancet*, **341**, 1–4.
28. Barker D. J. P., Bull A. R., *et al.* (1990). Fetal and placental size and risk of hypertension in adult life. *British Medical Journal*, **301**, 259–62.
29. Godfrey K. M., Redman C. W., Barker D. J., and Osmond C. (1991). The effect of maternal anaemia and iron deficiency on the ratio of fetal weight to placental weight, *British Journal of Obstetrics and Gynaecology*, **98**, 886–91.
30. Moore V. M., Miller A. G., *et al.* (1996). Placental weight, birth measurements and blood pressure at age 8 years. *Archives of Disease in Childhood*, **74**, 538–41.

31. Cook J. D. (1994). Iron-deficiency anaemia, *Baillieres Clinical Haematology*, **7**, 787–804.
32. Jacobs A. and Worwood M. (1982). Iron metabolism, iron deficiency and overload. In *Blood and its Disorders*, 2nd edn, (ed. R. M. Hardisty and D. J. Weatherall). Blackwell Scientific Publications, Oxford.
33. Finch C. A. and Huebers H. (1982). Perspectives in iron metabolism, *New England Journal of Medicine*, **306**, 1520–8.
34. Hallberg L. (1994). Prevention of iron deficiency, *Baillieres Clinical Haematology*, **7**, 805–14.
35. Chu T. W., Bowlus C., and Gruen J. R. (1996). Iron metabolism and related disorders. In *Emery's and Rimoin's Principles and Practice of Medical Genetics* (ed. D. L. Rimoin, J. M. Connor, and R. E. Pyeritz), 3rd edn, pp. 2047–70. Churchill Livingstone, New York.
36. Merryweather-Clarke A. T., Worwood M., Parkinson L., Mattock C., Poynton J. J., Shearman J. D., and Robson K. J. The effect of H. F. E mutation on serum ferritin and transferrin saturation in the Jersey population, *British Journal of Haematology.* **101**, 369–73
37. Jackson H. A., Worwood M., and Bentley D. P. (1998). Haemochromatosis mutations and iron stores in pregnancy. Abstract, Proceedings of British Society of Haematology, *British Journal of Haematology Suppl.* **101**, Suppl., 25.
38. Barrett J. F., Whittaker P. G., Williams J. G., and Lind T. (1994). Absorption of non-haem iron from food during normal pregnancy, *British Medical Journal*, **309**, 79–82.
39. Bentley D. P. (1985). Iron metabolism and anaemia in pregnancy, *Clinics in Haematology*, **14**, 613–28.
40. Thompson W. G. (1988). Comparison of tests for diagnosis of iron depletion in pregnancy, *American Journal of Obstetrics and Gynecology*, **159**, 1132–4.
41. Letsky E. A. (1995). Erythropoiesis in pregnancy, *Journal of Perinatal Medicine*, **23**, 39–45.
42. Kullander S. and Kallen B. (1976). A prospective study of drugs and pregnancy. 4. Miscellaneous drugs, *Acta Obstetrica et Gynecologica Scandinavica*, **55**, 287–95.
43. Stoltzfus R. J. and Dreyfuss M. L. (1998). *Guidelines for the Use of Iron Supplements to Prevent and Treat Iron Deficiency Anemia on behalf of the International Nutritional Anemia Consultative Group (INACG)*, International Life Sciences Institute Press, Washington.
44. Chanarin I. (1985). Folate and cobalamin, *Clinics in Haematology*, **14**, 629–41.
45. Van den Broek N. and Letsky E. A. (In press). The aetiology of anemia in pregnancy in South Malawi, *American Journal of Clinical Nutrition*.
46. Ibidapo D. and Letsky E. A. Ferritin vs. MCV as an indicator of iron deficiency in pregnancy, *Journal of Laboratory and Clinical Medicine*. (Submitted.)
47. Carriaga M. T., Skikne B. S., Finley B., Cutler B., and Cook J. D. (1991). Serum transferrin receptor for the detection of iron deficiency in pregnancy, *American Journal of Clinical Nutrition*, **54**, 1077–81.
48. Van den Broek N. R., Letsky E. A., *et al.* (1998). Iron status in pregnant women: which measurements are valid? *British Journal of Haematology*, **103**, 817–24.
49. Burrows R. F. and Kelton J. G. (1990). Low fetal risks in pregnancies associated with idiopathic thrombocytopenic purpura [see comments], *Am J Obstet Gynecol*, **163**, 1147–50.
50. Burrows R. F. and Kelton J. G. (1990). Thrombocytopenia at delivery: a prospective survey of 6715 deliveries, *American Journal of Obstetrics and Gynecology*, **162**, 731–4.
51. Letsky E. A. and Greaves M. (1996). Guidelines on the investigation and management of thrombocytopenia in pregnancy and neonatal alloimmune thrombocytopenia, *British Journal of Haematology*, **95**, 21–6.

52. Pillai M. (1993). Platelets and pregnancy, *British Journal of Obstetrics and Gynaecology*, **100**, 201–4.

53. Burrows R. F. and Kelton J. G. (1993). Fetal thrombocytopenia and its relation to maternal thrombocytopenia, *New England Journal of Medicine*, **329**, 1463–6.

54. Kaplan C., Morel-Kopp M. C., Kroll H., *et al.* (1991). HPA-5b(Br[a]) neonatal alloimmune thrombocytopenia: clinical and immunological analysis of 39 cases. *British Journal of Haematology*, **78**, 425–9.

55. Levine A. B. and Berkowitz R. L. (1991). Neonatal alloimmune thrombocytopenia, *Seminars in Perinatology*, **15**, 35–40.

56. Whittle M. J. (1994). Fetal thrombocytopenia, In *High Risk Pregnancy: Management Options*, (ed. D. K. James *et al.*). Saunders, London.

57. Williamson L. M., Hackett G., *et al.* (1998). The natural history of fetomaternal alloimmunization to the platelet-specific antigen HPA-1a (PL[A1], Zw[a]) as determined by antenatal screening. *Blood*, **92**, 2280–7.

58. Bussel J. B., Kaplan C., McFarland J. G., and the Working Party on Neonatal Alloimmune Thrombocytopenia of the Neonatal Hemostasis Subcommittee of the Scientific and Standardization Committee of the ISTH (1991). Recommendations for the evaluation and treatment of neonatal autoimmune and alloimmune thrombocytopenia, *Thrombosis and Haemostasis*, **65**, 631–4.

59. Khouzami A. N., Kickler T. S., Callan N. A., *et al.* (1996). Devastating sequelae of alloimmune thrombocytopenia: An entity that deserves more attention, *The Journal of Maternal-Fetal Medicine*, **5**, 137–41.

60. Bussel J. B., Skupski D. W., *et al.* (1996). Fetal alloimmune thrombocytopenia: consensus and controversy, *Journal of Maternal-Fetal Medicine*, **5**, 281–92.

61. Kaplan C., Murphy M. F., *et al.* (1998). Feto-maternal alloimmune thrombocytopenia: antenatal therapy with IvIgG and steroids – more questions than answers, *British Journal of Haematology*, **100**, 62–5.

62. Burrows R. F. and Kelton J. G. (1992). Thrombocytopenia during pregnancy, In *Haemostatis and Thrombosis in Obstetrics and Gynaecology*, (ed. I. A. Greer, A. G. Turpie, and C. D. Forbes), pp. 407–29. Chapman & Hall, London.

63. Hegde U. M. (1985). Immune thrombocytopenia in pregnancy and the newborn [editorial], *British Journal of Obstetrics and Gynaecology*, **92**, 657–9.

64. Kaplan C., Daffos F., Forestier F., *et al.* (1990). Fetal platelet counts in thrombocytopenic pregnancy [see comments], *Lancet*, **336**, 979–82.

65. Samuels P., Bussel J. B., Braitman L. E., *et al.* (1990). Estimation of the risk of thrombocytopenia in the offspring of pregnant women with presumed immune thrombocytopenic purpura [see comments], *New England Journal of Medicine*, **323**, 229–35.

66. Peleg D. and Hunter S. K. (1999). Perinatal management of women with immune thrombocytopenic purpura: survey of United States perinatologists, *American Journal of Obstetrics and Gynecology*, **180**, 645–9.

67. Bessos H., Mirza S., McGill A., Williamson L. M., Hadfield R., and Murphy W. (1996). A whole blood assay for platelet HPA-1 (PL[A1]) phenotyping applicable to large scale antenatal screening, *British Journal of Haematology*, **92**, 221–5.

68. Griffin H. M. and Ouwehand W. H. (1995). A human monoclonal antibody specific for the leucine-33 (Pl[A1], HPA 1a) form of platelet glycoprotein llla from a V gene phage display library, *Blood*, **86**, 4430–6.

Screening for specific disorders
(b) Antenatal and neonatal screening

11 *Genetic haematological disorders*

Sir David Weatherall and Elizabeth A. Letsky

INTRODUCTION

There are three main groups of inherited haematological disorders in which screening programmes are of importance. First, there are the genetic disorders of the structure or synthesis of haemoglobin (Hb), which are sufficiently common in many populations to justify antenatal or neonatal screening. Because of the severity of the homozygous states for these conditions, and the fact that their management is difficult, antenatal screening programmes are of particular importance so that parents can be offered the possibility of antenatal diagnosis and termination. Neonatal screening is of particular value in the sickling disorders because it is important to identify sickle cell disease in early life so that appropriate prophylactic measures can be established to prevent infection to which these babies are particularly prone.

The second group is comprised of red cell enzyme deficiencies of which only one, glucose-6-phosphate dehydrogenase deficiency, is particularly common in certain populations. Finally, there are rare genetic disorders of the blood for which screening is indicated if there is a history of a previously affected child. The most important disorders of this type are the hereditary bleeding diseases, particularly haemophilia and Christmas disease.

Rhesus haemolytic disease and other blood group disorders are considered separately in Chapter 12.

ANTENATAL SCREENING FOR GENETIC DISORDERS OF HAEMOGLOBIN

Nature of the disorders

The genetic disorders of the structure or synthesis of haemoglobin are the commonest single gene diseases in the world population. The WHO estimated that by the year 2000 approximately 7 per cent of the world's population would be carriers for these conditions.[1] They are made up of two main groups, the structural haemoglobin variants and disorders which result from inherited abnormalities of the synthesis of the globin chains of haemoglobin, the thalassaemias.

The structure of the normal human haemoglobins and the way that it is genetically determined is summarized in Fig. 11.1. All the normal human haemoglobins have the

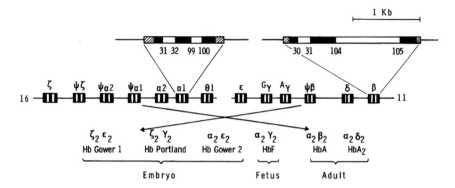

Fig. 11.1 The genetic control of human haemoglobin production. The α1 and β genes have been expanded to show their structure. The dark shading represents the coding regions or exons, the unshaded regions represent non-coding regions or introns, and the hatched regions represent the 5′ and 3′ non-coding regions respectively.

same basic structure.[2] They are made up of two different pairs of peptide chains, each of which has a haem molecule attached to it. Normal adults have major and minor haemoglobins, called haemoglobins A and A_2; their molecular formulae are represented as $\alpha_2\beta_2$ and $\alpha_2\delta_2$. In fetal life the main haemoglobin is haemoglobin F ($\alpha_2\gamma_2$) although small amounts of haemoglobin A are synthesized from as early as six weeks of gestation. Haemoglobin F is heterogeneous at all stages of human development. It consists of two different forms which have either glycine or alanine at position 136 in the γ chains. Gamma chains which have glycine at this position are called $^{G}\gamma$ chains, those with alanine $^{A}\gamma$ chains. These different types of γ chain are the products of distinct gene loci (Fig. 11.1). In addition to the fetal and adult haemoglobins there are several different embryonic haemoglobins which consist of different combinations of embryonic α-like chains, ζ chains, combined with embryonic non-α chains, ε chains. The embryonic haemoglobins disappear from the fetal blood by about the eighth week of development.

The α- and β-like globins are the products of gene clusters on chromosomes 16 and 11 respectively (Fig. 11.1). All the genes which make up these clusters, together with their flanking regions, have been sequenced. Both clusters contain many sites which are polymorphic, that is they show variation in nucleotide bases which may generate new sites or remove sites for cleavage by restriction enzymes. The arrangements of these restriction fragment length polymorphisms (RFLPs) are not random but occur in a limited number of arrangements, or haplotypes. These single-base RFLPs provide valuable markers for chromosomes carrying mutations of the globin genes. In addition, the α gene cluster contains several regions of minisatellite DNA which also are valuable polymorphic chromosomal markers.[2]

The inherited disorders of haemoglobin consist of the structural haemoglobin variants and the thalassaemias. The most important abnormal haemoglobins are haemoglobins S, C, and E. These all result from single amino acid substitutions in the globin chain genes which lead to the synthesis of a haemoglobin variant. The thalassaemias, on the other hand, result from defective synthesis of either the α or β globin chains.

The important structural haemoglobin variants

The most common structural haemoglobin variants are haemoglobins S, C, and E, all of which occur at high frequencies in different populations.[2]

The sickling disorders consist of the sickle cell trait (AS), the homozygous state for the sickle cell mutation, sickle cell anaemia (SS), and the compound hetero-zygous states for the sickle cell gene in association with β thalassaemia or structural haemoglobin variants such as haemoglobin C (sickle cell β thalassaemia; sickle cell haemoglobin C disease). Sickle cell *disease* is a collective term to include all geno-types that cause clinical sickling and are therefore clinically similar to sickle cell anaemia. The sickling disorders occur in a broad belt across tropical Africa and are found in any part of the world in which there has been migration from West Africa, notably the Caribbean, the United States and parts of South America. The sickling disorders also occur sporadically in Mediterranean populations such as those of Italy and Greece, in parts of the Middle East, and in isolated pockets in India.

The homozygous state for the sickle cell gene, sickle cell anaemia, is a condi-tion that runs a very variable course.[2] In many cases it is a severe disease char-acterized by lifelong anaemia and recurrent complications, or crises, in which there is widespread bone pain and damage to tissues. In addition there are other serious complications including life-threatening infections such as pneumococcal septicaemia, infarction of the lung or brain, transient bone marrow aplasia, pro-found anaemia due to sequestration of sickle cells in the spleen, and progressive renal failure. On the other hand some patients with this disorder have a very mild disease and remain symptom-free. Although some of the genetic factors responsible for these different types of sickle cell anaemia are beginning to be understood it is very difficult to prognosticate about the likely course in any individual patient.

Haemoglobin C is widespread in parts of West Africa. In the homozygous state it is associated with a mild haemolytic anaemia. Individuals who are compound het-erozygotes for the genes for haemoglobins S and C, haemoglobin SC disease, have a mild anaemia but occasionally severe complications occur, particularly widespread thromboses in pregnancy, aseptic necrosis of the femoral or humoral heads, and recurrent haematuria. Proliferative vascular disease involving the retinal vessels also occurs commonly and may lead to blindness.

Haemoglobin E is widespread throughout Southeast Asia and the eastern parts of the Indian subcontinent. In the homozygous state it causes a mild anaemia and its main importance is in its interactions with β thalassaemia (see next section).

The thalassaemias

The thalassaemias are an extremely heterogeneous group of genetic disorders of haemoglobin synthesis, all of which are characterized by a reduced rate of production of one or more of the globin genes of haemoglobin.[2-4] They are classified according to the chain which is inefficiently produced. Although there are many different forms

Table 11.1 The thalassaemias and related disorders

Type of disorder	Characteristics
α Thalassaemia	α^0
	α^+
	Deletion $(-\alpha)$
	Non-deletion (α^T)
β Thalassaemia	β^0
	β^+
	Normal Hb A_2
	'Silent'
$\delta\beta$ Thalassaemia	$(\delta\beta)^0$
	$(^A\gamma\delta\beta)^0$
	$(\delta\beta)^+$
γ Thalassaemia	
δ Thalassemia	δ^0
	δ^+
$\epsilon\gamma\delta\beta$ Thalassaemia	
Hereditary persistence of fetal haemoglobin	Deletion: $(\delta\beta)^0$ $(^A\gamma\delta\beta)^0$
	Non-deletion: linked to β globin genes
	$^G\gamma\beta^+$ $^A\gamma\beta^+$
	Non-deletion: unlinked to β globin genes

of thalassaemia they fall into three broad groups: α thalassaemia, β thalassaemia, and $\delta\beta$ thalassaemia (Table 11.1).

The α thalassaemias

These conditions are characterized by an inability to produce the α chains which are common to haemoglobins A, A_2, and F. In fetal life a deficiency of α chains results in the production of excess γ chains which form γ_4 molecules called haemoglobin Bart's. In adult life a deficiency of α chains leads to the overproduction of β chains which produce β_4 tetramers, or haemoglobin H.[4,5]

There are two main groups of α thalassaemias, the α^0 thalassaemias in which no α chains are produced, and the α^+ thalassaemias in which there is a reduced output of α chain production. There are more than 80 mutations causing the picture of α^+ and α^0 thalassaemia (cf. β thalassaemia, p. 250). The genetic basis for these conditions is illustrated in Fig. 11.2. The α^0 thalassaemias result from deletions of both linked α globin genes on chromosome 16. The α^+ thalassaemias result from the loss of one of the linked pair of α globin genes. This usually results from a deletion of one of the pair although it may also occur if there is a mutation which inactivates the particular α gene. Normal individuals have four α globin genes, two on each of the pairs of homologous chromosomes 16. Therefore their genotype can be written $\alpha\alpha/\alpha\alpha$. Heterozygotes for α^0 thalassaemia have the genotype $- -/\alpha\alpha$. Heterozygotes for the deletion forms of α^+ thalassaemia have the genotype $-\alpha/\alpha\alpha$, while that of those with non-deletion forms can be represented $\alpha^T\alpha/\alpha\alpha$.

The α thalassaemias occur widely in the Mediterranean populations, the Middle East, isolated pockets of the Indian subcontinent, and throughout Southeast Asia.[5] The heterozygote frequency in some of these populations is extremely high and in some Pacific islanders may reach over 80 per cent (Fig. 11.3).

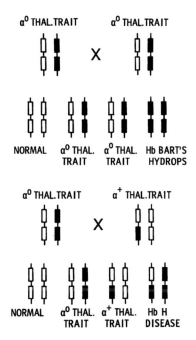

Fig. 11.2 The different forms of α thalassaemia and their interactions. The open boxes represent normal α globin genes and the shaded boxes represent α globin genes that have been inactivated by deletion or point mutation. In α⁰ thalassaemia both linked α globin genes are lost while in α⁺ thalassaemia one of the pair is lost or inactivated.

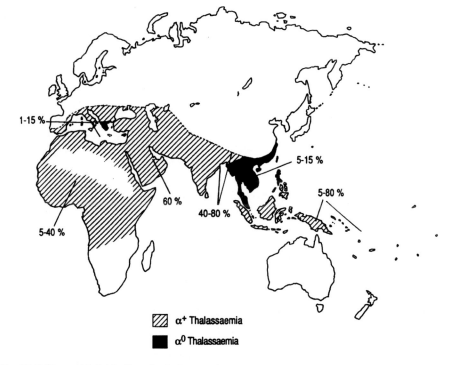

Fig. 11.3 The world distribution of α thalassaemia.

There are two important clinical forms of α thalassaemia, the haemoglobin Bart's hydrops syndrome and haemoglobin H disease. The former represents the homozygous state for α^0 thalassaemia while the latter is heterogeneous at the molecular level. It usually results from the inheritance of both α^0 and α^+ thalassaemia determinants (Fig. 11.2) although occasionally it may result from the homozygous inheritance of a non-deletion form of α thalassaemia. The haemoglobin Bart's hydrops syndrome is characterized by fetal death *in utero*, or, if the infant is liveborn, death within a few hours of birth. The clinical picture is severe hydrops fetalis with massive placental hypertrophy and the blood picture of thalassaemia. Women carrying babies with this syndrome have a high frequency of toxaemia of pregnancy and postpartum haemorrhage.[6]

Haemoglobin H disease is a moderately severe haemolytic anaemia with splenomegaly and a thalassaemic blood picture. It varies widely in its severity; some patients are relatively symptom-free while others are sufficiently anaemic to require intermittent blood transfusion.

One of the major difficulties in the α thalassaemia field is the clinical and laboratory definition of the various carrier states (see Table 11.2). In adult life α^0 thalassaemia carriers usually have thalassaemic red cell indices with a low MCH and MCV.[5,7] α^+ thalassaemia carriers have extremely mild red cell changes or their haematological pictures may be normal. These problems are compounded by the fact that the homozygous state for α^+ thalassaemia produces a clinical phenotype indistinguishable from the heterozygous state for α^0 thalassaemia (Fig. 11.4). Most of the α thalassaemia

Table 11.2   Haematological findings in α^0 or β thalassaemia heterozygotes, α^+ thalassaemia homozygotes, and αβ thalassaemia heterozygotes*

	Mean cell haemoglobin (pg) (± 2 SD)	Mean cell volume (fl) (± 2 SD)	Hb A₂ (%) (± 2 SD)
β thal trait	21±1	70±4	4.9±0.5
Normal Hb A₂ β thal trait†	22±2	73±6	3.2±0.6
α^0 thal trait (– –/αα)‡	22±4	70±8	1.9±0.4
Homozygous α^+ thal (–α/–α)§	23±1	72±5	2.0±0.5
β thal trait/homozygous α^+ thal	25±1	76±3	4.8±0.5
β thal trait/α^0 thal trait	na	na	?Raised
Normal values	30±3	90±10	2.6±0.5

* Data from refs 3, 7, 11, 13, 14. Only cases of α thalassaemia analysed by gene mapping are included.
† Heterozygous condition; a disorder with these findings interacts with β thalassaemia to produce thalassaemia major.
‡ Also known as α thalassaemia 1.
§ Also known as α thalassaemia 2.
na: Data not available on cases confirmed by mapping. Likely to be similar to β thal trait with homozygous α^+ thal.

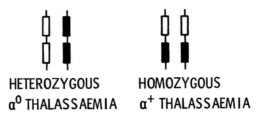

HETEROZYGOUS   HOMOZYGOUS
α^0 THALASSAEMIA α^+ THALASSAEMIA

Fig. 11.4 The arrangement of the globin genes in the heterozygous state for α^0 thalassaemia and the homozygous state for α^+ thalassaemia. Both arrangements are associated with an almost identical haematological phenotype.

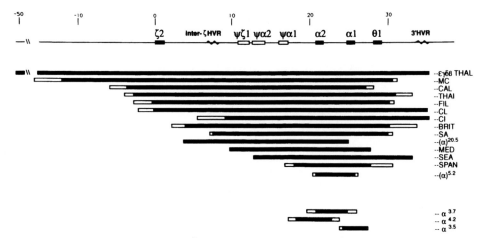

Fig. 11.5 Some deletions which cause α^0 and α^+ thalassaemia. The arrangement of the α globin genes is shown at the top of the figure. The deletions are shown in black with uncertainties about their extension in open boxes. The deletions are usually designated by the name of the country or region, BRIT = British and SEA = Southeast Asian, for example. Those that are designated - -(α) leave non-functional α globin genes.

traits are associated with elevated levels of haemoglobin Bart's in the neonatal period, but without DNA analysis there is no certain way of distinguishing them in adult life.[5] Their major haematological features are summarized in Table 11.2.

The molecular pathology of the α thalassaemias is now understood, at least in outline. All the α^0 thalassaemias result from long deletions involving the α globin gene cluster. Their length varies considerably (Fig. 11.5). In some cases only the α globin genes are lost and the ζ genes remain intact. In others the entire α globin gene cluster is deleted. In addition, there is a group of α^0 thalassaemias in which the α globin genes are intact but inactivated by deletions involving a major regulatory region for the α globin genes which is situated about 40 kb upstream from the cluster, the control region called HS40. By preparing appropriate gene probes, particularly the ζ genes, it is possible to identify many of these deletions in genomic DNA because of the new fragments that are generated as a result of the DNA which is lost in the deletion. However, because of the marked heterogeneity and normal variability of the α globin gene locus, and the fact that at least some of the deletions that cause α^0 thalassaemia remove the whole cluster or involve only the HS40, the identification of the α^0 thalassaemias is fraught with pitfalls.

The α^+ thalassaemias are also extremely heterogeneous at the molecular level. There are several common deletion forms which, again, can usually be identified by gene mapping using suitable probes. In addition there are several non-deletion forms of α^+ thalassaemia which result from mutations which interfere with either transcription or translation of α globin messenger RNA. These mutations can only be identified with appropriate oligonucleotide probes or by sequencing.

The molecular pathology of the α^0 and α^+ thalassaemias which are due to gene deletions are illustrated in Fig. 11.5.

β thalassaemia

The β thalassaemias occur commonly in the Mediterranean island populations, throughout the Middle East, in many parts of the Indian subcontinent, and throughout

Table 11.3   Molecular mechanisms leading to β thalassaemias. Full list of β thalassaemia mutations is given in refs 4 and 6

Defective transcription of β globin genes	Deletions Promotor mutations
Defective processing of mRNA precursor	Splice junction mutations Concensus sequence mutations Cryptic splice sites in exons Cryptic splice sites in introns Poly-A addition site mutations
Defective translation of β globin mRNA	Non-sense mutations in exons Frameshift mutations Initiation codon mutations CAP site mutations
Post-translational instability of β globin product	

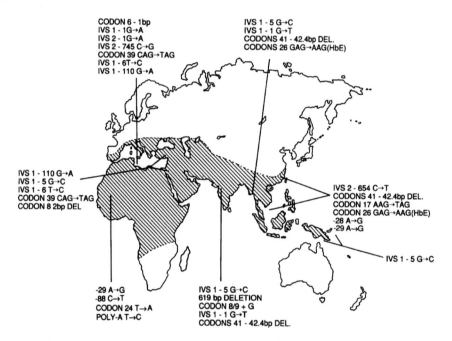

Fig. 11.6 The world distribution of β thalassaemia and some of the common molecular forms of the condition in different populations. IVS = intervening sequence; bp = basepair; poly-A = polyadenylation site; DEL = deletion. The various codon numbers represent the codons of the β globin gene.

Southeast Asia and the Pacific island populations (Fig. 11.6). The carrier rates in these populations range from 2 to 20 per cent.[3] The conditions leading to these disorders, which are quite heterogeneous, are classified in Table 11.3.

There are two main varieties of β thalassaemia, β^0 and β^+ thalassaemia, in which there is an absence or reduced output of β globin chain synthesis respectively. Over 180 different mutations have been identified in the β globin genes which produce the picture of β^0 or β^+ thalassaemia.[9] In some cases there are small deletions of the β globin genes but deletions are a much less common cause of β thalassaemia than is the case for the α thalassaemias. Most of the β thalassaemias are due to either non-sense or frameshift mutations involving the exons of the β globin gene or subtle mutations which interfere with the normal splicing and processing of β globin messenger RNA. Some of them involve the regulatory promoter regions of the β globin gene and others affect the non-coding sequences at the 3' end of the gene which are involved with polyadenylation of β globin messenger RNA.

The homozygous states for β^0 or β^+ thalassaemia or the compound heterozygous states for these conditions, are usually characterized by a transfusion-dependent life from the age of approximately 6–12 months.[3] If transfusion is inadequate there is severe anaemia, hepatosplenomegaly, serious deformities of the bones of the skull, proneness to infection, and numerous other complications with a high mortality during early childhood. With an adequate transfusion regime these children grow and develop normally with minimal splenomegaly but succumb to the effects of iron loading during the second or third decade.

The heterozygous states for β^0 and β^+ thalassaemia are characterized by hypochromic red cells, mild anaemia, reduced MCV and MCH values, and an elevated level of haemoglobin A_2. These findings are summarized in Table 11.2.

There are less common forms of β thalassaemia in which the haemoglobin A_2 level in heterozygotes is normal. Although these conditions are rare, and have been encountered most frequently in the Mediterranean populations, they are of considerable importance in screening and antenatal diagnosis programmes. These conditions are classified into type 1 and type 2 normal haemoglobin A_2 β thalassaemias. The first type is sometimes called 'silent' β thalassaemia because there are no haematological changes in heterozygotes. However, this condition can interact in the compound heterozygous state with β^+ or β^0 thalassaemia to produce a moderately severe thalassaemic disorder. Type 2 normal haemoglobin A_2 β thalassaemia is extremely heterogeneous. In many cases it represents the heterozygous state for both β and δ thalassaemia; a mutation in the δ globin gene prevents the elevation of haemoglobin A_2 which is usually found in β thalassaemia heterozygotes. There are some other rare causes of this type of β thalassaemia. The importance of the type 2 forms of normal A_2 β thalassaemia is that these conditions can interact with the more common forms of β thalassaemia to produce a severely affected child in the compound heterozygous state.

The δβ thalassaemias

These conditions are much less common than the α and β thalassaemias and many of them are associated with milder clinical disorders.[4] They consist of the $(\delta\beta)^+$ thalassaemias and the $(\delta\beta)^0$ thalassaemias. They are distributed unevenly throughout the world population and there are no high-frequency groups.

The $(\delta\beta)^+$ thalassaemias result from unequal crossing over between the δ and β globin genes with the production of δβ fusion genes which give rise to abnormal haemoglobins called the Lepore haemoglobins. In the homozygous state these conditions produce a condition similar to homozygous β thalassaemia. On the other hand the homozygous states for the $(\delta\beta)^0$ thalassaemias, which all result from deletions involving the δ and β globin genes, are much milder due to the high level of fetal haemoglobin production.

The heterozygous states for these conditions are easily identified. Haemoglobin Lepore carriers have thalassaemic blood pictures with 5–15 per cent haemoglobin Lepore. Heterozygotes for $(\delta\beta)^0$ thalassaemia have thalassaemic blood pictures and unusually high levels of haemoglobin F in the 5–20 per cent range with normal levels of haemoglobin A$_2$.

Antenatal screening for structural haemoglobin variants
Who should be screened?

All individuals of African or Mediterranean origin should be screened for haemoglobins S and C at their first antenatal visit. There are several reasons for this. Although the sickle cell trait causes no problems in an uncomplicated pregnancy it may be associated with the effects of intravascular sickling in periods of acute hypoxia or dehydration. Furthermore, if a woman is found to have the sickle cell trait it is very important to screen her partner because of the risk of the infant having sickle cell disease. Similarly, if a woman has the haemoglobin C trait her partner should be screened to make sure that the fetus is not at risk for haemoglobin SC disease. It is particularly important to identify sickle cell anaemia in pregnant women because this disorder is associated with a number of complications in pregnancy and requires extremely careful management. Similarly, haemoglobin SC disease is the cause of several serious complications in pregnancy.

It is equally important to screen women of Indian or Southeast Asian origin for haemoglobin E during pregnancy. Although the haemoglobin E trait causes no problems, if it is identified, it is very important to screen the woman's partner for β thalassaemia because the couple would then be at risk of having a baby with haemoglobin E thalassaemia which may be a very severe disorder.

Methods for screening

There are several simple sickling tests which can be used to screen for all the sickling disorders.[3] They depend on either the decreased solubility of haemoglobin S or on the fact that red cells sickle in conditions of reduced oxygen concentration. They do not distinguish between sickle cell trait and sickle cell disease and therefore they must be backed up by haemoglobin electrophoresis. Alternatively, haemoglobin electrophoresis can be the screening method for all structural haemoglobin variants. It will detect haemoglobins S, C, and E. Almost any form of haemoglobin electrophoresis at an alkaline pH will detect these haemoglobins. Most laboratories find cellulose acetate strips both rapid and convenient. The newer iso-electric focussing (IEF) or high performance liquid chromatography (HPLC) techniques are faster and more sensitive (see below). Appropriate controls should always be included in the analysis.

If haemoglobin electrophoresis is used as the initial screening test for structural haemoglobin variants it is important to subject any blood sample that produces the electrophoretic pattern of the sickle cell trait to a test for sickling. It should be remembered that there are other haemoglobin variants which migrate in the same position as haemoglobin S and therefore to be certain of the diagnosis of the sickle cell trait it is vital to perform a confirmatory analysis for sickling.

Using routine haemoglobin electrophoretic methods haemoglobins C and E have a rather similar rate of electrophoretic migration at alkaline pH. However, the racial background of the patient will usually distinguish between these variants; haemoglobin C is nearly always seen in persons of African or Mediterranean background while haemoglobin E is extremely rare in these populations and is only seen in individuals who originate from India or further east. They can also be distinguished biochemically. Citrate agar at acid pH (or acid agarose) electrophoresis can separate Hbs C, E, and O which run together on cellulose acetate at alkaline pH.

Two new techniques are also available.[10] First, automated high-performance liquid chromatography (HPLC) can be used to analyse both liquid and dried blood samples obtained from neonates, children, and adults. This technique requires only 5 µl of blood and will detect all the clinically important haemoglobins associated with sickle cell disease as well as β thalassaemia major, and it will also quantitate any peak it detects such as Hb A, A_2, F, S, C, E, D^{Punjab}, O^{Arab}, Lepore, and Hb A_2 variants. It can therefore replace Hb electrophoresis and the quantitation of Hb A_2 as tests for sickle cell disease and β thalassaemia major and their carrier states, although traditional electrophoretic methods will still be required to assist in the identification of some abnormal haemoglobins.

Second, monoclonal antibodies have recently been introduced as a means of identifying certain abnormal haemoglobins such as Hb S, C, and E and although they are expensive they are likely to have a useful role as confirmatory tests.

It is now possible to identify carriers for the common haemoglobin variants by DNA analysis. Oligonucleotide probes can be constructed that will identify the base changes that give rise to these abnormal haemoglobins, and in some cases the particular mutation alters a restriction enzyme site so that the variant can be identified directly on genomic DNA or on DNA amplified by the polymerase chain reaction (PCR).

Antenatal screening for thalassaemia

Who should be screened?

Ideally, antenatal screening programmes for thalassaemia should be established in all the high-incidence areas.[1] These include the entire Mediterranean region, the Middle East, the Indian subcontinent, Burma, and the whole of Southeast Asia. Although population screening programmes have been set up in some of these regions it is a massive undertaking, and in most countries antenatal screening for the haemoglobin disorders will be restricted to maternal screening at the first antenatal visit. If first trimester antenatal diagnosis becomes established, and women cannot be persuaded to present early in pregnancy, it may be necessary to set up population screening programmes, for school leavers for example. In high-incidence countries it is becoming routine to screen all pregnant women for thalassaemia or important haemoglobin variants depending on the particular population at risk. In countries with large immigrant populations it is equally important to screen women of appropriate racial backgrounds. The patient's name may not always give an indication of their race and in a busy antenatal clinic it is easy to miss patients who should be screened. This is not such a serious problem in the case of thalassaemia, since all pregnant women have an initial haematological screen, which, in most countries, includes an assessment of the red cell size on an automated blood cell counter.

Screening by estimation of red cell indices and haemoglobin A_2

The haematological findings in the carrier states for the common forms of thalassaemia are summarized in Table 11.2. The key red cell indices are the mean corpuscular haemoglobin (MCH) and mean corpuscular volume (MCV). If these are reduced, particularly if the haemoglobin level is normal or only slightly low, with a normal or raised red cell count, thalassaemia should be suspected. Although various mathematical treatments have been used to distinguish thalassaemia from iron deficiency they are not very reliable in practice and an independent method such as a serum iron or ferritin estimation should be used for assessing a woman's iron status. If the MCV and MCH are low, a haemoglobin A_2 estimation should be carried out. If the haemoglobin A_2 value is elevated (Table 11.2) the diagnosis is β thalassaemia trait and the woman's partner should be studied. If both are β thalassaemia carriers appropriate genetic counselling should be instituted. The key question is: 'below which values for the MCV and MCH should further investigations to confirm the diagnosis of thalassaemia be instigated?' Figures 11.7 and 11.8 show the distribution of MCV and MCH in pregnant women with or without β thalassaemia trait, based on a series of 54 carriers and 6314 non-carriers who attended the antenatal clinic at St Bartholomew's Hospital and 50 carriers who attended Queen Charlotte's Hospital, London (data provided by Dr A. Stephens and Dr E. Letsky), making 104 carriers in total. The MCH data are similar to those in Table 11.2; the mean MCV in carriers somewhat lower. Table 11.4 shows the observed detection and false-positive rates for β thalassaemia trait. Although it used to be recommended that an MCV of less than 70 femtolitres, or an MCH of less than 25 picograms were indications for further study, subsequent experience suggests that these values are too low (Table 11.2).[3,7,11–13] Ideally, the cut-off values should be 80 fl and 27 pg respectively if the aim is to detect virtually all affected pregnancies (as in Fig. 11.9). Although this will entail a large number of investigations (haemoglobin A_2 estimation) it may be justified in populations in which both α and β thalassaemia are common. We shall return later (p. 258) to the question of what screening methods to use in these populations.

Reducing the cut-off from 80 fl to, say, 70 fl results in one-tenth of affected fetuses

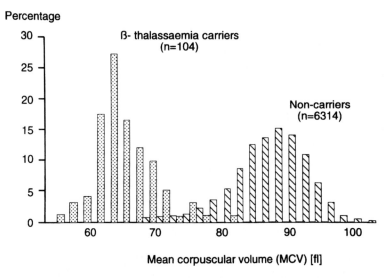

Fig. 11.7 The distribution of mean corpuscular volume (MCV) in pregnant women who are either β thalassaemia carriers or non-carriers. (Source: Antenatal clinics at St Bartholomew's Hospital and Queen Charlotte's Hospital.)

Table 11.4   Observed detection and false-positive rates using MCV or MCH as the screening test for β-thalassaemia trait in antenatal women

Test	Detection rate (%)	False-positive rate (%)
MCV (fl)		
≤55	0.0	0.0
≤60	7.7	0.2
≤62	25.0	0.5
≤63	42.3	0.7
≤64	51.9	0.9
≤66	68.3	1.1
≤67	74.0	1.8
≤70	89.4	2.7
≤72	94.2	3.7
≤74	95.2	5.1
≤75	96.2	5.9
≤76	98.1	7.1
≤78	99.0	10.2
≤80	99.0	15.5
No. of women	104	6314
MCH (pg)		
≤18	1.9	0.1
≤19	12.5	0.3
≤20	39.4	0.7
≤21	62.5	1.3
≤22	76.9	2.5
≤23	90.4	3.8
≤24	97.1	5.4
≤25	98.1	7.9
≤26	99.0	13.7
≤27	100.0	22.6
≤28	100.0	36.6
No. of women	104	6314

Source: Antenatal clinics at St Bartholomew's and Queen Charlotte's Hospitals.

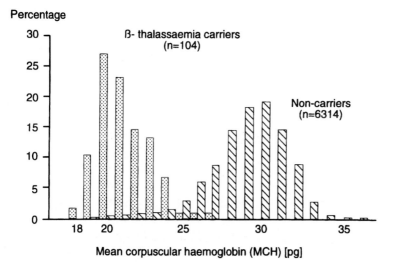

Fig. 11.8 The distribution of mean corpuscular haemoglobin (MCH) in pregnant women who are either β thalassaemia carriers or non-carriers. (Source: Antenatal clinics at St Bartholomew's Hospital and Queen Charlotte's Hospital.)

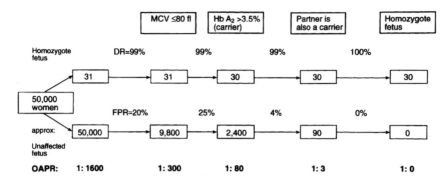

Fig. 11.9 Flow diagram illustrating screening for homozygote fetuses with β thalassaemia in 50 000 pregnancies. The odds of being affected given a positive result (OAPR) are indicated. All women with an MCV of 80 fl or less have an Hb A₂ estimation (i.e. 99 per cent of all female carriers and 15.5 per cent of all unaffected women, Table 7.4). It is assumed that 5 per cent of all women are carriers ($n = 2500$), of which 125 have partners who are also carriers (2500 × 5 per cent, assuming the same carrier prevalence in males) and there are 31 homozygote fetuses (1/4 × 125, assuming random mating). It is assumed that 99 per cent of women with Hb A₂ of 3.5 per cent or more are carriers.

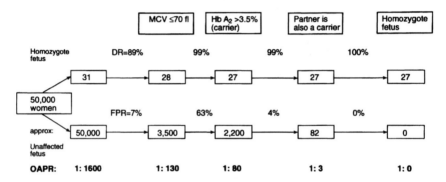

Fig. 11.10 Flow diagram illustrating screening for homozygote fetuses with β thalassaemia in 50 000 pregnancies (with same assumptions as in Fig. 11.9). All women with an MCV of 70 fl or less have an Hb A₂ estimation (i.e. 89.4 per cent of all female carriers and 2.7 per cent of all unaffected women, Table 11.4).

not being detected, but the false-positive rate is more than halved (7 per cent instead of 20 per cent) (see Fig. 11.10). It follows that less than half the number of haemoglobin A₂ estimations would be needed, with significant savings in cost and labour.

Overall, the estimation of Hb A₂ is an extremely reliable method of identifying the carrier state for all the different β thalassaemias.[14] Provided that recommended methods are used and that the laboratory carries out regular quality control of its method there are few practical problems. Whether the estimation is carried out by quantitative haemoglobin electrophoresis or chromatography over 98 per cent of β thalassaemia carriers have haemoglobin A₂ values of approximately twice normal, in the range 3.5 to 6.5 per cent (Table 11.2).[14] Occasionally, individuals are encountered with values in the 'grey area', that is just elevated in the range 3.2 to 3.8 per cent. If a value of this type is found in association with thalassaemic red cell indices it is important to confirm the diagnosis by globin chain synthesis analysis. There is increasing evidence that most of these cases are due to the inheritance of α and β thalassaemia mutations.[13]

The estimation of Hb F is not absolutely necessary when screening for β thalassaemia. It is only slightly elevated in about 50 per cent of β thalassaemia heterozygotes.[3] In δβ thalassaemia heterozygotes it is in the range of 5 to 15 per cent and can usually be identified on haemoglobin electrophoresis. However, in individuals with thalassaemic red cell indices and normal Hb A$_2$ levels it is useful to carry out an Hb F estimation to exclude δβ thalassaemia before embarking on the complex identification of the genotypes of thalassaemias with normal Hb A$_2$ values.

The two main practical problems which arise in antenatal screening of thalassaemia are the finding of a thalassaemic blood picture with a normal haemoglobin A$_2$ level, and the problem of identifying β thalassaemia in women who are heterozygous for both α and β thalassaemia.

If a woman is found to have a typical thalassaemic blood picture with a normal haemoglobin A$_2$ level the best approach in practice is to analyse the partner's blood. If it is normal the fetus is not at risk for a severe form of thalassaemia and the mother's thalassaemia genotype can be worked out at leisure. On the other hand, if the partner has a similar blood picture to his wife, or if he has β thalassaemia trait, the couple should be referred immediately to a laboratory which is able to sort out the different forms of α thalassaemia and the rare β thalassaemia variants.

A woman who has thalassaemic red cell indices with a normal haemoglobin A$_2$ level is likely to have α thalassaemia. Furthermore, if her red cell indices are similar to those of a β thalassaemia heterozygote, she is probably missing two out of the normal four α globin genes.[7] However, identification of the chromosomes from which the α genes are deleted has important implications for the prognosis of her children. As mentioned earlier, the normal α globin genotype can be written αα/αα. In the more severe form of α thalassaemia, α^0 thalassaemia, both α globin genes on the *same* chromosome 16 are deleted (– –/αα). In the deletion forms of α$^+$ thalassaemia only one of the α genes is lost; the heterozygous genotype is written –α/αα. Carriers for this condition are haematologically normal or have a very slight reduction in MCH and MCV values.[7] However, α$^+$ thalassaemia is so common that it is not unusual to encounter homozygotes with the genotype –α/–α (Fig. 11 4). As shown in Table 11.2, the red cell indices in such cases are indistinguishable from those of α^0 thalassaemia heterozygotes. However, Hb H inclusions are much more likely to be present after supravital staining in people heterozygous for α^0 thalassaemia than in people homozygous for α$^+$ thalassaemia. The deletion of two α genes produces the same phenotype, regardless of whether they are lost from the *same* or *opposite* pairs of homologous chromosomes 16.

The genetic counselling implications of the interactions of the different α thalassaemia determinants are shown in Fig. 11.2. A mating between two α^0 thalassaemia heterozygotes has a one in four chance of producing an infant with the haemoglobin Bart's hydrops syndrome. Apart from death in the third trimester or at term, this condition is also associated with a high incidence of toxaemia and post-partum haemorrhage. It is, therefore, a disorder for which antenatal diagnosis should be offered. On the other hand, an α$^+$ thalassaemia homozygote cannot have a child with haemoglobin Bart's hydrops: at worst they can have a child with haemoglobin H disease, which is relatively innocuous. The practical implication is that if a couple are both found to have thalassaemic red cell indices with a normal haemoglobin A$_2$

level it is important to sort out the arrangement of their missing α globin genes. Their racial background is helpful; α^0 thalassaemia is found in Orientals and some Mediterranean populations; it is very uncommon in other racial groups (Fig. 11.3). But the only certain way of defining these genotypes is by DNA analysis.[8] If a woman who is an α^0 thalasaemia carrier or α^+ thalassaemia homozygote has a partner who is a β thalassaemia heterozygote there are no risks for their children; $\alpha\beta$ thalassaemia is always an innocuous interaction.

As already noted (p. 251), a form of β thalassaemia in which the haemoglobin A_2 level is normal occurs in some populations,[12] and this heterogeneous disorder often results from heterozygosity for β and δ thalassaemia.[15] If one of a couple has this condition and the other has the high haemoglobin A_2 form of β thalassaemia, they may produce a child with thalassaemia major. This is why it is important to be sure that, if they have a partner with β thalassaemia, women who have the clinical picture of heterozygous thalassaemia and a normal haemoglobin A_2 are referred to a centre for globin chain synthesis analysis. The α/β globin chain synthesis ratio in the severe types of normal haemoglobin A_2 β thalassaemia is identical to that in high haemoglobin A_2 β thalassaemia.

Finally, it has become apparent in recent years that β thalassaemia heterozygotes who are also heterozygous for α^0 thalassaemia, or homozygous for α^+ thalassaemia, have MCH and MCV values which are very much higher than those of simple β thalassaemia heterozygotes (Table 11.2).[11,12] They always have elevated haemoglobin A_2 values. The practical implication of this observation is that in populations in which α thalassaemia and β thalassaemia occur together, such as those of Southeast Asia, the Middle East, and the Mediterranean region, a proportion of β thalassaemia heterozygotes may have much higher MCH and MCV values than is usually the case in other races. This is probably the basis for the condition which used to be called 'isolated high haemoglobin A_2'. If screening relies only on red cell indices such patients may be missed and yet they are at risk of having children with thalassaemia major. Thus in any population in which α and β thalassaemia occur together the best method of screening for thalassemia in pregnancy is to measure the haemoglobin A_2 level. If this is impractical, at least every women should have a haemoglobin A_2 estimation if her MCH is below 27 pg and her MCV below 80 fl.

In summary, the majority of β thalassaemia heterozygotes, α^0 thalassaemia heterozygotes, and α^+ thalassaemia homozygotes can easily be identified from studies of red cell indices and a haemoglobin A_2 estimation. Because of the common occurrence of α thalassaemia in populations where β thalassaemia is also common, a number of women will be encountered whose red cell indices are only just below normal because of the interaction of the two genes. Thus a strong case can be made for screening all women from these racial groups with a haemoglobin A_2 estimation. If this is impractical, they should have their haemoglobin A_2 level determined if their red cell indices are even slightly reduced.

Use of DNA analysis in screening

As mentioned later in this chapter, antenatal diagnosis using fetal DNA analysis is now widely applied for the inherited disorders of haemoglobin. This often entails the direct identification of particular β thalassaemia mutations in fetal DNA. Thus parental screening in the antenatal period to identify the particular mutations in each parent is now part of antenatal care in any centre that is running a programme of this type. It is beyond the scope of this chapter to describe the methodology in detail and readers who wish to learn more about the field are referred to several recent reviews.[9,10] It turns out that in most populations there are two or three common β thalassaemia mutations together with a varying number of rare ones (Fig. 11.6). In principle, these mutations are first identified by sequencing of the β globin genes after which specific oligonucleotide probes are constructed which will identify the mutation. Parental blood samples are then obtained to determine which mutations are present so that they can be identified subsequently in DNA obtained from an 'at risk' fetus.

Similarly, if a fetus is at risk for receiving one or more α^0 thalassaemia mutations the parents can be screened to see if either of them have α^0 thalassaemia of this type. The methods for screening for α^0 and α^+ thalassaemia using DNA probes have been reviewed recently.[8]

Another important aspect of antenatal screening for haemoglobin disorders relates to those families in which the mutation responsible for α or β thalassaemia cannot be identified by globin gene analysis. In these cases it may still be possible to offer antenatal diagnosis by genetic linkage analysis.[16] This is particularly valuable in the case of β thalassaemia. In the β globin gene cluster there are many restriction fragment length polymorphisms (RFLPs) which can act as useful linkage markers to identify which particular chromosomes carry the β thalassaemia mutations. Thus it may be valuable to screen the parents and other family members to see if an appropriate RFLP can be used as a linkage marker to determine whether a fetus has received chromosomes carrying β thalassaemia mutations. Several steps are involved. First, it is necessary to analyse both parents to see if they are heterozygous for RFLPs in the β globin gene cluster. If this is the case it is then necessary to examine another family member, ideally a previously born normal or affected child, to determine which chromosomes carry the particular markers. Using this approach it is often possible to determine which of the parental chromosomes carry the β thalassaemia mutations. This information can then be used to determine whether the fetus has received the affected chromosomes from each parent.

Comprehensive antenatal screening programme for thalassaemia

It is clear that antenatal screening for thalassaemia is a complex process which requires the availability of many different laboratory techniques.[14] At its simplest, the initial screen can be carried out by haematological analysis, provided that an electronic cell counter is available for measuring the size of the red cells. This has to be backed up by haemoglobin electrophoresis and a reliable method for measuring the haemoglobin A_2 level. This information, together with the racial origin of the patient, will be sufficient in the majority of cases to indicate the particular thalassaemia genotype in parents of children with the potential for having serious forms of thalassaemia.

In any screening programme there will be a small number of cases in which these simple techniques are insufficient to determine the parental genotype. Particularly in cases of α thalassaemia or suspected normal haemoglobin A_2 β thalassaemia it is necessary to analyse the relative rates of α and β chain production by *in vitro* labelling of the globin chains and their separation by chromatography.[14] The need for this technique may now be largely superceded by the availability of recombinant DNA technology which is able directly to identify the particular α and β thalassaemia mutations in the parents. A detailed account of the methods involved in these more specialized techniques will be found in several different reviews and manuals.[8–10,14] None of these reports deals with developments since the early 1990s, but the newer DNA technology is covered in a more recent monograph, as are the ethical aspects of antenatal diagnosis of the thalassaemias.[3]

As knowledge about the relationship between the genotypes and phenotypes of the thalassaemias has increased it has become possible to start to provide more sophisticated genetic counselling for these conditions. For example, it is now clear that the homozygous or compound heterozygous states for different β thalassaemia alleles may produce a clinical picture which varies from a condition which is lethal in the first year of life to an extremely mild, asymptomatic anaemia. This clinical heterogeneity reflects a number of factors including the type of β thalassaemia allele, or alleles, and the interaction of a number of other genetic factors including variability in the number of copies of the α globin genes and the action of several different genetic determinants which can modify the level of fetal haemoglobin in β thalassaemia.[4]

Antenatal screening for other genetic haematological disorders

Since other genetic blood disorders are so rare as to make routine antenatal screening impracticable, further haematological studies are only indicated in families in which there is a history of inherited blood disease.

Haemolytic anaemia

In women with a haemolytic anaemia an accurate diagnosis should be made in a laboratory capable of assaying the appropriate red cell enzymes; in cases with a dominant inheritance the risk to the fetus is 50 per cent. In recessive disorders in which heterozygotes can be identified, the partner should be studied at the same time. Most red cell enzymes can be assayed by fetal blood sampling, but gene probes for first trimester diagnosis of these conditions are becoming increasingly available. In fact, except for those which are associated with multisystem disease,[17] many genetic red cell enzyme deficiencies are so mild that most parents would not opt for antenatal diagnosis. There is no place for routine antenatal screening of G6PD deficiency.

Hereditary coagulation disorders[8,18]

The most important hereditary coagulation disorders are the sex-linked conditions haemophilia, due to the deficiency of plasma factor VIII coagulant activity (VIIIC), and Christmas disease which results from the deficiency of factor IXC. Haemophilia is a relatively uncommon disease. There are between 3000 and 4000 haemophiliacs in the United Kingdom; 1 in 25 000 of the population has the disease in its severe form. Christmas disease is even less common than haemophilia, the ratio of haemophilia to Christmas disease being in the region of 5:1. Thus antenatal screening for these conditions will be largely restricted to families in which there is a history of the disorder. It is usually indicated if a woman wishes to undergo antenatal diagnosis to determine whether her son has the disease.

Female carriers of haemophilia have, on average, 50 per cent of the normal mean level of factor VIIIC. However, because of the wide scatter of normal values, 50 to 150 per cent, and variability of Lyonization of the X chromosome, carriers often have factor VIIIC levels within the normal range. By measuring the level of von Willebrand factor antigen, the autosomally coded carrier protein for factor VIII, it is sometimes possible to improve discrimination, since carriers tend to have lower levels of factor VIII than von Willebrand's factor.[18] Even so there is still some overlap, which accounts for about 15 per cent between normals and carriers. This is due mainly to Lyonization of the X chromosome which, though random, can often cause unusually low or high values of mutant gene products in heterozygotes. Thus in recent years centres that are carrying out antenatal screening for these diseases are turning to DNA technology for diagnosis.

The factor VIII and IX genes have been isolated and sequenced, and many of the mutations that underlie haemophilia and Christmas disease have been determined.[8,18] These conditions result from both deletions and point mutations involving these genes. Furthermore, as is the case for the globin genes, many restriction fragment length polymorphisms have been found, both within and in the flanking regions of these genes.

There are, therefore, two approaches to antenatal screening for these conditions. First, it may be possible directly to identify the mutation responsible for haemophilia in female carriers, particularly if these involve major deletions of the factor VIII or IX genes. Second, as is the case for the haemoglobin disorders, by carrying out a family study using appropriate RFLP markers it may be possible to determine which X chromosome carries the particular mutation and hence to offer antenatal diagnosis. A number of intragenic RFLPs have been identified and several markers in the flanking region have been found to be particularly informative.[8,18] Because of genetic recombination, the flanking region RFLPs are associated with a small error in antenatal diagnosis due to their recombination distance from the factor VIII gene.

METHODS FOR ANTENATAL DIAGNOSIS OF HAEMATOLOGICAL DISORDERS

Cells or tissue for antenatal diagnosis can be obtained by fetal blood sampling, amniocentesis, or chorionic villus sampling. Fetal blood sampling can be used for the diagnosis of genetic disorders of red cells, white cells, or platelets, and for the identification of clotting factor deficiencies. The haemoglobin disorders can be identified by measuring the relative rates and patterns of globin chain synthesis; other conditions are diagnosed using micromethods for the assay of enzymes or clotting factors. Amniocentesis, chorionic villus sampling, and placental biopsy are all used to obtain cells for cytogenetic or biochemical analysis and to isolate fetal DNA.

Fetal blood sampling

Fetal blood can be obtained between 18 and 20 weeks of gestation by two methods.[19] The first involves aspiration of blood from the placenta under ultrasound guidance.[20] This usually produces a mixture of fetal and maternal cells and now that direct sampling from the cord is well developed this approach is used infrequently. The relative contribution of maternal and fetal blood can be determined by analysing the red cell size distribution using a Coulter Channelyzer.[21] It is often necessary to take multiple samples until an adequate number of fetal cells has been obtained. Several approaches have been used to isolate fetal cells from feto-maternal mixtures. The most useful is the Orskov procedure, which is based on the principle that adult cells, because they contain carbonic anhydrase, lyse in the presence of NH_4Cl and NH_4HCO_3, whereas fetal cells remain intact under these conditions.[22]

Purer fetal blood samples can be obtained by fetoscopy.[23,24] When this approach was first introduced blood was obtained from fetal vessels on the chorionic plate, but subsequently blood was aspirated directly from the umbilical vein at the placental insertion of the cord. Such samples contain pure fetal blood without contamination with maternal blood or amniotic fluid and hence are suitable for analyses requiring cells, serum, or plasma. More recent modifications of fetoscopy and other techniques for fetal blood sampling are the subject of an extensive review.[25]

Haemoglobin disorders

Although fetal blood samples have been used for antenatal identification of many haematological disorders, by far the most experience has been gained in the diagnosis of the structural haemoglobin variants and thalassaemias. Fetal cells are incubated with [^{3}H] leucine, globin chains separated by carboxymethylcellulose chromatography, and the relative amount of radioactivity incorporated into each chain determined.[26] For the antenatal diagnosis of β thalassaemia, the ratio of β to γ chain production is determined. The ratio increases slowly during the first and second trimesters in normal fetuses, and is $0.11 + 0.05$ at 16–23 weeks of gestation.[21,27] If a fetus is homozygous for β^0 thalassaemia there is no β chain synthesis; if it is homozygous for β^+ thalassaemia, or is a compound heterozygote for β^0 and β^+ thalassaemia, there is a reduced β/γ synthesis ratio, usually less than 0.035.[27] The precise diagnostic ratios have to be established for individual laboratories. Remarkably, the overall error rate in experienced laboratories is only about 0.8 per cent, and may be even lower.[21] The main source of error is maternal cell contamination or poor chromatographic technique. With an incomplete separation of γ and β chains it is difficult to distinguish homozygous from heterozygous β^+ thalassaemia. This technique can also be used for the diagnosis of the homozygous state for α^0 thalassaemia (haemoglobin Bart's hydrops syndrome), and structural haemoglobin variants such as haemoglobins S, C, E, O-Arab, and Lepore, the synthesis of which can be detected because of the charge difference of the abnormal globin chain. Fetal blood can also be analysed by sensitive electrophoretic techniques and related approaches.[14]

Other inherited haematological disorders

A variety of haemostatic and coagulation disorders can be identified *in utero* by fetal blood analysis (Table 11.5). Factors VIIIC and IXC can be assayed by immunological techniques even in the presence of amniotic fluid, thus allowing the antenatal recognition of haemophilia and Christmas disease.[8,28,29] Rarer haemostatic disorders that have been identified *in utero* include von Willebrand's disease,[29] autosomal recessive thrombocytopenia,[30] and the Wiskott–Aldrich syndrome.[31]

Potentially, many other red cell disorders can be identified by fetal blood sampling. Normal values for several red cell enzymes in fetal life have been established[32] and dis-

Table 11.5 Some of the disorders that can be identified by fetal blood sampling

Haemoglobinopathies	Structural haemoglobin variants S, C, E, Lepore β thalassaemia α thalassaemia, Hb Bart's hydrops
Coagulation and related disorders	Haemophilia Christmas disease von Willebrand's disease Other factor deficiencies Thrombocytopenia Wiskott–Aldrich syndrome α_1-antitrypsin deficiency
Other red cell disorders	Rhesus haemolytic disease Specific enzyme defects Hereditary erythroblastic multinuclearity with a positive acidified serum lysis test (HEMPAS)
White cell and related disorders	Chronic granulomatous disease Genetic neutropenia Immunodeficiency states
Cytogenetic analysis	Fanconi's anaemia Bloom's syndrome Xeroderma pigmentosum

orders such as triose phosphate isomerase deficiency have been identified in fetal blood.[33] It is also possible to grow erythroid colonies from fetal blood as an approach to the antenatal diagnosis of stem-cell disorders.[34]

Fetal white cells can also be used for antenatal diagnosis.[35] Chronic granulomatous disease can be diagnosed by the inability of the white cells of affected fetuses to reduce nitroblue tetrazolium.[36] Fetal cells have also been used for the antenatal diagnosis of the inherited immunodeficiency syndromes. For example, adenosine deaminase (ADA) deficiency has been identified *in utero* and severe combined immunodeficiency has been diagnosed by analysing T and B lymphocyte subsets.[37,38] Fetal white cells are particularly useful for cytogenetic studies; chromosomal analysis can be carried out within 72 hours, much quicker than using cultured amniotic fluid cells.

Amniocentesis

Although the main value of amniocentesis for the antenatal diagnosis of genetic disorders of the blood is for obtaining cells for DNA analysis (see below), cytogenetic and biochemical analysis of amniotic fluid cells can also be used for identifying haematological disorders. For example, patients with Fanconi's anaemia have increased chromosome fragility which is magnified after culture of their cells with diepoxybutane (DEB), a DNA cross-linker. Antenatal recognition of this condition has been carried out in this way using amniotic fluid cells.[19] Other fragile-chromosome syndromes which can be identified *in utero* include ataxia telangiectasia,[39] Bloom's syndrome,[19] and xeroderma pigmentosum.[19] Several conditions can be identified by enzyme analysis of amniotic fluid cells. These include glucose phosphate isomerase deficiency,[40] congenital methaemoglobinaemia due to NADH-linked methaemoglobin reductase deficiency,[41] and recessive erythropoietic porphyria.[42]

The diagnosis of metabolic disorders using amniotic fluid cells depends on the demonstration of reduced enzyme activity or the accumulation of a metabolite due to an enzyme deficiency. Thus this approach is only feasible for red or white cell enzyme deficiencies if these are expressed in other tissues, such as fibroblasts. Hecht and Cadien provide an extensive review of conditions which can be identified antenatally by biochemical analysis of amniotic fluid cells.[43] Valentine and Paglia have reviewed the increasing list of red cell enzyme defects which, as well as causing haemolytic anaemia, are associated with multisystem diseases.[17] These deficiencies are expressed widely in tissues other than the haemopoietic cells; at least some of them should be amenable to identification *in utero* by analysis of amniotic fluid cells.

It seems likely that in the future, cells obtained by chorion biopsy will be equally useful for cytogenetic and biochemical analysis.

Fetal DNA analysis

The development of techniques for DNA analysis has already revolutionized the antenatal diagnosis of genetic disease. So far this approach has been applied mainly to the antenatal diagnosis of the haemoglobin and coagulation disorders; this will not be the case for long.

Sources of Fetal DNA

Fetal DNA can be obtained either from amniotic fluid cells or chorionic villus sampling (CVS). Unfortunately, the yield of DNA from a conventional amniotic fluid tap is usually too small for DNA analysis, though this problem may be overcome by the new techniques for amplifying DNA (see below). If the precise defect is known and can be identified by restriction enzyme analysis (see below), it may be possible to obtain enough DNA by simply spinning down the amniotic fluid cells. If more extensive DNA analysis is required, the cells must be grown in culture for several weeks. In this case an antenatal diagnosis cannot be made until late in the second trimester.

Recently, CVS has been widely explored as an approach to obtaining fetal DNA in the first trimester,[25] and its safety has been analysed in several randomized clinical trials.[44-46] Although these trials indicate that it is less safe than second trimester amniocentesis, it appears likely to remain an acceptable procedure for diagnosing serious genetic disease at around three months of gestation. According to one of the clinical trials,[46] it is safer to sample chorionic villi transabdominally than transcervically. Amniocentesis and CVS are discussed in greater detail in Chapter 19.

The yield of DNA from chorion biopsy varies from 2 to 100 µg with an average of about 20–30 µg. There is good linear correlation between the weight of trophoblast tissue and the yield of DNA.

Methods for DNA analysis

The methods that can be used for analysing fetal DNA have been reviewed extensively and are summarized in Table 11.6.

Direct identification of mutant genes with restriction enzymes

Major gene deletions or rearrangements can be identified directly by gene mapping using appropriate DNA probes. For example, the homozygous state for α^0 thalassaemia (haemoglobin Bart's hydrops), or the Indian form of β^0 thalassaemia due to a deletion at the 3' end of the β globin gene, can be diagnosed in this way. Some of the

Table 11.6   Antenatal diagnosis by DNA analysis

Direct	Deletions and rearrangements by Southern blotting Point mutations that are identified by restriction enzymes; Southern blotting Oligonucleotide probes and Southern blotting Polymerase chain reaction (PCR): (1) identification with oligonucleotide probes, (2) electrophoresis or dot blot, (3) amplification refractory mutation system (ARMS)
Indirect (Southern blotting or PCR)	RFLP linkage—flanking or intragenic Allele-linked RFLP

Table 11.7   β thalassaemia mutations directly detectable by restriction analysis

Mutation	Restriction enzyme
β^0 thalassaemia	
1. Indian deletion	Various enzymes—619 bp
2. American Black deletion	Various enzymes—1.35\kb
3. Dutch deletion	Various enzymes—10 kb
4. Czech deletion	Various enzymes—4.2 kb
5. Turkish deletion	Various enzymes—300 bp
6. −1 codon 6	*Mst* II
7. IVS 2 splice junction	*Hph* I
8. IVS 1 (−25 bp)	*Fnu* 4H, *Mst* II
9. IVS 1 (−17 bp)	*Fnu* 4H, *Mst* II
10. IVS 1–position 116	*Mae* I
11. IVS 1 position 6	*Sfa* N1
12. IVS 2 3′ end AG → GG	*Alu* I
13. β^0 39	*Mae* I
14. β^0 17	*Mae* I
15. β^0 37	*Ava* II
16. β^0 121	*Eco* RI
β^+ thalassaemia	
17. IVS 2 position 745	*Rsa* I
18. −87 C → G	*Avr* II
19. Hb E	*Mnl* I

single base mutations which cause structural haemoglobin variants or thalassaemia alter restriction enzyme sites and hence can be identified directly with the appropriate enzyme (Table 11.7). For example, the difference between sickle cell haemoglobin and normal haemoglobin is a glutamic acid to valine substitution in the sixth position of the β chain. This reflects an A→T change in the DNA of the β globin gene. This substitution changes a sequence normally recognized and cleaved by three different restriction enzymes, *Dde* I, *Mnl* I, and *Mst* II; for technical reasons the latter is the most useful. Some varieties of β thalassaemia which can be analysed in this way are summarized in Table 11.7; other rare structural variants are amenable to diagnosis by the same approach.[47]

However, apart from the deletion forms of α thalassaemia, two types of non-deletion α thalassaemia, the Indian variety of deletion β^0 thalassaemia and a few other varieties of β^0 and β^+ thalassaemia (Table 11.7), most of the common forms of β thalassaemia are not amenable to diagnosis directly by restriction enzyme analysis because the mutations which cause them do not change the site of enzymatic cleavage.

RFLP linkage analysis

Scattered throughout human DNA every few hundred bases or so there are single base changes which produce either new restriction enzyme sites or remove previously existing ones.[48,49] These harmless polymorphisms, which are inherited in a simple Mendelian way, provide a wealth of genetic markers which, with appropriate gene probes, can be identified easily by gene mapping. A restriction fragment length polymorphism (RFLP) of this type which is close enough to a gene so that the two are not separated during meiosis can be used as a linkage marker to determine which chromosome carries the thalassaemia mutation in a particular family. Alternatively the polymorphism may be within the gene itself. The idea is to study the parents and previously born children or other relatives using several restriction enzymes and gene probes to see if an RFLP can be found on the chromosome carrying the mutant gene in each parent. If so, and if the fetus has inherited both the marker RFLPs, it must also be homozygous for the particular mutation, or a compound heterozygote for two different mutations.

The problem with this method is that is requires a previously born child or other family members to establish a linkage, and hence a considerable amount of laboratory work before the diagnosis can be made. Furthermore, the frequency of different RFLP markers varies between different racial groups. For example, studies in Britain suggest that this approach for the antenatal diagnosis of β thalassaemia will be feasible in about four-fifths of Cypriot and Asian families.[50,51]

The arrangement of RFLPs along the α and β globin gene clusters is not random; they exist in a series of patterns within individual populations, which are called haplotypes. Thus, within any particular racial group it is usual to find particular β thalassaemia mutations associated with a specific RFLP haplotype. However, this phenomenon cannot be used for antenatal diagnosis since the same haplotypes occur in *normal* members of the same population. Occasionally, however, mutations may be in so-called linkage disequilibrium with particular polymorphic sites. For example, it has been found that an *Hpa* I polymorphism is strongly associated with the β^S mutation in West Africans,[52] and a *Bam* HI polymorphism is associated with the common β^0 thalassaemia mutation in Sardinia.[53] However, examples of linkage disequilibria of this type are uncommon and it is usually necessary to establish linkages between a particular β globin mutation and an RFLP within an individual family.

Polymorphisms of this type may be useful, however. For example, a polymorphism for the restriction enzyme *Ava* II in the ψβ gene of the β globin gene cluster is found in Mediterranean populations. This site is absent in over 50 per cent of chromosomes carrying a common β thalassaemia mutation but in only 2–3 per cent of normal chromosomes.[54] This difference in frequency greatly increases the feasibility of antenatal diagnosis of β thalassaemia by DNA analysis in these populations. Indeed, it has been estimated that using it together with other RFLPs it should be possible to carry out antenatal diagnosis in over 90 per cent of families which have the common (Mediterranean) (IVS 110) β thalassaemia mutation.[54]

Oligonucleotide probes

The long DNA probes which are used for standard gene mapping analysis are not able to detect single base changes of the kind which cause many forms of thalassaemia and other single gene disorders. However, under appropriate conditions short synthetic

DNA fragments (oligonucleotides or oligomers) can be constructed which hybridize to their homologous sequences but not to heterologous sequences, that is those with *any* mismatch, even a single base difference.[55,56] For example, it is possible to construct short probes consisting of 19 nucleotides (19-mers), which contain the sequence of the normal β globin gene in the region of the β^S mutation, and which hybridize efficiently with the normal gene, but not with DNA that contains the sickle cell mutation.[56] Using high-specific-activity labelling of these synthetic probes normal and sickle sequences can be distinguished after hybridization of restriction-enzyme-digested total human DNA. Two 19-mers are made, one directed against the normal sequence, the other against the sequence with the altered base. Using both probes the genotype of an individual with respect to a specific mutation can be established.

As well as a specific oligonucleotide probe against the β^S mutation, similar probes have been made against all the common β thalassaemia mutations and are now used widely for the antenatal diagnosis of β thalassaemia.

More rapid identification of mutations

The 'classical' methods of gene analysis by Southern blotting take up to a week or more when used for diagnostic purposes. However, several new methods have been developed which have facilitated DNA analysis such that a diagnosis can easily be achieved in the same day. Most of the recent advances in this field have resulted from the development of a technique called the polymerase chain reaction (PCR) which allows the amplification of any short DNA sequence over a period of a few hours.[57,58]

The principle of PCR is to attach short DNA primers to the region containing a gene, or part of a gene, one on each of the opposite ends of the two pairs of homologous strands. These primers are used to direct the enzyme DNA polymerase to copy each of the strands in opposite directions. Repeated cycles of enzymatic amplification increase the quantity of the targetted DNA region more than 2000-fold. As the result of the development of a heat-stable DNA polymerase it is now possible to carry out repeated rounds of DNA synthesis at an elevated temperature thus greatly improving the amplification of targeted over background DNA.

The PCR technique permits the direct visualization of stained DNA fragments on gels, and thus radioactive probes are not needed to define specific gene fragments. Furthermore, it is possible to amplify DNA from blood or tissue samples without previous purification. By combining PCR amplification with the use of specific oligonucleotide probes, as described above, it is possible to identify single base mutations very rapidly[59,60] and, since sufficient DNA can be amplified for direct visualization on gels, it is possible to identify the RFLPs that cause alterations in restriction enzyme patterns without the use of radioactive probes.[61,62]

The development of PCR has also led to a variety of new approaches for rapid sequencing of human genes, all of which bypass the need to clone the particular gene of interest. Thus it is now becoming possible to identify mutations in individual families for diagnostic purposes. Another recent approach for the identification of mutations using PCR has been called the *a*mplification *r*efractory *m*utation *s*ystem (ARMS).[63] This is based on the observation that oligonucleotides with a 3' mismatched residue will, under appropriate conditions, not function as primers in the PCR. Hence this method makes use of two primers. The normal form is refractory to

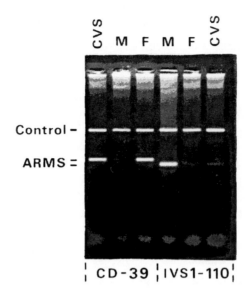

Fig. 11.11 The antenatal diagnosis of β thalassaemia in a fetus at risk for compound heterozygosity for two different β thalassaemia mutations. The diagnosis is carried out using the ARMS technique (see text). One parent has the common Mediterranean codon 39 (CD) mutation, the other the IVS-1–110-G→A mutation. The fetus is heterozygous for the codon 39 mutation. M = mother, F = father, CVS = fetal DNA from chorionic villus sampling.

PCR on mutant template DNA while the mutant form is refractory to PCR on normal DNA. The difference between normal DNA and that with a particular mutation is identified by size differences of the amplified fragments. This technique has a wide variety of applications for antenatal diagnosis and is turning out to be particularly useful for diagnosing compound heterozygosity for two different mutations in fetal DNA (Fig. 11.11).[64]

Hitherto the gene probes that we have described for isolating and studying human genes, or fragments thereof, have been radioactively labelled. This has several disadvantages. In particular it is expensive and, in the case of oligonucleoitide probes, requires radioactive isotopes with very high specific activity. These problems are being overcome by the use of non-radioactive sources of probe labelling.[65,66] For example, biotinylated nucleotides can be used as non-radioactive probes. Biotin-labelled analogues of TTP and UTP can be enzymatically incorporated into DNA or RNA. The biotin incorporated into the probe can be coupled to avadin, and antibodies that identify the biotin/avadin complexes can be raised and labelled by immunofluorescence, immunoperoxidase, or immunocolloidal gold. A variety of other ingenious approaches are being used for non-radioactive labelling of gene probes.

Finally, it is becoming feasible to amplify DNA so rapidly, and to define single point mutations in the amplified DNA with ologinucleotide probes, that it is now possible to analyse point mutations without the necessity of running DNA on gels.[9,10] The DNA is simply blotted onto a nylon filter and probed with appropriate oligonucleotides. Such 'dot blot' technology, if combined with non-radioactively labelled probes, provides a very rapid and simple laboratory approach to the diagnosis of genetic disease. Alternatively, the specific oligonucleotide probes can be immobilized on membranes and hybridized with PCR amplified DNA from the patient.[67]

Preimplantation and other approaches to antenatal diagnosis

The development of increasingly sophisticated microsurgical techniques together with the availability of PCR has raised the possibility that in the future it may be possible to identify genetic disease by biopsy procedures following *in vitro* fertilization. The principle of this approach is to obtain a number of fertilized ova and analyse them for a particular genetic disease before replacing one of the unaffected ones into the uterus. Couples with a one in four or one in two chance of producing a baby with a serious genetic disorder, particularly if they find abortion unacceptable, would bene-fit from this method. Experimental studies have shown that it is possible to obtain cells for PCR amplification of DNA at about the eight-cell stage and also a little later at the blastocyst stage of development.[68]

More work will need to be carried out to determine the safety of this approach, particularly with respect to the further development of pre-embryos that have been manipulated in this way. The technical problems of DNA analysis from one or two cells are considerable. Although PCR can generate enough DNA for a satisfactory analysis the problems of preventing contamination of the sample are considerable; it would only require a single cell from the skin or mucous membrane of an operator to confuse a diagnosis of this type. Thus it will be very important to build in techniques for defining the parental origin of cells treated in this way. There seems little doubt that this new approach will have an increasingly important place in clinical practice over the next few years. Recent successes suggest that it will be possible to overcome these problems.[69]

There has also been some progress towards developing antenatal diagnosis using fetal cells in the maternal circulation.[70]

OVERALL RESULTS OF SCREENING AND ANTENATAL DIAGNOSIS FOR HAEMATOLOGICAL DISORDERS

Fetal blood sampling

Up to the end of 1989 there were 13 291 reports of antenatal diagnosis for the major haemoglobinopathies, mainly β thalassaemia and sickle cell anaemia.[19] The overall fetal loss rate was 3.1 per cent, with 1.6 per cent maternal complications and 6.5 per cent premature deliveries. The error rate was 0.5 per cent. Perhaps most encouragingly, over the period covered by the report the birth-rate of infants with β thalassaemia major declined to between 10 and 50 per cent of the expected figures in north Italy, Cyprus, Greece, and Sardinia, and among British Cypriots (Fig. 11.12). Thus, fetal blood sampling for antenatal diagnosis of β thalassaemia has already made a major contribution to the public health burden posed by this disease. The results for ante-natal diagnosis of other genetic blood diseases, though based on smaller numbers, are equally encouraging. The majority of diagnoses were for coagulation disorders: 473 cases were at risk for haemophilia A, 46 for haemophilia B, and eight for von Wille-brand's disease. There were 10 reported errors: fetuses with haemophilia were not detected *in utero*. There were 60 fetal losses (1.3 per cent), which suggests that the risk

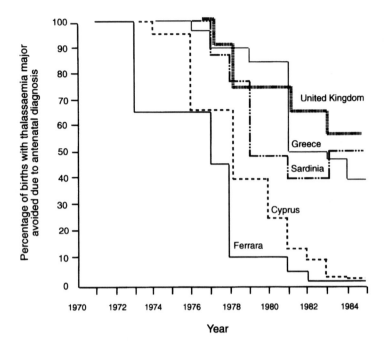

Fig. 11.12 The effects of the development of antenatal diagnosis programmes in different countries on the births of homozygous β thalassaemics. (Data from Modell and Bulyzhenkov.[1])

of haemophilia does not increase the likelihood of fetal loss following fetal blood sampling.

The total experience for the antenatal diagnosis of thalassaemia and the haemoglobinopathies in Greece between 1977 and 1988 has been summarized.[51] Altogether 3712 cases were diagnosed using fetal blood analysis. There were only 17 definite and three probable errors, and 33 instances in which it was impossible to obtain a sample. The overall fetal loss rate was approximately 2.5 per cent.

Thus it appears that fetal blood sampling is still associated with appreciable fetal loss, but that provided the laboratory techniques are well developed it is a remarkably successful approach to the antenatal diagnosis of common haemoglobin disorders. However, it has the major disadvantage of a long period of uncertainty for the mother and a difficult middle trimester termination of pregnancy, if indicated.

Fetal DNA analysis

Results for first trimester antenatal diagnosis of the haemoglobin disorders have been summarized by several groups.[19,51,71–73] In Sardinia, where the majority of cases of β thalassaemia result from one mutation, over 1000 antenatal diagnoses have been carried out using either direct detection of the mutation by oligonucleotide probes or, more recently, by dot blot analysis. There have been few mis-diagnoses and the fetal loss is in the region of 2 per cent. In the UK up to the end of 1995 over 2000 antenatal diagnoses have been carried out by DNA analysis. In this population the patients come from many different racial backgrounds and therefore many different β thalassaemia mutations have to be identified. The majority of cases of β thalassaemia were analysed by RFLP linkage studies with a smaller proportion being diagnosed using oligonucleotide probes. In this series there were 14 fetal losses and five mis-diagnoses with six failures. In both these series the failure rates were greater than if DNA was obtained from amniotic fluid.

It appears, therefore, that first trimester antenatal diagnosis is feasible and that it should be possible to achieve an error rate of less than 1 per cent. Possible sources of error include contamination of chorionic tissue with maternal tissue, plasmid contamination, failure of DNA digestion, recombination if RFLP probes that are not within a particular gene are used, and incorrect assignment of parental genotype. Studies in the author's (DJW) laboratory suggest that maternal contamination is present in less than 2 per cent of all samples received. Another important source of error is non-paternity, and it is becoming apparent that it will be necessary to run a paternity test using DNA fingerprinting technology if the overall error rates for DNA diagnosis are to be reduced to a minimum.

There has been less experience in first trimester antenatal diagnosis of other haematological disorders using DNA analysis. It has been possible to diagnose haemophilia and Christmas disease using either RFLP linkage analysis or PCR amplification.[8,61,74] A proportion of cases of haemophilia are due to new mutations and an ingenious approach to screening for mutations of large genes like those for factor VIII or dystrophin has been described.[75] Thus it seems likely that DNA analysis will be applied increasingly widely for both carrier detection and antenatal diagnosis of haemophilia and Christmas disease. The same approaches can be used for any haematological disorder for which a gene probe is available. The principles will be exactly the same as those outlined for the haemoglobin disorders and haemophilia. If the mutation is known an oligonucleotide probe can be constructed and the appropriate part of the gene amplified by PCR. If the mutation is not known the disorder can be identified by RFLP linkage analysis provided appropriate polymorphisms can be defined and the affected chromosomes determined by a previous family study.

STRATEGY FOR SCREENING AND ANTENATAL DIAGNOSIS PROGRAMMES

The pace of development of antenatal diagnosis technology has been so fast over the last few years that its role in clinical practice is still not fully defined. The field is still in a state of flux, and both sampling and analytical techniques require further evaluation. What should be done in practice during this uncertain period?

Haemoglobin disorders

As mentioned earlier, in most of the developed countries appropriate screening facilities for the common haemoglobin disorders are already established in haematology laboratories. It is essential that there is an adequate flow of information from laboratories to obstetricians, and that centres with expertise in counselling patients about the potential outcome of 'at risk' pregnancies are developed.

The importance of developing adequate counselling facilities cannot be overemphasized. In many ways the field of antenatal detection of genetic disease has run before it could walk. Thus while we have sophisticated methods for screening and antenatal detection of the major haemoglobin disorders the development of population programmes, both in the United States and in the United Kingdom, has been hampered by lack of adequate counselling facilities. It is no use developing all this powerful technology if patients are to be left confused and improperly educated about the diseases for which these methods are being applied.

It will have been clear from the description of these screening methods for the thalassaemias described earlier that any competent haematology laboratory can screen for the bulk of the common forms of thalassaemia and the other rarer genetic haematological disorders. However, because of the heterogeneity of the thalassaemias, and the complex interactions which may occur when individuals inherit one or more different forms of the condition, it is necessary to have at least one or two reference laboratories which are able to apply globin synthesis technology and DNA analysis for determining the genotypes in these cases.

Currently, it is clear that at least for the foreseeable future fetal DNA analysis following CVS will become the mainstay of antenatal diagnosis programmes. In determining the most cost-effective and simple laboratory technology a number of problems will have to be addressed. In particular it is turning out that many genetic diseases like thalassaemia and haemophilia are extremely heterogeneous at the molecular level. Thus while one gene probe or restriction enzyme is adequate for the diagnosis of sickle cell anaemia other technologies will have to be developed to cover the 180 or more β thalassaemia mutations that underlie this important disease. Such heterogeneity raises a number of practical issues. In the United Kingdom, for example, the thalassaemias are seen in individuals from Cyprus, other Mediterranean regions, the Middle East, the Indian subcontinent, Southeast Asia, and from many other parts of the world. Thus many different mutations will be encountered and many potentially affected children will be compound heterozygotes for different mutations. This problem is compounded by the fact that many women present late in the first trimester and there is very little time to determine parental genotypes and to carry out fetal DNA analysis.

Thus while it may be possible, in the long term, to identify the different mutations as part of a national screening programme, the provision of a comprehensive antenatal diagnosis service will, for the immediate future, require considerable flexibility of technical approach. And there is a further problem. To provide a fully comprehensive antenatal diagnosis programme it must be possible to give accurate genetic counselling to prospective parents. Children who receive two β thalassaemia genes may have a clinical disorder ranging from a life-threatening anaemia during the first year to an extremely mild condition that is compatible with normal development and survival. Recent studies have suggested that, by and large, it will be possible to determine many of the factors that cause either severe or mild β thalassaemia. But this type of analysis will have to be incorporated into antenatal diagnosis programmes in the future.

Given these problems how should a programme be established? First, it is important to determine the common thalassaemia mutations in a particular population. It turns out that most races have a handful of common mutations together with varying numbers of rare ones. Thus the ideal basis for an antenatal diagnosis programme will be to develop gene probes for the common mutations and to carry out fetal DNA analysis following CVS, using PCR with oligonucleotide probes or, if the mutation can be detected directly, using appropriate enzymes on amplified DNA. This technology can be converted to simple 'dot blot' analysis. Laboratories with a sufficient expertise may be able to develop rapid sequencing methods for identifying unusual β thalassaemia mutations. But it will still be necessary to carry out RFLP linkage studies in families in which the mutations cannot be identified. And it will also be necessary for laboratories with a large population of thalassaemics to retain their ability to carry out fetal blood sampling and globin chain synthesis for those rare cases in which DNA analysis is not possible, or if women present after the first trimester.

Ultimately this type of programme should be applicable to the large, rural populations of India and Southeast Asia. The best approach will be to set up diagnostic centres in various parts of the community as has already been done in Thailand for example. While expertise in CVS is being developed it should be possible to define the common mutations in the population. Once this has been done, it should be feasible to develop antenatal diagnosis programmes, particularly if simple dot blot technology can be used, perhaps in the form of a diagnostic kit.

Other haematological disorders

Antenatal detection of other haematological disorders will go along the same lines as the thalassaemias. While gene probes are being developed, fetal blood sampling will remain the mainstay for the antenatal detection of many red cell, white cell, and coagulation disorders. The rapid diagnostic techniques for determining mutations, such as have been applied to the factor VIII and IX genes, should make it possible to apply DNA technology widely for the detection of heterozygotes and for the antenatal diagnosis of haemophilia and Christmas disease. This can be carried out either by RFLP linkage analysis or by direct detection of the mutation as outlined in previous sections.

NEONATAL SCREENING

Overall, the major efforts for antenatal and neonatal screening for the serious genetic blood diseases are directed at developing antenatal diagnosis programmes. However, there are some disorders for which it is important to establish neonatal screening programmes. A proportion of women will not have wished to undergo antenatal diagnosis and it may be important to identify genetic blood diseases in the neonatal period so that prophylactic measures or therapy can be started early. Furthermore there are some conditions, particularly G6PD deficiency, which are associated with important complications in the neonatal period. Thus there is a place for neonatal screening although it is small compared with the major role of antenatal screening for genetic blood disease.

The haemoglobin disorders

The most important haemoglobin disorders for which neonatal screening is indicated are the sickling conditions. In fact, in many countries where sickle cell disorders are common, routine neonatal screening programmes are being carried out. There are several reasons for this development. First, any child of a women with the sickle cell trait should be screened at birth for a sickling disorder, particularly if it has not been possible to screen the father, as is often the case. Second, even if the parents have been screened and only one of them has the sickle cell trait it is important to identify the sickle cell trait in the neonatal period for future counselling purposes. Furthermore, because it has been established that the administration of prophylactic penicillin and careful clinical surveillance reduced the early mortality of sickle cell disease, it has become particularly important to identify both SS and SC disease as early as possible.

For these reasons neonatal screening programmes should be instituted in all countries where the sickle cell genes are common or in those with large immigrant populations which are made up of individuals from these high frequency countries.

The clinically important sickling genotypes (SS, SC, SD^{Punjab}, SO^{Arab}, S β thalassaemia) can easily be detected at birth by cellulose acetate electrophoresis at alkaline pH or by citrate agar electrophroesis at acid pH (or by commercial 'acid agarose' electrophoresis). These techniques can be used with umbilical cord blood or liquid capillary samples obtained in the neonatal period. The techniques were reviewed by the International Committee for Standardization in Haematology (ICSH) in 1988.[76] Isoelectric focusing and automated HPLC are also satisfactory for the analysis of such neonatal samples and they can also be used for dried blood spots on filter paper such as 'Guthrie cards'. However, many cases of α thalassaemia will be missed if dried spots are used since Hb Barts and Hb H are unstable and are much less likely to be detected on dried blood spots than when analysing liquid samples. In many clinical situations there is no need to screen for α thalassaemia at birth and then this disadvantage is not a problem. Neonatal screening to detect the sickling syndromes should be undertaken well before the infant is three months old because severe life-threatening crises can occur at any time after three months and have occasionally been described at eight to nine weeks after birth. Many paediatricians would plan to have all sickle cell disease babies on daily penicillin by the age of three months to avoid life-threatening crises infections.

Although it is possible to detect sickle cell disease at birth it is not possible to differentiate between certain genotypes such as between SS, S-β^0 thalassaemia, and S-HPFH, and it is therefore important to retest the infant later on during the first year of life, say six to 12 months, to determine the precise genotype. Similarly, it is not possible to differentiate between Hb EE and Hb E β^0 thalassaemia at birth and again it is important to retest at 6 to 12 months since these two conditions usually have quite different clinical implications.

It is quite difficult to diagnose homozygous β thalassaemia at birth, even using sensitive haemoglobin biosynthetic methods. It is therefore much better to carry out neonatal screening for β thalassaemia between the age of three and six months.[3] In homozygotes or compound heterozygotes for severe forms of β thalassaemia children are already anaemic by this time and have high levels of Hb F. The neonatal diagnosis of β thalassaemia trait is also best left until about six months at which time the raised level of Hb A$_2$ is established.

Glucose-6-phosphate dehydrogenase deficiency

In some but not all populations in which G6PD deficiency is common there is a high incidence of neonatal jaundice and kernicterus in affected babies.[77] This seems to be a particular problem in Southeast Asia. In populations where these complications of G6PD deficiency are common, neonatal screening for G6PD deficiency has become routine. A G6PD assay is carried out on cord blood or blood obtained immediately after birth and the affected babies are kept under close surveillance for several weeks with regular estimations of bilirubin levels. The precise mechanism for neonatal hyperbilirubinaemia associated with G6PD deficiency is still not clear, nor is it clear why this is only seen in certain races with G6PD deficiency.

Genetic bleeding disorders

There is no place for routine neonatal screening for the rare disorders of haemostasis and coagulation. If there is a strong family history and if the mother has not been evaluated for her carrier status with a view to antenatal diagnosis, it may be necessary to screen newborn infants, particularly if they are to undergo circumcision or other traumatic procedures. Furthermore it is useful to establish a diagnosis early so that appropriate prophylactic measures can be taken.

The principles for screening for these conditions are similar to those described earlier for identifying particular coagulation disorders in the antenatal period. Simple screening tests are carried out on citrated blood. The most important are the activated whole blood clotting time, partial thromboplastin time (PTT), which tests for the presence of all factors involved in intrinsic coagulation, and the prothrombin time, which tests mainly for factors synthesized in the liver, II, VII and X; that is, this combination of tests assesses the rapid intrinsic clotting mechanism.

Blood from male infants who may have inherited either haemophilia or Christmas disease will give normal prothrombin times with prolonged PTTs. Blood from those with severe von Willebrand's disease gives similar results as from those with factor XI deficiency. The specific abnormality can be confirmed by individual factor assays. As mentioned earlier, many of these conditions can now be identified at the DNA level.

SCREENING FOR HAEMOGLOBIN DISORDERS ASSOCIATED WITH MENTAL RETARDATION

Following the first description of the association between α thalassaemia and mental retardation[78] it has become apparent that this heterogeneous syndrome is of importance when screening families for otherwise unexplained mental retardation associated with dysmorphic features.[79]

The syndrome of α thalassaemia and mental retardation is heterogeneous and there are two major varieties.[80-82] First, there are cases associated with deletions involving the α globin gene cluster. In these cases there is mild mental retardation, variable dysmorphic features, and the haematological findings typical of α thalassaemia. The molecular pathology of this condition is heterogeneous and includes submicroscopic chromosomal translocations, truncations of the tip of chromosome 16 which contains the α globin genes, and otherwise unexplained long deletions involving the α globin genes and 1–2 kb of DNA adjacent to them. Because some of these conditions result from balanced chromosomal translocations in one parent it is extremely important to carry out detailed cytogenetic studies on the parents of infants of this type so that appropriate counselling can be given. In some cases microscopic chromosomal abnormalities can be detected but in others the translocations can only be demonstrated by *in situ* hybridization technology.[82]

Patients with the second variety of this syndrome have more severe mental retardation, a typical dysmorphic disorder, and a mild form of α thalassaemia associated with defective output from both pairs of α globin genes on chromosome 16.[81,82] Recent work has shown that this condition is determined by an X chromosome encoded locus, *XH2*[83], or *ATX*, the product of which is required for normal α globin chain production as well as for early development. Furthermore, studies suggest that the female carriers of children of this type have small red cell populations which carry haemoglobin H bodies thus making this haemoglobin H estimation a particularly valuable screening test for the presence of this syndrome.[84]

ACKNOWLEDGEMENTS

The authors wish to thank Dr Adrian Stephens and Allan Hackshaw for the Bart's data on β-thalassaemia.

REFERENCES

1. Modell C. B. and Bulyzhenkov V. (1988). Distribution and control of some genetic disorders. *World Health Statistics Quarterly*, **41**, 209–18.
2. Weatherall D. J., Clegg J. B., Higgs D. R., and Wood W. G. (1989). The hemoglobinopathies. In *The metabolic basis of inherited disease*, 6th edn, (ed. C. R. Scriver, A. L. Beaudet, W. S. Sly, and D. Valle), pp. 2281–366. McGraw Hill, New York.
3. Weatherall D. J. and Clegg J. B. (2000). *The thalassaemia syndromes*, 4th edn. Blackwell Scientific, Oxford. In press.
4. Weatherall D. J. (1993). Thalassemia. In *Molecular basis of blood diseases*, 2nd edn, (ed. G. Stamatoyannopoulos, A. W. Nienhuis, P. W. Majerus, and H. Varmus), pp. 157–206. Saunders, Philadelphia.
5. Higgs D. R., Vickers M. A., Wilkie A. O. M., Pretorius I.-M., Jarman A. P., and Weatherall D. J. (1989). A review of the molecular genetics of the human α globin gene cluster. *Blood*, **73**, 1081–104.
6. Liang S. T., Wong V. C.W, So W. W.K, Ma H. K., Chan V., and Todd D. (1985). Homozygous α-thalassaemia: Clinical presentation, diagnosis and management. A review of 46 cases. *British Journal of Obstetrics and Gynaecology*, **92**, 680–4.
7. Higgs D. R. and Weatherall D. J. (1983). α-thalassaemia. In *Current topics in hematology*, 4th edn. (ed. S. Piomelli and S. Yachnin), pp. 37–97. Liss, New York.
8. Old J. M. and Ludlam C. A. (1991). The haemoglobinopathies. *Baillière's Clinical Haematology*, **4**, 391–428.
9. Kazazian H. H. and Boehm C. D. (1988). Molecular basis and prenatal diagnosis of β-thalassemia. *Blood*, **72**, 1107–16.
10. Huisman T. H. J. (1993). The structure and function of normal and abnormal haemoglobins. *Clinical Haematology*, **6**, 1–30.
11. Kanavakis E., Wainscoat J. S., Wood W. G., Weatherall D. J., Cao A., Furbetta M., Galanello R., Georgiou D., and Sophocleous T. (1982). The interaction of α thalassaemia with heterozygous β thalassaemia. *British Journal of Haematology*, **52**, 465–73.

12. Kattamis C., Metaxatou-Mavromati A., Wood W. G., Nash J. R., and Weatherall D. J. (1979). The heterogeneity of normal Hb A₂-β thalassaemia in Greece. *British Journal of Haematology*, **42**, 109–23.

13. Rosatelli C., Falchi A. M., Scalas M. T., Tuveri T., Furbetta M., and Cao A. (1984). Hematological phenotype of the double heterozygous state for alpha and beta thalassemia. *Hemoglobin*, **8**, 25–35.

14. Weatherall D. J. (ed.) (1983). *Methods in haematology. The thalassaemias*. Churchill Livingstone, Edinburgh.

15. Pirastu M., Ristaldi M. S., Loudianos G., Murru S., Sciarratta G. V., Parodi M. I., Leone D., Agosti S., and Cao A. (1990). Molecular analysis of atypical β-thalassemia heterozygotes. *Annals of the New York Academy of Sciences*, **612**, 90–7.

16. Weatherall D. J. (1991). Prenatal diagnosis of haematological disease. In *Fetal and neonatal haematology*, (ed. I. M. Hann, B. E. S. Gibson, and E. A. Letsky), pp. 285–314. Bailliere Tindall, London.

17. Valentine W. N. and Paglia D. E. (1984). Erythrocyte enzymopathies, hemolytic anemia, and multisystem disease: an annotated review. *Blood*, **64**, 583–91.

18. Tuddenham E. G. D. (1989). Factor VIII and haemophilia A. *Baillière's Clinical Haematology*, **2**, 849–77.

19. Alter B. P. (1990). Antenatal diagnosis. Summary of results, *Annals of the New York Academy of Sciences*, **612**, 237–50.

20. Kan Y. W., Valenti C., Carnazza V., Guidotti R., and Reider R. F. (1974). Fetal blood-sampling in utero. *Lancet*, **i**, 79–80.

21. Alter B. P. (1980). Prenatal diagnosis of hemoglobinopathies. In *Progress in pediatric hematology/oncology*, Vol. III, (ed. E. Schwarz), pp. 123–46. P. S.G. Publishing, Littlejohn.

22. Alter B. P., Metzger J. B., Yock P. G., Rothchild S. D., and Dover G. J. (1979). Selective hemolysis of adult red blood cells: an aid to prenatal diagnosis of hemoglobinopathies. *Blood*, **53**, 279–87.

23. Hobbins J. C. and Mahoney M. J. (1974). *In utero* diagnosis of hemoglobinopathies. *New England Journal of Medicine*, **290**, 1065–7.

24. Rodeck C. H. (1980). Fetoscopy guided by real-time ultrasound for pure fetal blood samples, fetal skin samples, and examination of the fetus in utero. *British Journal of Obstetrics and Gynaecology*, **87**, 449–56.

25. Rodeck C. H. and Morsman J. M. (1983). First-trimester chorion biopsy. *British Medical Bulletin*, **39**, 338–42.

26. Weatherall D. J., Clegg J. B., and Naughton M. A. (1965). Globin synthesis in thalassemia: an *in vitro* study. *Nature*, **208**, 1061–5.

27. Cividalli G., Nathan D. G., Kan Y. W., Santamarina B., and Frigoletto F. (1974). Relation of beta to gamma synthesis during the first trimester: an approach to prenatal diagnosis of thalassemia. *Pediatric Research*, **80**, 553–60.

28. Mibashan R. S., Peake I. R., Rodeck C. H., Thumpston J. K., Furlong R. A., Gorser R., Bains L., and Bloom A. L. (1980). Dual diagnosis of prenatal haemophilia A by measurement of fetal factor VIIIC and VIIIC antigen (VIIIC Ag). *Lancet*, **ii**, 994–7.

29. Mibashan R. S., Rodeck C. H., and Thumpston J. K. (1982). Prenatal diagnosis of the hemophilias. In *Methods in hematology: the hemophilias*, (ed. A. L. Bloom), p. 176. Churchill Livingstone, Edinburgh.

30. Luthy D. A., Hall J. G., and Graham C. B. (1979). Prenatal diagnosis of thrombocytopenia with absent radii. *Clinical Genetics*, **15**, 495–9.

31. Holmberg L., Gustavii B., and Jonsson A. (1983). A prenatal study of fetal platelet count and size with application to fetus at risk fow Wiskott-Aldrich syndrome. *Journal of Pediatrics*, **102**, 773–6.

32. Lestas A. N., Rodeck C. H., and White J. M. (1982). Normal activities of glycolytic enzymes in the fetal erythrocytes. *British Journal of Haematology*, **50**, 439–44.

33. Rosa R., Prehu M. O., Calvin M. C., Forester F., Daffos F., Badoual J., Girod R., Alix D., and Galley J. C. (1984). New cases of hereditary triose-phosphate isomerase deficiency (TPI): possibility of prenatal diagnosis. *Blood*, **64**, 35a.

34. Linch D. C., Knott L. J., Rodeck C. H., and Huehna E. R. (1982). Studies of circulating hemopoietic progenitor cells in human fetal blood. *Blood*, **59**, 976–9.

35. Linch D. C., Beverley P. C., Levinsky R. J., and Rodeck C. H. (1982). Phenotypic analysis of fetal blood leukocytes: potential for prenatal diagnosis of immunodeficiency. *Prenatal Diagnosis*, **3**, 211–8.

36. Borregaard N., Bang J., Berthelsen J. G., Johansen K. S., Koch C., Philip J., Rasmussen K., Schwartz M., Therkelsen A. J., and Valerius N. H. (1982). Prenatal diagnosis of chronic granulomatous disease. *Lancet*, **i**, 114.

37. Durandy A., Oury C., Griscelli C., Dumez Y., Oury J. F., and Henrion R. (1982). Prenatal testing for inherited immune deficiencies by fetal blood sampling. *Prenatal Diagnosis*, **2**, 109–13.

38. Levinsky R. J., Linch D. C., and Rodeck C. H. (1982). Prenatal exclusion of severe combined immunodeficiency. *Archives of Disease in Childhood*, **57**, 958–60.

39. Shaham M., Voss R., Becker Y., Yarconi S., Ornoy A. S., and Kohn G. (1982). Prenatal diagnosis of ataxia telangiectasia. *Journal of Pediatrics*, **100**, 134–7.

40. Whitelaw A. G. L., Rogers P. A., Hopkinson F. D. A., Gordon H., Emerson P. M., Darley J. H., Reid C., and Crawfurd Md'A. (1979). Congenital haemolytic anaemia resulting from glucose phosphate isomerase deficiency: genetics, clinical picture, and prenatal diagnosis. *Journal of Medical Genetics*, **16**, 189–96.

41. Junien C., Lerous A., Lostanlen D., Reghis A., Boue J., Nicolas H., Boue A., and Caplan J. C. (1981). Prenatal diagnosis of congenital enzymopenic methaemoglobinaemia with mental retardation due to generalized cytochrome b_5 reductase deficiency: first report of two cases. *Prenatal Diagnosis*, **1**, 17–24.

42. Deybach J. Ch., Grandchamp B., Grelier M., Nordmann Y., Boue J., Boue A., and de Barringer P. (1980). Prenatal exclusion of congenital erythropoietic porphyria (Gunther's disease) in a fetus at risk. *Human Genetics*, **53**, 217–21.

43. Hecht F. and Cadien J. D. (1984). Tay–Sachs disease and other fatal metabolic disorders. In *Antenatal and neonatal screening*, 1st edn, (ed. N. Wald) pp. 129–54. Oxford University Press, Oxford.

44. MRC Working Party on the Evaluation of Chorionic Villus Sampling (1991). Medical Research Council European trial of chorionic villus sampling. *Lancet*, **337**, 1491–9.

45. Lippman A., Tomkins D. J., Shine J., and Hamilton J. L. (1992). Canadian multicentre randomised clinical trial of chorionic villus sampling and amniocentesis: final report. *Prenatal Diagnosis*, **12**, 385–476.

46. Smidt-Jensen S., Permin M., Philip J., Lundsteen C., Zachary M. J., Fowler S. E., *et al.* (1992). Randomised comparison of amniocentesis and transabdominal and transcervical chorionic villus sampling. *Lancet*, **340**, 1237–44.

47. Trent R. J., Davis B., Wilkinson T., and Kronenberg H. (1985). Identification of β variant hemoglobin by DNA restriction endonuclease mapping. *Hemoglobin*, **8**, 443–62.

48. Jeffreys A. J. (1979). DNA sequence variants in the $^G\gamma$-, $^A\gamma$-, γ- and β-globin genes of man. *Cell*, **18**, 1–10.

49. Orkin S. H., Antonarakis S. E., and Kazazian H. H. (1983). Polymorphism and molecular pathology of the human β-globin gene. *Progress in Hematology*, **13**, 49–73.

50. Old J. M., Petrou M., Modell B., and Weatherall D. J. (1984). Feasibility of antenatal diagnosis of β thalassaemia by DNA polymorphisms in Asian Indian and Cypriot populations. *British Journal of Haematology*, **57**, 255–64.

51. Old J. M., Thein S. L., Weatherall D. J., Cao A., and Loukopoulos D. (1989). Prenatal diagnosis of the major haemoglobin disorders. *Molecular Biology and Medicine*, **6**, 55–63.

52. Kan Y. W. and Dozy A. M. (1978). Antenatal diagnosis of sickle-cell anaemia by DNA analysis of amniotic-fluid cells. *Lancet*, **ii**, 910–12.

53. Kan Y. W., Lee K. Y., Furbetta M., Angius A., and Cao A. (1980). Polymorphism of DNA sequences in the beta globin gene region. Application to prenatal diagnosis of β^0 thalassemia in Sardinia. *New England Journal of Medicine*, **302**, 185–8.

54. Wainscoat J. S., Old J. M., Thein S. L., and Weatherall D. J. (1984). A new DNA polymorphism for prenatal diagnosis of β thalassaemia in Mediterranean populations. *Lancet*, **i**, 1299–301.

55. Wallace R. B., Schold M., Johnson M. J., Dembek P., and Itakura K. (1981). Oligonucleotide directed mutagenesis of the human β-globin gene: a general method for producing specific point mutations in cloned DNA. *Nucleic Acids Research*, **9**, 3647–56.

56. Conner B. J., Reyes A. A., Morin C., Itakura K., Teplitz R. L., and Wallace R. B. (1983). Detection of sickle cell β^S-globin allele by hybridization with synthetic oligonucleotides. *Proceedings of the National Academy of Sciences of the United States of America*, **80**, 278–82.

57. Saiki R. K., Gelfand D. H., Stoffel S., Scharf S. J., Higuchi R., Horn G. T., Mullis K. B., and Erlich H. A. (1988). Primer-directed enzymatic amplification of DNA with a thermostable DNA polymerase. *Science*, **239**, 487–91.

58. White T. J., Arnheim N., and Erlich H. A. (1989). The polymerase chain reaction. *Trends in Genetics*, **5**, 185–9.

59. Saiki R. K., Scharf S., Faloona F., Mullis K. B., Horn G. T., Erlich H. A., and Arnheim N. (1985). Enzymatic amplification of β-globin genomic sequences and restriction site analysis for diagnosis of sickle cell anemia. *Science*, **230**, 1350–4.

60. Pirastu M., Kan Y. W., Cao A., Conner B. J., Teplitz R. L., and Wallace R. B. (1983). Prenatal diagnosis of β-thalassemia: detection of a single nucleotide mutation in DNA. *New England Journal of Medicine*, **309**: 284–7.

61. Kogan S. C., Doherty M., and Gitschier J. (1987). An improved method for prenatal diagnosis of genetic diseases by analysis of amplified DNA sequences. *New England Journal of Medicine*, **317**, 985–90.

62. Chehab F., Doherty M., Cai S., Cooper S., and Rubin E. (1987). Detection of sickle cell anaemia and thalassaemia. *Nature*, **329**, 293–4.

63. Newton C. R., Graham A., Heptinstall L. E., Powell S. J., Summers C., Kalsheker N., Smith J. C., and Markham A. F. (1989). Analysis of any point mutation in DNA. The amplification refractory mutation system (ARMS). *Nucleic Acids Research*, **17**, 2503–16.

64. Old J. M., Varawalla N. Y., and Weatherall D. J. (1990). The rapid detection and prenatal

diagnosis of β-thalassaemia in the Asian Indian and Cypriot populations in the UK. *Lancet*, **336**, 834–7.

65. Cai S. P., Chang C. A., Zhang J. Z., Saiki R. K., Erlich H. A., and Kan Y. W. (1989). Rapid prenatal diagnosis of β-thalassemia using DNA amplification and nonradioactive probes. *Blood*, **73**, 372–4.

66. Saiki R. K., Chang C-A., Levenson C. H., Warren T. C., Boehm C. D., Kazazian H. H. Jr, and Erlich H. A. (1988). Diagnosis of sickle cell anemia and β-thalassemia with enzymatically amplified DNA and non-radioactive allele-specific oligonucleotide probes. *New England Journal of Medicine*, **319**, 537–41.

67. Saiki R. K., Walsh P. S., Levenson C. H., and Erlich H. A. (1989). Genetic analysis of amplified DNA with immobilized sequence-specific oligonucleotide probes. *Proceedings of the National Academy of Sciences of the United States of America*, **86**, 6230–4.

68. Handyside A. H., Pattinson J. K., Penketh R. J. A., Delahunty J. D., Winston R. M., and Tuddenham E. G. (1989). Biopsy of human preimplantation embryos and sexing by DNA amplification. *Lancet*, **i**, 347–9.

69. Kuliev, A., Rechitsky S., Verlinsky O., Ivakhnenko V., Evsikov S., Wolf G., Angastiniostis M., Georghiou D., Kukharenko V., Strom C., and Verlinsky Y. (1998). Preimplantation diagnosis of thalassemias. *Journal of Assisted Reproduction and Genetics*, **15**, 219–25.

70. Cheung M-C., Goldberg J. D., and Kan Y. W. (1996). Prenatal diagnosis of sickle cell anemia and thalassemia by analysis of fetal cells in maternal blood. *Nature Genetics*, **14**, 264–8.

71. Kazazian H. H. Jr, Phillips J. A. III, Boehm C. D., Vik T., Mahoney M. J., and Ritchey A. K. (1980). Prenatal diagnosis of β-thalassemia by amniocentesis: linkage analysis of multiple polymorphic restriction endonuclease sites. *Blood*, **56**, 926–30.

72. Cao A. and Rosatelli M. C. (1993). Screening and prenatal diagnosis of the haemoglobinopathies. *Clinical Haematology*, **6**, 263–86.

73. Old J. M., Fitches A., Heath C., Thein S. L., Weatherall D. J., Warren R., McKenzie C., Rodeck C. H., Modell B., Petrou M., and Ward R. H. T (1986). First trimester fetal diagnosis for haemoglobinopathies: report on 200 cases. *Lancet*, **ii**, 763–7.

74. Harper K., Winter R., Pembrey M., Hartley D., Davies K. E., and Tuddenham E. (1984). A clinically useful DNA probe closely linked to haemophilia A. *Lancet*, **ii**, 6–8.

75. Chamberlain J. S., Gibbs R. A., Ranier J. E., Nguyen P. N., and Caskey C. T. (1988). Deletion screening of the Duchenne muscular dystrophy locus via multiplex DNA amplification. *Nucleic Acids Research*, **16**, 1141–56.

76. International Committee for Standardization in Haematology—Expert Panel on Abnormal Haemoglobins (1988). Recommendations for neonatal screening for haemoglobinopathies. *Clinical and Laboratory Haematology*, **10**, 335–45.

77. Gibson B. E. S (1991). Inherited disorders. In *Fetal and neonatal haematology*, (ed. I. M. Hann, B. E. S. Gibson, and E. A. Letsky), pp. 219–75. Bailliere Tindall, London.

78. Weatherall D. J., Higgs D. R., Bunch C., Old J. B., Hunt D. M., Pressley L., Clegg J. B., Bethlenfalvay N. C., Sjolin S., Koler R. D., Magenic E., Francis J. L., and Bebbington D. (1981). Hemoglobin H disease and mental retardation. A new syndrome or a remarkable coincidence? *New England Journal of Medicine*, **305**, 607–12.

79. Bowcock A. M., Tonder S. V., and Jenkins T. (1984). The hemoglobin H disease mental retardation syndrome: molecular studies on the South African case. *British Journal of Haematology*, **56**, 69–78.

80. Wilkie A. O. M., Buckle V. J., Harris P. C., Lamb J., Bartin N. J., Reeders S. T., Lindenbaum R. H., Nicholls R. D., Barrow M., Bethlenfalvay N. C., Hutz M. H., Tolmie J. L., Weatherall D. J., and Higgs D. R. (1990). Clinical features and molecular analysis of the α thalassemia/mental retardation syndromes. I. Cases due to deletions involving chromosome band 16p13.3. *American Journal of Human Genetics*, **46**, 1112–26.

81. Wilkie A. O. M., Zeitlin H. C., Lindenbaum R. H., Buckle V. J., Fischel-Ghodsian N., Chui D. H. K., Gardner-Medwin D., MacGillivray M. H., Weatherall D. J., and Higgs D. R. (1990). Clinical features and molecular analysis of the α thalassemia/mental retardation syndromes. II. Cases without detectable abnormality of the α globin complex. *American Journal of Human Genetics*, **46**, 1127–40.

82. Gibbons R. J., Wilkie A. O. M., Weatherall D. J., and Higgs D. R. (1991). A newly defined X-linked mental retardation syndrome associated with α thalassaemia. *Journal of Medical Genetics*, **28**, 729–33.

83. Gibbons R. J., Picketts D. J., and Higgs D. R. (1995). Syndromal mental retardation due to mutations in a regulator of gene expression. *Human Molecular Genetics*, **4**, 1705–9.

84. Gibbons R. J., Breuton L., Buckle V. I., Burn J., Clayton-Smith J., Davison B. C. C., Gardner R. J. M., Homfray T., Kearney L., Kingston H. M., Newbury-Ecob R., Porteus M. E. P., Wilkie A. O. M., and Higgs D. R. (1995). Clinical and hematologic aspects of the X-linked α thalassemia/ mental retardation syndrome (ATR-X). *American Journal of Medical Genetics*, **55**, 288–99.

12 *Rhesus and other haemolytic diseases*

Elizabeth A. Letsky, Ian Leck, and John M. Bowman

INTRODUCTION

Without screening and appropriate treatment, fetal and neonatal haemolytic disease (generally referred to as haemolytic disease of the newborn or HDN) would be an important cause of perinatal death and brain damage. It occurs when maternal antibodies to fetal blood cell antigens (most notably the D-antigen of the Rh system) enter the fetal circulation. Women who produce these antibodies do so as a result of having been exposed to the antigen concerned, generally as a result of a fetomaternal haemorrhage in a previous pregnancy.

Effective measures are available both for preventing the development of these maternal antibodies and for treating HDN, but to enable these measures to reach those who need them it is necessary to identify (a) pregnancies at risk of HDN and (b) Rh D negative women who should receive anti-D immunoglobulin prophylaxis.

For these reasons, and to enable compatible blood to be supplied rapidly in obstetric emergencies, screening for blood group and antibodies in pregnant and newly delivered women and in neonates is required.

THE DISORDER

The Rh blood group system

In 1940, after production of a Rhesus monkey red cell antiserum in guinea pigs and rabbits, Landsteiner and Wiener[1] showed that 85 per cent of a New York City Caucasian population had the monkey red cell antigen (i.e. they were Rhesus or Rh-positive) and 15 per cent did not (i.e. they were Rhesus or Rh-negative). When Levine and co-workers[2] in the following year determined that a patient who had had multiple stillbirths was Rh-negative with a powerful antibody directed against her Rh-positive husband's red cells, the aetiology and pathogenesis of Rh haemolytic disease were elucidated.

Our knowledge of the Rh blood group system has advanced since Landsteiner and Wiener's original monkey experiments.[3] Until recently the system was widely supposed to involve six genetically inherited antigens, grouped in three pairs (Cc, Dd, Ee) and controlled by genes at three loci in very close proximity—a hypothesis introduced by

Fisher and Race. It has now been established that there is no d-antigen,[4] and the Rh system appears to be controlled by only two homologous structural genes. These genes are located on chromosome 1p34–p36. One encodes the D-antigen polypeptide and is missing in Rh(D)-negative individuals; the other encodes the Cc and Ee polypeptides, probably by alternate splicing of a primary transcript. These polypeptides have been cloned. The predicted translation of the Rh(D)mRNA is a 417 amino-acid product of molecular weight 45 000. The D and Cc/Ee polypeptides differ by 36 amino acid substitutions (8.4 per cent divergence).[5] The sequences of the two genes are 96 per cent identical, suggesting that they arose through duplication of a single ancestral gene.[6]

The D-antigen polypeptide is by far the most potent one in the Rh blood group system. Rh-negative individuals lack the Rh(D) gene and polypeptide, and Rh-positive people are either homozygous or heterozygous producers of this polypeptide (i.e. DD or Dd). All the fetuses of Rh-negative mothers and homozygous Rh-positive fathers are therefore heterozygous Rh-positive, as are half the fetuses of Rh-negative mothers and heterozygous Rh-positive fathers. Only an Rh-positive fetus can stimulate an Rh-negative mother to produce anti-D, and only Rh-positive fetuses will be affected by the anti-D produced.

Rh D immunization

Rh-negative women develop Rh D antibodies when exposed to Rh D-antigen. Although in the past such exposure was often due to an Rh incompatible blood transfusion, at present almost all such exposures are due to the transplacental passage of Rh-positive fetal red cells into the mother during a previous pregnancy and labour. Small numbers of fetal red cells cross the placenta into the maternal circulation

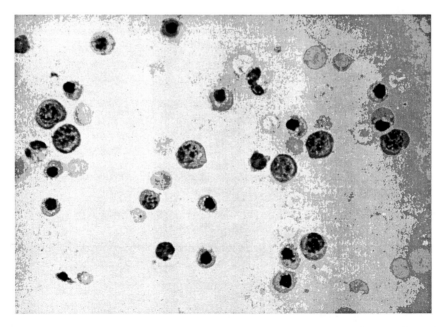

Fig. 12.1 Cord blood smear from infant with severe erythroblastosis; nucleated cells are in the erythroid series from normoblasts to early erythroblasts.

during normal healthy pregnancy. This may occur as early as 8–10 weeks of gestation, and the risk of it happening and the volume of cells involved increase as pregnancy advances, peaking with separation of the placenta at the end of labour. About 3/1000 women receive more than 15 ml of fetal red cells.[4]

Once the Rh-negative woman who has developed anti-D IgG antibody is pregnant, the antibody will cross the placenta into the fetal circulation. If the fetus is Rh-positive, the antibody will bind to the Rh-antigen in the red cell membrane (the only site where Rh-antigen is found) coating the red cell membrane and causing extravascular red cell destruction, primarily in the spleen. In about half of affected fetuses, the effects are not clinically significant, and no treatment is needed. In the remainder, anaemia with compensated erythropoiesis, both medullary and extramedullary, occurs. Hepatosplenomegaly develops and there is an outpouring of nucleated immature red cells (erythroblasts) (Fig. 12.1) into the fetal circulation. Universal oedema including pleural effusions, ascites, and anasarca (hydrops fetalis) develops before birth (primarily as a result of cardiac failure) in the most severe cases, and severe jaundice (icterus gravis) appears after birth in the remainder.

In hydrops fetalis, hepatosplenomegaly is extreme and the fetus usually dies *in utero*. Those born alive are waterlogged. Ventilation is frequently impossible because of pleural effusions and pulmonary hypoplasia. However, with modern tertiary level care, a significant number (at least 30 per cent) of liveborn hydropic infants can be salvaged.

In icterus gravis, the jaundice develops rapidly after birth, almost always within the first 24 hours of life. In these babies, if jaundice is looked for carefully, it is usually identifiable at birth or shortly after. Within the first two to four days jaundice becomes progressively more severe and is liable to culminate in death or severe sequelae (deafness, spasticity, and choreoathetosis) from brain damage (kernicterus) if appropriate treatment is not carried out.

The severity of Rh haemolytic disease tends to increase with successive pregnancies, although the increase is not fully predictable. If left untreated, 8–10 per cent of first pregnancies after Rh-immunization will end in stillbirth before term. On rare occasions, the pattern may reverse and a woman who has had a hydropic stillbirth will have a less severely affected fetus in her next pregnancy. Nevertheless, once hydrops has occurred, the risk of it recurring is at least 90 per cent, and the tendency is for hydrops to develop earlier in succeeding pregnancies.

The mother of an affected fetus usually has no symptoms. In the presence of severe Rh disease (hydrops or prehydrops), some women develop a pre-eclampsia-like syndrome, with excessive weight gain, oedema, and some albuminuria. After either delivery or successful treatment of the fetus *in utero*, these signs disappear. Once hydrops has developed, polyhydramnios is common, probably due to the inability of the oedematous fetus to swallow amniotic fluid. Although fetal movements may diminish as hydrops develops with impending fetal death, this is frequently not so. The mother may not notice any diminution until fetal death occurs.

Immunization by other blood group antigens

Sometimes maternal antibodies are produced in response to other fetal blood group antigens. Among these antibodies, anti-E, anti-c, anti-K, anti-A, and anti-B are of interest because of their frequency or serious effects.

Anti-E

Anti-E is one of the most frequent antibodies found in routine antenatal serology. The E-antigen is part of the Rh blood group system and develops most frequently in those Rh D positive women with the Rh genotype CDe/CDe (R_1R_1). This antibody can be naturally occurring or develop following pregnancy or transfusion. It never causes severe anaemia in the fetus and only rarely is associated with jaundice in the neonate, unless in combination with anti-c when severe anaemia *in utero* requiring transfusion has been reported.

Anti-c

This antibody, like anti-E, occurs most commonly in Rh D positive women with the genotype CDe/CDe (R_1R_1), but unlike anti-E, anti-c can cause very severe HDN,[4] and some pregnancies associated with this antibody may end in hydrops unless intrauterine transfusions are given. The pathogenesis of disease and management of women with this antibody are the same as for women with anti-D.

Anti-K

The Kell blood group system is associated with the development of IgG antibodies which occasionally cause severe allo-immune anaemia and hydrops *in utero* and may therefore require antenatal intervention. The system consists of at least 20 antigens, but only Kell (K_1) and occasionally Cellano (K_2), $Kp^a(K_3)$ and $Kp^b(K_4)$ are associated with HDN.[4] K_1 is by far the most important from a clinical point of view since the corresponding antibody is involved in transfusion reactions and in allo-immune disease of the fetus and newborn more frequently than any other antibody outside the Rh system. Ninety-one per cent of the British population are K_1 negative (kk) and 9.0 per cent are K positive, mostly heterozygous K/k. About 1 in 500 are KK homozygous. The antibody anti-K is usually detected in patients who have had transfusions from multiple donors, either as a single event to cover a traumatic incident or as recurrent supportive therapy over a long period of time.

When anti-K is found in antenatal sera the majority of women give a history of having had a blood transfusion. The partner's blood should be tested and will be found to be K negative in the vast majority of cases. Occasionally the partner is K positive but if so he is likely to be heterozygous for K-antigen.

Anti-K is the second most frequent antibody mediating severe fetal anaemia in most reported series.[7,8]

Kell allo-immune disease can be very severe and lead rapidly to intrauterine death. It is difficult to assess by indirect measures such as maternal antibody and amniotic fluid bilirubin. Recent clinical studies have confirmed anecdotal reports suggesting that the antibody results predominantly in erythroid suppression or ineffective erythropoiesis rather than haemolysis.[9,10] This has also been confirmed by recent *in vitro* studies demonstrating the suppressive effect of anti-K on erythroid progenitor cell growth.[11]

Anti-A and anti-B

During the first year of life, all group O individuals produce anti-A and anti-B; group A individuals, anti-B; and group B individuals, anti-A. In about one-third of ABO-incompatible pregnancies, the group O mother produces immune IgG anti-A or anti-B which is capable of crossing the placenta to the group A or B fetus. As a result, the direct antiglobulin (Coombs') test for antibody on cord red cells is weakly positive in 25–30 per cent of all infants from ABO-incompatible pregnancies.[4,12]

Even among antibody-exposed group A or B infants, only about 1 per cent develop severe ABO HDN; and its clinical features, significant haemolysis and hyperbilirubinaemia, only appear after birth, unlike some manifestations of Rh HDN.

There are several factors which explain why significant ABO HDN is relatively uncommon. A- and B-like substances are widespread in vegetable and animal life. The agglutinins, anti-A and anti-B, are often called naturally occurring antibodies, which is strictly a misnomer because they develop during the first few months of life, probably as a result of exposure to A- and B-like substances elaborated by gram-negative bacteria which colonize the gut. Naturally occurring anti-A and anti-B are usually IgM immunoglobulins which will not cross the placenta. The maternal antibody can only cause HDN if it is of the IgG type.

Cases of ABO HDN have only been reported in infants of group O mothers. This is because group O individuals make more avid antibody and are more likely to produce immune IgG antibody.

As well as developing IgG anti-A or anti-B as a result of an ABO-incompatible pregnancy, group O individuals who have been vaccinated or immunized with preparations derived from hog stomach or pneumococcal vaccine which contain an A substance may develop immune lytic IgG anti-A antibody which can persist for some years. (Hog pepsin is used in the preparation of TAB and diphtheria toxoid.) But even if the group O mother has a high titre of lytic IgG anti-A or anti-B antibody, it is unlikely to cause problems for the ABO incompatible fetus *in utero* because the A- and B-antigens, unlike Rh-antigens, are present not only on the fetal red cells but on cells of all other tissue and in body fluids. Neutralization of maternal antibody by soluble fetal antigens and by antigens carried on cells other than the red cells will help to protect the incompatible fetal red cells.

Another factor which may help to protect the fetal red cells is that the A- and B-antigens, although detectable in the five-week embryo, are present in smaller amounts on fetal red cells than on adult red cells and therefore do not react as strongly with antibody which crosses the placenta.[4] Unlike Rh disease, 40–50 per cent of cases occur in firstborn infants and the disease does not become more severe with each subsequent pregnancy.

Prevalence

Rh-negativity

In most Caucasian populations, the prevalence of Rh-negativity is approximately 16 per cent, in which case the expected proportion of Rh-incompatible pregnancies is 9.6 per cent (see Table 12.1). The prevalence of Rh-negativity is lower in Chinese and Japanese (0.1 per cent), in American Indians (1–2 per cent), and in American Blacks (7 per cent). The Basques of southern France and northern Spain have a prevalence of Rh-negativity of about 35 per cent, more than twice that of their Caucasian neighbours.

It is probable that the presence of Rh-negativity in races other than Caucasian is

Table 12.1 Frequency of Rh-incompatibility and related variables when the population prevalence of Rh-negativity is 16 per cent

Variable	Formula for frequency (where D = frequency of gene for the D-antigen)	Frequency
RhD-negative people	$(1 - D)^2$	16% (given)
Chromosomes without gene for D	$1 - D$	$\sqrt{0.16} = 40\%$
Chromosomes with gene for D	D	$1 - 0.4 = 60\%$
Homozygous Rh-positive people	D^2	$0.6^2 = 36\%$
Heterozygous Rh-positive people	$2D(1 - D)$	$2 \times 0.6 \times 0.4 = 48\%$
Rh-incompatible pregnancies (i.e. fetus Rh-positive, mother Rh-negative):		
Father homozygous Rh-positive	$D^2 (1 - D)^2$	$0.36 \times 0.16 = 5.76\%$
Father heterozygous Rh-positive	$2D(1 - D)(1 - D)^2/2*$	$(0.48 \times 0.16)/2 = 3.84\%$
		Total with Rh-positive father = 9.6%

* To obtain the frequency of Rh-positive fetuses with Rh-negative mothers and heterozygous Rh-positive fathers, the product of the frequencies of parents of these kinds is halved because only half the offspring of these parents are

Table 12.2 Approximate risk of Rh isoimmunization associated with pregnancy in D-negative women (modified from Bowman[13])

Rh isoimmunization	Risk (%)
1. Father D-negative, baby D-negative	0
2. Father D-positive homozygous and ABO-compatible with mother	16
3. Father D-positive homozygous and ABO-incompatible with mother, ABO of baby unknown	6
4. Baby D-positive and ABO-incompatible with mother	1.5
5. Father D-positive heterozygous and ABO-compatible with mother	8
6. Father D-positive heterozygous and ABO-incompatible with mother, ABO and Rh of baby unknown	3

due to the intermingling of Caucasian genes; the higher the prevalence the greater the degree and the longer the period of time that such intermingling has occurred.

Rh D immunization

In the absence of prophylaxis, the risk of Rh-immunization varies with the amount of Rh-antigen to which the Rh-negative mother has been exposed (i.e. the size of the fetal transplacental haemorrhage), and the ABO status of the mother and her fetus (Table 12.2). The overall risk of Rh-immunization for an Rh-negative mother carrying an ABO-compatible Rh-positive fetus is about 16 per cent:[14] 2.0 per cent during her pregnancy[15] and 14 per cent later. Anti-D appears within six months after delivery in half of the latter 14 per cent, whereas in the other half the fact that immunization has occurred does not become apparent until a subsequent Rh-positive pregnancy,[16] when the woman mounts a secondary immune response in the latter half of the second or early in the third trimester of pregnancy. Among the 2 per cent who become antibody-positive during the pregnancy in which they are exposed to the D-antigen, 7 per cent (i.e. 0.14 per cent of those exposed) develop anti-D at or before 28 weeks of gestation, and 93 per cent (1.86 per cent of those exposed) do so later in pregnancy.

Only the first of these two groups are likely to produce enough antibody to cause clinically significant haemolytic disease during the current pregnancy.

ABO incompatibility confers partial protection against primary Rh-immunization. The risk when the Rh-positive baby is ABO incompatible with his mother is reduced from about 16 per cent to about 1.5 per cent.[14] However, if maternal Rh-immunization does occur in the presence of fetal-maternal ABO incompatibility, this incompatibility has no ameliorating effect whatever upon the secondary immune response, or upon the severity of fetal haemolytic disease.

The risk for all Rh-negative women carrying Rh-positive fetuses therefore varies with the frequency of ABO incompatibility, which in turn depends on the A, B, and O gene frequencies. Where these are 0.25, 0.10, and 0.65 respectively (the approximate figures for people of white English origin), it can be estimated by methods similar to those used in Table 12.1 that mother–child ABO incompatibility will occur in 22 per cent of pregnancies. The overall risk of D-immunization for the Rhesus-negative mother carrying a Rhesus-positive fetus is therefore about 13 per cent (i.e. (22 × 0.015) + (78 × 0.16)) if there is no prophylaxis.

The proportions of all Rh-incompatible pregnancies in previously non-immune women that will give rise to D-immunization during different periods can therefore be estimated by multiplying the proportions given above for ABO-compatible pregnancies by 13/16 (since the risk of immunization in ABO-compatible pregnancies is 16 per cent). The resulting estimates are that antibody develops:

(1) during the first 28 weeks of the current pregnancy in 0.1 per cent of cases (i.e. 0.14 per cent × 13/16);

(2) between 28 weeks and delivery in 1.5 per cent (i.e. 1.86 × 13/16);

(3) after delivery in 11.4 per cent (i.e. 14 per cent × 13/16).

Rhesus haemolytic disease of the newborn

The effects of maternal Rh D-immunity on the Rh-positive fetus vary from no apparent abnormality at term to fetal death at 18–20 weeks of gestation (Table 12.3). The fetuses with no apparent abnormality at birth account for 45–50 per cent of all those exposed. Although they develop minimal to moderate hyperbilirubinaemia, they remain healthy without treatment. A further 25–30 per cent, although clinically well at birth, have some degree of hepatosplenomegaly and anaemia and rapidly develop icterus gravis, culminating in the brain damage due to kernicterus if treatment is not

Table 12.3 Classification of severity of erythroblastosis (from Bowman and Pollock[17])

Degree of severity	Features	Percentage of all cases
1. Mild	No treatment needed. Indirect bilirubin does not exceed 16–20 mg per 100 ml. No anaemia.	45–50
2. Moderate	Fetal hydrops will not develop. Anaemia moderate. Severe jaundice and risk of kernicterus unless treated after birth.	25–30
3. Severe	Fetal hydrops will develop *in utero*	20–25
	Before 33 weeks of gestation	8–10
	After 33 weeks of gestation	12–15

given. The remaining 20–25 per cent develop hydrops fetalis, half before 34 weeks of gestation and half between 34 weeks and term.

The proportion of all untreated Rh D-incompatible pregnancies in which the fetus would be affected by clinically significant haemolytic disease (as described above) increases with the number of these pregnancies that the mother has had. Among women in their third incompatible pregnancies, for example, more will have affected fetuses than did in their second pregnancies, for two reasons:

1. More will be antibody-positive, since those who have developed antibodies as a result of but following their second pregnancies, and those who develop them as a result of and during their third, will be added to those who were antibody-positive during their second pregnancies.

2. The antibody levels of women who were already antibody-positive during their second pregnancies will have been increased by further exposure to Rh-antigen at the end of their second pregnancies and during their third.

Estimates of the proportions of mothers with Rh-antibody at the end of successive Rh-incompatible pregnancies, and of the incidence of clinically significant Rh haemolytic disease in their fetuses, are given in Table 12.4. The proportions of antibody-positive mothers were estimated on the basis that every Rh-incompatible pregnancy carries a 13 per cent risk of inducing immunity in the mother (p. 288) and that one-eighth of these inductions occurs during, as opposed to after, the pregnancy by which it is caused (p. 287). In estimating the incidence of clinical disease, it was assumed that this would occur in all the Rh-positive fetuses of immunized women who had produced a clinically affected fetus in a previous pregnancy and in 45 per cent of the Rh-positive fetuses of other women who were anti-D positive at 28 weeks of gestation, which is consistent with the observation that 50–55 per cent of all immunized women's Rh-positive offspring are clinically affected (p. 288). The methods of calculation used are given in detail in Appendix 2 (pp. 313–316). The resulting estimates of the incidence of clinically significant Rh haemolytic disease in the absence of screening and prophylaxis rise from 0.05 per cent in the first Rh-incompatible pregnancy to 32 per cent in the fifth (see Table 12.4).

Table 12.4 Prevalence of maternal anti-D and of Rh haemolytic disease at the end of successive Rh-incompatible pregnancies, in the absence of prophylaxis. (See text and Appendix 2 for assumptions made and methods used.)

Number of Rh-incompatible pregnancies	Prevalence at end of specified pregnancy	
	Anti-D in mother	Clinically significant Rh haemolytic disease
1	1.6%	0.05%
2	14.4%	5.9%
3	25.5%	14.3%
4	35.2%	23.2%
5	43.6%	32.1%

Table 12.5 Antenatally detected maternal antibodies and outcome. Queen Charlotte's deliveries 1980–90 (4500–5000 deliveries per year)

	Anti-D	Anti-K	Anti-c	Anti-E+c	Anti-E	Other
No. of pregnancies	238	37	14	6	34	15
Amniocentesis	170	9	2	2	0	1
Intrauterine transfusion	86	12	0	1	0	0
Exchange transfusion	64	1	1	0	0	0
Intrauterine death	18	1	0	0	0	0
Neonatal death	4	1	1	0	0	0

Immunization by other blood group antigens

The frequency of maternal IgG antibodies detected antenatally by the indirect antiglobulin (Coombs') test is shown in Table 12.5, which covers 10 years of experience at Queen Charlotte's Hospital. Apart from anti-D, anti-c and anti-K either alone or in combination with other antibodies were the only antibodies shown which caused anaemia *in utero* of enough severity to lead to death and/or antenatal intervention. The relative prevalence of these antibodies in antenatal practice has been confirmed in other studies and reviewed recently.[7,8]

Maternal anti-A and anti-B are not listed in Table 12.5, since they are not screened for antenatally. The haemolysis they cause develops after birth, cannot be predicted by screening, and is rarely significant. Although it occurs in approximately 2 per cent of all births in Great Britain and the USA, it is only identified in 1 in 150 births, and only 1 in 3000 births is severely affected. Less than 5 per cent of affected newborns need phototherapy, and in only the very rare case is exchange transfusion required.

CONTROL MEASURES

Prevention

Following experimental work and clinical trials carried out in England[18] and North America,[19,20] it was shown that administration of Rh-antibody in the form of Rh-immune globulin (Rh IgG, Anti-D IgG) to the Rh-negative unimmunized woman carrying an Rh-positive fetus was very successful in preventing Rh-allo-immunization from developing. It would appear that prevention of Rh-immunization is always possible, provided that the anti-D IgG is given in sufficient dose and provided that it is given before Rh-immunization has begun.

The currently recommended dose for Rh-prophylaxis after delivery is 100 µg to 300 µg (500–1500 iu) of a standard intramuscular preparation or, where available, 120 µg of an ion-exchange prepared anti-D IgG given intravenously.[21–23] A dose of 300 µg of anti-D can be relied upon to protect against Rh-immunization up to a transplacental haemorrhage of about 15 ml of D-positive fetal red cells. In those rare instances of fetal transplacental haemorrhage of greater amount, which occur in about 0.3 per cent of Rh D-incompatible pregnancies,[4] there will be a 25–30 per cent failure rate if only one standard prophylactic dose is given. Full protection is possible in such a situation if the size of the transplacental haemorrhage is determined and larger doses of anti-D are given.

Although initially it was believed that Rh-immunization rarely developed before delivery, studies in Canada,[15,24] Sweden,[24] the UK[25] and elsewhere have shown that 1.5–2.0 per cent of unimmunized Rh-negative women bearing an Rh-positive child will be Rh-immunized during pregnancy, i.e. too early for post-delivery Rh prophylaxis to be effective. The failure rate of Rh prevention by post partum administration of Rh immune globulin is therefore $((1.5–2)/13) \times 100 = 12–15$) per cent, since the overall risk that an unimmunized Rh-negative women will be immunized if she bears a Rhesus-positive child is 13 per cent (p. 288). To prevent immunization developing before delivery, antenatal Rh-prophylaxis with anti-D IgG has been recommended and is standard practice in some centres,[22,23,26,27] Antenatal anti-D IgG is effective when given in one dose of 200 µg (1000 iu) at 28–30 weeks, or in two doses of 100 µg (500 iu), one at 28 weeks and one at 34.[27,28] Although prophylactic anti-D IgG can cross the placenta, this does not cause significant fetal haemolysis, because the amount of IgG reaching the fetus is very small in relation to the amount of D-antigen on the fetal red cells.

With Rh-prophylaxis for all Rh-negative women at 28 weeks of gestation (and earlier in cases of abortion and amniocentesis) and postnatally, and with the dose of anti-Rh IgG increased if tests show that there has been more transplacental haemorrhage than can be neutralized by the standard dose, it is possible to reduce the incidence of Rh-allo-immunization to less than 0.1 per cent of Rh-incompatible pregnancies.[15,25]

Comparable measures for preventing fetal disease due to other blood group incompatibilities have not been developed. Because anti-c and anti-K are capable of causing such severe disease *in utero*, there is a move afoot to provide K-negative and c-negative CDe/CDe (R^1R^1) typed blood for transfusion in all women in the reproductive years. This might be achieved by typing in the hospital blood bank or provision of appropriately typed units from the regional blood transfusion centre, but there are doubts about the logistical practicability of doing so.

Treatment

The treatment of haemolytic disease of the newborn depends more on its severity than on the blood group incompatibility to which it is due. The following methods of treating Rh D haemolytic disease are therefore also broadly applicable to cases of clinical disease due to other incompatibilities.

Exchange transfusion

Exchange transfusion[29,30] is the cornerstone of treatment of Rh-haemolytic disease. Replacement of coated haemolysing Rh-positive red cells with compatible Rh-negative red cells corrects anaemia, stops haemolysis, reduces bilirubin production, and, to a lesser extent, reduces already elevated bilirubin levels. Exchange transfusions performed promptly before brain damage has occurred will prevent kernicterus. By raising haemoglobin levels, exchange transfusion suppresses erythropoietin production and erythropoiesis. Provided the baby survives, the liver and spleen shrink in size, hydrops, if present, reverses, and death from severe anaemia is also prevented.

With the use of exchange transfusion, no infant with Rh-haemolytic disease, born alive and not hydropic, should die or be damaged by the disease.

Ancillary measures after birth

Measures such as phototherapy,[31] which bypasses the infant's immature bilirubin conjugation mechanism causing alteration of the bilirubin molecule to water-soluble bilirubin isomers, and phenobarbital,[32] which by enzyme induction hastens the maturation of the bilirubin conjugation system in the infant, are valuable adjuncts in reducing the degree of hyperbilirubinaemia. They reduce the need for multiple exchange transfusions once the haemoglobin of the infant has been raised, and in some instances of moderate haemolytic disease with only mild associated anaemia may remove the need for exchange transfusion altogether.

Early delivery

Although exchange transfusions completely altered the outlook for the affected baby born in relatively good condition, they may do little for the hydropic liveborn infant and can do nothing for the fetus that dies *in utero*. About 50 per cent of hydropic infants will become hydropic after 34 weeks of gestation and another 15–20 per cent between 30 and 34 weeks. Early delivery with subsequent exchange transfusions and ancillary intensive neonatal care measures will salvage a significant number of these fetuses who would otherwise die of their haemolytic disease. The risks of mortality and morbidity increase the earlier in gestation such babies are delivered. Ultimately one reaches a gestation where such risks outweigh any benefits one could hope to achieve. For this reason planned early delivery has rarely been undertaken prior to 32 weeks of gestation; and, in the authors' experience, the introduction of intrauterine transfusion make it generally inappropriate before 33.5 to 34 weeks of gestation. Although severe Rh-haemolytic disease added to prematurity increases mortality at every gestation, the outlook in the absence of hydrops is good: 95 per cent survival at 34 weeks of gestation, at least 80 to 90 per cent survival at 32 weeks. Occasional severely affected babies born spontaneously at 27–29 weeks of gestation have survived but the risks of death and damage are high.

In so far as they can be identified, only those fetuses who are likely to become hydropic and die within 7–14 days should be delivered prematurely; and the degree of prematurity should not be so great that there is less than a 90 per cent chance of survival.

Intrauterine fetal transfusions

Intrauterine transfusion by the intraperitoneal route, introduced by Sir William Liley in 1963,[33] revolutionized the outlook for the survival of fetuses with Rh-haemolytic disease otherwise doomed to become hydropic and die before 34 weeks of gestation. The procedure may be carried out successfully as early as 21 to 22 weeks of gestation. Four transfusions will maintain a fetus in good condition from 22 weeks to 34 weeks of gestation.

Intraperitoneal transfusion is, however, fraught with considerable risk if the placenta is anterior and must be traversed (7 per cent of procedures in one series).[34] Also, since absorption of red cells from the peritoneal cavity requires diaphragmatic movement (fetal breathing), intraperitoneal transfusion is of no value when an hydropic fetus is moribund and not breathing.[35] The survival rate of transfused fetuses, including cases of hydrops, was 76 per cent in one series.[34]

Since the late 1980s, it has been possible to carry out a fetal cord vessel puncture, obtain a fetal blood sample,[36] and then carry out a direct fetal intravascular transfusion if necessary. This has been a further major advance in management.[37-39] With direct intravascular transfusion, the moribund, hydropic, non-breathing fetus can be salvaged.[34,40] Survival rates, including cases with hydrops, are of the order of 85 to 90 per cent.[34,41]

Ancillary measures before birth

During or before the 1970s, the possibility of suppressing maternal immunity by various materials (Rh-hapten, corticosteroids, promethazine, and red cell stroma) was explored,[42-46] as was plasma exchange (replacement of large volumes of the mother's anti-D-containing plasma with Rh-negative normal plasma);[47-49] but these procedures were shown to be of limited or no value and in some cases to carry risks, and none has been generally adopted.

More recently, intravenous immune serum globulin (IGIV) has been used to ameliorate Rh-haemolytic disease, with partially but not totally encouraging results.[50-52] A maternally administered weekly dose of one gram per kg body weight is recommended. The procedure is of no value when a fetus is hydropic, and has not been generally adopted.[41]

SCREENING

A blood sample is obtained from every pregnant women at her first antenatal visit, preferably in the first trimester, for blood grouping and antibody screening; this procedure should be repeated between 28 and 36 weeks of gestation.[53] Testing is indicated no matter what previous grouping and screening tests have shown. An Rh-negative woman may have been incorrectly typed in the past, although mistyping is very rare—the precise frequency has not been reported. An Rh-positive woman will occasionally have developed 'atypical' blood-group antibodies (e.g. anti-c, anti-Kell) since a previous test, as a result of a former pregnancy or a blood transfusion.

Blood grouping

Blood grouping is carried out using appropriate specific anti-sera by the standard techniques followed in the laboratory to which the sample is sent.

When a pregnant woman has been determined to be Rh-negative, the Rh status of the father of her fetus should also be determined if possible. In the UK, this is not normally done unless the woman is Rh-negative with anti-D antibodies. If a father is Caucasian, there are about five chances in six that he will be Rh-positive. If he is, the case must be managed on the assumption that the fetus may also be Rh-positive. If, however, he is Rh-negative, the fetus will not be affected since it too will be Rh-negative. In this situation, if the mother has no Rh-antibodies, she is not at risk of Rh-immunization and not a candidate for Rh-prophylaxis. If she is already Rh-immunized, she is not a candidate for repeated antibody titrations, amniocentesis, early delivery, or intrauterine transfusion, if Rh-negative paternity is assured.

Blood group antibody screening

The blood group antibody screening tests carried out by the laboratory must be sensitive enough to detect very weak antibodies. This is of particular importance now that Rh haemolytic disease prevention is possible. Insensitive screening tests that fail to detect early Rh-immunization are responsible for a significant number of the reported failures of Rh-prophylaxis, the woman already being immunized at the time of injection of Rh IgG. A description of Rh-antibody screening tests is given in Appendix 1. These tests can be adapted for testing serum for antibodies to other blood group antigens, by using red cells with the relevant antigen instead of Rh D-positive cells.

The indirect antiglobulin test (Appendix 1) is the screening test recommended in UK hospital transfusion laboratories.[53] If an antibody is found, the serum is sent to the regional blood transfusion centre for confirmation and quantitation. The regional centres all use automated enzyme techniques for quantitation of the confirmed antibody.

Routine grouping and serological evaluation of antenatal sera will detect some women who have lytic IgG anti-A and/or anti-B in their plasma. These findings are not predictably associated with clinical disease, and it is therefore not relevant or cost-effective to report these antibodies or to evaluate infants born to mothers who have developed them.

All pregnant women (Rh D-positive and -negative) in whom no red cell allo-antibodies are detected at booking should be retested at 28–32 weeks of gestation. When no antibodies are found at 28–32 weeks, no further testing is required. Subse-

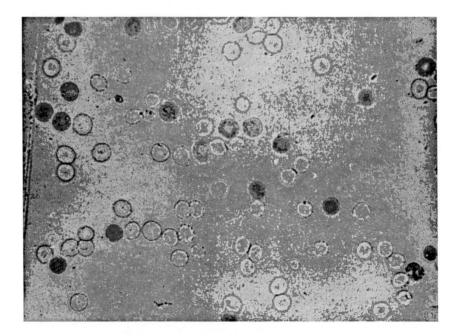

Fig. 12.2 Acid elution technique of Kleihauer.[54] Fetal red cells stain with eosin (appear dark), adult red cells do not stain (appear as ghosts). This maternal blood smear contained 11.2% fetal red cells, representing a transplacental haemorrhage of about 450 ml of blood.

quent detectable immunization is unlikely to result during the current pregnancy in antibody levels high enough to cause clinically significant disease.

Tests for fetomaternal transfusion

If antenatal prophylaxis with anti-D immunoglobulin is to be given to Rh-negative non-immunized women, it is recommended that the dose should be based on an estimate of how much feto-maternal haemorrhage has occurred. In the United States, this is commonly estimated by tests that specifically identify Rh-positive red cells in the mother's blood, but in Britain and Canada the Kleihauer test (which detects red cells containing fetal haemoglobin)[54] has generally been used. In the latter test, a blood film fixed in alcohol is suspended in an acid phosphate buffer (pH 3.2–3.3). At this pH, adult haemoglobin leaks through the red cell membrane (which remains intact) but fetal haemoglobin does not. After staining with eosin, adult red cells appear as unstained ghosts; fetal red cells retain their pink-staining characteristics (Fig. 12.2). This enables the extent of any feto-maternal haemorrhage to be estimated.

Although the Kleihauer test appears simple, experience, skill, and attention to detail as prescribed in published recommendations (for example those of the British blood transfusion service,[55] which regrettably are often ignored[56]) are essential if the test is to be carried out properly.

Increasingly, flow cytometry is being used in hospital blood banks and regional transfusion centres in place of the Kleihauer test. Flow cytometry identifies fetal cells in maternal blood samples with greater accuracy, and with increased efficiency in terms of labour.

Even if antenatal prophylaxis is not routine, fetal cell tests should be carried out on Rh-negative non-immunized pregnant women who have undergone procedures such as amniocentesis or external version. Whether or not fetal cells are found, Rh prophylaxis is indicated, but a higher than routine dose of IgG should be given if the number of fetal cells observed indicates a large bleed into the maternal circulation.

DIAGNOSIS AND ASSESSMENT

Antenatal assessment

Measurement of maternal antibody

Once a woman is found to have anti-D, anti-c, or anti-K antibody, the risk to her fetus is initially assessed by measuring the titre of the relevant IgG antibody. The IgG may be titrated using one or both of two methods: albumin titration and indirect antiglobulin titration. These methods (as used to titrate anti-D) are described in Appendix 1. The indirect antiglobulin method is, as a general rule, more sensitive than the albumin method. In JMB's laboratory, titres of 16 with the albumin method or of 32 with the indirect antiglobulin method are regarded as critical, except for anti-K which may cause severe HDN at lower titre. In the absence of a history of a previously affected fetus, a titre at or above the critical level suggests that there is a significant risk of fetal demise. If confirmed by retesting, it is therefore an indication for supplementary testing, or for prompt delivery if the fetus is mature. If the anti-D IgG titre with the albumin method is $\geqslant 16$ throughout pregnancy, the odds on the fetus needing treatment (or becoming hydropic) are probably between 3:1 and 9:1.

Although the indirect antiglobulin method is more costly in time and anti-sera than the albumin method, some workers prefer the indirect antiglobulin method because they believe it gives readings more closely related to the risk of HDN. Others consider that antibodies to Rh-antigens can be titrated just as well by the albumin method, although they too recommend using the indirect antiglobulin method when titrating antibodies to Kell or Duffy antigens.

Although not readily available, sophisticated radioimmune[57] and AutoAnalyzer methods[58] have been developed which enable anti-D to be directly measured in either anti-D international units (iu) or micrograms of anti-D per ml of maternal serum (5 iu = 1 μg of anti-D). These methods are more accurate than titration for predicting fetal risk. As a general rule, the risk of HDN is low at quantitative anti-D levels below 4 iu/ml (0.8 μg/ml), and moderate at 4–15 iu/ml (0.8–3.0 μg/ml). Above 15 iu/ml (3 μg/ml), the risk of hydrops fetalis is high.[53]

As with antibody screening of non-immunized Rh-negative women, antibody levels in women with anti-D, anti-c, or anti-K should be measured repeatedly during pregnancy, firstly so that if any supplementary testing becomes necessary this need can be recognized, and secondly to enable the timing of any such test to be delayed until as late in pregnancy as possible without jeopardizing the fetus. The first measurement should take place as soon as the mother is found to be immunized (preferably in the first trimester). Testing should be repeated at least monthly until 28 weeks of gestation and every two weeks thereafter.

Weekly measurement of antibody is indicated if an attempt is to be made to reduce the antibody levels and therefore degree of severity of haemolytic disease by the use of plasma exchange or intravenous immune serum globulin. The weekly antibody measurements should start just before treatment is initiated (preferably at 12–16 weeks of gestation).

None of the methods of measuring antibody that are described above can predict fetal risk with great accuracy, since all examine serum from the mother and not from the fetus. Whatever the mother's antibody titre, the fetus is not at risk if it does not have the relevant antigen. This is quite often the case. For example, if 16 per cent of a population is Rh-negative, the fetus and mother will both be Rh-negative in 6.4 per cent of all pregnancies (i.e. 16 per cent – 9.6 per cent; see Table 12.1), which is equivalent to 40 per cent of pregnancies in Rh-negative women (i.e. 6.4/16)—16 per cent in which the father is also Rh-negative and 24 per cent in which he is Rh-positive heterozygous. The only maternal anti-D test finding which even without other evidence makes it reasonably certain that the fetus is Rh-positive is a significant increase in antibody (e.g. a rise in titre of two double dilutions or a 50 per cent increase in quantitative anti-D level). It has, however, recently become possible to identify Rh D-positive fetuses by polymerase chain reaction (PCR) assays of fetal DNA. This approach is discussed in the next section.

Even in the 60 per cent of fetuses of Rh-negative women that are Rhesus-positive, the degree of risk cannot generally be accurately assessed by any method of maternal anti-D measurement, since none of these methods measures the avidity of the antibody for Rh-antigen or the ability of the fetus to compensate for red cell destruction without becoming hydropic. Even very severe disease is not always accompanied by a rising titre. In a series of cases which ended in stillbirth or neonatal death or in which premature delivery resulted in survival, assessments of severity based on history of previous pregnancies and serial Rh-antibody titres were reasonably accurate in only 62 per cent of cases.[17] Even when these two variables correctly predict severe disease, they do not give a sufficiently accurate prognosis to ensure that intervention takes place early enough to precede the onset of hydrops but late enough for the fetus not to be placed at unnecessary risk. It follows that when the maternal anti-D level is high or rising, the appropriate response is not generally to proceed directly to active treatment (e.g. transfusion), but to carry out supplementary tests and to decide in the light of their results how the case should be managed.

Determination of fetal D-antigen status

Now that the DNA of the Rh genes has been cloned (see p. 283), it is possible to determine the Rh(D) type of the fetus by DNA analysis. Bennett *et al.*[59] were able to do this with 100 per cent accuracy by polymerase chain reaction (PCR) assays on 30 samples of fetal cells obtained by chorionic villus sampling or amniocentesis. By this means, it is possible to determine the D status of a fetus whose mother has Rh(D) antibody and whose father appears to be heterozygous for D, which removes the need for further invasive tests if the fetus is D-negative. Fetal Kell status can be determined in the same way.[60]

One unresolved issue is whether it is acceptable in a PCR assay to target only one exon of the D-gene when testing whether fetuses are Rh-positive. Rarely, if only one exon is targeted, a deletion or other variation in that exon may cause a variant D-positive fetus to be classified as D-negative. In order to avoid this, the use of multiplex assays targeting more than one exon along the D-gene has been proposed.[61] However, the laboratory of one of us (JMB) has had 100 per cent success using a single exon probe alone to determine fetal D status in cells from amniotic fluid or chorionic villi.

It is now possible to determine fetal Rh D-group by a maternal blood sample PCR assay, using either the fetal nucleated erythroid precursors that are present in the maternal circulation early in pregnancy[62] or fetal DNA isolated from maternal plasma.[63] These methods have not yet reached a sufficient level of accuracy to be used clinically; but they will undoubtedly do so, replacing the use of cells from amniotic fluid and chorionic villi to determine fetal D-group when a mother has Rh(D) antibody.

Supplementary tests

Amniotic fluid spectrophotometry, ultrasonic fetal assessment, and percutaneous fetal blood sampling are the three most important supplementary tests in diagnosing the presence and the degree of severity of haemolytic disease. Fetal blood sampling has to some extent supplanted amniotic fluid spectrophotometry, but is more invasive and should be preceded by the latter if the placenta can be avoided by the amniocentesis needle. Cellular bioassays of maternal antibody may also be helpful.

Amniotic fluid spectrophotometry

Not all Rh-immunized pregnant women will require amniocentesis. If the immunized woman has had a previous stillborn infant or one requiring exchange transfusion, amniocentesis initially at 16–18 weeks of gestation is indicated irrespective of the Rh-antibody titre. In the absence of such a history, the normal practice has been to carry out amniocentesis if the titre or directly measured anti-D reaches a critical level as defined by the local laboratory (e.g. a titre of 16 in albumin or 32 by indirect antiglobulin test in JMB's laboratory, or directly measured anti-D >4 i.u. in EAL's laboratory). The initial amniocentesis is carried out at 16–18 weeks if a critical anti-body reading is reported at that time or earlier, and immediately after a critical reading is observed if this occurs later.

Further amniocenteses are carried out at 5–28-day intervals (usually 14 days), depending upon the spectrophotometric reading of the immediately preceding test. It is not uncommon for weekly amniocenteses to be necessary for five to six weeks or even longer before their frequency may be reduced or definitive treatment undertaken. Monitoring should also continue during antenatal treatment, even if anti-D levels fall, since in the presence of a past history of moderate to severe haemolytic disease, hydrops may develop despite lessening anti-D levels (<3 µg/ml).

The purpose of sampling the amniotic fluid is to measure its content of the yellow pigment bilirubin, which is present in cases of haemolytic disease. Because the amount present is relatively small, it can only be measured accurately by spectrophotometry. Its measurement was first introduced by Bevis[64] and refined by Liley.[65]

The bilirubin in the amniotic fluid is derived from the fetus. It may reach the amniotic fluid as a transudate from fetal vessels on the surface of the placenta, but it probably arises from fetal tracheal and bronchial secretions, which are quite yellow in infants with severe haemolytic disease.

Liley's method of amniotic fluid bilirubin analysis[65] is described in Appendix 1. The readings it yields are plotted against gestation length on a graph divided into three zones—zone 1 into which readings fall that are low enough to support a prediction that the fetus will not be anaemic at birth, zone 3 for readings high enough to predict intrauterine death if the fetus is not treated, and zone 2 for intermediate readings. Accuracies of 90–98 per cent have been achieved with these predictions, and less than half of the inaccuracies that occurred were life-threatening (Table 12.6). Accuracy is lowest in mid-trimester and when the bilirubin level is in zone 2.

It is beyond the scope of this chapter to describe all the methods of amniotic fluid bilirubin analysis that have been reported. However, a comparison by Bartsch[67] of the methods in use up to 1970 revealed no particular advantage of one over the other. Of greater importance than the method used is the expertise of the laboratory reporting and assessing the amniotic fluid spectrophotometric reading and the experience of the obstetrician to whom the readings are reported.

Table 12.6   Results of amniotic fluid spectrophotometry (Liley method) December 1971–February 1978. (Modified from Bowman[66])

Zone in which last bilirubin measurement fell (see text)	Predicted condition of infant at birth, based on bilirubin measurement	Number of women	Prediction inaccurate (%)	Life-threatening predictive inaccuracy* (%)
1	Not anaemic	231	2.6	1.3
2	Alive but anaemic	474	9.3	4.0
3	Stillborn if not treated	292	1.7	0.7
Total		997	5.5	2.4

* On the basis of the inaccurate amniotic fluid reading the treatment embarked on (early delivery or fetal transfusion) or withheld placed the life of the fetus in jeopardy.

Amniocentesis should be performed under ultrasound guidance (see p. 472). By using ultrasound, the placenta can usually (but not invariably) be avoided and the needle inserted in the proper direction and depth in order to obtain blood-free amniotic fluid. In the present fetal blood sampling era,[34] amniocentesis is not carried out if the placenta is implanted anteriorly and cannot be avoided by the amniocentesis needle.

Amniocentesis should be carried out with careful aseptic technique. One maternal clotted blood sample should be obtained before and another after the procedure. Kleihauer or flow cytometry fetal cell tests are carried out on both blood samples and the Rh-antibody titre is measured in the second. About 10 ml of amniotic fluid are withdrawn and sent for optical density measurement. The fluid is also examined for lecithin/sphingomyelin ratio and the presence of phosphatidyl-glycerol if gestation exceeds 32 weeks, in order to determine whether the lungs are mature enough for the fetus to be delivered.

The only maternal hazards associated with the screening and diagnosis of Rh-haemolytic disease are those associated with amniocentesis. These include infection, precipitation of labour, and *abruptio placentae*, all very rare.

Fetal hazards are greater. Direct needle trauma is a rare occurrence.[68] The major hazard is transplacental haemorrhage. Although this hazard is greatly reduced by the use of ultrasound to guide amniocentesis, it cannot be removed entirely.

Among pregnancies complicated by blood group antibodies other than anti-D, those with anti-c can usefully be investigated by amniotic fluid spectrophotometry as described above. This procedure is, however, not helpful and can be misleading in pregnancies with anti-K, because this leads to anaemia mainly through suppression of fetal haematopoiesis, rather than through haemolysis as with anti-D and anti-c.[9-11]

With newer developments in direct assessment the use of amniocentesis to assess the severity of haemolytic disease has become controversial, although it remains useful in a minority of cases.

Real time ultrasonography

As well as guiding amniocentesis, ultrasound has other uses in the assessment of severity of fetal haemolytic disease. Although not a substitute for amniotic fluid spectrophotometry or fetal blood sampling, it can determine placental and liver size and the presence or absence of generalized oedema and ascites in the fetus. The absence of placental thickening, hepatic hypertrophy, oedema, and ascites is reassuring. More subtle signs of increased marrow turnover and compensated anaemia may be indicated by blood flow measurements, e.g. increased velocity in the middle cerebral artery.[8]

Ultrasound is also necessary whenever cord blood sampling and fetal intravascular transfusion are carried out. Also, when intraperitoneal fetal transfusion is undertaken, ultrasound is a valuable ancillary measure in determining the presence of blood (fluid) in the fetal peritoneal cavity, observing its disappearance (absorption), and assuring the obstetrician by weekly monitoring that the fetus is in good condition up to the time of the next procedure (intrauterine transfusion or delivery).

In utero cord blood sampling

Fetal blood sampling is by far the most accurate means of determining the degree of severity of fetal haemolytic disease (in the absence of hydrops) and the need for fetal treatment measures. It allows the direct measurement of all blood variables that can be measured after birth (haemoglobin, haematocrit, blood groups, direct antiglobulin testing, serum bilirubin levels, and fetal blood gases). Fetal haemoglobin concentration is the main guide to severity. As a general rule, intra-uterine transfusion is recommended if the haemoglobin concentration is below 100–110 g/l at 33 weeks of gestation or earlier, and early delivery if the concentration is below 80–90 g/l at 34 weeks or later.

Fetal blood sampling from an umbilical vessel (preferably a vein) by a needle passed through the mother's abdominal wall under ultrasound guidance has been the preferred method since the mid-1980s,[36] and is described in Chapter 20. Sampling may be possible as early as 18 weeks of gestation; it is usually feasible by 20 to 21 weeks of gestation. One widely used sampling site is the placental insertion of the umbilical cord.

Fetal blood sampling carries with it a traumatic fetal mortality rate of less than one per cent,[36] but a high risk of fetomaternal haemorrhage, especially if the placenta is implanted on the anterior uterine wall. Because of this risk, its use is recommended only: (1) when the serial amniotic fluid bilirubin reading is in or above the top 35 per cent of zone 2, and (2) when an anterior placenta cannot be avoided at amniocentesis, and maternal pregnancy history and/or maternal allo-antibody titres show that the fetus is at risk.

In EAL's unit, the preferred site for both sampling and intrauterine transfusions is the hepatic vein, if easily accessible. This method does not usually induce an increase in maternal antibodies through fetomaternal haemorrhage.

Cellular bioassays of maternal antibody

In efforts to assess the state of the fetus more accurately without resorting to invasive procedures in the conceptus, various cellular bioassays have been developed.[69] These include antibody-dependent, cell-mediated cytotoxicity with monocytes or killer lymphocytes, monocyte-mediated chemiluminescence, and adherence to and phagocytosis by peripheral monocytes or cultured macrophages. These tests, particularly those of antibody-dependent cell-mediated cytotoxicity, may predict the severity of fetal haemolytic disease more accurately than antibody titres and antibody quantitations, and so reduce the need for more invasive tests,[69] but only to a modest extent. They are quite inaccurate in the presence of an antigen-negative unaffected fetus and are not readily available.

Postnatal assessment

Maternal blood tests

Immediately after delivery, the ABO and Rh status of any woman whose blood grouping is unknown (e.g. because of inadequate antenatal care) should be determined and her serum tested for Rh and atypical antibodies. Testing for anti-D (by a manual enzyme method) should also be carried out at this time in Rh D-negative women in whom antibody has not previously been reported. If a newly delivered D-negative woman is negative for anti-D in manual enzyme tests, and if her newborn infant is D-positive, she should be given prophylactic Rh IgG even if weak anti-D is detected by AutoAnalyzer, since the latter finding alone is not necessarily indicative of true Rh-immunization. If she has been given antenatal Rh-prophylaxis, even detection of a very weak anti-D by a manual enzyme method does not contraindicate Rh-prophy-laxis, since it is usually due to the persistence of passive anti-D.

Maternal Kleihauer[54] or flow cytometry testing for fetal cells (p. 295) is recommended after delivery in Rh-negative women with no demonstrable Rh-antibody, in order to detect those who have had too great a transplacental haemorrhage for its immunizing effect to be suppressed by the routine dose of anti-D IgG. If the routine dose is 300 µg, the proportion of Rh D-incompatible pregnancies that will fall into this category is rather less than one per 1000, i.e. between 25 and 30 per cent of the 3/1000 in which more than 15 ml of fetal red cells reach the mother (p. 290).

Cord blood tests

If a mother is D-negative or her blood contains clinically significant IgG red cell antibodies, blood grouping should be carried out on the cord blood, and cord red cells should be tested for antibody by suspending them in anti-human globulin serum (the direct antiglobulin (Coombs') test, which is positive if agglutination occurs). If Coombs' test is positive, the relevant red cell antigen must be identified by testing the maternal plasma for IgG antibodies to the infant's red cells if such antibodies have not already been detected.

The direct Coombs' test is invariably positive in the cord blood of babies with Rh or any other haemolytic disease, except for some infants born after intrauterine transfusion. In the past the test was sometimes negative in cases due to ABO antibodies; but with more sensitive reagents it is usual for the Coombs' test to be weakly positive in infants from ABO-incompatible pregnancies in which maternal immune IgG anti-A or anti-B has crossed the placenta (pp. 285–6). This condition accounts for most positive results in the offspring of women with negative Rh-antibody tests. Even when ABO incompatibility results in a weakly positive Coombs' test, the infant is usually unaffected clinically. If the mother of one of these infants is both Rh-negative and Rh-antibody-negative, she will not have been immunized to the D-antigen and should receive prophylactic Rh-immune globulin, since ABO incompatibility confers only partial protection against Rh- immunization.

The Coombs' test is negative in 60 per cent of babies born after intrauterine transfusion, because their circulating red cells are donor in origin; but this should not lull one into a false sense of security, since these babies frequently exhibit very marked continuing erythropoiesis with haemolysis and rapidly rising bilirubin levels.

If the Coombs' test of cord blood is positive, the extent to which the infant is affected by the antibody should be assessed by measuring the cord haemoglobin and bilirubin levels (total and direct). Immediate exchange transfusion must be considered if the cord haemoglobin level is below 110 g/l, or if the indirect bilirubin level is above 68 µmol/l (4 mg/100 ml) in the mature infant or above 55 µmol/l (3.0–3.5 mg/100 ml) in the premature infant. Other signs of severe haemolytic disease which can be observed in the cord blood include markedly elevated numbers of reticulocytes and nucleated erythrocyte precursors (Fig. 12.1), and a brownish discoloration of serum or plasma caused by the presence of haem pigment.

Because HDN occasionally arises unexpectedly as a result of maternal antibodies being missed, and because of the difficulties of anticipating significant HDN due to ABO incompatibility, some authorities consider that Coombs' tests should be carried out in all newborn infants. Ideally, the same might be said of Hb estimation and measurement of bilirubin concentration. Other experts dismiss this approach as impractical and not cost-effective. Testing is generally agreed to be necessary in neonates born to mothers who are Rh-negative or have IgG antibodies, those already known to have HDN, those with a history of HDN in an elder sib, and those who become jaundiced.

Other measures

If exchange transfusion is likely to be needed, the blood to be used should be cross-matched with maternal serum and be ABO compatible with both baby and mother so that there will be no maternal antibodies in the infant that will destroy the transfused red cells.

Serial capillary haemoglobin and bilirubin estimations at 8–12 hour intervals are valuable in following the course of haemolytic disease and determining the need for treatment. A serum indirect bilirubin rise exceeding 8 μmol/l/h (0.5 mg/dl/h) indicates the need for prompt exchange transfusion, as does a serum indirect bilirubin level of 340 μmol/l (⩾20 mg/dl) in the mature infant. In the preterm infant, lower thresholds for phototherapy and exchange transfusion are used depending on gestation. Administration of albumin, in order to reduce the risk of kernicterus developing by raising the albumin-binding capacity of the infant's plasma, is favoured in many Canadian units. It is not routine practice in the UK.

Serial platelet counts every 8–12 hours should be carried out in severe HDN, since this is frequently associated with thrombocytopenia. Platelet counts may drop below 30 000 per cm^3, in which case appropriate treatment should be given.

Diagnosis of ABO haemolytic disease

The diagnosis of ABO HDN must usually be based on the work-up of a mature infant who develops jaundice in the first 24 hours of life, because the majority of newborns do not have investigation of the cord blood. The diagnosis can be confirmed by finding lytic anti-A or anti-B in the mother's serum, but this is not usually deemed necessary. The main problem is that when apparently healthy term infants are quickly discharged from hospital, significant and potentially dangerous jaundice may develop at home. Midwives should be alerted to this possibility, and protocols instituted to ensure early examination of the infant so that prompt measures can be taken to prevent the devastating complications of hyperbilirubinaemia.

ORGANIZATION

As a result of the change in prevalence of Rh HDN, many obstetricians and paediatricians in training are never exposed to a severe or potentially severe case of red cell allo-immunization, and therefore gain no first-hand experience of the improvements in fetal and neonatal management. It is therefore important that women who have previously had an infant affected by HDN, or who are found to have antibodies to blood group antigens, are referred to a centre specializing in fetal medicine before 20 weeks of gestation for assessment, so that amniocentesis, fetal blood sampling and/or intrauterine transfusion can be considered. Women with anti-K antibodies, particularly those with no history of transfusion, should be referred to a specialist unit even earlier in pregnancy. Kell allo-immunization requires special attention, with early Kell-typing of the fetus either by fetal blood sampling or by DNA typing of amniotic fluid cells in cases considered to be at particular risk.

Centralization of laboratory testing for blood groups and antibodies is also desirable, to facilitate quality control and the collection of population-based blood group and antibody data.

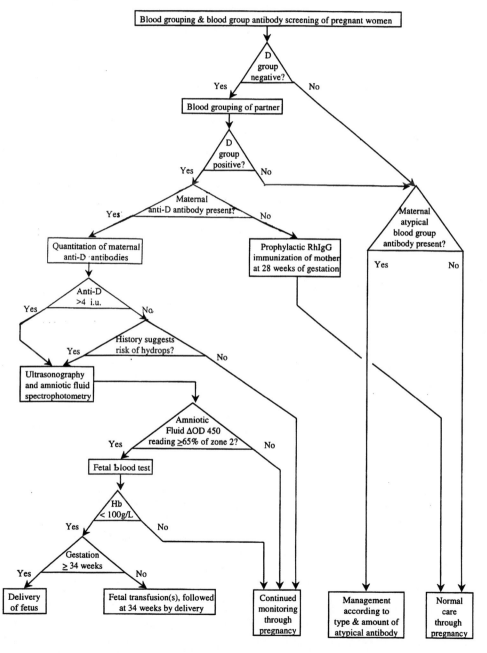

Fig. 12.3 Algorithm for antenatal HDN screening, diagnosis and treatment.

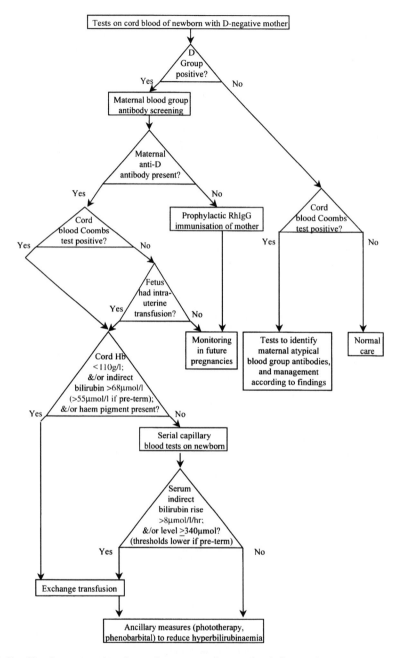

Fig. 12.4 Algorithm for postnatal testing and treatment when mother is D-negative.

The screening service should include all pregnant women early in pregnancy. Educational programmes directed both at the physician and at the pregnant patient can help in achieving this aim, as can collaborative arrangements for part of the blood sample taken at the first antenatal visit to be sent routinely to the appropriate laboratory for blood grouping and antibody screening.

CONCLUSION

The process of screening, diagnosis, and treatment for HDN is complex. The same is true of predicting the effects of screening. Figure 12.3 shows an algorithm summarizing antenatal screening, diagnosis and treatment. Figure 12.4 does the same for postnatal testing and treatment.

Figure 12.5 is a flow diagram of screening in first pregnancies to prevent HDN in second pregnancies. Among 100 000 women having second pregnancies, it is estimated that 454 would be affected by Rh HDN if anti-D were not given in the first pregnancy, and that 87 per cent of these could be prevented by giving anti-D after the first delivery and a further 11 per cent if it were also given in the first pregnancy at 28 weeks of gestation. It is assumed in Fig. 12.5 that all women who received anti-D in the first pregnancy would have a second, in which case the second-born children of one-thirtieth of these women would benefit (i.e. $(448 - 3)/(448 + 12\ 982)$).

In a similar way to Fig. 12.5, Fig. 12.6 outlines screening in second pregnancies to prevent HDN in third pregnancies. It is assumed that half the women receiving anti-D in their first and second pregnancies would have a third pregnancy. If so, 1 in 25 recipients would have a third child who benefited (i.e. $(531 - 2)/(531 + 12\ 889)$). The proportion of third-born children who would be affected if anti-D were not given is 1.1 per cent ($537/50\ 000$), of whom 57 per cent would be protected as a result of the anti-D given during and immediately after the first pregnancy and a further 42 per cent protected by giving anti-D during and after the second pregnancy (including 5 per cent who would not be protected if prophylaxis at 28 weeks of gestation were omitted).

As Figs. 12.5 and 12.6 illustrate, the proportion of children who can be expected to benefit from prophylaxis increases from 0.4 per cent (i.e. $(52 + 393)/100\ 000$) of all those who are second-born to 1.1 per cent (i.e. $(306 + 26 + 197)/50\ 000$) of all who are third-born. Among children of further pregnancies (not shown because there are relatively few of them), even higher proportions would benefit. Children of first pregnancies can derive very little benefit from prophylaxis, since they are very rarely affected by clinically significant Rh HDN: its estimated incidence in incompatible first pregnancies is only 0.05 per cent (Table 12.4), which corresponds to 0.005 per cent of all first pregnancies ($5/100\ 000$) in Caucasian populations where about 10 per cent of pregnancies are Rh-incompatible (see Table 12.1).

The value of the programme is confirmed by the decline in both the prevalence and the case-fatality of Rh HDN over time in places where screening has been instituted. In Manitoba, for example, the prevalence of Rh-allo-immunization declined from 10.6/1000 births in 1963 (before the introduction of prophylaxis) to 1.6/1000 in 1990.[70] The proportion of fetuses and infants affected by clinically significant HDN is therefore estimated to have declined from about 5 to 0.8/1000.

The relative decline in mortality has been greater. Prior to 1945, all of the estimated 45 per cent of fetuses with clinically significant HDN who developed hydrops died. Of the 55 per cent who developed kernicterus about 90 per cent died and the remaining 10 per cent were left severely damaged. Thus, the overall case fatality rate in clinically significant Rh-haemolytic disease before treatment measures developed was about 95 per cent. Subsequent to the introduction of exchange transfusions in 1945 for the management of liveborn non-hydropic infants,[29] the overall case fatality rate dropped

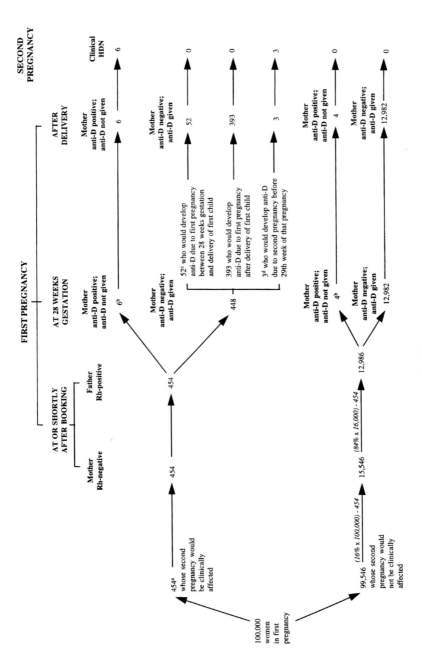

Fig. 12.5 Flow diagram of screening for anti-D in first pregnancies to prevent HDN in second pregnancies.

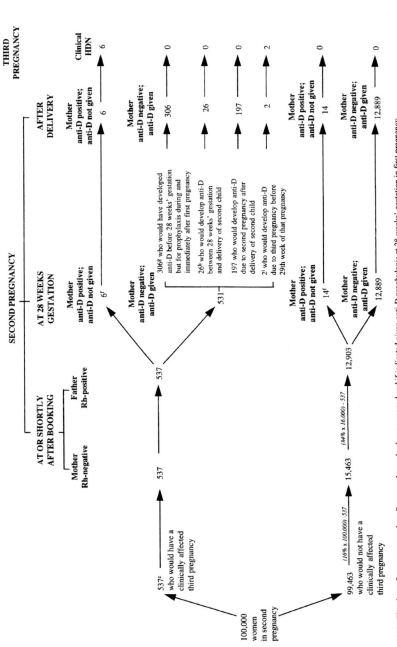

N.B. The above figures assume that all women have also been screened and if indicated given anti-D prophylaxis at 28 weeks' gestation in first pregnancy and after first delivery; that half of those having a second pregnancy have a third; and that none change their partners.

See Appendix 2 for footnotes e–i, which explain how the numbers to which they relate were derived.

Fig. 12.6 Flow diagram of screening for anti-D in second pregnancies to prevent HDN in third pregnancies.

to about 50 per cent. With the introduction of preterm delivery[17] ($\geq$32 weeks of gestation) in the mid-1950s, the rate was reduced to 30 per cent. With the introduction of amniotic fluid spectrophotometry in the early 1960s[65] it was reduced to 20–25 per cent. During the 20 years following the introduction of intrauterine fetal transfusion (IUT)[33,66] in the mid-1960s, the case fatality fell to less than 4 per cent of those affected in Manitoba, Canada.

Because of these improvements in both prevalence and case fatality, the perinatal mortality rate due to Rh HDN in Manitoba has declined from about 1.25/1000 to 0.02/1000 births since the early 1960s—a decline of 98 per cent. In England and Wales, 313 perinatal deaths related to HDN (45.8/100 000 births) were reported in 1973,[71] but only 33 (2.5/100 000) in 1984–5[72] and nine (1.3/100 000) in 1993[73]—a decline of 97 per cent. However, a recent study suggests that only one-fifth of all British deaths due to HDN are registered (partly because some result in miscarriage, which is not registrable).[74]

Anti-D antibodies still occur in an unacceptably high proportion of pregnancies. In Britain, where anti-D prophylaxis is generally given after delivery, antibodies appear in association with approximately 1.5 per cent of D-incompatible pregnancies,[23] or nearly one-eighth as many as would lead to the development of antibodies in the absence of prophylaxis (13 per cent, see p. 288). This has been attributed partly to early postnatal anti-D prophylaxis being omitted in some women at risk, and partly to failure to give prophylaxis during the antenatal period as well as after delivery.[23] Although antenatal prophylaxis can reduce the risk of antibodies developing to less than 0.1 per cent (see p. 291), some have argued that this is not enough to justify the cost of extending the use of anti-D from postnatal to antenatal prophylaxis,[75] and others have suggested a middle course in which antenatal prophylaxis would only be given in first pregnancies, thus leaving women at risk in subsequent ones.[76] In Manitoba in the early 1980s, it was estimated that the cost of routine prophylaxis at 28 weeks of gestation per case of clinical HDN prevented was $Canadian 6800.[77] In many communities, this cost would be regarded as acceptable. It is the authors' opinion that a programme including routine antenatal prophylaxis is the one to be recommended. A recent consensus meeting in the United Kingdom reached the same conclusion,[27] as is reflected in the most recent guidelines from the Royal College of Obstetricians and Gynaecologists.[78]

APPENDIX 1: LABORATORY METHODS

Rh-antibody screening tests
Saline agglutination[79]

When suspended in saline and treated with maternal serum, Rh-positive red cells agglutinate if the serum contains IgM anti-D, but they are not agglutinated by IgG anti-D. IgM anti-D is not always present in the serum of Rh-immunized women, so that a negative saline agglutination test result does not exclude the presence of active Rh-immunization. However, a positive result proves beyond doubt that a woman is actively Rh-immunized. The test is of value in cases in which prophylactic anti-D IgG (which contains minimal IgM) has been given. In these circumstances a weakly positive result in a test for IgG anti-D is not diagnostic of early active Rh-immunization since it may be due to the administered anti-D.

Colloid agglutination

Although IgG anti-D antibodies do not agglutinate Rh-positive red cells suspended in saline, they will agglutinate the same red cells when these are suspended in a more viscous medium. The more viscous media have higher dielectric constants, which reduce the negative electrical potential of the red cell membrane. The red cells then lie closer together. IgG anti-D can bridge the narrower gap and cause agglutination. The medium most frequently used is 30 per cent bovine serum albumin.[80] Although colloid (albumin) agglutination methods are frequently used for Rh-antibody titrations, they are too insensitive to be used to screen for the presence of very weak Rh-antibodies.

Anti-human globulin screening[81]

Anti-human globulin (Coombs' serum) is produced by injecting human serum (or purified human IgG) into other animal species. The animals recognize the serum (or IgG) as foreign and produce antibodies to it (i.e. anti-human globulin). The maternal serum to be screened for anti-D is incubated with Rh-positive red cells (usually for one hour). If anti-D is present, it will coat the red cells. The red cells are washed three or four times in isotonic saline and then suspended in anti-human globulin serum. The test (indirect antiglobulin test) is positive if agglutination occurs and denotes the presence of Rh-antibody in the maternal serum. In the UK this is the screening test used in hospital-based transfusion laboratories to detect significant IgG antibodies. If these are present, maternal serum is sent to regional transfusion centres for quantitation using autoanalysis and enzyme techniques.

Enzyme-treated red cell screening[82]

When Rh-positive red cells are incubated with enzymes such as trypsin, ficin, bromelin, or papain, membrane alterations occur, which reduce the negative electrical potential. When red cells treated in this manner are suspended in saline, they lie more closely together and are readily agglutinated by IgG anti-D. In experienced hands, properly carried out enzyme methods are the most sensitive manual techniques for detecting Rh-immunization. Manual enzyme methods are among the techniques used in Canada when screening Rh-negative maternal sera for the presence of anti-D.

Automated tests

Automated methods for Rh-antibody screening are now available using the AutoAnalyzer® (Technicon). Two methods in use are bromelin[83] and low ionic.[84] Automated equipment other than the AutoAnalyzer has also been used for antibody detection. Automated screening methods are extremely sensitive and should be reserved for the quantitation of antibodies. The AutoAnalyzer bromelin technique has been modified to allow very accurate quantitation of anti-D.[58]

Rh-antibody titration
Albumin titration

Doubling dilutions of maternal serum are mixed with Rh-positive red cells suspended in 30 per cent bovine serum albumin. Methods of carrying out the actual titration differ from laboratory to laboratory and vary in their sensitivity with consequent variation in the antibody titre reported in the same serum. The method used by JMB's laboratory[80] is to mix the serial dilutions of sera with the albumin suspended red cells in small-calibre glass test tubes. The tubes are centrifuged briefly. Agglutination is then observed by dislodging the button of red cells from the bottom of the test tube by gentle shaking. Agglutination is graded from solid (one clump of red cells), through 4+ to + to none at all. The highest dilution at which agglutination (+) is present is the albumin Rh-antibody titre. This method has largely been abandoned in the UK.

Indirect antiglobulin titration

Doubling dilutions of maternal serum under test are incubated with Rh-positive red cells (usually for about one hour). The temperature of incubation varies from laboratory to laboratory. Following incubation the red cells are washed four times with isotonic saline and mixed with anti-human globulin. A rapid and simple method of indirect anti-human globulin titration which uses very little anti-human globulin is the capillary method of Chown and Lewis.[85] The highest dilution at which agglutination of the Rh-positive red cells is observed is the indirect antiglobulin titre.

Liley's method of amniotic fluid bilirubin analysis[65]

Procedure

Amniotic fluid, protected from light (which decolorizes it), is centrifuged and filtered. Optical density measurements are made in a good quality spectrophotometer from wavelengths 700 to 350 nm. The readings are plotted manually or automatically and connected by a straight line on semilogarithmic graph paper on which the linear horizontal axis represents wavelength and the logarithmic vertical axis represents optical density (Fig. 12.7). The figure of prognostic importance is the deviation from linearity at 450 nm (ΔOD 450). This figure is derived by drawing a straight line

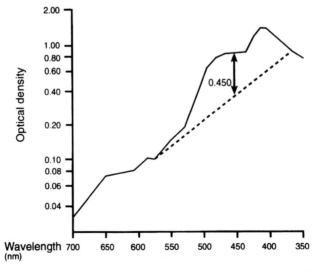

Fig. 12.7 Graph of optical density of an amniotic fluid speciman (measured by spectrophotometry) at different wavelengths. The dotted straight line connects the density readings at 550 and 365 nm. (Modified from Bowman.[66])

between the readings at 550 nm and 365 nm, and measuring the vertical distance between this line and the actual reading at 450 nm (Fig. 12.7). This distance is related to the severity of Rh disease.

Interpretation

ΔOD 450 measurements are commonly interpreted by plotting them against gestation length on graphs divided into three zones. The boundaries of these zones are drawn so as to discriminate as accurately as possible between readings so high that the fetus is likely to die from hydrops if untreated (zone 3); readings so low as to indicate that no treatment will be needed, except possibly for hyperbilirubinaemia after birth (zone 1); and intermediate readings (zone 2). The zone boundaries used by Liley[65] were straight lines which sloped down over the whole period when ΔOD 450 may be measured (from about 16 weeks of gestation onward). The downward slope took account of the fact that normal amniotic fluid bilirubin levels diminish during the last four mouths of pregnancy, so that a raised ΔOD 450 reading in late gestation is indicative of more severe haemolytic disease than an identical reading a few weeks earlier.

Although a single ΔOD 450 reading after 29–30 weeks is reasonably accurate in predicting severity of disease, this may not be so earlier in gestation (unless the ΔOD 450 reading is high in zone 3).[86] For this reason, and because amniotic fluid levels peak at 23–24 weeks of gestation in normal pregnancy,[86] JMB's laboratory now uses different boundaries before 24 weeks of gestation. These start lower and slope upwards as steeply as Liley's boundaries slope downwards. The two sets of boundaries meet at 24 weeks, beyond which Liley's boundaries are still used (Fig. 12.8). Fetal blood sampling is recommended when a ΔOD 450 reading is in or above the upper 35 per cent of zone 2 as defined by these revised boundaries.

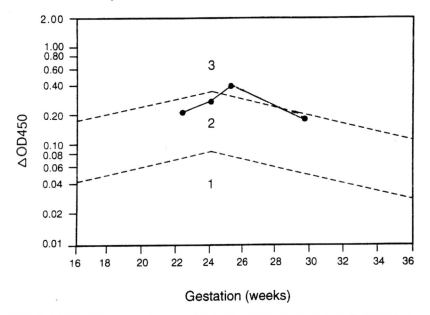

Fig. 12.8 Serial ΔOD 450 readings for a fetus given intrauterine transfusions for Rh haemolytic disease,[87] plotted against gestation length on a graph showing zone boundaries. Points for mild, moderate and severe cases are expected to fall in zones 1–3 respectively.

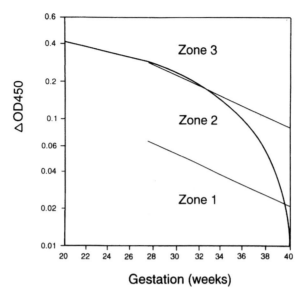

Fig. 12.9 Chart showing the Whitfield curved action line extrapolated to 20 weeks and Liley's zones from 27 weeks.

Serial ΔOD 450 readings, plotted on a graph which shows the three zones, give a more accurate assessment of severity of haemolytic disease than does a single ΔOD 450 reading. Figure 12.8 includes data of this kind for a fetus which was delivered at 33.5 weeks and survived after being given intrauterine transfusions in response to the second, third, and fourth ΔOD 450 readings.[87]

As an alternative to Liley's zones, Whitfield's action line (Fig. 12.9) has been proposed as a guideline for appropriate management based on ΔOD 450 and gestation. Intrauterine transfusion or delivery (followed by exchange transfusion if indicated) is considered when readings above the Whitfield line are obtained.[88]

Sources of error

Blood (maternal or fetal) in amniotic fluid produces optical density peaks at 580, 540, and 415 nm, which mask the ΔOD 450 reading and render the fluid valueless. Small amounts of blood, if removed promptly, will not vitiate the ΔOD 450 reading, but small amounts of fetal plasma will increase the ΔOD 450 reading and cause an incorrect interpretation of severity of disease. Haem (methaemalbumin) produces a sharp 405 nm peak that may mask the ΔOD 450 reading (Fig. 12.7) but is in itself an indication of very severe Rh disease.

Meconium in amniotic fluid causes a marked distortion of the ΔOD 450. Exposure of fluid to sunlight or fluorescent light reduces ΔOD 450 readings by disrupting the bilirubin molecules with production of colourless dipyrolles.

Aspiration of maternal urine or fetal ascitic fluid is another source of error. Maternal (or fetal) urine produces no 450 nm peak. Fetal ascitic fluid is clear, syrupy, and produces a very high pigment peak measurement at about 460 nm.

Congenital anomalies such as anencephaly and obstructive anomalies of the upper gastrointestinal tract (e.g. tracheo-oesophageal fistula) can produce high ΔOD 450 readings.

APPENDIX 2: STATISTICAL METHODS
prepared by Ian Leck

Derivation of Table 12.4

This section describes the estimation of prevalence of maternal anti-D and of clinically significant HDN, according to number of Rh-incompatible pregnancies.

Frequency of anti-D

The proportion of mothers expected to have anti-D in the absence of prophylaxis was estimated for each successive Rh-incompatible pregnancy by adding together two figures:

1. The proportion in which the mother would have anti-D as a result of previous incompatible pregnancies, given that each of these pregnancies would lead to the development of anti-D in 13 per cent of women in whom it was not already present (see p. 288).

2. The proportion in which the mother would develop anti-D during the current pregnancy as a result of this pregnancy. This was taken as 1.6 per cent (one-eighth of 13 per cent) of women who were not antibody-positive as a result of previous pregnancies, since only one-eighth of women who sero-convert as a result of an incompatible pregnancy do so during (as opposed to after) this pregnancy[15] (p. 287).

Table 12.7 shows the calculation in detail.

Frequency of clinically significant HDN

Using figures from Table 12.7, estimates were derived of the proportions of successive Rh-incompatible pregnancies in which clinically significant haemolytic disease would develop in the fetus in the absence of prophylaxis. Table 12.8 illustrates the method for third incompatible pregnancies.

The table was derived as follows. The first step was to estimate the prevalence of clinically significant HDN (the 'HDN rate') in pregnancies in which maternal anti-D was present at 28 weeks of gestation, according to which incompatible pregnancy (first, second, etc.) was the first in which the mother had anti-D at this stage. In pregnancies in which anti-D appears later than 28 weeks of gestation the fetus is not normally threatened, because relatively little anti-D is produced (see pp. 287–8). The HDN rates that were estimated were those that would occur if 100 per cent of mothers with anti-D at 28 weeks of gestation who had previously borne children with HDN and 45 per cent of those who had not done so were to produce children with HDN in the current pregnancy. Forty-five per cent is a reasonable estimate because it fits with the rate of 50–55 per cent reported in *all* Rh-positive fetuses of antibody-positive mothers (pp. 288–289). Column (*a*) of Table 12.8 shows the HDN rates for third pregnancies in women with anti-D according to when their anti-D appeared.

The second step (column (*b*) of Table 12.8) was to tabulate the proportions of *all* incompatible third pregnancies in which the mother had anti-D at 28 weeks, according

Table 12.7 Estimated proportions of Rh-incompatible pregnancies in which anti-D would be produced in the absence of prophylaxis, according to number of previous incompatible pregnancies. Every incompatible pregnancy is taken to carry a 13 per cent risk of immunizing the mother, and one-eighth of immunizations (equivalent to a risk of 1.6 per cent) are taken to occur during as opposed to after the pregnancy that causes them.

| Number of previous Rh-incompatible pregnancies (n) | Immunization due to previous pregnancies | | | | | Immunization due to current pregnancy [$0.016(1 - p_n)$] | Total with anti-D at end of current pregnancy |
	1st pregnancy ($p_1 = 0.13$)	2nd pregnancy [$p_2 = 0.13(1 - p_1)$]	3rd pregnancy [$p_3 = 0.13(1 - p_2)$]	4th pregnancy [$p_4 = 0.13(1 - p_3)$]	Total (p_n)		
0	–	–	–	–	–	0.016	0.016
1	0.130	–	–	–	0.130	0.014	0.144
2	0.130	0.113	–	–	0.243	0.012	0.255
3	0.130	0.113	0.098	–	0.341	0.011	0.352
4	0.130	0.113	0.098	0.086	0.427	0.009	0.436

Table 12.8 Estimation of the prevalence of clinically significant HDN—example of calculation for third Rh-incompatible pregnancies

First incompatible pregnancy in which fetus was at risk	Period in which immunization is estimated to have occurred	Prevalence of HDN in 3rd incompatible pregnancies with anti-D at 28 weeks (a)	Proportion of all 3rd incompatible pregnancies:	
			with anti-D at 28 weeks (b)	with HDN (c = a × b)
First	Before 29th week of first incompatible pregnancy	83%***	0.1%†	0.1%
Second	Between 29th week of first incompatible pregnancy and 28th week of second	70%**	13.0%††	9.1%
Third	Between 29th week of second incompatible pregnancy and 28th week of third	45%*	11.3%††††	5.1%
				Total: 14.3%

* Empirical.
** 0.45(1 − 0.45)+0.45.
*** 0.45(1 − 0.70)+0.70.
† See p. 288.
†† From Table 12.7 ('1st pregnancy' column).
††† From Table 12.7 ('2nd pregnancy' column).

to whether the incompatible pregnancy in which she *first* had anti-D at 28 weeks was the first, second, or third of these pregnancies. Only 0.1 per cent of mothers were estimated to have developed anti-D before the 29th week of their first incompatible pregnancy, since this is the proportion of previously non-immune women estimated to develop anti-D before the 29th week of any incompatible pregnancy (see p. 288). It was estimated that anti-D would have appeared in a further 13.0 per cent of mothers before the 29th week of their second incompatible pregnancy and in a further 11.3 per cent before the 29th week of their third. These estimates were derived from Table 12.7, in which 13.0 per cent of first and 11.3 per cent of second incompatible pregnancies had been estimated to initiate anti-D production (Table 12.7). The rationale for using the figures in Table 12.7 in this way is as follows. In incompatible pregnancies of each rank above the first, the proportion of pregnancies in which the fetus is at risk for the first time includes (1) pregnancies in which immunization was caused by the current fetus before 28 weeks and (2) pregnancies in women who were made immune by the fetus in their last incompatible pregnancy at a time beyond the 28th week of that pregnancy. The proportion in group (1) is so small, and so close to the corresponding proportion for the last incompatible pregnancy, that the proportion immunized at any time by the fetus in one incompatible pregnancy is likely to be the same (to an accuracy of 0.1 per cent) as the proportion who were first at risk of having an affected fetus in the next incompatible pregnancy.

The third and final step (column (*c*) of Table 12.8) was to estimate the proportion of all third incompatible pregnancies with HDN, by multiplying together the figures in columns (*a*) and (*b*) and summing the products to yield the answer of 14.3 per cent.

Derivation of various numbers in Figs. 12.5 and 12.6

This section consists of footnotes to the above figures. The letters preceding the text correspond to the superscripts in the figures.

(a). *Second pregnancies with clinical HDN*: 9.6 per cent of second pregnancies will be Rh-incompatible—5.76 per cent with homozygous Rh-positive fathers and 3.84 per cent with heterozygous Rh-positive fathers (see Table 12.1). All the 5.76 per cent and half of the 3.84 per cent would follow incompatible first pregnancies, and would have a 5.9 per cent prevalence of clinical HDN if anti-D was not given; the other half of the 3.84 per cent would follow a compatible first pregnancy and have a 0.05 per cent prevalence of clinical HDN (see Table 12.4). The proportion of all second pregnancies with clinical HDN would therefore be: $0.059 (0.0576 + 0.0384/2) + (0.0005 \times 0.0384/2) = 454/100\,000$.

(b). *Women who develop anti-D before the 29th week of their first pregnancy*: 9.6 per cent of first pregnancies will be Rh-incompatible (see Table 12.1). Anti-D would develop before the 29th week of gestation in 0.1 per cent of these (see p. 288), i.e. in $10/100\,000$ first pregnancies. Incompatibility recurs in 80 per cent of second pregnancies following incompatible first pregnancies (i.e. in all the 60 per cent in which the father is D-homozygous and in half of the 40 per cent in which he is D-heterozygous, see Table 12.1). If one incompatible pregnancy is followed by another and anti-D has appeared before the 29th week of the first of these two pregnancies, the chance of the second resulting in HDN is estimated to be 70 per cent (i.e. [0.45 + 0.45(1 − 0.45)]; see p. 313). Among 100 000 first pregnancies, it can therefore be estimated that six of the 10 with anti-D at 28 weeks (i.e. 10 × 0.8 × 0.7) would be followed by HDN in the second pregnancy and that four would not.

(c). *Women who would develop anti-D during their first pregnancy after 28 weeks of gestation*: If prophylactic anti-D was not given, natural anti-D antibody would develop between 28 weeks of gestation and delivery in 1.5 per cent of the 9.6 per cent of first pregnancies that are Rh-incompatible (see p. 288), i.e. in 144/100 000 first pregnancies. Incompatibility would recur in 80 per cent of the second pregnancies that followed these first pregnancies (see note b), and it is estimated that there is a 45 per cent chance of HDN occurring in the second of a pair of incompatible pregnancies when anti-D has appeared during the first of the pair between 28 weeks and delivery (p. 313). Among all first pregnancies, the number with anti-D appearing between 28 weeks and delivery which would be expected to be followed by HDN in the second pregnancy is therefore the product of 144/100 000, 0.8 and 0.45, i.e. 52/100 000.

(d). *Second pregnancies with clinical HDN caused by anti-D produced in response to the second pregnancy before its 29th week*: These cases of HDN would not be prevented by giving anti-D during and immediately after the first pregnancy. The affected pregnancies that followed compatible first pregnancies (i.e. 0.0005 × 0.0384/2, or 1/100 000) would be of this kind, as would some of the 5760/100 000 second pregnancies in which incompatibility occurred for the second time (see note a). The number affected among the 5760 can be estimated by multiplying together 5760, 87 per cent (the proportion of incompatible first pregnancies which would not lead to the development of anti-D, see p. 288), 0.1 per cent (the proportion of incompatible second pregnancies leading to the development of anti-D before 28 weeks of gestation, see p. 288), and 45 per cent (the estimated prevalence of HDN in pregnancies in which anti-D is present before the 29th week without there being any history of HDN in a previous pregnancy, see p. 313). The product of these figures is 2. Adding this product to the figure for HDN in incompatible second pregnancies following compatible first ones yields an estimate of 3/100 000 for the total number of second pregnancies in which HDN would be caused by antibody produced in response to the same pregnancy.

(e). *Third pregnancies with clinical HDN*: Among 50 000 third pregnancies, 4800 (i.e. 9.6 per cent) will be incompatible—2880 (5.76 per cent) with homozygous Rh-positive fathers and 1920 (3.84 per cent) with heterozygous Rh-positive fathers (see Table 12.1). The two pregnancies preceding each of the 2880 with homozygous fathers will also have been incompatible. Among the 1920 incompatible third pregnancies with heterozygous fathers, 480 (one-quarter) will have been preceded by two incompatible pregnancies, 480 by two compatible, 480 by an incompatible first and a compatible second, and 480 by a compatible first and an incompatible second. The prevalence of clinical HDN would be 0.05 per cent in the 480 first incompatible pregnancies, 5.9 per cent in the 960 second, and 14.3 per cent in the 3360 third (see Table 12.4). The number of third pregnancies with clinical HDN would therefore be: (480 × 0.0005) + (960 × 0.059) + (3360 × 0.143) = 537.

(f). *Women who develop anti-D as a result of their second pregnancy before its 29th*

Table 12.9   Numbers of women in their second pregnancy in whom anti-D would be present at 28 weeks of gestation, among 100 000 pregnant for the second time after being screened and (if appropriate) given anti-D prophylaxis at 28 weeks of gestation in first pregnancy and after first delivery

	Number of women[1] (a)	Prevalence of incompatability in 3rd pregnancy (b)	Prevalence of HDN in incompatible 3rd pregnancies[2] (c)	Number of 3rd pregnancies with HDN[3] (d = abc/2)
Incompatibility in both of first two pregnancies:				
Anti-D appeared in 1st pregnancy before 28 weeks	8*	0.875†	0.83	3
Anti-D appeared in 2nd pregnancy before 28 weeks	8**	0.875†	0.70	3
Incompatibility in one of first two pregnancies:				
Anti-D appeared in 1st pregnancy before 28 weeks	2***	0.5††	0.70	0
Anti-D appeared in 2nd pregnancy before 28 weeks	2***	0.5††	0.70	0
Total	20	–	–	6

[1] Given that 0.1 per cent of women with an incompatible pregnancy who have not previously developed anti-D will do so by 28 weeks of gestation (see p. 288).
[2] See Table 12.8, column (a).
[3] The product of the figures in columns a, b, and c (i.e. the number of cases of HDN to be expected in the third pregnancies of the women specified if all became pregnant for the third time) is halved on the assumption that only half would become pregnant again.
* 0.1 per cent of 7680. 7680 is the number of women whose first two pregnancies would both be incompatible, i.e. all the 5 760 with homozygous Rh-positive partners and half of the 3 840 with heterozygous partners whose first pregnancies were incompatible (see Table 12.1).
** 0.1 per cent of 7672. 7672 is the number of women whose first two pregnancies would both be incompatible and who would not have developed anti-D before the second pregnancy (i.e. 7680 – 8).
*** 0.1 per cent of 1920. 1920 is the number of women with compatible second pregnancies among the 3840 with heterozygous partners whose first pregnancies were incompatible (see Table 12.1) and also the number with first compatible and second incompatible pregnancies.
† Among the 7680 women whose first two pregnancies are both incompatible, all the 5760 with homozygous Rh-positive partners and half of the 1 920 with heterozygous partners (a total of 6720) will have incompatible third pregnancies. 6720/7680 = 87.5 per cent.
†† A woman who has had both compatible and incompatible pregnancies will have a heterozygous Rh-positive partner and therefore a 50 per cent chance of incompatibility in every pregnancy.
NB: The above figures assume no changes of partner.

week: These women are estimated to number 20, of whom six would have a third pregnancy with HDN and 14 would not (see Table 12.9).

(g). *Women prevented from developing anti-D before the 29th week of a second pregnancy by giving anti-D during/immediately after first pregnancy*: Giving anti-D during and immediately after the first pregnancy would prevent some cases of HDN in two groups of incompatible third pregnancies: (1) the 3360 in women whose first and second pregnancies were also incompatible and (2) the 480 in women who had incompatible first and compatible second pregnancies (see note e). If none of these women were given prophylactic anti-D, their first pregnancies would cause anti-D to develop beyond 28 weeks of gestation in 12.9 per cent of each group (i.e. 433 of the 3360 and 62 of the 480, see p. 288); and HDN would complicate the third pregnancies of 331 of these 495 women (45 per cent of the 62 with incompatible first and compatible second pregnancies and 70 per cent (i.e.

Table 12.10 Numbers of women in their second pregnancy who would develop anti-D between 28 weeks of gestation and delivery if not given prophylactic anti-D at 28 weeks, among 100 000 pregnant for the second time after being screened and (if appropriate) given anti-D prophylaxis at 28 weeks of gestation in first pregnancy and after first delivery

	Number of women[1] (a)	Prevalence of incompatibility in 3rd pregnancy[2] (b)	Number of 3rd pregnancies with HDN[3] (c = ab × 0.45/2)
Both of first two pregnancies incompatible	115*	0.875	23
First pregnancy compatible, second incompatible	29**	0.5	3
Total	144	–	26

[1] Given that 1.5 per cent of women with an incompatible pregnancy who have not developed anti-D as a result of a previous pregnancy will do so between 28 weeks of gestation and delivery (see p. 288).
[2] See footnotes to Table 12.9, column (b), for derivation of figures.
[3] The product of the figures in columns (a) and (b) (i.e. the number of incompatible third pregnancies to be expected in the women specified if all became pregnant for the third time) is multiplied by 0.45 because the next incompatible pregnancy to one in which anti-D appears after 28 weeks of gestation is estimated to have a 45 per cent chance of being complicated by HDN (see p. 289). The resulting figure is halved on the assumption that only half of the women with a second pregnancy would become pregnant again.
* 1.5 per cent of 7672. 7672 is the number of women whose first two pregnancies would both be incompatible and who would not have developed anti-D before the second pregnancy (see Table 12.9, footnote **).
** 1.5 per cent of 1920. 1920 is the number of women with compatible first and incompatible second pregnancies.
NB: The above figures assume no changes of partner.

$[0.45 + 0.45(1 - 0.45)]$) of the 433 whose first and second pregnancies were both incompatible). If anti-D were given during and immediately after their first pregnancies, none of the 495 would develop anti-D as a result of these pregnancies; if no further prophylactic anti-D was given, natural anti-D would be expected to develop as a result of the second pregnancies of 56 of the 495, i.e. in 13 per cent (see p. 288) of the 433 whose second pregnancies were incompatible and in none of the 62 with compatible second pregnancies; and HDN would be expected to occur in the third pregnancies of 25 (45 per cent of the 56). It follows that giving anti-D during the first pregnancy alone would prevent 306 (i.e. 331 – 25) of the 537 cases of HDN expected to occur in 50 000 third pregnancies in the total absence of prophylaxis (see note e).

(h). *Women who would develop anti-D during second pregnancy beyond 28 weeks of gestation*: If no anti-D was given during the second pregnancy, these women would be expected to number 144, of whom 26 would have third pregnancies in which HDN would occur (see Table 12.10).

(i). *Third pregnancies with clinical HDN caused by anti-D produced in response to the third pregnancy before its 29th week*: These cases of HDN would not be prevented by giving anti-D during and immediately after the first two pregnancies. The first incompatible pregnancies with HDN (i.e. 480 × 0.0005) would be of this kind, as would some of the 960 second incompatible pregnancies and of the 3360 third (see note e). The number of cases of this kind among the 960 can be estimated by multiplying together 960, 87 per cent (the proportion of first incompatible pregnancies which would not lead to the development of anti-D), 0.1 per cent (the proportion of second incompatible pregnancies leading to the development of anti-D before 28 weeks of gestation, see p. 288), and 45 per cent (the estimated prevalence of HDN in pregnancies in which anti-D is present before the 29th week without there being any history of HDN in a previous pregnancy, see p. 289). The number of cases among the 3360 third incompatible pregnancies can be estimated by multiplying together 3360, 76 per cent (the proportion of women remaining without anti-D after two consecutive incompatible pregnancies, which is obtained by squaring 87 per cent), 0.1 per cent and 45 per cent. Summing the estimates for first, second, and third incompatible pregnancies yields a figure of 2/100 000 for the total number of third pregnancies in which HDN would be caused by antibody produced in response to the same pregnancy.

REFERENCES

1. Landsteiner, K. and Weiner, A. (1940). An agglutinable factor in human blood recognized by immune sera for rhesus blood. *Proceedings of the Society for Experimental Biology and Medicine*, **43**, 223.

2. Levine, P, Katzin, E, and Burnham, L. (1941). Isoimmunization in pregnancy: its possible bearing on the etiology of erythroblastosis fetalis. *Journal of the American Medical Association*, **116**, 825–7.

3. Bowman, J.M. (1998). RhD hemolytic disease of the newborn. *New England Journal of Medicine*, **339**, 1775–7.

4. Mollison, P.L., Engelfriet, C.P., and Contreras, M. (1997). *Blood Transfusion in Clinical Medicine,* 10th edn. Blackwell Science, Oxford.

5. Le Van Kim, C., Mouro, I., Cherif-Zahar, B., *et al.* (1992). Molecular cloning and primary structure of the human blood group RhD polypeptide. *Proceedings of the National Academy of Science of the USA,* **89**, 10925–9.

6. Avent, N.D. and M.E. Reid (2000). The Rh blood group system: a review. *Blood,* **95**, 375–87.

7. Geifman-Holtzman, O., Wojtowycz, M., Kosmas, E., and Artal, R. (1997). Female alloimmunization with antibodies known to cause hemolytic disease. *Obstetrics and Gynecology*, **89**, 272–5.

8. Mari, G. and for the Collaborative Group for Doppler Assessment of the Blood Velocity in Anemic Fetuses (2000). Noninvasive diagnosis by Doppler ultrasonography of fetal anaemia due to maternal red-cell alloimmunization. *New England Journal of Medicine*, **342**, 9–14.

9. Vaughan, J.I., Warwick, R., Letsky, E.A., Nicolini, U., Rodeck, C.H., and Fisk, N.M. (1994). Erythropoietic suppression in fetal anemia because of Kell alloimmunization. *American Journal of Obstetrics and Gynecology*, **171**, 247–52.

10. Wiener, C.P. and Widness, J.A. (1996). Decreased fetal erythropoiesis and hemolysis in Kell hemolytic anemia. *American Journal of Obstetrics and Gynecology*, **174**, 547–51.

11. Vaughan, J.I., Manning, M., Warwick, R.M., Letsky, E.A., Murray, N.A., and Roberts, I.A.G. (1998). Inhibition of erythroid progenitor cells by anti-Kell antibodies in alloimmune anemia. *New England Journal of Medicine*, **338**, 798–803.

12. Bowman, J.M. (1977). Neonatal management. In *Modern Management of the Rh Problem*, 2nd edn, (ed J.T. Queenan), p. 233. Harper and Row, Hagerstown, MD.

13. Bowman, J.M. and Friesen, R.F. (1976). Rh-isoimmunization. In *Perinatal Medicine*. (ed J. Goodwin, J. Godden, and G. Chance), pp. 92–107. Williams and Wilkins, Baltimore.

14. Woodrow, J. (1970). Rh-immunization and its prevention. *Series Hematologica* (**3**):1–151.
15. Bowman, J., Chown, B., Lewis, M., and Pollock, J. (1978). Rh-immunization during pregnancy: antenatal prophylaxis. *Canadian Medical Association Journal*, **118**, 623–7.
16. Nevanlinna, H. (1953). Factors affecting maternal Rh-immunization. *Annales Medicinae Experimentalis et Biologiae Fenniae (Suppl 2)*, **31**, 1–80.
17. Bowman, J. and Pollock, J. (1965). Amniotic fluid spectrophotometry and early delivery in the management of erythroblastosis fetalis. *Pediatrics*, **35**, 815–35.
18. Clarke, C., Donohoe, W., McConnell, R., Woodrow, J., Finn, R., Krevans, J., *et al.* (1963). Further experimental studies in the prevention of Rh-haemolytic disease. *British Medical Journal*, **i**, 979–84.
19. Freda, V., Gorman, J., and Pollack, W. (1964). Successful prevention of experimental Rh sensitization in man with an anti-Rh gamma 2-globulin antibody preparation: a preliminary report. *Transfusion*, **4**, 26–32.
20. Chown, B., Duff, A., James, J., Nation, E., Ellement, M., Buchanan, D., *et al.* (1969). Prevention of primary Rh-immunization: first report of the Western Canadian Trial, 1966–1968. *Canadian Medical Association Journal*, **100**, 1021–4.
21. Hoppe, H., Mester, T., Hennig, W., and Krebs, H. (1973). Prevention of Rh-immunization: modified production of IgG anti-Rh for intravenous application by ion exchange chromatography (IEC). *Vox Sanguinis*, **25**, 308–16.
22. Bowman, J., Friesen, A., Pollock, J., and Taylor, W. (1980). WinRho: Rh immune globulin prepared by ion exchange for intravenous use. *Canadian Medical Association Journal*, **123**, 1121–5.
23. Letsky, E.A. and de Silva M. (1994). Preventing Rh immunization—much scope for improvement. *British Medical Journal*, **309**, 213–15.
24. Anon. (1979). McMaster Conference on Prevention of Rh Immunization, 28–30 September 1977. *Vox Sanguinis*, **36**, 50–64.
25. Tovey, L.A.D., Townley, A., Stevenson, B.J., and Taverner, J. (1983). The Yorkshire antenatal anti-D immunoglobulin trial in primigravidae. *Lancet*, **ii**, 244–6.
26. Bowman, J. and Pollock, J. (1978). Antenatal Rh prophylaxis: 28 week gestation service program. *Canadian Medical Association Journal*, **118**, 627–30.
27. Robson, S.C., Lee, D., and Urbaniak, S. (1998). Anti-D immunoglobulin in Rh prophylaxis. *British Journal of Obstetrics and Gynaecology*, **105**, 129–34.
28. van Dijk, B. (1997). Preventing RhD haemolytic diesase of the newborn. *British Medical Journal*, **315**, 1480–1.
29. Wallerstein, H. (1946). Treatment of severe erythroblasosis by simultaneous removal and replacement of blood of the newborn. *Science*, **103**, 583–4.
30. Diamond, L., Allen, F., and Thomas, W. (1951). Erythroblastosis fetalis. VII. Treatment with exchange transfusion. *New England Journal of Medicine*, **244**, 39–49.
31. Lucey, J. (1972). Neonatal jaudice and phototherapy. *Pediatric Clinics of North America*, **19**, 827–39.
32. Trolle, D. (1968). Decrease of total serum bilirubin concentration in newborn infants after phenobarbitone treatment. *Lancet*, **ii**, 705–8.
33. Liley, A. (1963). Intrauterine transfusion of fetus in haemolytic disease. *British Medical Journal*, **ii**, 1107–9.
34. Bowman, J., (1990). Treatment options for the fetus with allo-immune hemolytic disease. *Transfusion Medicine Reviews*, **IV**, 191–207.

35. Menticoglou, S., Harman, C., and Manning, F. (1987). Intraperitoneal fetal transfusion: Paralysis inhibits red cell absorption. *Fetal Therapy*, **2**, 154–9.
36. Daffos, F., Capella-Pavlovsky, M., and Forestier, F. (1985). Fetal blood sampling during pregnancy with use of a needle guided by ultrasound: A study of 606 consecutive cases. *American Journal of Obstetrics and Gynecology*, **153**, 655–60.
37. De Crespigny, L., Robinson, H., and Quinn, M. (1985). Ultrasound-guided blood transfusion for severe rhesus isoimmunization. *Obstetrics and Gynecology*, **66**, 529–32.
38. Berkowitz, R., Chitkara, U., and Goldberg, J. (1986). Intrauterine intravascular transfusions for severe red blood cell isoimmunization: Ultrasound-guided percutaneous approach. *American Journal of Obstetrics and Gynecology*, **153**, 574–81.
39. Nicolaides, K., Soothill, P., and Clewell, W. (1986). Rh disease: Intravascular fetal blood transfusion by cordocentesis. *Fetal Therapy*, **1**, 185–92.
40. Harman, C., Bowman, J., Menticoglou, S., and Manning, F. (1988). Profound fetal thrombocytopenia in Rhesus disease: Serious hazard at intravascular transfusion. *Lancet*, **2**, 741–2.
41. Schumacher, B. and Moise, K.J. Jr (1996). Fetal transfusion for red blood cell alloimmunization in pregnancy. *Obstetrics and Gynecology*, **88**, 137–50.
42. Carter, B. (1947). Preliminary report on a substance which inhibits anti-Rh serum. *American Journal of Clinical Pathology*, **17**, 646–9.
43. Gusdon, J., Caudle, M., Herbst, G., and Iannuzzi, N. (1976). Phagocytosis and erythroblastosis: I. Modification of the neonatal response by promethazine hydrochloride. *American Journal of Obstetrics and Gynecology*, **125**, 224–6.
44. Bierme, S., Blanc, M., Abbal, M., and Fournie, A. (1979). Oral Rh treatment for severely immunized mothers. *Lancet*, **i**, 604–5.
45. Rubinstein, A., Eidelman, A., Melamed, J., Gartner, L., Kandall, S., and Schulman, H. (1976). Possible effect of maternal promethazine therapy on neonatal immunologic functions. *Journal of Pediatrics*, **89**, 136–8.
46. Gold, W. Jr, Queenan, J., and Woody, J. (1983). Oral desensitization in Rh disease. *American Journal of Obstetrics and Gynecology*, **146**, 980–1.
47. Bowman, J., Peddle, L., and Anderson, C. (1968). Plasmapheresis in severe Rh-isoimmunization. *Vox Sanguinis*, **15**, 272–7.
48. Graham-Pole, J., Barr, W., and Willoughby, M. (1977). Continuous flow plasmapheresis in management of severe Rhesus disease. *British Medical Journal*, **i**, 1185–8.
49. Isbister, J., Ting, A., and Seeto, K. (1977). Development of Rh-specific maternal auto-antibodies following intensive plasmapheresis for Rh-immunization during pregnancy. *Vox Sanguinis*, **33**, 353–8.
50. Berlin, G., Selbing, A., and Ryden, G. (1985). Rhesus haemolytic disease treated with high dose intravenous immunoglobulin. *Lancet*, **1**, 1153.
51. De la Camara, C., Arrieta, R., Gonzalez, A., Iglesias, E., and Omenaca, F. (1988). High-dose intravenous immunoglobulin as the sole prenatal treatment for severe Rh-immunization. *New England Journal of Medicine*, **318**, 519–20.
52. Margulies, M., Voto, L., Mathet, E., and Margulies, M. (1991). High dose intravenous IgG for the treatment of severe Rhesus alloimmunization. *Vox Sanguinis*, **61**, 181–9.
53. Mitchell, R., Bowell, P., Letsky, E., de Silva, M., and Whittle, M. (1996). Working party of the British Committee for Standards in Haematology Blood Transfusion Task Force. Guidelines for blood grouping and red cell antibody testing during pregnancy. *Transfusion Medicine*, **6**, 71–4.

54. Kleihauer, E., Braun, H., and Betke, K. (1957). Demonstration von fetalem haemoglobin in dem erythrozyten eines blutausstriches. *Klinische Wochenschrifte*, **35**, 637–8.

55. National Blood Transfusion Service Immunoglobulin Working Party (1991). Recommendations for the use of anti-D immunoglobulin. *Prescribers' Journal*, **31**, 137–45.

56. Duguid, J.K.M. and Bromilow, I. (1994). Value of Kleihauer testing after administration of anti-D immunoglobulin. *British Medical Journal*, **309**, 240.

57. Hughes-Jones, N. (1967). The estimation of the concentration and equilibrium constant of anti-D. *Immunology*, **12**, 565–71.

58. Moore, B. (1969). Automation in the blood transfusion laboratory: I. Antibody detection and quantitation in the Technicon AutoAnalyzer. *Canadian Medical Association Journal*, **100**, 381–7.

59. Bennett, P.R., Le Van Kim, C., Colin, Y., *et al.* (1993). Prenatal determination of fetal RhD type by DNA amplification. *New England Journal of Medicine*, **329**, 607–10.

60. Avent, N.D. and Martin, P.G. (1996). Kell typing by allele-specific PCR (ASP). *British Journal of Haematology*, **93**, 728.

61. Hyland, C.A., Wolter, L.C., and Saul, A. (1995). Identification and analysis of Rh genes: application of PCR and RFLP typing tests. *Transfusion Medicine Review*, **IX**, 289–301.

62. Lo, Y-M.D., Bowell, P.J., Selinger, M., *et al.* (1993). Prenatal determination of fetal RhD status by analysis of peripheral blood of rhesus negative mothers. *Lancet*, **341**, 1147–8.

63. Lo, Y.M.D., Corbetta, N., *et al.* (1997). Presence of fetal DNA in maternal plasma and serum. *Lancet*, **350**, 485–7.

64. Bevis, D. (1956). Blood pigments in haemolytic disease of the newborn. *Journal of Obstetrics and Gynaecology of the British Empire*, **63**, 68–75.

65. Liley, A. (1961). Liquor amnii analysis in management of the pregnancy complicated by rhesus sensitization. *American Journal of Obstetrics and Gynecology*, **82**, 1359–71.

66. Bowman, J. (1978). Management of Rh-isoimmunization. *Obstetrics and Gynecology*, **52**, 1–16.

67. Bartsch, F. (1971). Bilirubin in the amniotic fluid. A review. *Annals of Obstetrics and Gynecology*, **92**, 482–92.

68. Rehder, H. and Weitzel, H. (1978). Intrauterine amputations after amniocentesis. *Lancet*, **i**, 382.

69. Mollison, P. (1991). Results of tests with different cellular bioassays in relation to severity of RhD haemolytic disease. Report from nine collaborating laboratories. *Vox Sanguinis*, **60**, 225–9.

70. Bowman, J. and Pollock, J. *Annual Report of the Winnipeg Rh Laboratory to the Health Sciences Centre and Provincial Department of Health*. Manitoba Government, 1 Nov 1989—31 Oct 1990.

71. DHSS (1976). *Haemolytic Disease of the Newborn*. Department of Health and Social Security, London.

72. Clarke, C.A., Whitfield, A.G.W., and Mollison, P.L. (1987). Deaths from Rh haemolytic disease in England and Wales in 1984 and 1985. *British Medical Journal*, **294**, 1001.

73. CESDI (1995). *Confidential Enquiry into Stillbirths and Deaths in Infancy*. Department of Health, London.

74. Whitfield, C.R., Raafat, A., and Urbaniak, S.J. (1997). Underreporting of mortality from RhD haemolytic disease in Scotland and its implications: retrospective review. *British Medical Journal*, **315**, 1504–5.

75. Tovey, G. (1980). Should anti-D immunoglobulin be given antenatally? *Lancet*, **ii**, 466–8.
76. Tovey, L. and Taverner, J. (1981). A case for the antenatal administration of anti-D immunoglobulin to primigravidae. *Lancet*, **i**, 878–81.
77. Bowman, J.M. and Pollock, J.M. (1987). Failures of intravenous Rh immune prophylaxis: an analysis of the reasons for such failures. *Transfusion Medicine Review*, **1**, 101–12.
78. Royal College of Obstetricians and Gynaecologists (1999). Use of anti-D immunoglobulin for Rh prophylaxis. *Green Top Guidelines No. 22*. London, The Royal College of Obstetricians and Gynaecologists.
79. Race, R. and Sanger, R. (1950). Introduction. In: *Blood Groups in Man*. Blackwell Scientific, Oxford, 1950, 2–3.
80. Lewis, M. and Chown, B. (1957). A short albumin method for the determination of isohemagglutinins, particularly incomplete Rh antibodies. *Journal of Laboratory and Clinical Medicine*, **50**, 494–7.
81. Coombs, R., Mourant, A., and Race, R. (1945). A new test for the detection of weak and 'incomplete' Rh agglutinins. *British Journal of Experimental Pathology*, **26**, 255–60.
82. Lewis, M. and Kaita, H. Two stage papain capillary method. Unpublished.
83. Rosenfield, R. and Haber, G. (1965). Detection and measurement of homologous human hemagglutinins. Automation in analytical chemistry. *Technicon Symposia*, 503–6.
84. Lalezari, P. (1968). A new method for detection of red blood cell antibodies. *Transfusion*, **8**, 372–80.
85. Lewis, M., Kaita, H., and Chown, B. (1958). Kell typing in the capillary tube. *Journal of Laboratory and Clinical Medicine*, **50**, 163–8.
86. Nicolaides, K., Rodeck, C., Mibashan, M., and Kemp, J. (1986). Have Liley charts outlived their usefulness? *American Journal of Obstetrics and Gynecology*, **155**, 90–4
87. Bowman, J. (1977). Rh-isoimmunization. *Modern Medicine of Canada*, **32**, 17–25.
88. Letsky, E.A. (1995). Haematological disorders. In: *Prenatal Diagnosis in Obstetric Practice*, (ed. M.J. Whittle and J.M. Connor), 2nd edn, pp. 74–7. Blackwell Scientific, Oxford.

13 *Cystic fibrosis*

David J. H. Brock

INTRODUCTION

Cystic fibrosis (CF) is the most common life-shortening Mendelian disorder found in children and in young adults of Caucasian descent. It was first clearly described by Anderson[1] as 'cystic fibrosis of the pancreas', although the name was subsequently shortened to cystic fibrosis. An autosomal recessive mode of inheritance was suggested in the late 1940s[2] and is now universally accepted.

Attempts to locate the primary defect in CF by comparison of protein differences in affected and non-affected tissues were routinely unsuccessful over a 40-year period of intense investigation. Despite these failures it was still possible to develop practical methods of both neonatal screening[3] and second trimester antenatal diagnosis,[4] based on quite specific but secondary disturbances in the biochemistry of affected tissues. However, it was the application of molecular genetic techniques, and in particular the powerful technology of positional cloning, that led to the successful identification of the CF gene in 1989.[5-7]

THE DISORDER

On the basis of anatomical findings, cystic fibrosis was at first thought to involve primarily the pancreas and secondarily the pulmonary system. With the demonstration of consistent abnormalities of sweat and salivary gland excretions in 1953,[8] it became evident that the disease was in reality based on a more generalized disorder of most, and perhaps all, exocrine glands. The triad of chronic pulmonary disease, pancreatic insufficiency, and abnormally elevated sweat electrolytes is present in most patients. Major clinical findings are progressive bronchiolar obstruction with complicating pulmonary infection, meconium ileus, steatorrhoea, and growth retardation. Hepatic cirrhosis, intestinal obstruction, nasal polyps, and rectal prolapse may further complicate the picture. The majority of clinically significant abnormalities are thought to be due to obstruction of organ ducts (bronchioles, pancreatic ducts, and biliary ductules) by abnormal secretions.[9]

Description

CF presents in a variety of ways, and although usually diagnosed within the first few years of life, may escape detection until the second or later decades. In early infancy a majority of patients present with a combination of respiratory symptoms, failure to thrive, and steatorrhea. Some 10 to 15 per cent of newborns with CF have meconium ileus, and this is virtually diagnostic. A family history of the disorder should alert the paediatrician to search for more subtle presenting features. Isolation of *P. aeruginosa*, particularly in the mucoid form, from the lower respiratory tract of a child or young adult almost always signals CF.[9]

Abnormally high concentrations of sodium and chloride ions in the sweat of CF patients were first noted by di Sant'Agnese *et al.*[8] Although the sweat test is not without problems, a standard procedure in which sweating is stimulated by pilocarpine iontophoresis has become the primary laboratory test for CF. A sweat chloride concentration greater than 60 mEq/l., when found in association with other pulmonary manifestations, gastrointestinal symptoms, or history of CF in the immediate family, constitutes a certain diagnosis of the disorder.

The cloning of the CF gene[5-7] introduced a new laboratory method of diagnosis which can be absolutely definitive. However, as outlined below, there are a large number of mutant CF alleles, not all of which have been identified. The most prevalent of these, ΔF508, is found on 70 to 85 per cent of CF chromosomes in populations of north European ancestry.[10] Homozygosity for this allele makes a diagnosis of CF inescapable. Homozygosity or compound heterozygosity for any other defined CF mutant allele (or alleles) is equally definitive. However, the inability to detect two copies of a defined mutant allele in an individual thought to have CF does not constitute a diagnostic exclusion.

Birth prevalence

For a genetic disorder, CF is unusually common in Caucasian populations. Epidemiological surveys show a birth prevalence ranging from about 1 in 1700 to about 1 in 6500,[9] but many of these are bedevilled by incomplete ascertainment. Newborn screening using the serum immunoreactive trypsin (IRT) method is thought to have a sensitivity of 90 to 95 per cent and has tended to show slightly higher birth prevalences.[11] There is now abundant evidence that the disease is caused by mutant alleles at a single genetic locus.[12] Thus if the birth prevalence in the UK population is assumed to be 1 in 2500,[13] the gene frequency is 0.02 and the heterozygote frequency 0.04 or 1 in 25. This accords with data emerging from recently completed pilot trials of population carrier detection[14] (see, for example, Tables 13.4, and 13.5).

Prognosis

The prognosis for an individual born with CF is variable, ranging from death due to complications of meconium ileus in the neonatal period through to survival to age 40 or 50. A survey made by the British Paediatric Association covering 1977 to 1985 suggested a median survival in the UK for boys of 21 years and for girls of 19 years.[13] Statistics from the Cystic Fibrosis Foundation indicate that in 1991 the median survival age in the USA was 30.6 years for males and 28.2 years for females.[9] An analysis of mortality data has projected that a child born with CF in the UK in 1990 may have a life expectancy of 40 years.[15]

Molecular biology

The CF gene is localized on the long arm of chromosome 7. It spans some 230 kb of genomic DNA and contains 27 exons. The gene product, the cystic fibrosis trans-membrane conductance regulator (CFTR), is expressed in those tissues primarily involved in the disease process, such as pancreas, nasal polyps, lung, colon, sweat glands, placenta, liver, and parotid gland. It is a protein with a calculated molecular mass of 170 000, showing strong homology with a class of ATP-dependent membrane transport proteins.[5-7] Unfortunately, CFTR is not expressed in accessible tissues such as red or white blood cells, and this means that tracking the CF gene through protein assays is impractical.

The predominant mutant allele at the CF locus is a three base-pair deletion in exon 10, which removes a phenylalanine residue at position 508 of the 1480 amino acid sequence of CFTR. This allele, known as ΔF508 (F is the single letter code for pheny-lalanine), makes up 50 to 90 per cent of mutations in Caucasian populations (Table 13.1).[10,16] In the British Isles published figures are England (76 per cent), Scotland (74 per cent), Republic of Ireland (76 per cent), and Northern Ireland (54 per cent). It must be noted that these are the proportions of ΔF508 on single CF chromosomes, and that figures for homozygosity (i.e. affected individuals with both chromosomes carrying ΔF508) are obtained by squaring the ΔF508 proportions.

It is now known that CF is an extremely heterogeneous condition at the DNA level. Over 500 different mutant alleles have been described.[17] Many are extremely rare and have been found in one or a handful of patients. With the exception of ΔF508 only a

Table 13.1 Worldwide geographic distribution of the ΔF508 mutant allele[10,16]

Country	CF chromosomes	
	Total	ΔF508 (%)
North America		
Caucasian, non-Ashkenazi	3193	2240 (70)
Black	169	60 (36)
Ashkenazi	95	30 (32)
Europe		
Denmark	586	511 (87)
Netherlands	1043	804 (77)
England	6085	4560 (75)
Belgium	982	734 (75)
Wales	341	245 (72)
Germany	3046	2166 (71)
France	5158	3595 (70)
Czechoslovakia	490	336 (69)
Scotland	836	571 (68)
Republic of Ireland	292	199 (68)
Switzerland	402	270 (67)
Northern Ireland	456	258 (57)
Bulgaria	202	112 (55)
Greece	326	173 (53)
Spain	1308	695 (53)
Italy	2331	1146 (49)

few have been found at frequencies of more than 1 per cent in the British population. Table 13.2, showing data for Scotland,[18] is probably representative of most of the UK.

SCREENING AND DIAGNOSIS

The tests

It is possible to detect both normal and mutant CF alleles on any tissue which contains nucleated cells; in practice this means any tissue with the exception of mature red blood cells. Adequate amounts of DNA for the purpose of diagnosis can be extracted from 10 ml of whole blood or from 10 mg of a chorionic villus biopsy. For screening, a mouthwash sample, obtained by swilling out the mouth with 10 to 20 ml of isotonic saline, isotonic sucrose, distilled, or even tap water, provides enough buccal cells for subsequent amplification of the DNA content. A mouthwash sample is in effect a self-administered buccal scrape and may sometimes fail; for this reason a spatula scrape gives more reliable material. DNA may also be amplified from dried blood spots or exfoliated cells in urine samples, and (if need be) from histological and archival specimens.

Laboratory detection of CF alleles is nearly always performed after prior amplification of the portion of the CF gene in which the relevant mutation lies. The standard technique used is the polymerase chain reaction (PCR), which employs a heat-stable DNA polymerase to produce between 10^7 and 10^9 copies of the target DNA sequence in a few hours. Commercial PCR-based kits for detection of the more common CF alleles (especially ΔF508) are now marketed. Not only is the PCR a quick and easy procedure, but it may also be applied to samples with an extremely low DNA content.

A disadvantage of the PCR is that it is most efficiently carried out when the target DNA sequence is comparatively small, ideally not more than 500 base pairs. The CF gene, in common with most other genes in higher organisms, is made up of small exons separated by large intervening sequences (introns) which are spliced out during RNA processing and therefore not translated into the amino acids of the CFTR protein. Mutant CF alleles are scattered through the different exons and also at the beginnings and endings of introns (where they interfere with correct RNA processing) in such a way that no single PCR amplification can cover all the points of mutation. In

Table 13.2   Percentage frequency of the more common CF alleles in the Scottish population[18]

Allele	Frequency
ΔF508	74.2
G551D	5.9
G542X	3.7
R117H	1.2
1717–1G→A	1.0
A455E	0.6
N1303K	0.4
621+1G→T	0.4
ΔI507	0.4
R560T	0.2
W1282X	0.2
S549N	0.2

fact it is generally appropriate to amplify each exon (and if appropriate the adjacent intronic regions) in a separate PCR reaction, before searching for the presence or absence of a specific mutation.

Once the target DNA sequence has been amplified, the mutant CF allele may be detected by a number of procedures. In the case of the predominant ΔF508 allele (which encompasses a three base pair deletion), the amplified material will be smaller than the normal allele by three nucleotides, and this difference can be directly visualized after electrophoresis and staining of products on an acrylamide gel.[19-21] There is a further advantage in this technique. Individuals who are ΔF508/normal heterozygotes not only show both ΔF508 and normal bands on the gel, but also a characteristic pair of heteroduplex bands which migrate more slowly (Fig. 8.1).[22] These are non-covalent interactions between the different DNA fragments, with conformational changes resulting from incomplete annealing of the non-identical strands. A slightly different heteroduplex band is seen in the amplified DNA of an individual who is heterozygous for the ΔI507 and normal alleles.[18] Thus although it is not possible, by gel electrophoresis alone, to distinguish ΔF508/ΔF508 homozygotes from ΔI507/ΔI507 homozygotes or from ΔF508/ΔI507 compound heterozygotes, it is possible to distinguish ΔF508/normal and ΔI507/normal heterozygotes (Fig. 13.1). This is particularly useful when screening for CF carrier status.

A second procedure for detecting CF mutations employs the precise specificity of restriction enzyme digestion. If a mutation either destroys an existing restriction endonuclease recognition site, or alternatively creates a new one, it is possible to generate different size fragments from the normal and mutant alleles. An example is shown in Fig. 13.2 of detection of three specific mutations in exon 11.[23] The PCR amplification produces a product of 425 base pairs, which in normal alleles can be cleaved by both *Dde*I and *Hinc*II. In the S549N mutation the *Dde*I restriction site is

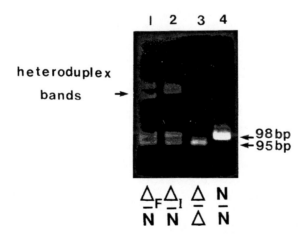

Fig. 13.1 Amplication of a portion of exon 10 to show the ΔF508 (ΔF) and ΔI507 (ΔI) mutations. The two different heterozygous states (ΔF/N and ΔI/N) can be distinguished by the different appearance of heteroduplex bands. Homozygotes for either deletion can be distinguished from homozygotes for the normal allele (N/N), but not from one another or from the ΔF/ΔI compound heterozygote; hence Δ/Δ in the figure. (Courtesy of Dr A Shrimpton.)

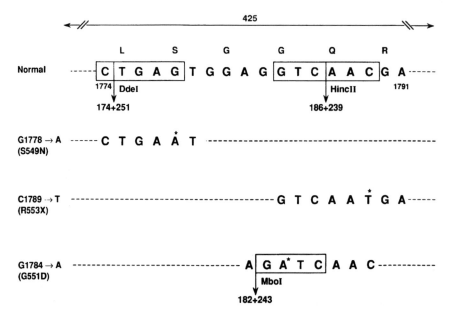

Fig. 13.2 Use of differential restriction enzyme digestion to detect mutations in exon 11 of the CF gene. The normal sequence contains recognition sites for *Dde*I and *Hinc*II (boxes). In the S549N mutation a G→A change abolishes the *Dde*I site and in R553X a C→T change abolishes the *Hinc*II site. In the G551D mutation a G→A change also abolishes the *Hinc*II site but creates a new cleavage site for *Mbo*I.

abolished by a G→A change at nucleotide 1778. In both R553X and G551D mutations the *Hinc*II restriction site is destroyed, the former by a C→T change at nucleotide 1789, and the latter by a G→A change at nucleotide 1784. However, in the latter the G→A change creates a novel *Mbo*I restriction site, which is not present in either the normal or the S549N and R553X alleles. Thus if exon 11 is amplified and the resulting sample digested with *Dde*I, *Hinc*II, and *Mbo*I, the size of the fragments will reveal the presence or absence of these three mutant alleles.

A third method of detection uses hybridization to allele-specific oligonucleotides. For each specific mutation it is necessary to synthesize two short oligonucleotides, one exactly complementary to the region surrounding the mutation and the other exactly complementary to the equivalent region in the normal allele. Under conditions of high stringency (i.e. designed to permit hybridization when sequences are exactly complementary), the oligonucleotides will only anneal to their respective counterparts. Most individuals in a screened population will show a hybridization signal with the normal oligonucleotide, while heterozygotes for the specific mutation will produce signals with both oligonucleotides.

It is also possible to detect mutations by altering the specificity of the PCR in such a way that only the normal or only the mutant allele is amplified. This is referred to either as the amplification refractory mutation system (ARMS)[24] or as allele-specific amplification. The method requires synthesis of three amplification primers, one reverse primer complementary to the normal allele, one reverse primer complementary to the mutant allele, and one forward primer complementary to both alleles

(Fig. 13.3). Two separate amplifications are carried out, differing in the forward primer used, but each having the common reverse primer. DNA from normal homozygotes is only amplified in the reaction containing the complementary forward primer. The same is true for DNA from individuals homozygous for the mutation, although one would not expect to encounter these in screening a general population. DNA from individuals heterozygous for the specific mutation would be amplified in both reactions. Amplification products are inspected after electrophoresis on agarose gels and ethidium bromide staining.

It will be apparent from the above discussion that attempts to detect more than just the predominant ΔF508 allele are likely to become quite complicated. Two simplifying procedures are available. The first is to amplify several exons simultaneously (multiplexing) and then to sort out the products by electrophoresis, restriction enzyme digestion, or allele-specific hybridization. The second is to concentrate on those CF alleles at highest frequency in the population being screened, and to design ARMS primers capable of selective amplification. The latter procedure—multiplex ARMS—has the virtue of being suitable for commercial kits. An example of a multiplex ARMS,[25] designed to detect ΔF508, G551D, G542X, and 621+1G→T, is shown in Fig. 13.4. It must be noted, however, that multiplex ARMS can only detect the specific

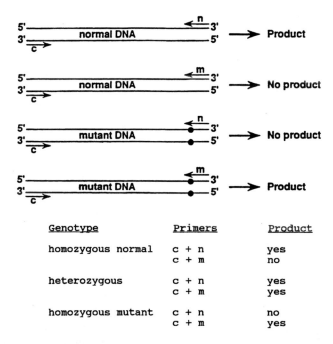

Genotype	Primers	Product
homozygous normal	c + n	yes
	c + m	no
heterozygous	c + n	yes
	c + m	yes
homozygous mutant	c + n	no
	c + m	yes

Fig. 13.3 Principle of the allele-specific amplification or ARMS technique. The common primer is marked by 'c', the normal primer by 'n' and the mutant primer by 'm'. Since it will not be known whether the target DNA is normal or mutant, two reactions are carried out, one having 'c' and 'n' primers and the other 'c' and 'm' primers. 5' and 3' indicate different ends of the DNA strand.

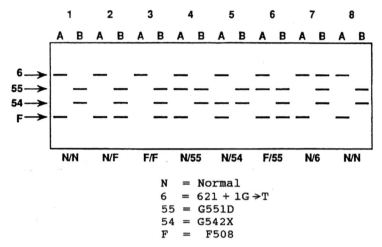

Fig. 13.4 A multiplex ARMS system for the detection of four CF mutant alleles: 621+1G→T (6), G551D (55), G542X (54), and ΔF508 (F). Each sample is run in two tubes, A and B, both of which contain a set of forward primers that will amplify the segments of DNA that include the four specified alleles when complementary reverse primers are present. Tube A contains reverse primers complementary to the 621+1G→T and ΔF508 *normal* sequences and reverse primers complementary to the G551D and G542X *mutant* sequences. Tube B contains reverse primers complementary to the G551D and G542X *normal* sequences and reverse primers complementary to the ΔF508 and 621+1G→T *mutant* sequences. Thus samples 1 and 8 show a pattern of four bands indicating normality at each of the four sequences, i.e. a normal homozygote. The appearance of extra bands in either tube A or B signals a heterozygote (samples 2, 4, 5, and 7). For an affected homozygote (e.g. sample 3) there are both additional and missing bands. For a compound heterozygote (e.g sample 6), there are additional bands in both tubes.

mutations for which it is designed. In contrast exon multiplexing can in theory detect any mutation in the amplified exons.

Antenatal screening

Objectives of screening

There is considerable confusion and some disagreement about the objectives of screening for CF, and indeed for any other serious disorder inherited as an autosomal recessive trait. Many geneticists take the view that screening programmes should be set up in such a way as to offer 'reproductive options' to heterozygous carriers of a single mutant gene.[26] This means that testing must be carried out at an early enough stage for carriers to be able to contemplate and select one of a number of choices, which include foregoing reproduction altogether, selecting a partner who is not a carrier of a mutant gene at the same locus, or embarking on a pregnancy as a result of artificial insemination by a screened donor. In practice, experience with other screening programmes, such as β thalassamia[27] or Tay–Sachs disease,[28] points strongly to the fact that very few heterozygotes select any of these somewhat idealized reproductive options. The desire to have a child by a partner chosen for non-genetic reasons is sufficiently strong for most heterozygous couples to accept their high-risk status and to seek to avoid the birth of an affected child through antenatal diagnosis and termination of pregnancy.[29]

If this is indeed the case, the primary objective of screening becomes allowing high-risk couples the opportunity of avoiding the birth of an affected child. Some couples may choose to close their eyes to their 1 in 4 risk and simply take a chance; such behaviour may be important in communities where religious beliefs forbid termination of pregnancy or where there is controversy about the long-term burden of the disease in question. Screening must reflect the choice of parents—if a large proportion choose not to be screened, a programme may need to be abandoned. No government would be prepared to finance screening programmes where a substantial proportion of heterozygous couples did not take the opportunities offered by prenatal diagnosis.

From a practical point of view there are therefore two closely-linked aims to screening—allowing couples to choose not to have an affected child and reducing the birth prevalence of the disorder. Stating the objectives in this way makes it easier to plan a screening programme and to assess its impact. Not only must the option of avoiding the birth of affected children be realistically presented, but the option must be as widely available to the targeted group as is practical.[29] Presenting a programme to a limited group of participants, selected by social class or educational advantage, should be avoided. Screening of this kind is by its nature inequitable and in the long run likely to be invalidated by its failure to reach a substantial portion of the population.

When to screen

There are several potential groups within the population at whom screening for CF could be targeted. A distinction must be made between screening at any stage *before* pregnancy, when the initial objective is to identify heterozygotes, and screening *during* pregnancy, when the initial objective is to identify heterozygous couples. As the end-goal is detection of a CF fetus, screening during pregnancy will inevitably be a more efficient process. Nonetheless, since any well-directed programme of screening before pregnancy could lead to identification of at-risk couples within a partnership planning a pregnancy, this approach is worth serious consideration.

Some thought has been given to the idea of screening neonates to identify heterozygotes. It is a superficially attractive idea since birth and death are the only universal turnstiles through which everyone passes and the entire target population could be easily reached. Detection of CF heterozygotes could be added to neonatal Guthrie card screening for phenylketonuria and thus carried on the back of an existing collection, analysis, and reporting system. However, it would create formidable problems in counselling, since CF heterozygosity is not a disorder and only of consequence in certain limited situations. Furthermore, the benefits of such screening would not be realized for several decades, and there would be inevitable problems in ensuring that knowledge of CF heterozygote status was transmitted to the screened child and retained until deemed useful. There are intractable ethical problems in even contemplating such screening, an issue which is already troubling directors of programmes of neonatal CF homozygote screening (see the section on neonatal screening for CF).

One of the models of screening for an autosomal recessive disorder, Tay–Sachs disease, has selected young people in secondary schools as the initial target for heterozygote detection.[30] Participation in this programme was enthusiastic and some 80 per cent of the target group (Ashkenazi Jews) elected to be tested. However, although a follow-up study[31] some eight years later suggested that screened individuals had positive attitudes to their earlier testing and were making appropriate use of the information, the response rate was low (42 per cent), presumably due to population mobility. This programme has attracted adverse comment, not all of it well informed.[32,33] Nonetheless, many doubts must remain about the suitability of this target group for screening. Parental consent would be needed for those under 16, and as there is a pronounced social class bias towards early school-leaving, there would inevitably be a large majority of tested candidates in the educationally (and probably socially) advantaged groups.

Another model for screening is to offer carrier testing through community health services such as general practitioners, family planning clinics, or (in the USA) health maintenence organizations. Several reports of trials of this form of delivery for CF screening have appeared.[34–36] In each case it was found that the take-up of screening depended on whether the offer was made by personal intervention or by a postal invitation (Table 13.3). Acceptance rates of around 70 per cent were achieved when there was face-to-face explanation of the purposes and scope of screening to the targeted group by a dedicated researcher. Mail-shots elicited responses of below 10 per cent. These trials confirm that an offer of screening is best received when made in person and particularly in the context of planned reproduction. However, the resource implications are considerable if every general practice, family planning clinic, or health maintenace organization needs a dedicated counsellor to present the advantages and disadvantages. It is also difficult to get a realistic idea of the outreach of this form of delivery.

Cascade 'screening'

Most genetic centres now offer testing for CF heterozygosity to relatives of affected individuals. In general such programmes are reactive, and respond to requests for such tests. Super and colleagues[37] have proposed a more proactive approach, taking screening out into the population by focussing on the relatives of index cases. They argue

Table 13.3   Take-up rates of CF heterozygote testing in primary care

Approach to identified target group	Take-up (%)
Watson et al.[34]	
Opportunistic screening, general practice	340/513 (66)
Opportunistic screening, family planning clinics	371/431 (87)
Invitation letter, general practice	87/852 (10)
Bekker et al.[35]	
Letter at beginning of trial in one general practice	59/502 (12)
Letter and booklet	47/496 (9)
Passive opportunistic	81/471 (17)
Active opportunistic—test now	453/649 (70)
Active opportunistic—test at return visit	22/88 (25)
Letter at end of trial	128/2953 (4)
Tambor et al.[36]	
Mailed invitation	101/2713 (4)
On-site invitation	143/608 (24)

that the ratio of carriers detected to people tested will be higher this way, that only one or two mutant alleles need be screened for, and that less anxiety would be generated among the screened population.

In a pilot trial Super *et al.*[37] tested 1563 relatives and partners of subjects in 129 index families in which CF was segregating. In the group of 1563 they identified 15 heterozygous couples (1 per cent), in eight of whom prenatal diagnosis was carried out. By extrapolating to a total of 10 000 relatives and partners, it was suggested that 100 heterozygous couples would be detected and 25 affected fetuses found. It was claimed that this was equal to the number of CF children born annually in the region, and that proactive cascade testing was a genuine substitute for what they call 'unfocussed' screening.

There is no doubt that CF cascade testing is an effective way of identifying large numbers of carriers and carrier couples with a great deal less effort than in any standard population screening. However, it is not screening in any conventional sense of the word, nor can it have a major impact on the birth prevalence of affected cases. Inspection of the data presented by Super *et al.* shows why this is so. Among the relatives tested no fewer than 427/1122 (38 per cent) were carriers. Thus the study was concentrating predominantly on close relatives. In the next phase, as the cascade moves to more distant relatives of the index case, the proportion of carriers detected will drop. It is thus misleading to extrapolate the figure of 1 per cent for heterozygous couples found in the easy part of the programme to more difficult parts. Furthermore, it cannot be assumed that all heterozygous couples would be planning pregnancies, or that all would seek antenatal diagnosis and act on the results. In fact of the 15 heterozygous couples reported by Super *et al.*, one had completed their family and another five did not request antenatal diagnosis. This contrasts with the 22 heterozygous couples detected through our antenatal screening programmes, all of whom have requested prenatal diagnosis.[14]

It is impossible to measure the theoretical effectiveness of cascade testing by simple extrapolation. It is necessary to create models with family size distributions and alternative testing stategies. Our projections,[38] using such modelling, suggest that fewer than 25 per cent of heterozygous couples could be detected by cascading to the second cousin level. In contrast, we have already shown that over 50 per cent of heterozygous couples can be detected by either of the two major forms of antenatal screening. Thus cascade testing may be seen as a useful adjunct to population screening but certainly not as a substitute for it.

Screening during pregnancy

Two different forms of wide-scale screening during pregnancy have been tested in trial projects. For convenience they will be referred to as 'two-step' (or 'sequential') and 'couple' screening. In both forms the objective is to identify heterozygous couples who can be offered antenatal diagnosis and (if necessary) termination of pregnancy. However, the two forms differ considerably in their mode of delivery, their use of resources, and in their side-effects.

Two-step screening

In this form of screening the primary target is the pregnant woman. In the UK she is most easily identified when she attends a hospital antenatal clinic, although in other countries such as the USA the obstetrician's office will be a more suitable venue. In view of the fact that CF is a disorder with highest incidence in groups of Caucasian background, it is possible to introduce a pre-screening step which seeks information on the woman's (and her partner's) ethnic antecedents. However, in view of our relative ignorance about CF heterozygote frequencies in non-Caucasian populations, it is probably unwise to exclude women from testing simply because they are not Caucasians. In the Edinburgh screening trial[39] the offer of testing was only *not* made when the woman's command of the English language was inadequate for her to understand all the possible consequences of screening. Obviously if a woman is unable to identify the biological father of her child, the offer of heterozygote testing must be seen as having a different aim.

Women who elect to be screened are tested for the more prevalent mutant CF alleles in the population. It is comparatively easy in the UK to exclude about 85 per cent of CF alleles by concentrating on six of the mutations listed in Table 13.2. Figure 13.5 is a flow chart of the results to be expected with this approach. A woman who is negative on the primary screen has a risk of bearing a CF child which has reduced from 1 in 2500 to 1 in 16 100 (i.e. (400–340)/(1 000 000—34 000)). Such women are reassured and no attempt made to test their partners.

A woman who is positive on the primary screen is, of course, a CF carrier, with an immediate 1 in 100 (i.e. 340/34 000) chance of bearing an affected child. Testing her partner and finding him to be negative reduces the risk to about 1 in 650 (i.e. (340–289)/34 000). If her partner is positive, the couple's risk of bearing a CF child is 1 in 4, and an offer of prenatal diagnosis is immediately made. If 85 per cent of CF alleles are detectable it is theoretically possible to identify 72 per cent (85 per cent × 85 per cent) of affected fetuses.

When screening during pregnancy was first contemplated there was some discussion of the problem of couples in which the woman tested as a carrier and the man as a non-carrier. It was pointed out that the residual risk of a CF child was greater than

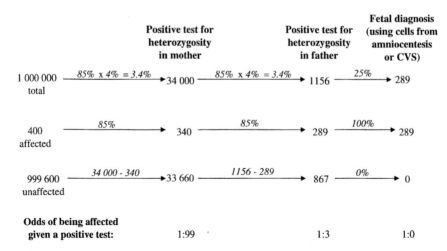

Fig. 13.5 Flow diagram for two-step screening for CF during pregnancy, using a procedure which tests for the six most frequent mutations.

the pre-testing population risk of 1 in 2500. For example, if 15 per cent of male carriers were missed, the prevalence of missed carriers among all males would be 0.6 per cent (i.e. 15 per cent of 4 per cent), and the proportion of carrier women's children who would be affected as a result of having a missed carrier father would be 0.15 per cent (i.e. one-quarter of 0.6 per cent). The term 'genetic limbo' was coined for positive/negative couples,[40] and it was suggested that screening should be delayed until at least 96 per cent of CF alleles were detectable.[41] At this point positive/negative couples would have a residual risk of 1 in 2500, and directors of screening programmes could be satisfied that no couples had been disadvantaged by the screening process.

A number of ideas have been floated in an attempt to deal with the problem of positive/negative couples. One is the concept of couple screening,[42] discussed in the next section. Another is the possibility of offering positive/negative couples second-trimester amniocentesis either with microvillar enzyme testing alone or with microvillar enzyme testing combined with mutation analysis on amniotic fluid cells. Unfortunately, the imperfect sensitivity (about 95 per cent) and specificity (about 92 per cent) of microvillar enzyme testing[3] makes this ancillary procedure unsatisfactory in pregnancies with relatively low risks of affected outcome. It is, of course, possible to exclude the risk of CF in half such pregnancies by demonstrating that the fetus has not inherited the maternal mutant allele. However, over 3 per cent of all pregnancies would have to undergo amniocentesis, and this would constitute an unacceptable burden for obstetric services.

In the Edinburgh two-step trial the issue of positive/negative couples was approached by changing the emphasis of the preliminary information leaflet. It was pointed out that any woman found to be a carrier had a CF gene segregating in her immediate family, and that her sibs and more distant relatives might wish to avail themselves of carrier testing.[43] The carrier herself was reminded that she had a 1 in 100 risk of bearing an affected child, but that the risk could be reduced some six-fold by testing her partner. Although this is a less than ideal approach to the problem, the carrier women identified reported that they were quite satisfied by their relative reduction in risk. Data on anxiety testing, using a series of well-established instruments, confirmed that the reported sense of reassurance was quite genuine.[44,45]

Four different trials of two-step antenatal screening have been reported. Jung *et al.*[46] recorded a take-up of 99 per cent among 638 women in East Berlin, Miedzybrodszka *et al.*[47] a take-up of 91 per cent among 1641 women in Aberdeen, Schwartz *et al.*[48] a take-up of 80 per cent among 3054 women in Copenhagen, and Mennie *et al.*[39] a take-up of 71 per cent among 7011 women in Edinburgh (Table 13.4).

Couple screening

The concept of couple screening was first proposed by Wald.[42] Since a CF fetus can arise only when each partner contributes a mutant allele, the screening unit should be seen as the couple rather than the individual parent. Testing is only carried out when samples are received from both parents. Analysis is performed initially on only one of the two samples (either maternal or paternal), and if it is negative for CF alleles the other sample is not tested. If the sample is positive the partner is also tested. However, positive/negative couples are treated as low risk, and their residual chance of carrying

Table 13.4 Completed results of Edinburgh two-step antenatal screening trial[39]

	No.	% of total	% of those offered screening
Woman attending clinics	7011	100	
Not eligible for screening	981	14	
Late gestation	701		
Abnormal pregnancy	125		
Partner unavailable	124		
Other	31		
Eligible for screening	6030	86	100
Declined screening	1052	15	17
Screened	4978	71	83
Carrier women identified	190[1]		
Carrier partners screened	189		
Heterozygous couples	7		
Affected fetuses	2		

[1] At 85 per cent detection rate this indicates a true carrier frequency of 4.5 per cent, or 1 in 22 (i.e. $190/4978 \times 100/85$).

a CF fetus not reported as such, but rather 'buried' in the composite risk to couples who are not heterogyzous for the mutations covered by the test. All couples are therefore divided into two classes: those with a 1 in 4 risk who are offered prenatal diagnosis and those with a composite risk for whom no further action is needed. Figure 8.6 is a flow chart of the results to be expected with this approach, and suggests that the risk to those not offered fetal diagnosis is 1 in 9000 (i.e. $(400-289)/(1000\,000-1156)$).

When the idea of couple screening was first proposed, it met with some hostility. Some of the opposition was based on disagreements about the purpose of antenatal screening; whether it was designed to identify CF heterozygotes or CF fetuses. There were also some worries about the deliberate withholding of information about CF heterozygote status from individuals in the positive/negative couples. However, it now seems to be generally accepted that the primary purpose of antenatal screening is to offer heterozygous couples the chance of avoiding the birth of a child with a serious disorder and that identification of individual parental heterozygosity is a secondary feature of uncertain benefit. Furthermore, since it has become clear that there are no practical actions that can be taken to reduce the risk of affected fetuses in positive/negative couples, it can hardly be claimed that they are harmed by withholding information which is likely to be anxiety-provoking.

Couple screening has considerable advantages in terms of the resources needed for such programmes. Experience in the Edinburgh two-step trial showed that the counselling of women identified as heterozygotes was time-consuming and that some became anxious while waiting for their partners to be tested. Several women needed more than one counselling session in this interim period, and there was great pressure on staff to collect the partner's sample and test it as quickly as possible. This problem is avoided when the couple is treated as a unit.

Another objection to couple screening was that the take-up of testing might be much lower than that experienced in the two-step model. In the Edinburgh two-step

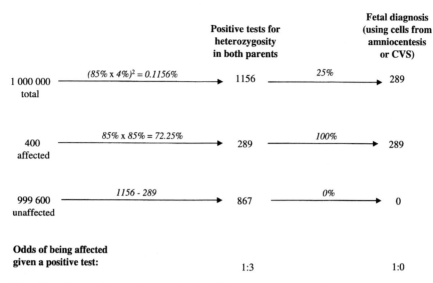

Fig. 13.6 Flow diagram for couple screening for CF during pregnancy, using a procedure which tests for the six most frequent mutations.

trial some 86 per cent of eligible pregnant women attending the antenatal clinics accepted the offer of screening (Table 13.4). Of these 40 per cent claimed to have made the decision to opt into the trial without reference to their partner.[43] Nonetheless, of the 190 female heterozygotes identified, all but one produced a partner or a partner's sample within a week of the test result. This suggests that female motivation is a powerful factor in antenatal screening and that if the decision to be screened were to be made jointly by the couple the take-up might be substantially less.

These problems have now been answered by a number of practical screening trials. The largest, carried out in Edinburgh, is summarized in Table 13.5. The offer of screening was made to 16 571 women of 18 211 attending two antenatal clinics, the 9 per

Table 13.5 Edinburgh couple screening results[14]

	No.	% of total	% of those offered screening
Woman attending clinics	18 211	100	
Not eligible for screening	1 640	9	
Eligible for screening	16 571	91	100
Declined screening	4 005	22	24
Screened	12 566	69	76
Carrier couples identified	17[1]		
Carrier couples opting for antenatal diagnosis	15		
Number of antenatal diagnoses	19		
Affected fetuses identified	6		
Terminations of pregnancy	6		

[1] At 85 per cent detection this represents a true carrier frequency of 4.3 per cent, or 1 in 23 (i.e .$\sqrt{(17/12\ 566)} \times 100/85$).

cent who were not offered screening representing mainly those who booked after 18 weeks of gestation. Another 22 per cent declined the offer, so that screening was actually delivered to 69 per cent, a figure that compares very favourably with the 71 per cent delivery in two-step screening. Another couple screening trial in Aberdeen[47] gave a much higher take-up figure of 89 per cent (321/361). However, the 67 per cent take-up among 810 couples in the demonstration trial reported by Wald *et al.*[49] is much closer to the Edinburgh hall-mark.

Other issues

The models of two-step and couple screening have been presented here in somewhat idealized form. In practice the operation of screening will have blurred edges. In the Edinburgh two-step trial samples were occasionally collected from partners who attended the antenatal clinic, and then held in storage against the chance that the woman was a heterozygote. In such cases no result was released until both partners had been tested, thus sparing the anxiety of the waiting period. However, it was not practical to collect partners' samples from all women under this system. It was also not possible to withhold information on carrier status for positive/negative couples in a model where the information leaflet stated the two-step nature of the procedure.

In couple screening some participants will inevitably ask for information on whether one or other of them is a carrier. Although such queries are not encouraged, it would be unwise to deny the information, and therefore some provision must be made for direct counselling. In the recently-reported Edinburgh couple trial[50] only 1.5 per cent of participants requested information on their individual carrier status. It is thus unlikely that counselling will have major resource implications.

In the USA, where antenatal care is usually managed by private physicians, there has been a brief trial of delivering CF couple screening. This was to counter the suggestion that the couple concept, with non-disclosure of individuals' carrier status, was unacceptable in an American context. Doherty *et al.*[51,52] reported that the take-up of screening in a decentralized primary care setting was greater than 50 per cent. None of the screened individuals requested information on their individual carrier status.

One of the problems of screening in antenatal clinics is that the time of first booking may be too late to allow necessary action to be taken in the first trimester of pregnancy. Harris *et al.*[53] have suggested that this problem can be circumvented if general practitioners offer heterozygote testing to women at the time of a positive pregnancy test. A pilot trial claimed that this was a viable option, although no data on take-up rates were provided. However, it was pointed out that there are 33 839 general practitioners in the United Kingdom, and the chance of persuading a reasonable number of these to participate in CF screening seems improbable. At best, such screening must be seen as a useful adjunct to more generally applicable programmes.

Despite its problems, it seems that antenatal CF screening can be highly effective in reducing birth prevalence. In the maternity units of Edinburgh (the only British city with an established routine programme of this kind), the mean number of affected children born per year was 4.6 in 1984–90, the last seven years in which antenatal screening (two-step or couple) was not offered to most pregnant women. The corresponding figure for 1991–5 was 1.8—only two-fifths of the former figure. This change was not due to a change in the total birth rate, and is statistically significant ($p<0.02$).[54] In the United States, an NIH consensus development expert panel has recommended that antenatal preconceptional screening for cystic fibrosis be implemented.[55] A conference was subsequently convened in Scarborough, Maine, USA to examine issues related to implementation.[56] It was determined that considerable experience and materials exist to guide screening by either the two step or couple model and that screening can proceed as soon as any given program has assembled the critical elements.

Economic aspects of antenatal screening

Two recent publications have estimated the costs of heterozygote screening for cystic fibrosis. Morris and Oppenheimer[57] examined screening carried out in antenatal clinics, in GP surgeries (both antenatal and general) and in the work place, using two-step, couple, and individual-oriented models. The least expensive forms of screening were those carried out in hospital antenatal clinics; couple screening was estimated at £142 900 and two-step screening at £146 500 per affected fetus identified. Antenatal screening in a GP surgery was also relatively economical. However, Cuckle *et al.*[58] came to rather different conclusions, and estimated couple screening to be about 13 per cent more expensive than the two-step model. The probable reasons for this unexpected result were the failure of Cuckle *et al.* to include the costs of genetic counselling in the two-step model and also the assumption that 10 per cent to 30 per cent of women change partners between pregnancies. As someone who has run field trials of both two-step and couple antenatal screening, I can testify that Cuckle *et al.* are not correct.

Neonatal screening

Screening tests

Until very recently the tests used in neonatal screening for CF were indirect measures of physiological malfunction of the newborn infant rather than direct tests for mutant genes or gene products. Inevitably, such tests were characterized by relatively high false-positive and false-negative rates. Since most of these tests detected the consequences of pancreatic insufficiency in the newborn, they were prone to miss affected infants with normal pancreatic function.

The most widely used neonatal screening method for CF remains the serum immunoreactive trypsin(ogen) (IRT) test on dried blood spots taken between three and five days after birth. The rationale for IRT testing is that when pancreatic ducts are blocked or partially blocked in the newborn, there is a back-leakage of acinar products, including trypsin and trypsinogen, into the vascular system.[59,60] IRT is usually measured by radioimmunoassay with poyclona or monoclonal antibodies directed against serum trypsinogen. The test is not effective if the infant is born with meconium ileus[61] (this does not matter since meconium ileus in a newborn is virtually diagnostic of CF), but appears to work even when neonates have substantial residual pancreatic function.[62] The main problem with IRT testing is that in order to achieve high detection rates, cut-off levels need to be set at a point where the initial false-positive rate is quite high. Positive results are followed by repeat testing at three to five weeks, and where necessary, by a sweat test at about five to seven weeks. The prolonged period between initial testing and the final confirmatory test may be a time of great anxiety for the parents of a suspect case.

It is now possible to combine IRT and DNA testing on the same dried blood spot sample. However, as indicated earlier, DNA testing is complicated by the plethora of mutant CF alleles and is still a relatively expensive laboratory procedure. It therefore tends to be used as a confirmatory test on infants with raised IRT levels. Although this can reduce the proportion of false positives in the initial IRT screen, there are disadvantages. The most important of these is the inadvertent detection of CF heterozygotes and the problems that arise in devising suitable information protocols and counselling procedures for the parents of these children.

Screening programmes

Screening by IRT alone

Methodologies of neonatal IRT screening for CF continue to evolve and it is thus difficult to make exact comparisons between different programmes, some of which may have changed the initial cut-off level during the survey. It has become obvious that there are a number of inherent problems in both sample collection and processing and in the assay itself.[63] Improperly dried samples and contamination with faecal material are common difficulties. There is a decline in extractable IRT with age of sample, and significant differences in median IRT for populations in different areas (e.g. Tasmania, South Australia) which seem unlikely to be ethnically-determined. It is possible that these derive from slightly earlier times of sample collection in some areas, since it is known that the highest IRT values are found in the first few days of life. Another problem is the question of what exactly is being measured—trypsin, cationic or anionic trypsinogen, trypsin-α_1-antitrypsin complex, or some mixture of the four. The answer probably depends on the antibody used and perhaps on the source of the radiolabelled trypsin. Thus different commercial assays give extraordinarily different IRT values.

Most of the screening trials reported to date have chosen an initial IRT cut-off designed to give a fixed percentage recall rate of between 0.3 per cent and 0.6 per cent. Wilcken *et al.*[64] screened 75 000 infants in New South Wales with a recall rate of 0.58 per cent, and claimed to have detected 35 of 36 CF infants. Chatfield *et al.*[65] tested 227 183 infants in Wales and the West Midlands with an initial recall rate of 0.42 per cent. There were 98 positive second IRT tests (0.043 per cent) and of these 65 were confirmed as having CF. There were 13 cases of CF missed on screening, although three had meconium ileus. The false-negative rate for IRT testing (excluding all six infants presenting with meconium ileus) was 14 per cent. Hammond *et al.*[66] screened 279 399 newborns in Colorado with a recall rate of 0.32 per cent, and a repeat positive rate of 0.046 per cent. They missed 7 of 61 CF infants (11.5 per cent), most of these being attributable to laboratory errors or changes of procedure during testing. Hammond *et al.*[66] claim that an achievable false-negative rate for IRT screening (excluding meconium ileus) is of the order of 5 per cent. This conclusion is often repeated, even though its origins are obscure.

IRT combined with DNA

Obviously considerable doubts remain about how to balance sensitivity and specificity of neonatal IRT testing. With the cloning of the CF gene an alternative strategy became possible. The cut-off level of the initial IRT test is reduced to a point of improved potential sensitivity, and samples from infants with elevated values scanned for the presence of detectable CF alleles before further action is contemplated. In the absence of detectable CF alleles, no recall is made and the infant reported as 'CF not indicated'. If the infant is a homozygote or a compound heterozygote for a CF allele, the diagnosis of CF is confirmed at the time of the first report. When only one CF allele is detectable, a sweat test is carried out at age five to seven weeks to confirm or exclude a diagnosis of the disorder.[67]

An illustrative flow chart of this type of screening is presented in Fig. 13.7 for a population of 1 000 000 newborns among whom 1 in 2500 is affected by CF. It may be expected that about 15 per cent of these cases will present with meconium ileus and will not need IRT testing. Based on experience in New South Wales,[68] it is also assumed that an IRT cut-off at the 99th percentile will detect 98.5 per cent of cases—i.e. 335 of the 340 in the primary screen.

If DNA testing is carried out only for the ΔF508 allele, and if this represents 75 per cent of mutant alleles, 56.25 per cent of the 335 (i.e. 188) will be homozygotes detected at the time of DNA testing, and 6.25 per cent (i.e. 21) will have no ΔF508 on either chromosome and will thus be missed. The remaining 37.5 per cent (i.e. 126) will have ΔF508 on one chromosome and another undetected CF allele on the other chromosome, and will be indistinguishable in the DNA test from the ΔF508/normal heterozygotes among the 9605 unaffected infants tested. ΔF508/normal heterozygosity is assumed to be present in 588 of these 9605 infants, in accordance with Australian experience that it occurs in one-seventeenth of all infants who are positive in the IRT test.[63] This is twice as high as the expected prevalence of ΔF508/normal heterozygosity in the general population ($0.015 \times 0.980 \times 2$, or 1 in 34), which is consistent with other evidence that the distribution of IRT values is shifted to the right in ΔF508/normal heterozygotes.[63]

All the infants who are heterozygous for ΔF508 will need to undergo sweat testing a few weeks after birth. Again on the basis of Australian experience,[63] it is assumed in Fig. 13.7 that chloride levels in the sweat test would be at or above the 60 mEq/1 threshold in 90 per cent of the 126 cases with combinations of ΔF508 and another abnormal allele, and in none of the 588 unaffected heterozygotes. In this case, the overall detection rate for the screening programme would also be 90 per cent (i.e. 361/400), and the false-positive rate would be zero. With the threshold at 35 mEq/1 instead of 60, the Australian data suggest that positive results would be recorded in 100 per cent of cases and 1.3 per cent of ΔF508/normal heterozygotes, which is equivalent to a detection rate of 93.5 per cent (i.e. 374/400) and a false-positive rate of 0.0008 per cent (i.e. 8/999 600) for the whole programme.

Is neonatal screening for CF justified?

There have been two major arguments against implementing wide-scale neonatal screening programmes for CF. The first follows from the comparatively high false-positive rate which is necessary if the primary IRT cut-off is set at a level which detects a satisfactory proportion of affected newborns. There is a fairly long wait before confirmatory sweat testing can be implemented, and parents may become very anxious during this period. However, the data from trials of combined IRT and DNA testing[63] now show that this particular problem has been satisfactorily addressed. But combined testing has created a new problem, in the higher-than-expected proportion

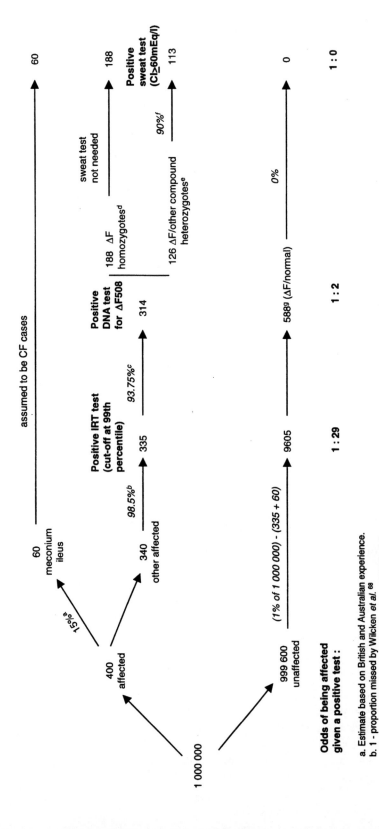

Fig. 13.7 Flow diagram for combined IRT and DNA-based neonatal screening for CF. See text for details.

(5 to 10 per cent) of CF heterozygotes amongst the IRT positive, sweat test negative cohort. It is obviously necessary to design the primary information leaflet in such a way as to take this into account, but also to have on hand trained genetic counsellors who can explain the significance of CF heterozygosity to parents who believe their carrier infants to be genetically abnormal. The need for counselling will have resource implications for programmes of newborn screening. One possible way around the problem would be to carry out a second IRT test at five to six weeks on those with first positive values and a positive mutation test. If the second IRT test is normal the parents can be reassured that CF has been excluded without the need for a sweat test.[63] However, this protocol is not very different to the original IRT-alone systems, where second testing was found to be upsetting to parents.

A more serious objection to neonatal CF screening is that its benefits have not yet been demonstrated. It can be argued that detection of CF in the newborn period permits genetic counselling of heterozygous parents and the prevention of recurrence (when so desired) by antenatal diagnosis. However, in developed countries where neonatal screening is most likely to occur, the average number of children per family is close to two, and a CF child is as likely to be the second (and final one) as the first. Thus the maximum possible reduction in birth prevalence of CF, from a neonatal screening programme where all counselled parents availed themselves of antenatal diagnosis and termination of pregnancy, would be 12.5 per cent. In the absence of screening, some 10 per cent of infants with CF would present at birth with meconium ileus, while some 60 to 70 per cent would be ascertained clinically in the first year of life. If second pregnancies were not started until a year after the birth of the first child, as many as 80 per cent of heterozygous couples would know that they were at risk. One could therefore reasonably expect a reduction in birth prevalence (assuming again that all counselled parents availed themselves of antenatal diagnosis) of 10 per cent. The marginally greater reduction achievable by neonatal screening hardly justifies the expense and inevitable problems of such programmes.

The case for neonatal screening must therefore rest on whether or not it improves the prognosis. Several studies have addressed this point, but as yet with unconvincing results. A trial in the UK, in which screening was carried out on alternate weeks, was followed by assessment of both screened and unscreened groups for the first four years of life.[65] CF children detected by screening spent a significantly shorter time in hospital in the first year of life compared to the unscreened group. However, there were no significant differences between the groups in mean height or mean weight, and it is often pointed out that nutritional deficiency is a potent indicator of poor prognosis in CF. Other studies have been more successful in the diagnosis and treatment of unsuspected protein malnutrition and deficiencies of fat-soluble vitamins in CF infants detected early by screening.[69]

The value of newborn screening for CF, if any, is unlikely to be conclusively demonstrated without sustained follow-up of controlled trials, using either random assignment or alternative week methodologies. It is natural for paediatricians to feel that there *must* be benefits in early detection of this disorder. However, it is dangerous to conclude that the case for neonatal screening has been made, and important to resist the pressure for wide-scale implementation until adequate data on the benefits have been presented.

REFERENCES

1. Anderson, D.H. (1988). Cystic fibrosis of the pancreas and its relation to celiac disease: clinical and pathological study. *Am. J. Dis. Child.*, **56**, 344–99.
2. Anderson, D.H. and Hodges, R.G.V. (1946). Genetics of cystic fibrosis of the pancreas with a consideration of etiology. *Am. J. Dis. Child.*, **72**, 62–8.
3. Crossley, J.R., Elliott, R.B., and Smith, P.A. (1979). Dried-blood spot screening for cystic fibrosis in the newborn. *Lancet*, **i**, 472–4.
4. Brock, D.J.H., Clarke, H.A.K., and Barron, L. (1988). Prenatal diagnosis of cystic fibrosis by microvillar enzyme assay on a sequence of 258 pregnancies. *Hum. Genet.*, **78**, 271–5.
5. Rommens, J.M., Iannuzzi, M.C., Kerem, B. *et al.* (1989). Identification of the cystic fibrosis gene; chromosome walking and jumping. *Science*, **245**, 1059–65.
6. Riordan, J.R., Rommens, J.M., Kerem, B. *et al.* (1989). Identification of the cystic fibrosis gene: cloning and characterization of complementary DNA. *Science*, **245**, 1066–73.
7. Kerem, B., Rommens, J.M., Buchanan, J.A. *et al.* (1989). Identification of the cystic fibrosis gene: genetic analysis. *Science*, **245**, 1073–80.
8. Di Sant'Agnese, P.A., Darling, R.C., Perera, G.A., and Shea, E. (1955). Abnormal electrolyte composition of sweat in cystic fibrosis of the pancreas: clinical significance and relationship to disease. *Pediatrics*, **12**, 549–63.
9. Welsh, M.J., Tsui, L.P., Boat, T.F., and Beaudet, A.L. (1995). Cystic fibrosis. In: *The metabolic and molecular bases of inherited disease*, 7th edn, (ed. C.R. Scriver, A.L. Beaudet, W.S. Sly, and D. Valle), pp. 3799–877. McGraw Hill, New York,.
10. The Cystic Fibrosis Genetic Analysis Consortium (1990). Worldwide survey of the ΔF508 mutation. *Am. J. Hum. Genet.*, **47**, 354–9.
11. Brock, D.J.H. (1992). Cystic fibrosis. In: *Prenatal diagnosis and screening*, (eds. D.J.H. Brock, C.H. Rodeck, and M.A. Ferguson-Smith), pp. 520–46. Churchill-Livingstone, Edinburgh.
12. Beaudet, A., Bowcock, A., Buchwald, M. *et al.* (1986). Linkage of cystic fibrosis to two tightly linked DNA markers: joint report from a collaborative study. *Am. J. Hum. Genet.*, **39**, 681–93.
13. British Paediatric Association Working Party on Cystic Fibrosis (1988). Cystic fibrosis in the United Kingdom 1977–1985: an improving picture. *Br. Med. J.*, **297**, 1599–602.
14. Brock, D.J.H. (1996). Prenatal screening for cystic fibrosis: five years experience reviewed. *Lancet*, **347**, 148–51.
15. Elborn, J.S., Shale, D.J., Britton, J.R. (1991). Cystic fibrosis: current survival and population estimates to the year 2000. *Thorax*, **46**, 881–5.
16. Schwarz, M.J., Malone, G.M., Hayworth, A., *et al.* (1995). Cystic fibrosis mutation analysis: report from 22 UK regional genetics laboratories. *Hum. Mut.*, **6**, 326–33.
17. Tsui, L.C., personal communication.
18. Shrimpton, A.E., McIntosh, I., and Brock, D.J.H. (1991). The incidence of different cystic fibrosis mutations in the Scottish population: effects on prenatal diagnosis and genetic counselling. *J. Med. Genet.*, **28**, 317–21.
19. Taylor, G.R., Noble, J.S., Hall, J.L. *et al.* (1989). Rapid screening for ΔF508 deletion in cystic fibrosis. *Lancet*, **ii**, 1345.
20. Scheffer, H., Verlind, E., Penninga, T. *et al.* (1989). Rapid screening for ΔF508 deletion in cystic fibrosis. *Lancet*, **ii**, 1345–6.

21. Matthew, C.J., Roberts, R.J., Harris, A., Bentley, D.R., and Bobrow, M. (1989). Rapid screening for ΔF508 deletion in cystic fibrosis. *Lancet*, **ii**, 1346.
22. Rommens, J.M., Kerem, B., Grier, W. *et al.* (1990). Rapid non-radioactive detection of the major cystic fibrosis mutation. *Am. J. Hum. Genet.*, **46**, 395–6.
23. Cutting, G.R., Kasch, L.M., Rosenstein, B.J. *et al.* (1990). A cluster of cystic fibrosis mutations in the first nucleotide binding fold of the cystic fibrosis conductance regulator protein. *Nature*, **345**, 366–9.
24. Newton, C.R., Graham, A., Heptonstall, L.E. *et al.* (1989). Analysis of any point mutation in DNA. The amplification refractory mutation system. *Nucleic Acids Res.*, **17**, 2503–16.
25. Ferrie, R.M., Schwarz, M. J., Robertson, N.H. *et al.* (1992). Development, multiplexing and amplification of ARMS tests for common mutations in the CFTR gene. *Amer. J. Hum. Genet.*, **51**, 251–62.
26. Wilfond, B.S., and Fost, N. (1990). The cystic fibrosis gene: medical and social implications for heterozygote detection. *J. Am. Med. Assoc.*, **263**, 2777–83.
27. Angastiniotis, M.A., Kyriakidou, S., and Hadjiminas, M. (1990). How thalassaemia was controlled in Cyprus. *World Health Forum*, **7**, 291–7.
28. Shapiro, D.A., and Shapiro, L.R. (1989). Pitfalls in Tay–Sachs carrier detection: physician referral patterns and patient ignorance. *N. Y. State J. Med.*, **89**, 317–19.
29. Modell, B. (1990). Cystic fibrosis screening and community genetics. *J. Med. Genet.*, **27**, 475–9.
30. Clow, C.L. and Scriver, C.R. (1977). Knowledge about and attitudes towards genetic screening among high school students: Tay–Sachs experience. *Pediatrics*, **59**, 86–91.
31. Zeesman, S., Clow, C.L., Cartier, L., and Scriver, C.R. (1984). A private view of heterozygosity: eight-year follow up study on carriers of Tay–Sachs gene detected by high school screening in Montreal. *Am. J. Med. Genet.*, **18**, 769–78.
32. Ten Kate, L.P., and Tyjmstra, T. (1989). Carrier screening for cystic fibrosis. *Lancet*, **ii**, 973–4.
33. Holtzman, N.A. (1989). *Proceed with caution: predicting genetic risks in the recombinant DNA era*, pp. 217–18. Johns Hopkins University Press, Baltimore.
34. Watson, E.K., Mayall, E., Chappell, J. *et al.* (1991). Screening for carriers of cystic fibrosis through primary health care services. *Br. Med. J.*, **303**, 504–7.
35. Bekker, H., Modell, M., Denniss, G. *et al.* (1993). Uptake of cystic fibrosis testing in primary care: supply push or demand pull? *Br. Med. J.*, **306**, 1584–6.
36 Tambor, E.S., Bernhardt, B.A., Chase, G.A. *et al.* (1994). Offering cystic fibrosis screening in an HMO population: factors affecting utilization. *Am. J. Hum. Genet.*, **55**, 626–37.
37. Super, M., Schwarz, M.J., Malone, G. *et al.* (1994). Active cascade testing for carriers of cystic fibrosis gene. *Br. Med. J.*, **308**, 1462–8.
38. Holloway, S. and Brock, D.J.H. (1994). Cascade testing for identification of carriers of cystic fibrosis. *J. Med. Screening*, **1**, 159–64.
39. Mennie, M., Gilfillan, A., Compton, M. *et al.* (1992). Prenatal screening for cystic fibrosis. *Lancet*, **340**, 214–16.
40. Gilbert, F. (1990). Is population screening for cystic fibrosis appropriate now? *Am. J. Hum. Genet.*, **46**, 394–5.
41. Ten Kate, L.P. (1990). Carrier screening for cystic fibrosis and other autosomal recessive diseases. *Am. J. Hum. Genet.*, **47**, 359–61.
42. Wald, N.J. (1991). Couple screening for cystic fibrosis. *Lancet*, **338**, 1318–19.

43. Mennie, M., Liston, W.A., and Brock, D.J.H. (1992). Prenatal cystic fibrosis carrier testing: designing an information leaflet to meet the specific needs of the target population. *J. Med. Genet.*, **29**, 308–12.

44. Mennie, M.E., Compton, M.E., Gilfillan, A. *et al.* (1993). Prenatal screening for cystic fibrosis: psychological effects on carriers and their partners. *J. Med. Genet.*, **30**, 543–8.

45. Mennie, M.E., Gilfillan, A., Compton, M.E., Liston, W.A., and Brock, D.J.H. (1993). Prenatal cystic fibrosis carrier screening: factors in a woman's decision to decline testing. *Prenat. Diag.*, **13**, 807–14.

46. Jung, U., Urner, U., Grade, K., and Coutelle, C. (1994). Acceptability of carrier screening for cystic fibrosis during pregnancy in a German population. *Hum. Genet.*, **94**, 19–24.

47. Miedzybrodzka, J.H., Hall, M.H., Mollison, J. *et al.* (1995). Antenatal screening for carriers of cystic fibrosis: randomised trial of stepwise vs couple screening. *Br. Med. J.*, **310**, 353–7 .

48. Schwartz, M., Brandt, N.J., and Skovby, F. (1993). Screening for carriers of cystic fibrosis among pregnant women: a pilot study. *Eur. J. Hum. Genet.*, **1**, 239–44.

49. Wald, N.J., George, L., Wald, N., and Mackenzie, I.Z. (1995). Letter to the editor. Further observations in connection with couple screening for cystic fibrosis. *Prenat. Diag.*, **15**, 589–90.

50. Livingstone, J., Axton, R.A., Mennie, M.E., Gilfillan, A., and Brock, D.J.H. (1993). A preliminary trial of couple screening for cystic fibrosis: designing an appropriate information leaflet. *Clin. Genet.*, **43**, 57–62.

51. Doherty, R.A., Palomaki, G.E., Kloza, E.M. *et al.* (1994). Prenatal screening for cystic fibrosis. *Lancet*, **343**, 172.

52. Doherty, R.A., Palomaki, G.E., Kloza, E.M., Erikson, J.L., and Haddow, J.E. (1996). Couple-based prenatal screening for cystic fibrosis in primary care settings. *Prenat. Diag.*, **16**, 397–404.

53. Harris, H., Scotcher, D., Hartlie, N. *et al.* (1993). Cystic fibrosis carrier testing in early pregnancy by general practitioners. *Br. Med. J.*, **306**, 1580–3.

54. Cunningham, S. and Marshall, T. (1998). Influence of five years of antenatal screening on the paediatric cystic fibrosis population in one region. *Arch. Dis. Child.*, **78**, 345–8.

55. Genetic Testing for Cystic Fibrosis. NIH Consensus Statement Online 1997 Apr 14–16 [cited April 20, 2000]; **15**, 1–37.

56. Haddow, J.F., Bradley, L.A., Palomaki, G.E., Doherty, R.A. *et al.* (1999). Issues in implementing prenatal screening for cystic fibrosis: results of a working conference. *J. Med. Screen.*, **6**, 60–6.

57. Morris, J.K. and Oppenheimer, P.M. (1995). Cost comparisons of different methods of screening for cystic fibrosis. *J. Med. Screen.*, **2**, 22–7.

58. Cuckle, H.S., Richardson, G.A., Sheldon, T.A., and Quirke, P. (1995). Cost effectiveness of antenatal screening for cystic fibrosis. *Br. Med. J.*, **311**, 1460–4.

59. Crossley, J.R., Smith, P.A., Edgar, B.W., Gluckman, P.D., and Elliott, R.B. (1981). Neonatal screening for cystic fibrosis using immunoreactive trypsin assay in dried blood spots. *Clin. Chim. Acta.*, **113**, 111–21.

60. Kirby, L.T., Applegarth, D.A., Davidson, A.G.F. *et al.* (1981). Use of a dried blood spot in immunoreactive trypsin assay for detection of cystic fibrosis in infants. *Clin. Chem.*, **27**, 678–80.

61. Roberts, G., Stanfield, M., Black, A., and Redmond, A. (1988). Screening for cystic fibrosis: a four-year regional experience. *Arch. Dis. Child.*, **63**, 1438–43.

62. Watters, D.L., Dorney, S.F.A., Gaskin, K. *et al.* (1990). Pancreatic function in infants identified as having cystic fibrosis in a neonatal screening programme. *New Engl. J. Med. Genet.*, **322**, 303–8.

63. Ranieri, E., Lewis, B.D., Morris, C.P., and Wilcken, B. (1996). Neonatal screening using combined biochemical and DNA-based techniques. In: *Cystic fibrosis: current topics*, Vol. III, (ed. J. Dodge, D. J. H. Brock, and J. H. Widdicombe). Chichester, Wiley.

64. Wilcken, B., Towns, S.J., and Mellis, C.M. (1983). Diagnostic delay in cystic fibrosis: lessons from newborn screening. *Arch. Dis. Child.*, **58**, 863–6.

65. Chatfield, S., Owen, G., Ryley, H.C. *et al.* (1991). Neonatal screening for cystic fibrosis in Wales and the West Midlands: clinical assessment after five years of screening. *Arch. Dis. Child.*, **66**, 29–33.

66. Hammond, K.B., Abman, S.H., Sokol, R.J., and Accurso, F.J. (1991). Efficacy of statewide neonatal screening for cystic fibrosis by assay of trypsinogen concentrations. *New Engl. J. Med.*, **325**, 769–74.

67. Ranieri, E., Ryall, R.G., Morris, C.P. *et al.* (1991). Neonatal screening strategy for cystic fibrosis using immunoreactive trypsinogen and direct gene analysis. *Br. Med. J.*, **302**, 1237–40.

68. Wilcken, B., Wylie, V., Sherry, G., and Bayliss, U. (1995). Neonatal screening for cystic fibrosis: a comparison of two strategies for case detection in 1.2 million babies. *J. Pediatr.*, **127**, 965–70.

69. Holtzman, N.A. (1991). What drives neonatal screening programmes? *New Engl. J. Med.*, **325**, 802–4.

Screening for specific disorders
(c) Neonatal screening

14 *Phenylketonuria and other inherited metabolic defects*

George C. Cunningham

INTRODUCTION

Phenylketonuria has been described as the epitome of metabolic disease screening.[1] As such it will be discussed in some detail because it raises many issues applicable to screening for metabolic disorders in general. Since the measurement used to detect phenylketonuria by screening is the level of phenylalanine in the blood, it is more correct to refer to this group of disorders as hyperphenylalaninaemias. The chapter will include, however, a brief commentary on other, similar metabolic disorders for which screening has been proposed.

PHENYLKETONURIA: THE DISORDER

Description

Phenylketonuria (PKU) is a disorder of amino acid metabolism due to failure of phenylalanine hydroxylation which results in elevation of the plasma phenylalanine and excretion of phenylketoacids. So-called 'classical' PKU was first described by Folling in 1934.[2] The affected individuals almost always suffer severe mental retardation. There are few physical findings. An eczematous rash, microcephaly, growth retardation, decreased pigmentation of hair and skin, and vomiting are common, but non-specific symptoms. More rarely, hyperkinesis and seizures are observed in untreated cases. In the absence of preventive treatment there is reduced life expectancy.[3] Although there is a rough correlation of the severity of symptoms with blood phenylalanine, the exact metabolites responsible for the neuropathology have not been identified.

Since the original report, it has become clear that there are other forms of hyperphenylalaninaemia with differing clinical implications. These phenotypes are clearly unique defects in a multi-stage metabolic pathway which in turn are related to a variety of mutational haplotypes which have since been identified. This accounts for rare descriptions of seemingly 'classical' cases with normal or near normal mental abilities.[4-7]

Investigators have conventionally classified cases in four general categories.[8,9] First, classical PKU is defined as a case in which the plasma phenylalanine is persistently over 1.0 mM/l (16.5 mg/dl), dietary intakes greater than 20 mg/kg/day lead to rapid elevation of plasma phenylalanine, and there is less than one per cent of normal phenylalanine hydroxylase (PAH) activity. This threshold for plasma phenylalanine is somewhat arbitrary since brain damage has been reported at lower levels. Second, non-phenylketonuric hyperphenylalaninaemic variants, also referred to as variant or atypical PKU, are defined as persistent plasma phenylalanine elevations between 0.60 mM/l (10 mg/dl) and 1.0 mM/l (16.5 mg/dl), toleration of 20–50 mg/kg/day of phenylalanine in the diet without marked plasma elevation, and 1–3 per cent of normal PAH activity.[9,10] The third category is benign hyperphenylalaninaemia, where plasma phenylalanine is persistently higher than the normal range but never exceeds 0.60 mM/l (10 mg/dl) and PAH activity is over 3 per cent of normal. This group, which is classified as a type of false-positive, is rarely treated with dietary restrictions. The adoption of screening and effective dietary intervention revealed a fourth category of 'malignant phenylketonuria' which was not responsive to low-phenylalanine dietary treatment. This form of PKU proved to be due to defects in tetrahydrobiopterin cofactor metabolism rather than PAH.[11–13]

Diagnosis frequently requires assessment of pterin metabolism, urinary ketoacids, serum tyrosine levels, and response to protein challenge diets. Based on current knowledge of the genetics of the disorder, an improved clinical phenotype assignment

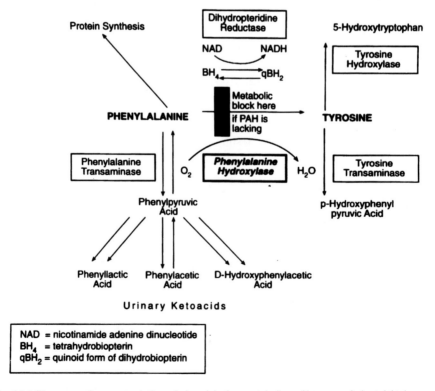

Fig. 14.1 Diagrammatic representation of phenylalanine metabolism. Absence of phenylalanine hydroxylase in PKU prevents conversion to tyrosine.

based on haplotypes may soon be part of the follow-up of newborn screening programmes.

Biochemistry

The biochemistry of phenylalanine has been described in detail in several reviews.[9,11] Briefly, phenylalanine cannot be synthesized by the body and is therefore an essential amino acid. Phenylalanine is normally converted by the hepatic enzyme l-phenylalanine hydroxylase (PAH) to tyrosine in the presence of a cofactor tetrahydrobiopterin (BH_4) and oxygen. This pathway is disrupted in PKU individuals who lack PAH. The pathways are outlined in Fig. 14.1. Hyperphenylalaninaemia can also result because of a deficiency in the enzymes controlling BH_4 metabolism. This is the basis of various metabolic defects, four of which [dihydropteridine reductase deficiency (DHPR), guanosine triphosphate cyclohydrolase deficiency (GTPCH), -6-pyruvoyl-tetrahydropterin synthase (6 PTS) deficiency, and primapterinuria] have been investigated and described.[12,13] PKU due to BH_4 deficiency has been called 'malignant' or 'unresponsive' PKU because the metabolic defects can also lead to a lack of other essential metabolites such as l-dihydrophenylalanine and 5 hydroxytryptophan which must be given, in addition to a low-phenylalanine diet, to avoid or mitigate adverse effects.

Genetics

PKU is an autosomal recessive disorder. More than 300 mutations have already been identified[14-16] and most but not all are associated with classical PKU, usually as compound heterozygotes. Many more mutations are expected since a large number of cases worldwide have not been associated with a specific mutation. For example, the gene for dihydropteridine reductase (DHPR) is on chromosome 4 (p 15.1–16.1) and two distinct mutations have been described.[17] The genes for GTPCH and 6 PTS are as yet unmapped. The gene responsible for production of phenylalanine hydroxylase (PAH) is on chromosome 12 (q 22–q 24.1). The coding reading frame includes 1353 base pairs and produces an enzyme monomer of 452 amino acids. Human PAH is considered to be a homopolymer. The gene is about 90 000 nucleotide base pairs with 13 exons. Restriction fragment length polymorphism (RFLP) analysis, when applied to PKU families, has identified at least 70 haplotypes.[14,15] Six of these haplotypes (1 to 6) account for over 90 per cent of most European families with classical PKU. When informative, i.e., a family has haplotype heterozygosity and an affected proband, the RFLP technique can provide antenatal risk figures. Ninety-five percent of families have informative haplotypes.

These investigations have revealed that PKU originated, by independent mutations, in different founder populations, so while the phenotype, i.e., the clinical picture, may be similar, Scandinavians, Jews, Italians, Turks, Chinese, and West Africans each have a different genetic disorder (genotype).

Birth prevalence

There is a 20-fold ethnic and geographical range in the prevalence rates of hyperphenylalaninaemia. Data reported in the literature are based on newborn screening and frequently fail to distinguish between classical PKU and non-PKU hyper-

Table 14.1   Birth prevalence of hyperphenylalaninaemia

Group tested	Prevalence of hyperphenylalaninaemia per million births
Turkey[18]	385
Ireland[19]	249
Yemenite Jews[20]	190
Germany[21]	149
Poland[22]	142
Scotland[19]	127
Yugoslavia[23]	127
England[19]	102
Wales[19]	99
Hungary[24]	88
Denmark[8]	85
China[25]	74
Norway[26]	73
New Zealand[27]	60
France[28]	59
Greece[29]	50
United States[30]	50
Canada[31]	45
Sweden[32]	26
Japan[33]	7
Ashkenazi Jews[34]	5

Table 14.2   Classical PKU birth prevalence by ethnic group in California (February 1982 to May 1991—4 551 666 births)

Ethnic group	No. of newborns	Prevalence per million births
White, non-hispanic	2 086 536	57
Hispanic	1 630 016	25
Black	354 874	3
Asian	303 138	16
Other	126 712	32

All four 'other' cases were either Middle Eastern or Armenian, but there is no denominator for this group.

phenylalaninaemia. These apparently occur in different proportions in different ethnic groups. With this reservation in mind, data have been combined from several sources in Table 14.1. The highest prevalence is in the Irish, and the lowest in the Ashkenazi Jews. Based on experience of the Californian programme, the prevalence is also low in blacks and hispanics (Table 14.2). Classical PKU represents about 67 per cent, hyperphenylalaninaemic variants 33 per cent, and biopterin deficient forms, 1 to 3 per cent of the total cases in Caucasian populations.

SCREENING

Prior to 1961, the only method of screening was testing the urine for phenylketoacids using ferric chloride. This method had serious shortcomings and no longer has general acceptance as a screening method in public health.[35] In 1963, Guthrie and Susi published a microbiological inhibition assay (MIA) for phenylalanine that could be performed on dried spots of blood collected on special filter paper.[35,36] This major contribution made population-based screening possible. It is a semiquantitative test with a standard deviation of ± 0.06 mM/l (1 mg/dl) at the cut-off of 0.24 mM/l (4 mg/dl). The method's chief advantage is its low cost. It has persisted virtually unchanged for over 30 years as the most widely used method.[36] Another semiquantitative method which was used on a limited basis in the United Kingdom and Europe is paper chromatography.[37] The fluorometric method[38] which is quantitative and has a within-run standard deviation of ± 0.01 mM/l (0.2 mg/dl) and a day to day standard deviation of 0.015 mM/l (0.3 mg/dl) when the plasma phenylalanine is 0.24 mM/l (4 mg/dl) is gradually replacing the older techniques. This method permits finer adjustment of cut-off and is easier to quality control. Although initial outlay for automated equipment is expensive, in practice the cost per test is quite competitive. Another method gaining in popularity uses an enzyme linked immuno-absorbent assay in a microtiter plate system.[39,40] Phenylalanine is oxidized in the presence of PAH to tyrosine, simultaneously reducing nicotinamide adenine dinucleotide (NAD). The reduced NAD becomes an electron donor reacting with tetrazolium salt to produce a coloured compound which is measured in a colorimiter.

Some have proposed that DNA testing may replace biochemical tests but this appears to be an unlikely prospect. An ideal screening test is inexpensive, has a high detection rate, and a low false-positive rate. DNA testing is relatively expensive. Because of the multiple genotypes associated with the disease and the extreme specificity of DNA testing, it is difficult to maintain a high detection rate without using multiple DNA techniques. DNA based tests, however, can be used to make specific diagnosis after biochemical screening and can be performed using amplification of DNA on the initial filter paper specimen.[41-43]

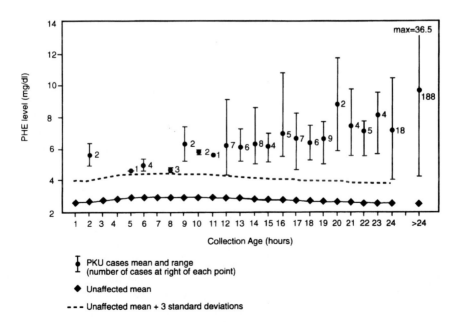

Fig. 14.2 Mean phenylalanine levels by time of collection: unaffected (*n* = 563 813) and confirmed PKU (*n* = 288).

Timing of screening

There has been considerable debate in the past on when to screen.[44–47] When screening was first instituted in the 1960s, it was widely believed that the plasma phenylalanine would not be raised to positive levels until sufficient phenylalanine had been ingested. While mean cord plasma phenylalanine of PKU infants is significantly higher than normal,[46,48–51] the distribution of values of PKU newborns is not sufficiently different from unaffected newborns to use cord blood as a reliable screening specimen. It is now clear that the negative nitrogen balance of a newborn with PKU will produce sufficient endogenous phenylalanine to give a positive result with fluorometry in almost all cases with specimens collected after 24 hours of age.[50–54] This response to negative nitrogen balance is also seen in older patients who are not eating as a result of illness. Protein ingestion, while not critical,[53] will accentuate the rise. The phenylalanine levels of affected neonates increases with time (Fig. 14.2). The optimal compromise is to obtain the specimen in the hospital of birth as close to discharge as possible. The tendency for early discharge makes this an important consideration. Attempts to obtain the initial specimen after discharge generally miss many babies and requires a well established universal home visiting programme. Delay in testing for four or five days does not produce a better yield of cases, has higher false-positive rates, and delays treatment. In over 10 000 000 tests, more than 2 500 000 of which were under 24 hours of age, the Californian programme, using a quantitative assay, has missed only two cases of PKU while 351 classical and 334 non-PKU hyperphenylalaninaemias were detected.

Values of screening test in affected and unaffected subjects

Cut-off level

When screening was started in the U.S., the positive level for the Guthrie method was set at 0.7 mM/l (12 mg/dl), but this was soon lowered to 0.36 mM/l (6 mg/dl) and, again on the basis of experience of missed cases, to 0.24 mM/l (4 mg/dl). The test has an average initial positive rate of approximately one positive for each 1286 tests or 7.77 per 1 000 000 tests[30] in the U.S. where most programmes use 0.24 mM/l. The Guthrie MIA technique, however, may not be sensitive enough at this cut-off level to be used reliably for screening, especially screening of early discharges from hospital. Because of the trend in the U.S. toward early discharge at under 24 hours from birth, the use of a lower cut-off, to 0.12 mM/l (2 mg/dl) has therefore been proposed.[9,44–46] With the fluorometric method, a 0.26 mM/l cut-off is used in California.

Detection rate

The detection rate, i.e. the proportion of newborns affected by significant hyperphenylalaninaemia who are classified as positive when screened, is influenced by several variables. The most critical are proper specimen collection, quality control of the laboratory, cut-off selected, and age of newborns at time of testing (see 'Timing of screening' above). To a lesser extent the sex of the newborn and feeding history can modify results. Most missed cases are due to poorly designed programmes, failure to follow protocol, or laboratory errors. 'Biological' false-negatives (defined as cases in which phenylketonuria is eventually diagnosed after a confirmed plasma phenylalanine reading of less than 0.18 mM/l (3 mg/dl) with the Guthrie method or less than

0.24 mM/l (4 mg/dl) with the fluorometric method) do occur but are extremely rare; in the worldwide experience of over 100 million tests, few cases are well documented in the literature.[19,21,22,24,45,46,48,50]

The detection rates reported in various programmes are shown in Table 14.3. Except in the early years of screening, most programmes using the Guthrie test reported detection rates above 99 per cent. No cases were missed using fluorometric or chromatographic methods in the United Kingdom.[19] Two cases with negative test at two hours of age were the only missed cases identified in California, mainly by fluoro-metry with a cut-off of 0.26 mM/l, in 1980–1999. Both occurred in one hospital. This gives a detection rate of 99.7 per cent. The extensive follow-up and frequent con-tact with practitioners and mental retardation services agencies, and the litigious ten-dencies in the States, decrease the likelihood that cases missed at screening would not be identified later. Even if under-reporting of missed cases is postulated, it appears unlikely that there would be enough to lead to a detection rate below 99 per cent.

False-positive rate

Since the disorder being screened for is *clinically* significant hyperphenylalaninaemia, transient elevations of phenylalanine and some persistent but low elevations should be regarded as false-positives. There is no agreement on where to draw the line on the phenylalanine concentrations with respect to time from birth (see Fig 14.2). Therefore each program must provide its own policy.

There is noteworthy variability between the false-positive rates observed in different screening programmes and from year to year within screening programmes. This variability as well as that exhibited by detection rates is illustrated in Table 14.3. The variability of the rates reported during the first few years when the Guthrie test was used led Hansen to conclude that 'traditional indices of programme validity cannot be estimated with confidence'.[47]

In the programmes listed in Table 14.3 that used the Guthrie test alone with a cut-off of 0.24 mM/l, the false-positive rate varied from 0.02 per cent to 0.07 per cent. Lowering the cut-off to 0.12 mM/l resulted in Massachusetts in only a slightly higher false-positive rate for the Guthrie test, 0.16 per cent. However, experience in California shows that using this cut-off with the more accurate fluorometric test would result in an extremely high false-positive rate (84 per cent). This indicates the inaccuracy of the Guthrie test at low concentrations. The false-positive rate when the fluorometric test was used with a cut-off of 0.26 mM/l was 0.22 per cent in California.

Recall of initial positives

Newborns positive on the first test are retested as soon as possible. Untreated PKU will have rapidly rising plasma phenylalanine. Most initial positive tests will prove to be normal on repeated testing. Prematurity contributes the largest number of these false-positive results. Any infant with persistent hyperphenylalaninaemia, i.e. 0.26 mM/l (4.3 mg/dl) or higher, should be referred for diagnostic evaluation.

Routine repeat tests

The concern over inadequate feeding and early discharge has led many programs to require a second test on initially negative newborns some weeks after birth. The yield of new cases is appallingly low.[30,56] The cost per case detected is extremely high. Most

Table 14.3 Detection and false positive rates

Test method	Newborns tested	Cut-off (mM/l)	Detection rate (%)	False-positive rate (%)
California 1965–80	Guthrie[a] and fluorometric	5 190 782	0.24	94.3	10–12.0
California 1985–90	Fluorometric	4 304 964	0.12[b]	100.0	84.0
California 1985–90	Fluorometric	4 304 964	0.24[b]	100.0	0.36
California 1985–90	Fluorometric	4 304 964	0.26[c]	100.0	0.22
California 1985–90	Fluorometric	4 304 964	0.36[c]	87.0	0.02
USA[55] 1962–63	Guthrie	408 568	0.36	94.0	0.06
USA[44] 1968–70	Guthrie	1 167 000	0.24[d]	91.7	0.05
West Germany[21] 1969–84	Guthrie	9 901 432	0.25	99.4	0.31
Hungary[24] 1973–84	Guthrie	800 000	0.24	98.7	–
United Kingdom[19] 1974–88	Guthrie 43% Fluorometry 23% Chromatography 34%	11 850 000 (est)	0.20 (8%), 0.24 (76%), 0.30 (3%), 0.48 (3%)	98.7[e]	–
Manchester[54] 1979–80	Guthrie	122 488	0.24	100.0	0.02
Poland[22] 1979–91	Guthrie	8 267 190	0.24	97.6	–
Massachusetts[30] 1989	Guthrie	92 923	0.12	100.0	0.16
New York[30] 1989	Guthrie	288 878	0.18	100.0	0.08
Texas[30] 1989	Guthrie	312 279	0.24	–	0.07

[a] There were approximately 70 Guthrie laboratories and 50 fluorometric laboratories.
[b] Calculated based on hypothetical cut-off.
[c] Actual experience.
[d] Reports from 23 states; one state used 0.12 mM/l and another 0.36 mM/l as the cut-off, the rest used 0.24 mM/l.
[e] All missed cases were tested by Guthrie test.

missed cases are the result of errors of omission or commission in the initial screening protocols, rather than true biological false-negatives.[9,52] Resources directed to improvement of the primary screening are a better investment than a repeat testing programme.

DIAGNOSIS

All initially positive screening tests need to be quickly repeated. Many initially positive tests are due to immaturity and gradual activation of the PAH system. Repeat tests in these cases will be in the normal range. Persistent elevation of plasma phenlyalanine over 16.5 mg/dl measured by a quantitative technique is diagnostic. All newborns with elevations should also have a urine specimen collected for pterin metabolites to detect biopterin defects. The diagnostic tests used to distinguish these disorders are BH$_4$ loading, high-pressure liquid chromatographic pterin analysis of urine, and direct analysis of cofactor activity in the blood (see Table 14.4).[57] Direct measurement of enzymatic activity is possible but is only available in research centres and is rarely needed.

Low-level elevations that show a slowly declining trend or plateau below 16.5 mg/dl and are normal on pterin testing are classified as non-PKU hyperphenylalaninaemias. Most clinicians do not treat such cases with a low-phenylalanine diet but monitor physical and mental development closely. Protein may be restricted to the minimum needed for normal development. The recent description of abnormal magnetic resonance findings on brain scans in PKU patients might provide a guide to when to use the low-phenylalanine diet in this group.[58-60] The amount of phenylalanine restriction needed is usually less than that needed with classical PKU.

To rule out transient defects some clinicians will challenge the PKU child after completion of myelination, e.g., at age one year, with phenylalanine or protein ingestion. Rapid rise of phenylalanine confirms the diagnosis.

SUMMARY OF NEONATAL SCREENING AND DIAGNOSIS

Figure 14.3 summarizes the screening and diagnostic process. The figures it includes are examples of what can be achieved by a systematically planned population-based screening programme administered by a public health agency, integrated with follow-up, diagnosis, and treatment facilities. Most experts favour this kind of centrally organized programme, and experience in California supports them. From 1965 to 1980, PKU screening in California was performed in about 120 private hospital and

Table 14.4 Differential diagnostic patterns for biopterin (BH$_4$) defects and classical PKU

Defect	Test		
	BH$_4$ loading	Urinary pterins	Cofactor
DHPR deficiency	PP lowered (unreliable)	N/B ratio ↓ (N↑B↑)	BH$_4$ decreased
GTPCH deficiency	PP lowered	N/B ratio normal (N↓B↓)	BH$_4$ decreased
6PTS deficiency	PP lowered	N/B ratio ↑ (N↑B↓)	BH$_4$ decreased
Primapterinuria	PP lowered	N/B ratio ↑ (N↑B↑)	BH$_4$ decreased
PKU (classical)	PP unchanged	N/B ratio normal (N↑B↑)	BH$_4$ normal

PP = plasma phenylalanine, N = neopterin, B = biopterin, ↑ = increased value, ↓ = decreased value

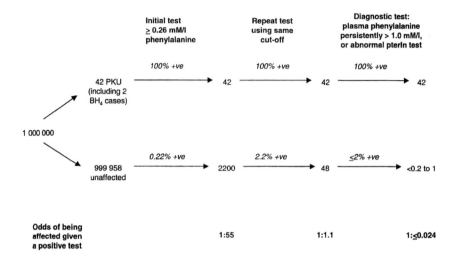

Fig. 14.3 Flow chart of screening for phenylketonuria based on Californian experience with the automated fluorometric method.

outpatient laboratories. Positive results were reported to local physicians or health agencies for follow-up. During this period, 5 190 782 newborns were screened, 267 cases of PKU found, and 16 cases missed. The mean age at time of treatment was 22 days. In 1980, the state health department took direct responsibility and adopted statewide uniform automated testing in eight quality controlled regional laboratories in a computer monitored system with 14 dedicated regional follow-up facilities. As of December 1990, 4 841 171 newborns have been screened and 194 classical PKU cases found. No cases have been missed following the state protocol and treatment was started at a mean age of 9.8 days.

TREATMENT

The mainstay of treatment is restriction of phenylalanine in the diet. On a daily allowance of 250–500 mg phenylalanine per day, positive nitrogen balance and plasma phenylalanine levels within the desired range of 0.25 mM/l and 0.6 mM/l can be maintained. Evidence now favours beginning treatment as soon after birth as possible and continuing restriction for as long as the patient can be persuaded to endure it.[26,27,61,62] The initial period of vulnerability to irreversible damage is during the completion of brain growth and myelination, approximately birth to age ten. Premature termination of the diet after this point will frequently depress cognitive function and may adversely affect behaviour by toxic mechanisms that are apparently not reversible. While brief exposure to phenylalanine will result in transient toxic effects, persistently elevated levels in older children and adults, however, can result in permanent damage and symptoms such as seizures.[59,63,64]

While treatment is undoubtedly effective in promoting normal growth and in preserving near normal IQ, minor defects in conceptual, visual—spatial and language development have been reported. While these may affect school performance, they do not constitute a major problem for adults in terms of social adjustment and work performance.

Treatment of 'malignant PKU' most commonly due to 6 PTS or DHPR deficiency consists of reduction of plasma phenylalanine by dietary control, combined with oral L-dihydrophenylalanine (dopa) (12 mg/kg/day) and 5 hydroxytryptophan (10 mg/kg/day) to replace missing neurotransmitters. Carbidopa prevents rapid degradation of L-dopa and can be used to lower the dose. Folinic acid (12.5 mg/kg/day) is used to restore tissue folate levels.

Maternal PKU

The success of newborn screening for PKU has exposed another related problem, maternal PKU. Females affected by PKU, because of early dietary treatment, will now join the general population as potential mothers. They will expose any fetus to their elevated plasma phenylalanine levels. This *in utero* exposure results in mental retardation in 90 per cent of the live births. Frequently, such infants are microcephalic, have cardiac and other anomalies, and low birth weight.[32,65,66] Reports of improved outcome when such women were placed on a low-phenylalanine diet have prompted efforts to find and treat them.[67,68] Several long-term studies on the effectiveness and optimum conditions for treatment of maternal hyperphenylalaninaemia are in progress.[69] From these studies it appears that both classic PKU, and non-PKU HPA, where plasma phenylalanine is 0.6 mM/l (10 mg/dl) or greater occur, are at risk. Treatment must begin before conception to achieve optimal outcomes. Some screening programmes have developed registries of female cases[70,71] and attempt to follow them through the child-bearing years. Others have proposed selective or universal antenatal screening.[72] There is a critical need to analyze the cost-effectiveness of these various approaches and aggressively address this issue if the benefits of newborn screening are to be preserved.[73,74]

Difficulties with diet compliance in this group of women prompted the suggestion that use of intestinal bacterial phenylalanine ammonia lysase (PAL) to reduce plasma phenylalanine, either alone or in addition to dietary control, might be a more acceptable alternative.[11]

COSTS

The costs of screening programmes vary depending on their structure and the economies of the locale in which they operate. They are frequently under-estimated by being limited to the cost of laboratory personnel, equipment and supplies. The true costs should include the costs of collection, laboratory quality control, repeat tests, reporting and follow-up activities, data collection, and programme evaluation. The cost of PKU testing is also difficult to separate when a panel of tests is performed. Estimates at 1993 prices based on the California programme (which pays for all costs except the collection of specimens) are provided in Table 14.5.

There have been many cost/benefit analyses of varying degrees of sophistication appropriate to specific programme designs and jurisdictions.[75-80] The conclusion of all such studies is that PKU screening is cost beneficial to varying degrees. A detailed cost analysis is a laborious effort and is applicable only to the particular service costs in the region studied. Using costs in California, the following estimate of the PKU testing component was made.

Table 14.5   Cost estimates of PKU only based on California programme

Item	Cost (US$) per test
Filter paper forms	0.20
Collection costs	6.00
Postage	0.40
Laboratory personnel	3.60
Laboratory operating costs	0.50
Laboratory quality control	0.50
Reagents and supplies	1.00
Follow-up costs (salaries, letters, telephone)	3.00
Data processing	0.25
Administrative costs (fee collection, regulations, personnel, contract admin.)	1.30
Total	16.75

The frequency of detection of classic PKU is one in 25 000. Therefore, the estimated cost of detection of one case is $16.75 × 25 000 = $418 750. The cost of diagnosis, diet, and clinic visits for 10 years is approximately $15 000 for a net cost of $433 750 per case.

The costs of services to an untreated case which includes home care for six years with admission to a state institution thereafter are approximately $50 000 per year for 60 years, or $3 000 000. The approximate cost avoidance per dollar spent in screening is $6.92.

OTHER METABOLIC DISORDERS

There are many metabolic disorders that have been proposed to be added to the basic PKU blood spot programme. Analysis of programmes in the US as of 1989 found that 41 states screen for galactosaemia, 21 for maple syrup urine disease, 20 for homocystinuria, and 14 for biotinidase deficiency.[30]

Galactosaemia has been discussed in more detail elsewhere and will only be briefly reviewed.[81,82] Galactosaemia is an autosomal recessive disorder of galactose metabolism due to absence of galactose-1-phosphate uridyl transferase. This leads to accumulation of galactose-1-phosphate in body tissues resulting in cataracts, hepatic failure, and mental retardation. The newborns are susceptible to overwhelming infection which makes early identification and treatment critical. The substitution of meat or soy-based formulas and avoidance of galactose is effective in prevention of most of these problems, although recent reviews have documented persistent problems.[83,84] The disorder can be screened by direct assay of the transferase enzyme by fluorometry or by microbiological assay for galactose or galactose-1-phosphate.[85] The birth prevalence is 1:60 000 to 80 000. False-positives occur if the enzyme is inactivated by heat or mishandling of specimens. Missed cases are rare and usually occur when galactose or galactose-1-phosphate are assayed in the absence of milk feeding. The disorder is generally felt to meet the criteria for population screening previously discussed. Based on Californian experience, there will be 800 false positives and 12 cases for every million newborns screened. (Fig. 14.4).

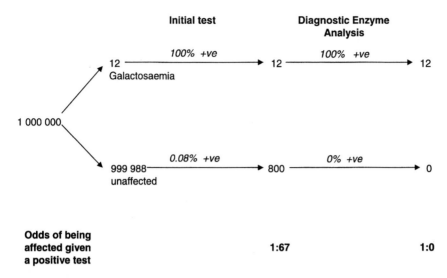

Fig. 14.4 Flow chart of screening for galactosaemia based on Californian experience with the quantitative fluorometric G-1–P-U transferase method.

The case for screening for maple syrup urine disease (MSUD) is less compelling. This is another mixed group of autosomal recessive disorders of branch chain alpha keto acid dehydrogenase enzyme complex which results in inability to metabolize leucine isoleucine and valine.[86] The birth prevalence has been reported as 1:200 000 but in practice the figure of 1:500 000 is more typical. This may be due to intermittent appearance of the branch chain amino acids used as a screening indicator. Some cases may die as newborns undiagnosed and untested. The test is inexpensive and has a tolerably small false-positive rate. The detection rate, however, is less satisfactory. Treatment is difficult, requiring a special synthetic diet and careful monitoring to avoid acidosis and excessively high or low blood amino acid levels. Infections and stress will produce dramatic metabolic changes and apparently cause cumulative injury to the brain. Long-term follow-up has reported premature death and less than optimum mental development in a disturbing number of cases. There has been limited publication of long-term results, however, and information on the screening, diagnosis, and treatment of this disorder needs to be pooled and analyzed to reach any conclusion about the value of screening.

REFERENCES

1. Scriver C. R., and Clow C. L. (1980). Phenylketonuria. Epitome of biochemical genetics. *New Engl. J. Med.*, **303**, 1336–1400.
2. Folling A. (1934). Excretion of urinary phenylpyruvic acid as a metabolic anomaly in connection with imbecility. *Hoppe Seyler's Z Physiol. Cl Chem*, **227**, 169–76.
3. Eyman R. K. *et al.* (1989). The life expectancy of profoundly handicapped people with mental retardation. *New Engl. J. Med.*, **323**, 584–9.

4. Allen R. A., and Gibson R. M. (1961). Phenylketonuria with normal intelligence. *Am. J. Dis. Child.*, **102**, 145.
5. Hsia D. Y.-Y. *et al.* (1968). Atypical phenylketonuria with borderline or normal intelligence. *Am. J. Dis. Child.*, **116**, 143–57.
6. Knox W. E. (1974). Phenylketonuria. In: *The metabolic basis of inherited disease*, 3rd edn. (ed: J. B. Stanbury, J. B. Wyngaargen, and D. S. Fredrickson), p. 258. McGraw-Hill, New York.
7. Primrose D. A. (1983). Phenylketonuria with normal intelligence. *J. Ment. Defic. Res.*, **27**, 239–46.
8. Guttler F. (1980). Hyperphenylalaninaemia: diagnosis and classification of the various types of phenylalanine hydroxylase deficiency in childhood. *Acta Paediat. Scand.*, **280**, (Suppl.), 1–80.
9. Scriver C. R. *et al.* (1995). The hyperphenylalaninaemias. In: *The metabolic basis of inherited disease*, Vol. 1, 7th edn. (ed: C. Scriver, A. Beaudet, W. Sly, and D. Valle), pp. 1015–75. McGraw-Hill, New York.
10. Guttler F. (1989). Modern techniques of differentiating the various phenotypes of phenylketonuria. *Postgrad. Med. J.*, **65** (Suppl. 2), 52–6.
11. Scriver C. R. *et al.* (1989). The hyperphenylalaninaemias. In: *The metabolic basis of inherited disease*, Vol. 1, 6th edn. (ed: C. Scriver, A. Beaudet, W. Sly, and D. Valle), pp. 495–546. McGraw-Hill, New York.
12. Dhondt J. L. (1984). Tetrahydrobiopterin deficiencies: preliminary analysis from an international survey. *J. Pediatrics*, **104**, 501–8.
13. Blau N. *et al.* (1989). Primapterinuria: a new variant of atypical phenylketonuria. *J. Inher. Metab. Dis.*, **12** (Suppl. 2), 335–8.
14. Scriver C. R. *et al.* (1994). PAH gene mutation analysis. *Consortium Newsletter* (April).
15. Eisensmith R., and Woo S. L. C. (1992). Updated listing of haplotypes at the human phenylalanine hydroxylase (PAH) locus. *Am. J. Hum. Genet.*, **51**, 1445–8.
16. Rey F., and Rey J. (eds) (1990). *Abstracts of the International PKU Workshop*, Hôpital des Enfants Malades. Hôpital des Enfants Malades, Paris.
17. Lyonnet S. *et al.* (1989). Molecular genetics of phenylketonuria in Mediterranean countries: a mutation associated with partial phenylalanine hydroxylase deficiency. *Am. J. Hum. Genet.*, **44**, 511–17.
18. Özalp J. *et al.* (1986). Incidence of phenylketonuria and hyperphenylalaninaemia in a sample of the newborn population. *J. Inher. Metab. Dis.*, **9** (Suppl. 2), 237.
19. Smith I. *et al.* (1991). Review of neonatal screening programme for phenylketonuria. *Br. Med. J.*, **303**, 333–5.
20. Avigad S. *et al.* (1985). A single origin of phenylketonuria in Yemenite Jews. *Nature*, **334**, 168–70.
21. Mathias D., and Bickel H. (1986). Follow-up study of 16 years neonatal screening for inborn error of metabolism in West Germany. *Eur. Pediatr.*, **145**, 310–12.
22. Cabalsky B. *et al.* (1993). Twenty-five years' experience with newborn screening for phenylketonuria (PKU) in Poland. *Screening*, **2**, 29–32.
23. Guthrie R. (1967). Laboratory screening and diagnosis. In: *Proceedings of the International Conference on Inborn Errors of Metabolism*, May 30–June 3, 1966, Dubrovnik, Yugoslavia., p.17. Department of Health, Education and Welfare.
24. Szabó L. *et al.* (1985). Experience based on 800,000 newborn screening tests of the Budapest Phenylketonuria Centre. *Acta Ped. Hung.*, **26**, 113–25.

25. Wang T. *et al.* (1989). Molecular genetics of phenylketonuria in orientals: linkage disequilibrium between a termination, mutation and haplotype 4 of the phenylalanine hydroxylase gene. *Am. Hum. Gen.*, **45**, 675–80.

26. Halvorsen S., and Skjelkväk L. (1974). Screeninggundersokelser pä fenylketouri med en papirkkromatographick methodik. *Läkartedningen*, **71**, 1166–7.

27. Becroft D. M., and Horn C. R. (1969). The Guthrie screening test for phenylketonuria: a report on two years participation in the national programme. *N. Z. Med. J.*, **69**, 212–5.

28. Frézal J. *et al.* (1990). The French program of systematic neonatal screening. I: Organization and results. In: *Genetic screening from newborns to DNA typing.* (ed: B. M. Knoppers, and C. M. Laberge), pp. 41–64, Excerpta Medica, Amsterdam.

29. Missiou-Tsagaraki S. *et al.* (1988). Phenylketonuria in Greece: 12 years' experience. *J. Ment. Defic. Res.*, **32**, 271–87.

30. Cunningham G. C., and Riggle S. (1989). *Council of Regional Networks for Genetic Services. Newborn Screening Report.*

31. Laberge C. *et al.* (1987). Hyperphenylalaninemies: experience canadienne et québecoise. *Arch. Fr. Pediatr.*, **44**, 643–7.

32. Bodegärd G., and Zetterström R. (1974). Erfarenheter av diagnostik och behandling av fenylketouric. *Lakartedningen*, **71**, 1163–85.

33. Aoki K., and Wada Y. (1988). Outcome of the patients detected by newborn screening in Japan. *Acta Pediatr. Jap.* **30**, 429–34.

34. Cohen B. E. *et al.* (1973). The hyperphenylalaninemias in Israel. *Israel J. Med. Sci.*, **9**, 1393.

35. Cunningham G. C. (1971). Phenylketonuria testing: its role in pediatrics and public health. *CRC. Critical Reviews in Clin. Lab. Sci.*, **2**, 1. Chemical Rubber Company.

36. Guthrie R., and Susi A. (1963). A simple phenylalanine method for detecting phenylketonuria in large populations òf newborn infants. *Pediatrics*, **32**, 338–43.

37. Efron M. L. *et al.* (1964). A simple chromatographic screening test for the detection of disorders of amino acid metabolism. *New Engl. J. Med.*, **270**, 1378.

38. McCaman M. N., and Robins E. (1962). Fluorometric method for the determination of phenylalanine in serum. *J. Lab. Clin. Med.*, **59**, 885.

39. Wendel U. *et al.* (1989). Monitoring of phenylketonuria. A colormetric method for determination of plasma phenylalanine using L-phenylalanine dehydrogenase. *Anal. Biochem.*, **180**, 91–4.

40. Naruse H. *et al.* (1992). A method of PKU screening using phenylalanine dehydrogenase and microplate system. *Screening*, **1**, 63–6.

41. Ponzone A. *et al.* (1988). Two mutations of dihydropteridine reductase deficiency. *Arch. Dis. Child.*, **63**, 154–7.

42. Lyonnet S. *et al.* (1988). Guthrie cards for detection of point mutations in phenylketonuria (letter). *Lancet*, **2**, 507.

43. Schwartz E. I. *et al.* (1990). Polymerase chain reaction amplification from dried blood spots on Guthrie cards. *Lancet*, **336**, 639–40.

44. Holtzmann N. A. *et al.* (1974). Neonatal screening for phenylketonuria: effectiveness. *J. Am. Med. Assoc.*, **229**, 667–75.

45. Doherty L. B. *et al.* (1991). Detection of phenylketonuria in the very early newborn specimen. *Pediatrics*, **87**, 240–4.

46. McCabe E. R. B. *et al.* (1983). Newborn screening for phenylketonuria: predictive validity as a function of age. *Pediatrics*, **72**, 390–8.

47. Hansen H. (1975). Prevention of mental retardation due to PKU: selected aspects of program validity. *Prev. Med.*, **4**, 310–21.
48. Komrower G. M. (1984). Phenylketonuria and other inherited metabolic defects. In: *Antenatal and neonatal screening.*, 1st edn, (ed:. N. J. Wald), pp. 221–8, Oxford University Press, Oxford.
49. Guthrie R. I., and Whitney S. (1964). *Phenylketonuria: Detection in the newborn as a routine hospital procedure.* Children's Bureau Publication 419.
50. Scriver C. R. *et al.* (1980). Cord blood tyrosine levels in the full term phenylketonuric fetus and the 'justification hypothesis'. *Proc. Natl. Acad. of Sci. USA*, **77**, 6175–8.
51. Schneider A. J. (1983). Newborn phenylalanine/tyrosine metabolism: implications for screening for phenylketonuria. *Am. J. Dis. Child.*, **137**, 427–32.
52. Cunningham G. C. *et al.* (1987). Phenylalanine level of newborns in their first few days of life. In: *Advances in neonatal screening.*, Excerpta Medica International Congress Series 741., (ed:. B. L. Therrell), pp. 179–81, Elsevier Science, Amsterdam.
53. Schoen E. J. *et al.* (1983). More on newborn screening for phenylketonuria: recommendations of the Committee on Genetics. *Pediatrics*, **72**, 390–8.
54. Holzman C. *et al.* (1986). Descriptive epidemiology of missed cases of phenylketonuria and congenital hypothyroidism. *Pediatrics*, **78**, 553–8.
55. Dontanville V. K., and Cunningham G. C. (1973). Effect of feeding on screening for PKU in infants. *Pediatrics*, **51**, 531–8.
56. Sepe S. J. *et al.* (1979). An evaluation of routine follow-up blood screening of infants for phenylketonuria. *New Engl. J. Med.*, **300**, 606–9.
57. Dhondt J. L. (1991). Strategy for screening of tetrahydrobiopterin deficiency among hyperphenylalaninaemic patients: 15 years' experience. *J. Inher. Metab. Dis.*, **14**, 117–27.
58. Cleary M. A. *et al.* (1994). Magnetic resonance imaging of the brain in phenylketonuria. *Lancet*, **344**, 87–90.
59. Thompson A. J. *et al.* (1990). Neurological deterioration in young adults with phenylketonuria. *Lancet*, **366**, 602–5.
60. Thompson A. J. *et al.* (1991). Magnetic resonance imagining changes in early treated patients with phenylketonuria. *Lancet*, **337**, 1224.
61. Azen C. G. *et al.* (1991). Intellectual development in 12 year old children treated for phenylketonuria. *Am. J. Dis. Child.*, **145**, 35–9.
62. Editorial (1991). Phenylketonuria grows up. *Lancet*, **337**, 1256–7.
63. Villasana D. *et al.* (1989). Neurological deterioration in adult phenylketonuria. *J. Inher. Metab. Dis.*, **12**, 451–7.
64. Ris M.D. *et al.* (1994). Early treated phenylketonuria: adult neuropsychologic outcome. *J. Pediat.*, **124**, 388–92.
65. Mabry C. *et al.* (1969). Maternal phenylketonuria. *New Engl. J. Med.*, **269**, 1505.
66. Levy H. L., and Waisbren W. E. (1983). Effect of untreated maternal phenylketonuria and hyperphenylalaninaemia on the fetus. *New Engl. J. Med.*, **309**, 1269–74.
67. Drogari E. *et al.* (1987). Timing of strict diet in relation to fetal damage in maternal phenylketonuria. An International Collaborative Study by the MRC/DHSS Phenylketonuria Register. *Lancet*, **2**, 927–30.
68. Rohr F. J. *et al.* (1987). New England Maternal PKU Project: Prospective study of untreated and treated pregnancies and their outcomes. *J. Pediatr.*, **110**, 391–8.

69. Koch R. *et al.* (1986). The maternal PKU collaborative study. *J. Inher. Metab. Dis.*, **9**, (suppl. 2), 159–68.

70. Friedman J. M. *et al.* (1987). ReCAP, the Registry of Cytogenetic Abnormalities and Phenylketonuria. *Am. J. Med. Genet.*, **27**, 325–36.

71. Cartier L. *et al.* (1982). Prevention of mental retardation in offspring of hyperphenylalaninaemic mothers. *Am. J. Public Health*, **72**, 1386–90.

72. Luke B., and Keith L. G. (1990). The challenge of maternal phenylketonuria screening and treatment. *J. Reprod. Med.*, **35**, 667–73.

73. Guthrie R. (1988). Maternal PKU. A continuing problem. *Am. J. Public Health*, **78**, 771.

74. Luder A. S., and Greene C. L. (1989). Maternal phenylketonuria and hyperphenylalaninaemia. Implications for medical practice in the United States. *Am. J. Obstet. Gynecol.*, **161**, 1102–5.

75. Bush J. W. *et al.* (1973). Health status index in cost effectiveness: Analysis of PKU program. In: *Health status indexes*, pp. 172–209, (ed: R. L. Berg). Chicago Hospital Research and Educational Trust, Chicago.

76. Dagenais D. L. *et al.* (1985). A cost benefit analysis of the Québec Network of Genetic Medicine. *Soc. Sci. Med.*, **20**, 601–7.

77. Van Pelt A., and Levy H. L. (1974). Cost-benefit analysis of newborn screening for metabolic disorders. *New Engl. J. Med.*, **291**, 1414–6.

78. Steiner K. C. and Smith H. A. (1973). Application of cost benefit analysis to a PKU screening program. *Inquiry*, **10**, 34.

79. U.S. Congress Office of Technology Assessment (1988). *Healthy children: investing in the future in newborn screening for congenital disorders.* Washington, D.C.:U.S. Congress Office of Technology Assessment, p. 93.

80. Alm J. *et al.* (1982). Health economic analysis of the Swedish neonatal metabolic screening programme. (A method of optimizing routines). *Med. Decis. Making*, **2**, 33–45.

81. Segal S., and Berry G. T. (1995). Disorders of galactose metabolism. In: *The metabolic basis of inherited disease.*, Vol. 1, 7th edn. (ed:. C. Scriver, A. Beaudet, W. Sly, and D. Valle). pp. 967–1000. McGraw Hill, New York.

82. Donnell G. N. (ed.) (1993). *Galactosemia: new frontiers in research.* U.S. Department of Health and Human Services, Washington, DC. National Institutes of Health Publication No. 93–3438.

83. Donnell G. N. *et al.*. (1969). Observations on results of management of galactosemic patients. In: *Galactosemia.*, (ed:. D. Y. Y. Hsia). p. 247, Charles C Thomas, Springfield, IL.

84. Komrower G. M., and Lee D. H. (1970). Long term follow-up of galactosemia. *Arch. Dis. Child.*, **45**, 367–73.

85. Guthrie R. *et al.* (1983). A comparison of three newborn screening tests for galactosemia. In: *Neonatal Screening. Proceedings of the Second International Conference on Neonatal Screening*, p. 243 (ed: N. Naruse and M.H, Irie). Excerpta Medica Amsterdam, Tokyo.

86. Chuang D. T., and Shih V. E. (1989). Disorder of branch chain amino acid and keto acid metabolism. In: *The metabolic basis of inherited disease*, Vol. 1, 6th edn. (ed:. C. Scriver, A. Beaudet, W. Sly, and D. Valle), pp. 1239–77. McGraw-Hill, New York.

15 *Congenital hypothyroidism*

Joseph G. Hollowell, Bradford L. Therrell, and W. Harry Hannon

INTRODUCTION

Congenital hypothyroidism (CH) is a well-established cause of mental retardation. Before neonatal screening for CH was available, ascertainment was based on clinical findings, and treatment was generally delayed until the infants were three to six months old.[1-4] Children with CH identified through clinical findings had a median IQ of roughly 80; 40 per cent had an IQ below 70.[5] Neonatal screening has nearly eliminated the associated mental retardation in many parts of the world since it was first introduced in the 1970s.[6,7] Screening for CH fulfils the requirements for population based screening programmes, since (1) untreated infants with CH are at great risk for mental retardation and developmental delay; (2) CH can be detected inexpensively at birth; (3) there is a relatively high incidence rate; and (4) safe and inexpensive treatment will effectively change the course of the disease.[5] Screening programmes for CH must include mechanisms for blood sampling; laboratory testing and reporting; early diagnosis, treatment, and follow-up for the entire group at risk; and there must be systems of quality assurance throughout.

THE DISORDER

Description

CH results from a deficiency of serum concentrations of 'free' thyroxine. CH has few signs and symptoms at birth. A study of one-week-old infants found only a few discriminating characteristics, namely, decreased linear growth and delayed skeletal maturation for gestational age, jaundice, enlarged tongue, abdominal distention, mottled skin, and muscle hypotonia. Increased head size was a borderline discriminant. The signs, when present, are non-specific, and some infants with CH have none of these characteristics.[8]

Postnatally, thyroid hormone has its greatest effect during infancy and early childhood, the period when most postnatal thyroid-dependent brain and bone growth occurs and a time critical for thyroid replacement treatment. If CH is left untreated during this period, it progresses to lethargy, constipation, prolonged neonatal jaundice, poor feeding, hypothermia, growth retardation, and neurologic damage.[5,9] Because of their passivity, hypothyroid infants are often considered 'good babies' and fail to elicit particular medical attention.

Physiology of thyroid hormone production

All of the components necessary to regulate thyroid hormone production appear to function adequately in early fetal life (Fig. 15.1). The hypothalamus produces thyrotropin-releasing hormone (TRH), which causes the release of thyrotropin (thyroid stimulating hormone–TSH) from the pituitary gland. TSH, a glycoprotein, stimulates the thyroid gland to increase production of thyroxine (tetra-iodothyronine– T4), which is converted primarily outside the thyroid into the active form triiodo- thyronine (T3). Thyroid hormone feedback to the hypothalamus and pituitary decreases TSH synthesis thus modulating thyroid hormone production.[10] In addition, maternal T4 crosses the placenta and contributes to the fetal pool.[11]

There is a brief surge in the TSH level during the first few hours after birth. Whether this is from thermal challenge or stress of parturition is unknown. T4 and T3 also increase shortly after birth (Fig. 15.2) and decrease more slowly than TSH during the next few weeks.[12] In primary hypothyroidism, the primary hormonal abnormality is

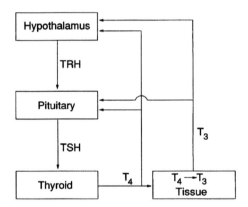

Fig. 15.1 Regulation of thyroid hormone secretion.

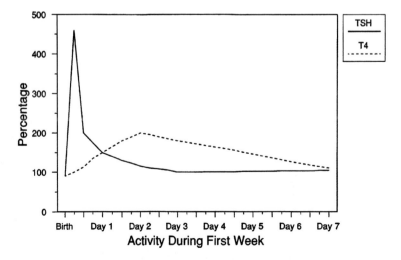

Fig. 15.2 Thyroid function tests among euthyroid neonates as a function of age. The mean values at each age are expressed as percentages of mean normal values at 90 days of age.

low T4, with the result that T3 is also low and TSH is high. In secondary hypothyroidism and tertiary hypothyroidism, the low T4 is secondary to insufficient TSH
production.

Aetiology

The causes of CH include: (1) dysplasia or structural abnormalities of the gland
(aplasia and hypoplasia); (2) abnormal location of the gland (ectopic gland); (3)
inborn errors of thyroid gland metabolism (dyshormonogenesis); (4) hypothalamic or
pituitary insufficiency; and (5) transient hypothyroidism. The first three of these are
primary hypothyroidism. The fourth is secondary hypothyroidism when the pituitary
is involved or tertiary hypothyroidism when the hypothalamus fails. Transient
hypothyroidism occurs more commonly in Europe and Japan than in North America.

**Table 15.1   Birth prevalence of congenital
hypothyroidism in Europe before and after
screening programmes**

Country	Rate per 100 000	
	Before screening	After screening
Sweden[2]	14.5	38.5
Netherlands[4]	16	23.8
Denmark[3]	16.4	45.4

Table 15.2   Birth prevalence of congenital hypothyroidism

Country	Total screened	Cases of CH	Rate per 100 000	Years screened
Australia[18]	1 812 683	436	24.1	1977–85
Austria[16]	346 185	63	18.2	1985–88
Belgium[16]	360 264	109	30.3	1985–88
Canada[19]	874 000	209	23.9	1973–83
China, Hong Kong[20]	14 411	5	34.7	1982–84
China, Shanghai[21]	18 926	3	15.9	1981–82
Czechoslovakia[16]	773 593	136	17.6	1985–88
Denmark[16]	224 189	76	33.9	1985–88
Finland[16]	246 752	58	23.5	1985–88
France[16]	3 216 596	750	23.3	1985–88
Germany (FRG)[16]	1 148 415	279	24.3	1985–88
Greece[16]	412 714	135	32.7	1985–88
Hungary[22]	306 265	56	18.3	1982–88
Israel[16]	393 304	159	40.4	1985–88
Italy[16,23]	5 018 241	1647	32.8	1977–91
Japan[24]	8 846 297	1151	13.0	1979–85
Kuwait[14]	86 910	25	28.8	1981–87
New Zealand[21]	228 783	47	20.5	up to1983
Norway[16]	215 124	68	31.6	1985–88
Pakistan[25]	5000	5	100.0	1987–88
Portugal[16]	431 536	98	22.7	1985–88
Saudi Arabia[15]	44 033	21	47.7	1985–91
Spain[16]	1 400 279	433	30.9	1985–88
Sweden[16]	413 616	131	31.7	1985–88
Switzerland[16]	314 599	85	27.0	1985–88
The Netherlands[16,26]	1 601 603	481	30.0	1985–88
United Kingdom[16]	2 784 603	840	30.2	1985–88
United States[27]	4 095 092	1180	28.8	1992

Table 15.3 Screening results for CH in the United States

Racial/ethnic groups	Number screened	Cases of CH	Rate per 100 000	95% CI
Total[27]	4 095 092	1180	28.8	(27.2–30.5)
Whites				
California[28]	1 497 971	359	24.0	(21.6–26.6)
Georgia*	337 746	93	27.5	(22.2–33.7)
New Mexico[29]	75 660	14	18.5	(8.8–28.2)
Texas**	668 736	198	29.6	(25.6–34.0)
Blacks				
California[28]	249 415	23	9.2	(5.8–13.8)
Georgia*	196 873	22	11.2	(7.0–16.9)
Texas**	171 069	25	14.6	(9.5–21.6)
Hispanics				
California[28]	1 042 518	367	35.4	(31.7–39.8)
New Mexico[29]	66 610	28	42.0	(26.5–57.6)
Texas**	398 604	161	40.4	(34.4–47.1)
Native Americans				
New Mexico[29]	21 010	18	85.7	(46.1–125.2)

* Unpublished data, Ann Brown, Division of Medical Genetics, Department of Pediatrics, Emory University School of Medicine, Atlanta, Georgia, July 1991.
** Unpublished data, B. L. Therrell, Texas Department of Health, Austin, Texas, 1991.

The predominant cause of CH varies by population group. Among Hispanics in San Diego dysplastic glands is the most important cause.[13] In Finland, France, Germany, Australia, and Japan, ectopic glands is the predominant cause. In Kuwait and Saudi Arabia, 46 and 47 per cent of infants with CH respectively were found to have dyshormonogenesis, a genetic cause related to the parental consanguinity present in those countries.[14,15] The severity of CH can vary considerably and is related to the type of disorder. More severe symptoms are found with thyroid aplasia, while other forms such as ectopic gland, hypoplasia, or dyshormongenesis are associated with less severe disturbances.[9]

Birth prevalence (incidence)

In Sweden, Denmark, and The Netherlands[2–4,16] the prevalence of CH ascertained clinically before newborn screening began was lower than the birth prevalence reported with screening (Table 15.1). This was substantiated in another Swedish study in which TSH levels measured retrospectively in dried blood spots collected at birth from 31 five-year-old children were found to be greater than 40 µU/mL. Nine of these children were euthyroid. Twenty-two were hypothyroid, of whom 15 had been clinically detected. The seven children not detected had developmental scores which were 'normal', but significantly lower than in those clinically detected and treated.[17] It is likely that many of the increased numbers of infants detected with population screening are infants with less severe disease. This study makes the point that without detection and treatment, children with milder disease can have demonstrable developmental impairment.

In studies based on screened populations of 100 000 or more, the birth prevalence of CH has ranged from 13/100 000 in Japan to 40/100 000 in Israel (Table 15.2). There are also racial and ethnic differences in the CH rate within populations (Table 15.3). The reported rate for black infants in the United States is about half the rate for white infants. For Hispanics the rate is about 40 per cent higher than for white infants. Data from New Mexico suggest that the rate in Native Americans is even higher.[29] Most studies have found a greater prevalence of CH in females.

Reports from both England and South Africa indicate that CH is several times more common in children whose forebears came from the Indian subcontinent than in white children.[21,30] Screening programs report small additional increases in incidence rates as screening approaches 100 per cent of the newborn population. In Japan, for example, the incidence in 1979–80 was 12.2/100 000 and in 1985–6, 15.4/100 000.[24] In Georgia, reported incidence rose by 100 per cent in black and 40 per cent in white infants between 1981 and 1985[31] and 1986–90 (personal communication, Ann Brown, 1991). The observed increases in birth prevalence with screening experience can be explained by improvement in screening systems and procedures and by the detection at birth of less severely affected children.

All the above findings were based mainly on cases of primary hypothyroidism. Only programmes that measure T4 or a combination of TSH and T4 in the total population can detect secondary and tertiary hypothyroidism. Most European and Japanese programmes measure TSH alone for the initial screen. Measurement of T4 followed by TSH has been widely used as the primary method of screening in the United States and The Netherlands.[26] In the United States the reported birth prevalence of secondary and tertiary CH is 0.7–1.5/100 000.[32]

SCREENING TESTS

Markers of thyroid metabolism

Sensitive, semi-automated micromethods for measuring T4 and TSH in dried blood-spot samples have made newborn screening for CH feasible for large populations.[6] The tests can be carried out on punches from the same dried blood spot sample routinely collected to screen for phenylketonuria.

Before discussing the rationale for different approaches to screening for CH, the thyroid hormones and various proteins that may be analysed during screening or diagnosis will be described.

Thyroid stimulating hormone (TSH)

TSH is the pituitary glycoprotein responsible for stimulating production of the active thyroid hormones T4 and T3. Secretion of TSH occurs through stimulation by thyrotropin-releasing hormone in response to lowered levels of the circulating thyroid hormones. The serum TSH concentration is considered to be the best indicator of thyroid function.

Thyroxine (T4)

T4 commonly circulates at a concentration of approximately 6.5 to 16.3 µg/dL at birth. Proteins in serum (thyroxine-binding globulin, serum albumin, and thyroxine-binding pre-albumin) effectively bind more than 99 per cent of the circulating T4 and T3, which is in equilibrium with a pool of 'free T4'.[33] Free T4 reflects the bio-availability of T4 and determines the metabolic status of the infant. The total measurable T4 (or T3) is the total of the bound and 'free' fractions. Abnormal concentrations of binding proteins can mislead the interpretation of screening results. Measurement of these proteins and of free T4 may therefore be needed to properly interpret the findings.

Binding proteins

Thyroxine-binding globulin, a glycoprotein, contains one binding site per molecule and reversibly binds about 75 per cent of the circulating T4 and 60 per cent of the circulating T3. A patient's thyroxine-binding globulin level can be measured directly in cases where the thyroid hormone levels do not correlate well with the apparent signs or symptoms of hypothyroidism.[34] Excessive amounts of thyroxine-binding pre-albumin may also decrease the concentration of free T4 and must be considered during diagnosis and follow-up.[35,36]

Free thyroxine

Patients in whom it is important to measure free T4 levels include those where levels of binding proteins are outside the normal range. The correct technique for free T4 analysis and its clinical interpretation is controversial.[37,38] In cases in which analytical techniques are not available, free T4 may be estimated indirectly by measuring total T4 and the 'T3-uptake'.

T3-uptake

The T3-uptake is commonly used in conjunction with total T4 as a means of correcting for the influence of circulating thyroid-binding proteins on the total T4 concentration. When isotopically labeled T3 is added to a mixture of serum and erythrocytes (RBCs) or resin, it distributes itself between binding sites on serum proteins and binding sites on RBCs or resin. If the binding protein has few binding sites because of increased T4 or because of deficient protein, the uptake of the T3 tracer by RBCs or resin will be increased. The uptake of T3 tracer will be decreased with low T4 or increased binding sites.

Free thyroxine index

The product of the T3-uptake and the total T4 when divided by 100 gives the free thyroxine index, an indirect measure of free T4. An independent evaluation of the T4 and T3-uptake is useful in some instances. High T4 combined with low T3-uptake suggests an increase in the thyroid-binding proteins, which may occur with pregnancy, use of oral contraceptives, hyperproteinemia, acute liver disease, or hereditary TBG increases. A low T4 combined with a high T3-uptake indicates lowered concentrations of thyroid-binding proteins and may be associated with elevated androgens, stress, hypoproteinemia, or drugs such as salicylates, which occupy binding sites on the protein.

The use of markers in screening

The major CH screening approaches rely on either TSH testing alone (TSH-Programmes) or on T4 testing with supplementary TSH testing in infants with low or borderline T4 values (T4/TSH-Programmes). In this section we will discuss these alternative approaches in terms of laboratory technique, detection and false-positive rates, the proportion of samples requiring retesting, and the proportion of infants recalled for definitive diagnostic testing. A problem, however, is that data on the detailed distributions of TSH and T4 levels in affected and unaffected neonates are only beginning to be collected and analysed.[26,39] Also, the influence of the background nutritional levels of iodine on these distributions is still not well understood.

The choice between a TSH-Programme for screening and a T4/TSH-Programme varies with the experience and history of specific screening programmes. The advantages of TSH screening include less variable results for infants at five days of age with fewer false-positive screening findings than are found with T4 at five days of age.[40] Most infants in the United States have samples collected from 24 to 72 hours after birth. TSH blood levels, unlike those of T4, are not influenced by thyroxin binding globulin deficiency; thus, measuring TSH alone will not detect this relatively common and benign sex-linked condition and further reduces the rate of false-positives.

Cases of secondary and tertiary congenital hypothyroidism are also not detected by TSH screening alone. T4 screening, on the other hand, can detect these cases. When newborn screening for CH began, T4 screening was found to be technically less difficult, less expensive, and well suited for large regionalized programmes.[41] The costs for both T4 and TSH tests are now much more comparable although TSH testing may require a slightly larger sample. Because of the TSH surge after birth, TSH-programmes have experienced very high false-positive rates during the first 12 hours after birth.

Sample collection

The age at which screening is performed is important because of the predictable variation in the TSH and T4 concentrations after birth (Fig. 15.2.) In particular, the TSH concentration is highly unstable during the first two days—especially the first 12 hours. Because of this, any screening done in the first two days should use T4 followed by TSH.

Testing at three to five days of life is ideal, but because newborns are often discharged from hospital before three days of age, this ideal may not be realized. It is essential, however, that testing be done before discharge because of the uncertainty that testing will be done later. In the United States all screening programmes recommend sample collection before discharge, regardless of how early that occurs.[42]

The primary sample matrix used in newborn CH screening is whole blood collected at the birthing facility one to five days after delivery depending on the medical facility. The procedure involves a heel stick of the newborn and collecting the blood directly onto special ('filter') paper. The blood spots are dried at ambient temperature and mailed to the testing laboratory within 24 hours of collection. Since testing is quantitative, special paper specifically designed, tested, and approved for its effectiveness for newborn screening must be used.[43] This paper does not have the same construction as paper used for filtration, although it is routinely referred to as 'filter' paper. The blood-spot punches used in thyroid assays, usually 1/8 inch (3.175 mm) in diameter for T4 or 3/16 inch (4.76 mm) in diameter for TSH, equate to whole blood volumetric measurements of 2.9 μL and 6.5 μL respectively.[44] Other less often used sample sources are cord or venipuncture blood, which is applied to filter paper and dried. Liquid serum from cord or venipuncture blood has also been used.[45,46] Differences in analyte values have been reported for blood-spot samples obtained from venous and capillary sources.[47]

In the United States a standard that is applicable to all techniques involving collection of blood on filter paper has been developed and published.[43] This standard specifies proper collection procedures and defines an adequate sample. The sample collection card usually consists of an information section and an attached piece of filter paper. The information requested relates, at a minimum, to specifics about the birth, the parents, and the physician or birthing attendant. If a specimen is inadequate or unsatisfactory for analysis, that fact is recorded at the testing laboratory and conveyed to the sample submitter along with a request for collection of a new sample. If inadequate or unsatisfactory specimens are submitted frequently by a particular collection center, the programme can provide training assistance to the collection personnel. A training video has been prepared in conjunction with the published specimen collection standard.[43]

Programmes and tests

Using a variety of dose-response indicators, laboratories can use immunoassays to quantify either T4 or TSH for CH screening. The dose-response indicator can be an isotope,[48,49] enzyme,[50] or fluorophore.[51] In general, these assays are referred to as radioimmunoassays (RIA), enzyme-linked immunoassays (EIA), immunochemiluminometric assays,[52] or fluoroimmunoassays. The dose-response indicators must have a high specific activity because of the small volume of sample available for the screening tests. Test kits are widely available commercially, or tests can be developed from bulk reagents by the laboratory. The detection limit of dried blood-spot assays must be <1.0 µg/dL for T4 and <5.0 µIU/mL for TSH. The reported coefficients of variation for assay precision of these screening tests are usually 5 to 20 per cent for T4 and 10 to 25 per cent for TSH.[53–55] Most screening programmes use commercial immunoassay kits for T4 and TSH measurements.

In the United States, most screening programmes use a primary T4 analysis by RIA, and most use a floating cut-off of 0.5 to 3 SD below the daily mean values of the screened population. All samples below the designated cut-off or below a predefined fixed value (e.g. 3 to 8 µg/dL according to programme) are followed by a repeat T4 and TSH analysis in duplicate.[56] TSH assays generally use a fixed cut-off value >20 µIU/mL (whole blood) or higher, depending on the iodine deficiency status of the population in a particular region, and samples that exceed this are classified as 'presumptive positive'. Programmes in the United States use various cut-off procedures because manufactured kits and product performance vary and because there has been no national concensus as to a uniform screening protocol.

Most programmes outside North America analyse TSH by EIA for primary CH screening.[53] In a Japanese study, 734 000 infants were tested simultaneously for T4 and TSH by using dried blood specimens collected on the fourth to the seventh day after birth. Of the 94 infants with primary CH, 64 were found to have high TSH and low T4, and 30 had high TSH and normal T4. No case of CH was found with normal TSH and low T4. Because of these findings, the Japanese programme uses TSH for the initial CH screening.[24]

In Texas, where the initial screening measures T4, a second routine screen after one week of age detected an additional 7.4 per cent of cases of CH in 1990.[27] Re-examination of the original filter paper specimens in these cases indicated that half of these infants would have been detected had TSH been used for the initial test.[57]

Programmes that do not do a second screen should consider using TSH as the initial test either alone or in combination with T4 for all specimens. This decision must be weighed against the number of false-positive tests on specimens collected during the TSH surge period and the ability of the programme to follow these infants without the medical community losing confidence in the programme.

Some laboratories in the United States are currently considering the shift to primary TSH screening. Seven states have already changed their protocols to TSH analysis only. Illinois is using T4 with repeat testing after a primary TSH screen. Others are carrying out pilot testing. From 1990 to 1995 the State of Missouri screened 401 679 newborns using both T4 and TSH assays on all specimens. Of the 87 infants with confirmed CH, five would not have been detected had the TSH assay been performed on only the lowest 10 per cent of T4 tests. An additional affected infant was detected on a repeat screen after one week.[39] On the other hand, TSH analysis alone will miss secondary CH cases. Free T4 assays have been used for CH screening,[37] but in one study, this method did not improve the detection rate or the false-positive rate of the screening when compared with T4 alone.[58] The optimal test would combine both T4 and TSH assays for all specimens.[56] Presumptive CH identified by screening must be confirmed by diagnostic testing with venipuncture serum and other clinical procedures.

Quality assurance

Several programmes exist internationally to help ensure the quality of newborn screening for CH.[59-65] Standards of practice are written for the laboratory outlining the best practice, potential errors, and corrective actions.[66] A two-component national external quality assurance programme is operated by the Centers for Disease Control and Prevention (CDC) in Atlanta, Georgia for all screening laboratories in the United States[61] and with some laboratories in 28 other countries. One component of this programme is the production of dried blood-spot quality control materials for T4 and TSH assays. These quality control specimens provide laboratories with an extra level of control– beyond the kit or laboratory prepared control specimens—which transcends changes in test kit lots and other control materials. Laboratories are encouraged to keep daily quality control charts on the analytic performance for each procedure in the laboratory.[66] The other component of the CDC programme is proficiency evaluation. On a quarterly basis, a panel of blind-coded dried blood spots that simulate blood spots for normal and presumptive hypothyroid infants are sent to participating laboratories. These proficiency evaluation specimens provide an external check on the ability of the laboratory to identify and classify abnormal and normal specimens using coded identifiers. CDC issues quarterly reports indicating the performance of each laboratory and distributes them to the screening laboratories.

Discrimination between affected and unaffected infants

The detection rate and false-positive rate of screening tests for CH are heavily influenced by the procedures being used for screening, by the age at which screening occurs, and by background environmental levels of influences on thyroid metabolism. In particular, geographical variations in iodine intake complicate screening for CH.[67] In areas where iodine intake is adequate, the positive predictive value for a given TSH level is higher than where iodine deficiency is endemic. The proportion of TSH readings exceeding standardized cut-off levels has been proposed as a method of assessing the background iodine levels of an area.[68,69]

Most programmes that screen initially by measuring T4 are designed to incorporate an initial positive rate of 0.5–1.0 per cent. Therefore, with a CH rate of 0.3/1000, between 17 and 33 persons would require a follow-up test for every case of CH detected, even if the detection rate were 100 per cent.

Where a programme is designed to have a large number of false-positive results, several problems can arise. Such a situation may produce loss of credibility and apathy among physicians,[70] and compliance with criteria for rescreening may suffer. Follow-up and retesting are expensive. The family and child may have long-term psychological problems because of unnecessary worry.[71] However, direct and clear information given to parents militates against serious problems.[72,73]

Primary TSH screening

Surprisingly little has been published about the detection and false-positive rates observed with this procedure. Among a total of 25/100 000 French infants in whom hypothyroidism was reported, the detection rate was 94.7 per cent when the lower limit for a positive TSH reading was set at >50 μU/mL, and 96.4 per cent when this limit was reduced to >30 μU/mL.[74] The false-positive rate was not reported; but with a cut-off of 30 μU/mL, it would have been at least 0.13 per cent, since this was the proportion of unaffected infants whose TSH readings were estimated to lie between 30 and 50 μU/mL. It was estimated that among infants with readings of 30–50 μU/mL, 310 would be unaffected for every one with hypothyroidism. The report concluded

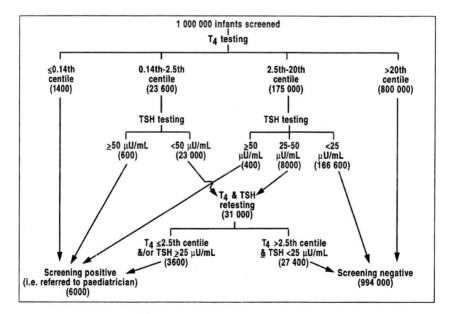

Fig. 15.3 Algorithm for T4/TSH screening in The Netherlands.[26] Distributions shown for results of initial tests for TSH, and for retests, are hypothetical.

that the cost of retesting this number of infants with false-positive results was out-weighed by the benefit of finding one true positive.

Primary T4 screening, with TSH testing if T4 is low

Reports on the performance of programmes of this type sometimes focus specifically on the initial T4 screen, and sometimes on the outcome of this combined if the initial T4 reading is low with further tests including measurement of TSH. Both approaches can be illustrated using the experience of a nationwide programme in The Netherlands in which infants whose T4 readings were among the lowest 20 per cent underwent measurement of TSH and in some circumstances a repeat measurement of T4 analysis, using the algorithm shown in Fig. 15.3. Hypothyroidism was eventually diagnosed in 30/100 000 of the infants in this programme.[26]

Estimates of the performance of the *initial* measurement of T4 in the Dutch programme are given in Table 15.4. As the T4 cut-off point is raised, the detection rate increases such that about half the cases missed at each cut-off level are detected at the next level shown.

However, since the disorder occurs with a frequency of only about 30/100 000, the odds of being affected given a positive result (OAPR) are very low in the additional infants classified as positive when the cut-off point is raised from one of the lower centiles listed to one of the higher. For example, those between the tenth and twentieth centiles have an OAPR of less than 1:25 000.

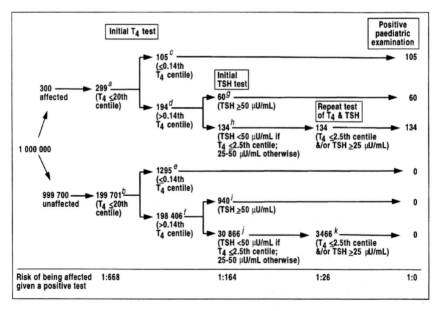

Fig. 15.4 Flow diagram for combined T₄ and TSH screening for CH. It is based on the estimates in Table 15.4 and Fig. 15.3. It is assumed that the risk of being affected for infants referred to a pediatrician (5 per cent overall) is 7.5 per cent in those in the lowest 0.14th T₄ centile at initial screening and in those between the 0.14th and 2.5th T₄ centiles who have a TSH value of < 50 μU/ml when first screened, but that it is only half as much (3.75 per cent) in all others referred. Key: a, 300 × 99.8 per cent (99.8 per cent is the proportion of cases at or below 20th centile reported by Verkerk et al.[26]); b, (20 per cent of 100 000)–299; c, 1400 × 0.075; d, 299–105; e, 1400 × (1–0.075); f, 199 701–1295; g, (600 × 0.075) + (400 × 0.0375); h, 194–60; i, 600 + 400–60; j, 31 000–134; k, 3600–134.

Table 15.4 Detection and false positive rates, and odds of being affected given a positive result (OAPR), to be expected with primary T4 screening, using various definitions of a positive test[26]

T4 cut-off (centile)	Detection rate (%)	False positive rate (%)	OAPR
2.5th	92.1	2.47	1:89
5th	96.5	4.97	1:172
10th	98.5	9.97	1:337
15th	99.4	14.97	1:502
20th	99.8	19.98	1:667

Table 15.5 shows the results to be expected from the whole programme of tests shown in Fig. 15.3. The results regarded as positive are those leading to referral to a pediatrician. The findings indicate that at each T4 centile, with the secondary tests shown the false-positive rate is reduced to between 0.5 per cent and 0.6 per cent, the detection rate is maintained, and the OAPR is about 1:19. This does not of course mean that the case for the secondary tests is as strong for subjects near to the 20th centile as for those below the 2.5th centile, given that far more of the former than of the latter must be screened in order to detect one case. The authors of the Dutch report questioned whether a cut-off point above the 10th centile was justified. However, if the secondary tests were relatively inexpensive, even testing 25 000 infants between the 10th and 20th centiles to find one with CH might be worthwhile. A flow diagram of the outcome in affected and unaffected infants to be expected with the Dutch programme, including secondary screening for all those below the 20th T4 centile, is given in Fig. 15.4.

In the T4-TSH programme used in California, secondary screening for TSH was confined to infants in the lowest 7–10 centiles.[75] The proportions of infants classified as true-positives (270/million) and false-positives (400/million) were lower than the corresponding figures for the Dutch programme (300 and 5700/million respectively), and the OAPR was consequently higher (1:1.5 as compared with 1:19). These differences would probably have been even greater but for the fact that 17 per cent of the Californians but none of the Dutch were screened before 24 hours, when the false-positive rate is reported to be higher: the Californians of normal birth-weight tested

Table 15.5 Detection and false positive rates, and odds of being affected given a positive result (OAPR), to be expected in a programme where primary T4 screening is followed by secondary TSH and other screening if primary test result is regarded as positive.[26] In this table, any outcome that satisfied protocol for referral to a paediatrician* is counted as a positive test result.

T4 cut-off (centile)	Detection rate (%)	False positive rate (%)	OAPR
2.5th	92.1	0.52	1:19
5th	96.5	0.54	1:19
10th	98.5	0.55	1:19
15th	99.4	0.55	1:19
20th	99.8	0.56	1:19

* Referral to a paediatrician was prescribed (a) for all subjects with T4 readings at least 3 SDs below the mean and/or TSH readings of at least 50 µU/ml, and (b) for other subjects with T4 readings at least 2 SDs below the mean and/or TSH readings of at least 25 µU/ml provided that these findings were confirmed on a repeat heel stick blood sample.

before 24 hours showed an OAPR of 1:4.2, compared with a ratio of 1:0.4 for infants tested after 24 hours of age.[75]

As noted earlier, one source of false-positive results in screening for T4 (although not for TSH) is thyroxin-binding globulin deficiency. This has been reported in 23.2 per 100 000 births,[76] which makes it not much less common than CH.

A 1986 survey of screening programmes in the United States found that cases missed because of systems error occurred once for every 120 cases of CH detected. Of these errors, 14 per cent occurred during collection, 45 per cent during laboratory procedures, 16 per cent during follow-up, 11 per cent because of biological variation, and 14 per cent for unknown reasons.[77] A programme in France estimated that 3.6 per cent of infants with CH were initially false-negative, more than half due to technical errors.[78] Another study found that administrative deficiencies were predominantly responsible for inefficiencies in screening.[79] These figures point out the need for system safeguards and for monitoring a system's efficacy.

Value of repeat tests

To minimize the number of missed cases, some screening programmes in the United States and Europe (e.g. Switzerland) require or recommend second screening routinely at one to four weeks of age.[27] These programmes rescreen 60 to 95 per cent of children at risk by the T4 and TSH combination and find an additional 8 to 12 per cent of infants with CH.[57,80–82] There appears to be a trend among state screening programmes in the United States to incorporate second tests either voluntarily or through statutory requirement. At least 10 programmes have repeated screening on over 80 per cent of the target population. At present this is being driven by the discharge of mothers and infants from the hospital within a few hours of birth and the concern that biological false-negative results will occur in this group. In the United States all but one screening programme recommends a repeat specimen for infants initially screened less than 24 hours after birth.[42]

The Pacific Northwest Regional Screening Program (PNRSP)[81] in the United States reported a detection rate of 3.9/100 000 on second specimens with a rate of 22.4/100 000 on the initial specimen. The Texas programme[80] reported a detection rate of 2.5/100 000 on second specimens with a rate of 27.8/100 000 on initial testing. Patients detected by second tests in the Pacific Northwest Regional Screening Program were more likely to have some residual thyroid tissue, greater skeletal maturation, and a milder form of the disease spectrum.[32]

DIAGNOSTIC TESTS

Tests on a second heel-stick blood sample (as carried out in the Dutch programme described above[26]) may be enough to exclude CH in infants with abnormal T4 but normal TSH concentrations, and in those with slightly elevated TSH but normal T4 levels. When, however, a newborn screening result shows a combined low T4 and elevated TSH or an extremely elevated concentration of TSH alone, serum must be collected, because of the greater acceptability of serum test results. Patient evaluation should include a complete physical examination, and it may include testing all or part of the available clinical thyroid panel (profile), T4, T3, TSH, T3-uptake, free T4 index, free T4, free T3, thyroid-binding globulin, thyroglobulin, calcitonin, and maternal blocking and other thyroid antibodies. A thyroid scan with isotopic iodine or technetium gives diagnostic information on the function and structure of the thyroid.[38,56] Bone age determinations may also be useful.[56,83]

Diagnostic testing for CH must proceed rapidly if treatment is to start before the infant is three weeks of age (a goal of most screening programmes related to outcome studies of mental retardation). If delays are expected, treatment should start at the first physician's visit pending confirmatory testing results.

Serum testing

Serum TSH, generally accepted as the best indicator of thyroid function, is the most frequent measurement used to confirm primary hypothyroidism. But the physician should measure serum concentration of both T4 and TSH and estimate the concentration of free T4. At present, most laboratories use serum RIA methods, which have high accuracy and precision. Non-isotopic assays are displacing some of these RIA procedures.[56] For infants with a family history of thyroiditis, thyroid antibody measurements and a urine measurement for iodine can identify iodine-induced hypothyroidism.

Low T4 and elevated TSH

(Serum T4 <6.5 µg/dL or <84 nmol/L, and serum TSH>10 µU/mL or >10 mU/L.) When a screening laboratory reports low T4 and high TSH concentrations that are presumptively positive for CH, blood drawn to measure serum T4, free T4, and TSH will provide confirmatory information. The low T4 and high TSH pattern is evidence that the thyroid gland fails to produce adequate amounts of T4. All infants with low T4 and high TSH are considered to have permanent CH, and treatment should start immediately following diagnostic testing.

Low T4, normal TSH

(Serum T4 <6.5 µg/dL or <84 nmol/L, and serum TSH<10 µU/mL or <10 mU/L.) Findings of low T4 and normal TSH occur most commonly among premature infants, but should not be ignored.[84,85] In the New England screening programme, of 71 infants with CH, nine (13 per cent), who weighed less than 1300 g at birth, were characterized by low T4 and normal TSH. TSH in this group did not become grossly elevated for weeks to months after birth.[86] Infants suspected of having a delay in TSH elevation should be retested in two to six weeks and followed closely. Some states have been prompted to initiate routine second screening because of the concern of missing these children.[27] Low T4 combined with normal TSH may also be a result of TBG deficiency or hypothyroidism secondary to hypothalamic or pituitary deficiency. Physicians can distinguish among these possibilities by measuring free T4, thyroid-binding globulin concentrations, and the effect of thyrotropin-releasing hormone and by specifically looking for other clinical evidence of pituitary failure such as micropenis or hypoglycemia. Except for pituitary failure (secondary or tertiary CH), usually no treatment is warranted. In the case of secondary or tertiary hypothyroidism, treatment with T4 should be cautiously started only after the status of other pituitary hormones has been determined. Some infants with delayed TSH rise may also require treatment.

Normal T4, high TSH

(Serum T4 >6.5 µg/dL or >84 nmol/L, and serum TSH >10 µU/mL or >10 mU/L.) The finding of normal T4 and elevated TSH means adequate, but inefficient, T4 production (compensated hypothyroidism). Such a finding may also be caused by a less severe structural abnormality of the thyroid gland (dysplasia or ectopia), by inborn errors of metabolism, or may be due to transient hypothyroidism from perinatal exposure to iodine, other goitrogens, maternal anti-thyroid medication, or maternal blocking antibodies.[69,87] In iodine-deficient areas, transient CH is fairly common. The condition may progress in severity. Japanese children with persistent elevation of TSH for several years[88] had no maternal antithyroid antibodies or hypothyroidism. Some of the children later developed small diffuse goiters. Another report from Japan found that infants with mildly elevated concentrations of TSH were later confimed to have primary CH.[89] When children are discovered to have high TSH, they should be monitored closely. If elevated TSH concentrations persist or increase, treatment should be instituted for at least two years. At that time L-thyroxine can be withdrawn for re-evaluation and definitive diagnosis by imaging tests to determine the permanence of the hypothyroidism.[69]

Quality assurance, diagnostic testing

Proficiency testing programmes are available in most countries for evaluation of clinical laboratories performing diagnostic testing on serum samples for thyroid function. In the United States, the College of American Pathologists (Northfield, Illinois) and the American Association of Bioanalysts Proficiency Testing Services (Brownsville, Texas) operate national evaluation programmes for clinical laboratory tests. Participation in these external quality control programmes is strongly encouraged. In some countries it is legally mandated.

Clinical evaluation

The detection of infants with CH that were missed by a screening programme or the discovery of infants and young children with acquired hypothyroidism requires a high index of suspicion. Physicians should not relax their clinical diligence because of screening programs and test results. Without chemical screening tests, detection of CH must rely on observations of non-specific signs and symptoms. The clinical features of CH must be considered during the newborn examination and during subsequent well-child visits for any infant with prolonged jaundice, transient hypothermia, posterior fontanelle larger than 1 cm in the newborn, failure to feed, or respiratory distress on feeding. At term, infants with CH tend to be heavier and longer than average. The classic signs appear during the first weeks after birth with myxoedema of the subcutaneous tissues and tongue resulting in coarse features and protuberant tongue. The cry becomes hoarse, due to myxoedema of the vocal cords. These findings may not be fully obvious until after several months of life.[10] Care should be taken not to overlook a diagnosis of acquired hypothyroidism in older infants.[90]

Infants with CH are at greater risk for other congenital anomalies[15,24,30,31,91,92] which can interfere with timely screening and diagnosis. Delaying diagnosis and treatment puts the infant with a congenital anomaly at even higher risk and may explain the high mortality rate among infants with CH.[30,93] Infants with Down's syndrome are at higher risk for CH with a rate of 709/100 000[94] and require close follow-up and retesting if CH was not identified at birth. Because of the additional risk of acquired hypothyroidism in children with Down's syndrome, periodic testing should continue into later childhood.[95]

Anatomical evaluation

Testing for etiology is desirable, but not essential during the newborn period.[96] L-thyroxine in physiologic dosage is effective and safe.[97,98] Treatment should not be delayed until etiologic tests are done. Etiologic or functional diagnosis can wait until the child is three years of age when thyroid hormone treatment can be safely withdrawn for the time needed to confirm the original assumption of disease.

Some clinicians recommend cervical ultrasound and thyroid scintigraphy routinely for etiologic diagnosis and prognosis.[99,100] Cervical ultrasonography can provide valuable information on size and location of thyroid tissue[101–103] but may lack the sensitivity to detect small ectopic glands; it is not useful with dyshormonogenesis and requires experienced interpreters. Radionuclide scanning is more reliable for etiology.[104,105]

Aplasia of the thyroid gland will require lifelong replacement treatment. Hypoplastic or ectopic glands may require lifelong treatment, but withdrawal of treatment at age three years for retesting will establish the degree of impairment. The concentrations of thyroglobulin[106] and calcitonin[106,107] can also give information on the amount and activity of residual thyroid tissue, but these have limited value for following up on patients with CH.[103,107]

TREATMENT

Medication

The goal is to begin treatment for infants before they are three weeks of age. Mental retardation for the most part is thought to be a postnatal consequence of late or inadequate treatment. Accumulated data show that given an appropriate replacement dose of the sodium salt of L-thyroxine, hypothyroid infants can be expected to grow[108] and develop normally.[109,110] Exceptions include babies severely hypothyroid at birth with mothers who also have hypothyroidism. Since brain cell T3 derives from serum T4, L-thyroxine is the treatment of choice for CH.[111] Treatment should be designed to elevate serum T4 and FT4 to normal concentrations quickly after diagnosis. Study results show that doses between 10 and 14 µg/kg/day of L-thyroxine normalize the serum T4 concentrations within the first week of therapy and appear to be a safe and effective treatment for CH.[111,112] For a normal 3–4.5 kg infant, 50 µg per day usually supplies an adequate amount. Beginning with a lower dose for the first week of treatment only delays the start of effective treatment.[113] The dosage should keep the concentrations of circulating T4 and FT4 in the upper half or upper third of the normal range.[5,99] Serum TSH should be suppressed to the normal range.[99,114] Although the first two to three years of life are the most critical time, subsequent therapy must maintain T4 in a range that allows for optimal development and growth.

Complications of treatment

Premature craniosynostosis has been associated with excessive L-thyroxine dosages in the range of 200 to 300 μg/day given through most of infancy.[115] This is much higher than the dose currently recommended.

Follow-up and monitoring of infants

Careful monitoring and adjustment of dosage is important during the early weeks and months of treatment. Repeat T4 and TSH measurements at two weeks and four to six weeks after starting treatment and four weeks after any change in treatment will give information on adequacy of treatment. Subsequent testing should occur every two months for the first year, every three months for the second and third years and every four months after the third year.[5] The necessity for prompt normalization and adequate T4 replacement during the first and second years of life dictates that personnel with adequate experience to recognize the pitfalls accompanying diagnosis and treatment– optimally experienced pediatric endocrinologists—must initiate treatment and guide follow-up of infants with CH and educate their primary physicians, who may only rarely see such patients. This plan will set the stage for effective treatment and follow-up.

In a few cases TSH may remain persistently elevated despite seemingly adequate doses of L-thyroxine. It has been reported that children with dyshormonogenesis do not exhibit this apparent delay in the feedback inhibition of TSH by thyroid hormones[112] and require less L-thyroxine to normalize the serum T4 and free T4 concentrations. When using T4 measurements for follow-up, one must know the contribution of binding proteins to the serum T4 to ensure adequate free T4 concentrations. The relative amount of L-thyroxine needed for growth and development will decrease to 5–6 μg/kg/day by 12 months of age. When sensitive EIA methods are used for measuring TSH, failure to detect it may be an indication to reduce the dosage of L- thyroxine.[114]

Giving the infant a careful clinical examination, measuring its growth and development, measuring TSH and T4, and looking for evidence of hyperthyroidism are the components of monitoring. Coordinated follow-up is essential for the first two to three years of life, the critical period of brain and organ development. Parents must be given information early so that they have a thorough understanding of the screening and confirmation procedures, the meaning of laboratory findings, and the child's diagnosis and treatment regimen. This knowledge will generally allay their anxieties about their child's diagnosis.[73,116]

Developmental outcomes

Earlier diagnosis, treatment, and follow-up of infants with CH have resulted in a major improvement in their mental development and may completely overcome the effect of antenatal hypothyroidism,[117] although this hypothesis has not been confirmed in all studies.[109,118] The intelligence of children with CH detected through screening is typically within normal limits, and few children exhibit mental retardation, although their IQ scores may be slightly, though significantly, lower than in normal, comparison children.[119] Some children may show developmental delays later or persisting impairments in language, neuromotor,[120–122] and perceptomotor areas.[118,123]

At greatest risk appear to be children with thyroid aplasia or severe hypothyroidism at the time of diagnosis.[122] Children who are not treated adequately during the first year of life may have delayed development.[124]

COST ANALYSIS

Cost can be measured in many ways. The cost of each T4 and TSH laboratory test was reported in 1989 to be $1.50. Fees charged for the screening service in 44 US programs ranged from no charge (14 programs) to $56.00.[27] The cost of treatment varies by country. A 1979 analysis in the United States showed that the cost of detecting and treating a case of CH was $11 800 with an economic benefit of $105 000, a cost savings of $93 000 per case detected early and treated compared with the cost per case with no screening.[125,126] Many programmes have chosen to detect mild cases and avoid false-negative outcomes despite the greater costs. The additional costs that milder CH impairments may have on learning, working, and other individual achievements are important to the individual and, in the long run, to society. These costs and the benefits achieved by avoiding these impairments are more difficult to measure in financial terms. The 'cost benefit' from adding to, or fine-tuning, a system to assure no missed cases, early and adequate treatment, and satisfactory clinical follow-up will be less dramatic in the next generation of laboratory and systems enhancements than the benefits achieved over the past 20 years.

OTHER ASPECTS

Iodine deficiency

The thyroid gland of a fetus is more susceptible to iodine deficiency than the gland of an adolescent or adult. The requirement for high T4 production during the first six months of life and small capacity for storing iodine in the neonatal thyroid (0.5 to 1 per cent of adult capacity) make newborn infants a population at risk for diseases resulting from goitrogenic factors in the environment. Any interference with thyroid iodine accumulation, including iodine deficiency, will affect the thyroid function of the fetus and neonate more critically than it will affect the adult function. Endemic iodine deficiency with no iodine supplementation becomes a major problem for the neonate. TSH increases in the fetus and newborn to compensate for the transient impairment in thyroid production, and false-positive screening results can occur. The collective results of neonatal screening provide a sensitive indicator for iodine deficiency in a population.[68]

The effect of iodine deficiency on the fetus and developing newborn can vary. In regions with severe endemic iodine deficiency, many newborns may be affected (250 to 10 000/100 000). Severe iodine deficiency in both mother and fetus can cause severe mental retardation.[67] Less severe cases of iodine deficiency can lead to clinical and chemical evidence of hypothyroidism.[127] Such hypothyroidism can be transient and can be compensated for by adequate L-thyroxine and iodine supplementation thereby restoring normal thyroid function. Milder cases of iodine deficiency such as those observed in Europe may appear to be transient CH. In communities endemically deficient in iodine it is important to supplement the population with dietary sources of iodine.[67]

Antenatal testing

Early postnatal therapy has effected normal growth and development for nearly all infants with CH. Exceptions include infants with evidence at birth of severe prenatal hypothyroidism, which usually occurs when the mother also has thyroid disease or when there is severe iodine deficiency. Other subtle effects of fetal hypothyroidism have not been uniformly demonstrated, but concern continues about central nervous system sequelae resulting from untreated intrauterine hypothyroidism.

Fetuses who may be at risk for the developmental effects of T4 deficiency include those whose mothers have thyroid disease,[128–130] are taking antithyroid medications, or have had other infants with CH.[131] Two cases of CH in infants of mothers with unexplained elevated serum alphafetoprotein have also been reported.[132] Other risk factors are environments that contain goiterogens or that are severely deficient in iodine.[133] Determinations of fetal TSH and T4 levels may be appropriate in some such cases, since antenatal treatment of infants with CH has been successfully attempted in sporadic cases,[134,135] usually when repeated CH has occurred among infants of mothers with histories of severe thyroid disease. Many women with hypothyroidism require increased amounts of T4 during pregnancy and should be monitored closely.[136,137] When iodine deficiency is present in pregnancy, it should be treated.

CONCLUSIONS

Population-based screening for CH has positively influenced the health of many children in the developed world. When sensitive screening tests are coupled with systems of early diagnosis, treatment and follow-up, an increased number of infants are detected–some with transient CH and some who might have been diagnosed with acquired hypothyroidism at an older age. Because of screening, treatment can begin at an earlier age–weeks after birth instead of months or years. The preponderance of evidence now suggests that in most cases profound developmental failure associated with CH results from inadequate treatment of the condition during the first few years of life, the first year being the most important.

Specific etiologic diagnosis is interesting but unnecessary for the decisions of treatment and should not unnecessarily delay the onset of treatment. Effective doses of T4 should initially equal 10 to 15 µg/kg/day for the newborn.

For samples collected two days or later after birth, TSH appears to be a sensitive and more specific initial screening test for CH than T4 although it does not detect secondary and tertiary hypothyroidism. For infants less than two days of age screening with T4 and TSH is recommended.

RESEARCH QUESTIONS

Studies to understand the etiology of dysplastic CH are needed. What are the genetic or environmental factors that may be protecting certain infants such as Japanese or black infants from CH or that appear to increase the risk for Hispanic, American Indian, and Pakistani infants? We need to understand the relative contributions of T4 deficiency during the antenatal, neonatal, and post neonatal periods to any abnormal development seen in childhood. It will be important to know whether those cases of CH requiring a second screening for detection have less severe CH and consequently a decreased risk for developmental abnormality. What is the relation between maternal thyroid disease during the infant's gestation and cognitive and learning outcomes in the child? The etiologic relationships between CH and the increased risk for congenital malformations, chromosomal abnormalities, and infant mortality should be studied. Researchers should extend the screening and study of newborns for resistance to thyroid hormone, commonly associated with attention deficit hyperactivity disorder.[138]

Given the availability of more reliable and analytically sensitive methods to measure TSH and the reduction in test costs, researchers also need to determine whether simultaneous testing for both T4 and TSH in all infants would perform better than measuring only one of these as a primary screening test.

Technological research is being directed toward rapid EIA systems for microtiter plate configurations for T4 and TSH measurements on dried blood spots. These advances include not only improved EIA kits, but modifications of the automated punching devices and other instruments for a network system that could handle the microtiter plate and enhance automated laboratory facilities for all newborn screening tests. These new approaches may conserve the newborn specimen for new tests and lead to the elimination of the use of isotopes in CH screening.

ACKNOWLEDGEMENTS

The authors would like to thank Dr Jose Cordero, CDC for review of the text and recommendations and Dr Glen F. Maberly, Emory University, Atlanta, Georgia, for insights on iodine deficiency. We appreciate the assistance of Fred Lorey, Department of Public Health, California, Ann Brown, Emory Univerity, Atlanta, Georgia, and Holly Nyerges, Department of Public Health, Santa Fe, New Mexico in releasing advance data from their state screening programs in 1991. The Lorey data have been published since. We are grateful to Dr Joanne F. Rovet, Hospital for Sick Children, Toronto, Canada, for reviewing and making suggestions on the section on developmental outcomes. We thank Connie Woodall for assistance with graphics. Helen McClintock, CDC, gave expert editorial advice.

REFERENCES

1. Alm, J., Larsson, A., and Zetterstrom, R. (1978). Congenital hypothyroidism in Sweden: Incidence and age at diagnosis. *Acta Paediatrica Scandinavica*, **67**, 1–3.
2. de Jonge, G.A. (1976). Congenital hypothyroidism in the Netherlands. *Lancet,* **ii**, 143.
3. Jacobsen, B.B. and Brandt, N.J. (1981). Congenital hypothyroidism in Denmark. *Archives of Disease in Childhood*, **56**, 134–6.
4. Klein, A., Meltzer, S., and Kenny, F. (1972). Improved prognosis in congenital hypothyroidism treated before age three months. *Journal of Pediatrics*, **81**, 912–15.
5. Klein, R.Z. (1985). Infantile hypothyroidism then and now: the results of neonatal screening. *Current Problems in Pediatrics*, **15**, 1–58.

6. Klein, A.H., Agustin, A.V., and Foley, T.P. Jr (1974). Successful laboratory screening for congenital hypothyroidism. *Lancet,* **ii**, 77–9.

7. Dussault, J.H., Coulombe, P., Laberge, C., Letarte, J., Guyda, H., and Khoury, K. (1975). Preliminary report on a mass screening program for neonatal hypothyroidism. *Journal of Pediatrics*, **86**, 670–4.

8. Virtanen, M. (1988). Manifestations of congenital hypothyroidism during the 1st week of life. *European Journal of Pediatrics*, **147**, 270–4.

9. Grant, D.B., Smith, I., Fuggle, P.W., Tokar, S., and Chapple, J. (1992). Congenital hypothyroidism detected by neonatal screening: relationship between biochemical severity and early clinical features. *Archives of Disease in Childhood*, **67**, 87–90.

10. Fisher, D.A. (1990). The thyroid. In *Clinical pediatric endocrinology*, revised edn, (ed. S.A. Kaplan). Saunders, Philadelphia.

11. Vulsma, T., Gons, M., and Vijlder, J. (1989). Maternal-fetal transfer of thyroxine in congenital hypothyroidism due to a total organification defect or thyroid agenesis. *New England Journal of Medicine*, **321**, 13–16.

12. Fisher, D.A. and Klein, A.H. (1981). Thyroid development and disorders of thyroid function in the newborn. *New England Journal of Medicine*, **304**, 702–12.

13. Penny, R., Hoffman, P., and Barton, L. (1989). Congenital hypothyroidism in Spanish-surnamed infants in southern California: increased incidence and clustering of occurrence. *American Journal of Diseases of Children*, **143**, 640–1.

14. Daoud, A.S., Zaki, M., Al-Saleh, Q.A., Teebi, A.S., and Al-Awadi, S.A. (1989). Congenital hypothyroidism in Kuwait. *Journal of Tropical Pediatrics*, **35**, 312–14.

15. Majeed-Saidan, M.A., Joyce, J., Khan, M., and Hamam, H.D. (1993). Congenital hypothyroidism: the Riyadh Military Hospital experience. *Clinical Endocrinology*, **38**, 191–5.

16. Working group on congenital hypothyroidism of the European society for Paediatric Endocrinology (1990). Epidemiological inquiry on congenital hypothyroidism in Europe (1985–1988). *Hormone Research*, **34**, 1–3.

17. Alm, J., Hagenfeldt, L., Larsson, A., and Lundberg, K. (1984). Incidence of congenital hypothyroidism: retrospective study of neonatal laboratory screening versus clinical symptoms as indicators leading to diagnosis. *British Medical Journal*, **289**, 1171–5.

18. Connelly, J. (1987). Australian experience in neonatal thyroid screening 1977–1985. In *Advances in neonatal screening*, (ed. B.L. Therrell, Jr), pp. 31–4, Elsevier, Amsterdam.

19. Dussault, J. (1985). An update on screening for congenital hypothyroidism. *Thyroid Today*, **8**, 1–5.

20. Low, L.C., Lin, H.J., Cheung, P.T., Lee, F.T., Chu, S. Y., Kwok, T.L., *et al.* (1986). Screening for congenital hypothyroidism in Hong Kong. *Australian Paediatric Journal*, **22**, 53–6.

21. Bernstein, R.E., Op't Hof, J., and Hitzeroth, H.W. (1988). Neonatal screening for congenital hypothyroidism: a decades review, including South Africa. *South African Medical Journal*, **73**, 339–43.

22. Peter, F., Blatniczky, L., Kovacs, L., and Tar, A. (1989). Experience with neonatal screening for congenital hypothyroidism in Hungary. *Endocrinologia Experimentalis*, **23**, 143–51.

23. Sorcini, M., Balestrazzi, P., Grandolfo, M.E., Carta, S., and Giovannelli, G. (1993). The national register of infants with congenital hypothyroidism detected by neonatal screening in Italy. *Journal of Endocrinological Investigation*, **16**, 573–7.

24. Irie, M., Nakajima, H., Inomata, H., Naruse, H., Suwa, S., and Takasugi, N. (1987).

Screening of neonatal hypothyroidism in Japan. In *Advances in neonatal screening*, (ed. B.L. Therrell), pp. 41–7, Elsevier, Amsterdam.

25. Lakhani, M., Khurshid, M., Naqvi, S. H., and Akber, M. (1989). Neonatal screening for congenital hypothyroidism in Pakistan. *Journal of the Pakistan Medical Association*, **39**, 282–4.

26. VerKerk, P.H., Buitendijk, S.E., and Verloove-Vanhorick, S.P. (1993). Congenital hypothyroidism screening and the cutoff for thyrotropin measurement: recommendations from the Netherlands. *American Journal of Public Health*, **83**, 868–71.

27. Newborn Screening Committee, The Council for Regional Networks for Genetic Services (CORN), 1995. *Newborn Screening Report—1992*, CORN, Atlanta, GA.

28. Lorey, F.W. and Cunningham, G.C. (1992). Birth prevalence of primary congenital hypothyroidism by sex and ethnicity. *Human Biology*, **64**, 531–8.

29. Harrison-Davis, J., Buchanan, I., Nyerges, H., and Padilla, D. (1988). Racial differences in the incidence of congenital hypothyroidism in New Mexico. *Program and Abstracts of the 116th Annual Meeting of the American Public Health Association*, Boston, Massachusetts, November 13–17, 1988.

30. Rosenthal, M., Addison, G.M., and Price, D.A. (1988). Congenital hypothyroidism: increased incidence in Asian families. *Archives of Disease in Childhood*, **63**, 790–3.

31. Fernhoff, P., Brown, A., and Elsas, L. (1987). Congenital hypothyroidism: increased risk of neonatal morbidity results in delayed treatment. *Lancet*, **i**, 490–1.

32. LaFranchi, S.H., Hanna, C.E., Krainz, P.L., Skeels, M. R., Miyagira, R.S., and Sesser, D.E. (1985). Screening for congenital hypothyroidism with specimen collection at two time periods: results of the Northwest Regional Screening Program. *Pediatrics*, **76**, 734–40.

33. Murphy, B. and Pattee, C.J. (1964). Determination of thyroxine utilizing the property of protein binding. *Journal of Clinical Endocrinology and Metabolism*, **24**, 187.

34. Glinoer, D., Fernandez-Deville, M., and Ermans, A. M. (1978). Use of direct thyroxine-binding globulin measurements in the evaluation of thyroid function. *Journal of Endocrinological Investigation*, **1**, 329.

35. Drop, S.L.S., Krenning, E.P., Docter, R., deMuinck Keizer-Schrama, S.M.P.F., Visser, T.J., and Hennemann, G. (1989). Congenital hypothyroidism and partial thyroid hormone unresponsiveness of the pituitary in a patient with congenital thyroxine binding albumin elevation. *European Journal of Pediatrics*, **149**, 90–3.

36. Leung, A.K.C. and McArthur, R.G. (1989). Hypothyroidism with thyroxine-binding globulin excess. *Pediatrics*, **83**, 147–8.

37. Arakawa, H., Maeda, M., and Tsuji, A. (1987). Enzyme immunoassay of total and free thyroxin in dried blood spots on filter paper. In *Advances in neonatal screening*, (ed. B.L. Therrell), pp. 157–8, Elsevier, Amsterdam.

38. Bakerman, S. (1984). *ABC's of interpretive laboratory data*, 2nd edn, pp. 408–19. Interpretive Laboratory Data, Inc., Greenville, NC.

39. Baumgartner, J.H. and Haibach, H. (1995). Screening for primary hypothyroidism in Missouri, using thyroxine and TSH assay for all specimens: a five-year experience. *Proceedings of the 11th National Neonatal Screening Symposium, Corpus Cristi, Texas.* ASTPHLD, Washington, DC.

40. Delange, F., Camus, M., Winkler, M., Dodion, J., and Ermans, A-M. (1977). Serum thyrotropin determination on day 5 of life as screening procedure for congenital hypothyroidism. *Archives of Disease in Childhood*, **52**, 89–96.

41. Fisher, D., Dussault, J., Foley, T., Klein, A., LaFranchi, S., Larson, P. R., *et al.* (1979). Screening for congenital hypothyroidism: results of screening one million North American infants. *Journal of Pediatrics*, **94**, 700–5.

42. Walraven, C., Sorrentino, J.E., Levy, H.L., and Grady, G.F. (1995). Early newborn specimen: survey of practices among newborn screening programs in the United States. *Screening*, **4**, 1–8.

43. Hannon, W.H., Aziz, K.J., Collier, F.C., Fisher, D.A., Fafara, C., Knight, W., *et al.* (1988). *Blood collection on filter paper for neonatal screening programs; approved standard.* NCCLS Document LA4-A, 8, No.9., National Committee for Clinical Laboratory Standards, pp. 163–82, Vilanova, PA.

44. Slazyk, W.E., Phillips, D.L., Therrell, B.L., and Hannon, W. H. (1988). Effects of lot-to-lot variability in filter paper on the quantification of thyroxin, thyrotropin and phenylalanine in dried blood specimens. *Clinical Chemistry*, **34**, 53–8.

45. Foley, T.P. Jr, Foley, B., and Klein, A.H. (1978). Four-year experience with cord thyrotropin screening for congenital hypothyroidism. *Journal of Pediatrics*, **93**, 310.

46. Clagg, M.E. (1989). Venous sample collection from neonates using dorsal hand veins. *Laboratory Medicine*, April, 248–50.

47. Lorey, F.W. and Cunningham, G.C. (1994). Effect of specimen collection method on newborn screening for PKU. *Screening*, **3**, 57–65.

48. Dussault, J.H. and Laberge, C. (1973). Thyroxine (T4) determination in dried blood by radioimmunoassay: a screening method for neonatal hypothyroidism. *Union Medicale du Canada*, **102**, 2062–4.

49. Larsen, P.R., Merker, A., and Parlow, A.F. (1976). Immunoassay of human TSH using dried blood samples. *Journal of Clinical Endocrinology and Metabolism*, **42**, 987–90.

50. Irie, M., Enomoto, K., and Naruse, H. (1975). Measurement of thyroid stimulation hormone in dried blood spot. *Lancet*, **ii**, 1233–7.

51. Torresani, T.E. and Scherz, R. (1986). Thyroid screening of neonates without use of radioactivity: evaluation of time-resolved fluoroimmunoassay of thyrotropin. *Clinical Chemistry*, **32**, 1013–16.

52. Woodhead, J.S., Siddle, K., and Weeks, I. (1987). Immunochemilumnometric assay of thyrotrophin in filter paper blood spots. In *Advances in neonatal screening*, (ed. B.L. Therrell), pp. 149–52, Elsevier, Amsterdam.

53. Naruse, H., Nakajima, H., Irie, M., Takasugi, N., and Suwa, S. (1986). Comparison of primary TSH and T4 screening for congenital hypothyroidism. In *Genetic diseases: screening and management*, (ed. T.P. Carter), pp. 253–79, Liss, New York.

54. Jewell, S.E., Slazyk, W.E., Smith, S.J., and Hannon, W.H. (1989). Sources of imprecision in laboratories screening for congenital hypothyroidism: analysis of nine years of performance data. *Clinical Chemistry*, **35**, 1701–5.

55. Miyai, K., Ishibashi, K., and Kawashima, M. (1981). Two site immunoenzymometric assay for thyrotropin in dried blood spot samples on filter paper. *Clinical Chemistry*, **27**, 1421–3.

56. American Academy of Pediatrics, Committee on Genetics (1989). Newborn screening fact sheets. *Pediatrics*, **83**, 449–64.

57. Therrell, B.L. Jr, Brown, L.O., and Borgfeld, L. (1989). Importance of second screen in diagnosis of hypothyroid cases. In *Proceedings of the 7th National Neonatal Screening Symposium*, (ed. H.B. Bradford, W.H. Hannon, and B. L. Therrell), pp. 189–91, AST-PHLD, New Orleans.

58. Joseph, R., Aw, T.C., and Tan, K.L. (1993). Free thyroxine as a supplement to thyrotropin

in cord screening for hypothyroidism. *Annals of the Academy of Medicine, Singapore*, **22**, 549–52.

59. Farriaux, J-P. and Dhondt, J-L. (1988). French screening programs for congenital hypothyroidism. *American Journal of Diseases of Children*, **142**, 1137–8.

60. Amino, Y. (1987). Quality control in Japan. In *Advances in neonatal screening*, (ed. B.L. Therrell, Jr), pp. 531–6, Elsevier, Amsterdam.

61. Hannon, W.H. and Slazyk, W.E. (1987). Quality control of newborn screening for inborn metabolic errors. In *Advances in neonatal screening*, (ed. B.L. Therrell, Jr), pp. 537–40, Elsevier, Amsterdam.

62. Mathias, D. (1987). Results of external quality control in neonatal screening for West Germany and centers in other countries. In *Advances in Neonatal Screening*, (ed. B.L. Therrell, Jr), pp. 541–4, Elsevier, Amsterdam.

63. Webster, D. and Lyon, I. (1987). Australasian quality assurance program 1986: preliminary report. In *Advances in neonatal screening*, (ed. B.L. Therrell, Jr), pp. 545–8, Elsevier, Amsterdam.

64. Arends, J. (1987). Methodologic factors which contribute to imprecision. In *Advances in neonatal screening*, (ed. B.L. Therrell, Jr), p. 549, Elsevier, Amsterdam.

65. Dhondt, J.L., Farriaux, J.P., and Pollitt, R.J. (1993). Neonatal screening for congenital hypothyroidism: analysis of interlaboratory quality control. *Screening*, **2**, 187–99.

66. Council of Regional Networks for Genetic Service (1990). *Newborn screening system guidelines*, pp. 1–9. CORN, Phoenix, AZ.

67. Delange, F. and Burgi, H. (1989). Iodine deficiency disorders in Europe. *World Health Organization Bulletin*, **67**, 317–25.

68. Nordenberg, D.F., Ratajczak, R., Tulck, D., Sullivan, K., Wiley, V., Wilcken, B., *et al.* (1993). TSH levels among newborns: an indicator for community based iodine status. *Abstracts of the Newborn Screening Meeting*, France.

69. Working group on congenital hypothyroidism of the European Society for Paediatric Endocrinology (1993). Guidelines for neonatal screening programs for congenital hypothyroidism. *European Journal of Paediatrics*, **152**, 974–5.

70. Allen, D., Hendricks, S.A., Sieger, J., Hassemer, D., Katcher, M., Maby, S., *et al.* (1988). Screening programs for congenital hypothyroidism. *American Journal of Diseases of Children*, **142**, 232–6.

71. Fyro, K. and Bodegard, G. (1987). Four-year follow-up of psychological reactions to false-positive screening tests for congenital hypothyroidism. *Acta Paediatrica Scandinavica*, **76**, 107–14.

72. Clemens, P.C. and Neumann, R.S.J. (1989). Psychological adjustment to the results of neonatal hypothyroid screening. *Acta Paediatrica Scandinavica*, **78**, 447–8.

73. Wacht, M.A. and Hintz, R.L. (1989). Follow-up of diagnosed cases of hypothyroidism at Stanford University. *Proceedings of the 7th National Neonatal Screening Symposium*, (ed. H.B. Bradford, W.H. Hannon, and B.L. Therrell), pp. 64–6. ASTPHLD, New Orleans.

74. Leger, J., Lemerrer, M., Briard, M.L., and Czernichow, P. (1987). Hypothyroidism in children with filterpaper TSH of 30 to 50 uU/ml at initial screening. Implication of the TSH cut-off point for recalling infants. *Acta Paediatrica Scandinavica*, **76**, 599–602.

75. Foley, B.L., Fisher, D.A., Shapiro, L.J., and Cunningham, G. C. (1987). Early neonatal discharge and its effects on thyroid screening results in Southern California. In *Advances in neonatal screening*, (ed. B.L. Therrell, Jr), pp. 65–6, Elsevier, Amsterdam.

76. Mandel, S., Hanna, C., Boston, B., Sesser, D., and LaFranchi, S. (1993). Thyroxine-binding globulin deficiency detected by newborn screening. *Journal of Pediatrics*, **122**, 227–30.

77. Holtzman, C., Slazyk, W., Cordero, J., and Hannon, W.H. (1986). Descriptive epidemiology of missed cases of phenylketonuria and congenital hypothyroidism. *Pediatrics*, **78**, 553–8.

78. Leger, J. (1990). Screening for congenital hypothyroidism in France. Misdiagnosed cases: collaborative study of screening centres in France. *European Journal of Pediatrics*, **149**, 605–7.

79. Pharoah, P.O.D. and Madden, M.P. (1992). Audit of screening for congenital hypothyroidism. *Archives of Disease in Childhood*, **67**, 1073–6.

80. Levine, G.D. and Therrell, B.L. (1986). Second testing for hypothyroidism. *Pediatrics*, **78**, 375.

81. Tuerck, J. (1989). Routine rescreening, 1985–88; Pacific Northwest Regional newborn screening: Oregon, Idaho, Nevada, Alaska. In *Proceedings of the 7th National Neonatal Screening Symposium*, (ed. H.B. Bradford, W.H. Hannon, and B.L. Therrell), p. 204. AST-PHLD, New Orleans.

82. Panny, S., Szuch, W., Corcoran, L., and Gordon, S. (1989). Usefulness of a second specimen in screening infants for hypothyroidism in Maryland FY 1978–1989. In *Proceedings of the 7th National Neonatal Screening Symposium*, (ed. H. B. Bradford, W.H. Hannon, and B.L. Therrell), pp 194–8. ASTPHLD, New Orleans.

83. Newland, C.J., Swift, P.G.F., and Lamont, A.C. (1991). Congenital hypothyroidism–correlation between radiographic appearances of the knee epiphyses and biochemical data. *Postgraduate Medical Journal*, **67**, 553–6.

84. Delange, F., Dalhem, A., Bourdoux, P., Lagasse, R., Glinoer, D., Fisher, D.A., *et al.* (1984). Increased risk of primary hypothyroidism in preterm infants. *Journal of Pediatrics*, **105**, 462–9.

85. Hadeed, A.J., Asay, L.D., Klein, A.H., and Fisher, D.A. (1981). Significance of transient postnatal hypothyroxinemia in premature infants with and without respiratory distress syndrome. *Pediatrics*, **68**, 318–19.

86. Mitchell, M.L., Walraven, C., Rojas, D.A., McIntosh, K.F., and Hermos, R.J. (1994). Screening very-low-birthweight infants for congenital hypothyroidism. *Lancet*, **343**, 60–1.

87. Chanoine, J.P., Boulvain, M., Bourdoux, P., Pardou, A., Van Thi, H.V., Ermans, A.M., *et al.* (1988). Increased recall rate at screening for congenital hypothyroidism in breast fed infants born to iodine overloaded mothers. *Archives of Disease in Childhood*, **63**, 1207–10.

88. Miki, K., Nose, O., Milyai, K., Yaabuuchi, H., and Harada, T. (1989). Transient infantile hyperthyrotrophinaemia. *Archives of Disease in Childhood*, **64**, 1177–82.

89. Harada, S., Ichihara, N., Arai, J., Honma, H., Natsuura, N., Fujieda, K., *et al.* (1995). Later manifestations of congenital hypothyroidism predicted by slightly elevated thyrotropin levels in neonatal screening. *Screening*, **3**, 181–92.

90. Foley, T.P., Jr, Abbassi, V., Copeland, K.C., and Draznin, M.B. (1994). Brief report: hypothyroidism caused by chronic autoimmune thyroiditis in very young infants. *New England Journal of Medicine*, **330**, 466–8.

91. Siebner, R., Merlob, P., Kaiserman, I., and Sack, J. (1992). Congenital anomalies concomitant with persistent primary congenital hypothyroidism. *American Journal of Medical Genetics*, **44**, 57–60.

92. Cassio, A., Tato, L., Colli, C., Spolettini, E., Costantini, E., and Cacciari, E. (1994). Incidence of congenital malformations in congenital hypothyroidism. *Screening*, **3**, 125–30.

93. Marsh, T.D., Freeman, D., McKeown, R.E., and Bowyer, F.P. (1993). Increased mortality in neonates with low thyroxine values. *Journal of Perinatology*, **13**, 201–4.

94. Fort, P., Lifshitz, F., Bellisario, R., Davis, J., Lanes, R., Pugliese, M., *et al.* (1984). Abnormalities of thyroid function in infants with Down syndrome. *Journal of Pediatrics*, **104**, 545–9.

95. American Academy of Pediatrics (1993). Newborn screening for congenital hypothyroidism: recommended guidelines. *Pediatrics*, **91**, 1203–9.

96. Rosenbloom, A.L., Schatz, D.A., and Silverstein, J.H. (1990). To scan or not to scan in congenital hypothyroidism, Editorial. *Clinical Pediatrics*, **29**, 733–4.

97. Leger, J. and Czernichow, P. (1990). Secretion of hormones by ectopic thyroid glands after prolonged thyroxine therapy. *Journal of Pediatrics*, **116**, 111–17.

98. Cavallo, L., Laforgia, N., DeBellis, T., DeLuca, B., and Mele, M. (1990). Thyroid function after prolonged treatment of congenital hypothyroidism. *Journal of Pediatrics*, **117**, 1004.

99. Fisher, D.A. (1991). Clinical review 19: Management of congenital hypothyroidism. *Journal of Clinical Endocrinology and Metabolism*, **72**, 523–9.

100. Schoen, E.J. and Weber, P.M. (1990). Proposed classification of congenital primary hypothyroidism. *Clinical Pediatrics*, **29**, 731–2.

101. Ehrlich, R. (1988). Thyroid scanning, ultrasound, and serum thyroglobulin in determining the origin of congenital hypothyroidism. *American Journal of Diseases of Children*, **142**, 1023–4.

102. Chanoine, J.P., Toppet, V., Lagasse, R., Spehl, M., and Delange, F. (1991). Determination of thyroid volume by ultrasound from the neonatal period to late adolescence. *European Journal of Pediatrics*, **150**, 395–9.

103. Chanoine, J.P., Toppet, V., Body, J.J., Van Vliet, G., Lagsse, R., Boudoux, P., *et al.* (1990). Contribution of thyroid ultrasound and serum calcitonin diagnosis of congenital hypothyroidism. *Journal of Endocrinological Investigation*, **13**, 103–9.

104. Muir, A., Daneman, D., Daneman, A., and Ehrlich, R. (1988). Thyroid scanning, ultrasound, and serum thyroglobulin in determining the origin of congenital hypothyroidism. *American Journal of Diseases of Children*, **142**, 214–16.

105. De Bruyn, R., Ng, W.K., Taylor, J., Campbell, F., Mitton, S.G., Dicks-Mireaux, C. *et al.* (1990). Neonatal hypothyroidism: comparison of radioisotope and ultrasound imaging in 54 cases. *Acta Paediatrica Scandinavica*, **79**, 1194–8.

106. Ilicki, A., Ericsson, U., Larsson, A., Mortensson, W., and Thorell, J. (1990). The value of neonatal serum thyroglobulin determinations in the follow-up of patients with congenital hypothyroidism. *Acta Paediatrica Scandinavica*, **79**, 769–75.

107. Zamboni, G., Avanzini, S., Giavarina, D., and Tato, L. (1989). Monomeric calcitonin secretion in infants with congenital hypothyroidism. *Acta Paediatrica Scandinavica*, **78**, 885–8.

108. Aronson, R., Ehrlich, R., Bailey, J., and Rovet, J. (1990). Growth in children with congenital hypothyroidism detected by neonatal screening. *Journal of Pediatrics*, **116**, 33–7.

109. Rovet, J., Ehrlich, R., and Sorbara, D. (1987). Longitudinal prospective investigations of hypothyroid children detected by neonatal thyroid screening in Ontario. In *Advances in neonatal screening*, (ed. B. L. Therrell), pp. 99–106. Elsevier, Amsterdam.

110. Grant, D.B. (1995). Congenital hypothyroidism: optimal management in the light of 5 years experience of screening. *Archives of Disease in Childhood*, **72**, 85–9.

111. Fisher, D.A. and Foley, B.L. (1989). Early treatment of congenital hypothyroidism. *Pediatrics*, **83**, 785–9.

112. Germak, J. and Foley, T. (1990). Longitudinal assessment of L-thyroxine therapy for congenital hypothyroidism. *Journal of Pediatrics*, **117**, 211–19.

113. Sato, H., Inomata, H., Sasaki, N., Niimi, H., and Nakajima, H. (1987). Recovery period of hypersecretion of thyroid-stimulating hormone in patients with congenital hypothyroidism treated with thyroid hormone. *Acta Paediatrica Japonica*, **29**, 833–6.

114. Sato, H., Inomata, H., Sasaki, N., Nimi, H., andNakajuma, H. (1988). Optimum replacement dose of thyroid hormone assessed by highly sensitive TSH determination in patients with congenital hypothyroidism. *Endocrinology Japan*, **35**, 531–6.

115. Penfold, J. and Simpson, D. (1975). Premature craniosynostosis: a complication of thyroid replacement therapy. *Journal of Pediatrics*, **86**, 360–3.

116. Lorenson, J.R., Levy, H.L., Mangione, T.W., and Sepe, S.J. (1984). Parental response to repeat testing of infants with 'false-positive' results in a newborn screening program. *Pediatrics*, **73**, 183–7.

117. Ilicki, A., Larsson, A., and Mortensson, W. (1990). Neonatal skeletal maturation in congenital hypothyroidism and its prognostic value for psychomotor development at 3 years in patients treated early. *Hormone Research*, **33**, 260–4.

118. Virtanen, M., Santavuori, P., Hirvonen, E., and Perheentupa, J. (1989). Multivariate analysis of psychomotor development in congenital hypothyroidism. *Acta Paediatrica Scandinavica*, **78**, 405–11.

119. Rovet, J.F. (1990). Congenital hypothyroidism; intellectual and neuropsychological functioning. In *Psychoneuroendocrinology: brain, behavior, and hormonal interactions*, (ed. C.S. Holmes), pp. 273–322. Springer, New York.

120. Fuggle, P., Grant, D.B., Smith, I., and Murphy, G. (1991). Intelligence, motor skills, and behavioral 5 years in early-treated congenital hypothyroidism. *European Journal of Pediatrics*, **150**, 570–4.

121. Rochiccioli, P., Alexandre, F., and Roge, B. (1989). Neurological development in congenital hypothyroidism. In *Research in congenital hypothyroidism*, (ed. F. Delange, D. Fisher, and D. Glinoer), pp. 301–8. Plenum, New York.

122. Rovet, J.F. (1991). Neuromotor deficiencies in six year old hypothyroid children identified by newborn screening. 8th National Neonatal Screening and XXI Birth Defects Symposium Proceedings, January 29 to February 2, 1991, Saratoga Springs, NY, ASTPHD, pp. 378–81.

123. Heyerdahl, S., Kase, B.F., and Lie, S.O. (1991). Intellectual development in children with congenital hypothyroidism in relation to recommended thyroxine treatment. *Journal of Pediatrics*, **118**, 850–7.

124. Murphy, G.H., Hulse, J.A., Smith, I., and Grant, D.B. (1990). Congenital hypothyroidism:physiological and psychological factors in early development. *Journal of Child Psychology and Psychiatry*, **31**, 711–25.

125. Layde, P., Von Allmen, S.D., and Oakley, G.P. (1984). Congenital hypothyroidism control programs. *Journal of the American Medical Association*, **243**, 119–20.

126. Office of Technology Assessment (1988). *Healthy children: Investing in the future.* OTA–H–35, pp. 91–116. US Government Printing Office, Washington DC.

127. Boyages, S., Collins, J., Maberly, G., Jupp, J., Morris, J., and Eastman, C. (1989). Iodine deficiency impairs intellectual and neuromotor development in apparently normal persons. *The Medical Journal of Australia*, **150**, 676–82.

128. Root, A.W. (1992). The role of maternal autoimmune thyroid disease in neonatal hypothyroidism. *American Journal of Diseases of Children*, **146**, 1029–30.

129. Man, E., Brown, J.F., and Serunian, S.A. (1991). Maternal hypothyroxinemia: psychological deficits of progeny. *Annals of Clinical and Laboratory Science*, **21**, 227–39.

130. Carr, E.A., Beierwaltes, W.H., Raman, G. *et al.* (1959). The effect of maternal thyroid function on fetal thyroid function and development. *Journal of Clinical Endocrinology and Metabolism*, **19**, 1–17.

131. Yano, K., Itoh, Y., Inyaku, F., Taguchi, T., Takimoto, M., and Okuno, A. (1992). Athyreotic congenital hypothyroidism in two sisters. *Folia Endocrinologica*, **68**, 1197–204.

132. Ben-Neriah, Z., Yagel, S., Zelikoviz, B., and Bach, G. (1991). Increased maternal serum alpha fetoprotein in congenital hypothyroidism. *Lancet*, **i**, 337, 437.

133. Hollowell, J.G. and Hannon, W.H. (1997). Teratogen update: iodine deficiency, a community teratogen. *Teratology*, **55**, 389–405.

134. Hirsch, M., Josefsberg, Z., Schoenfeld, A., Pertzlan, A., Merlob, P., Leiba, S., *et al.* (1990). Congenital hereditary hypothyroidism—prenatal diagnosis and treatment. *Prenatal Diagnosis*, **10**, 491–6.

135. Perelman, A.H., Johnson, R.L., Clemons, R.D., Finberg, H. J., Clewell, W.H., and Trujillo, L. (1990). Intrauterine diagnosis and treatment of fetal goitrous hypothyroidism. *Journal of Clinical Endocrinology and Metabolism*, **71**, 618–21.

136. Mandel, S.J., Larsen, P.R., Seely, E.W., and Brent, G.A. (1990). Increased need for thyroxine during pregnancy in women with primary hypothyroidism. *New England Journal of Medicine*, **323**, 91–6.

137. Glinoer, D., Soto, M.F., Bourdoux, P., Lejeune, B., Delange, F., Lemone, M., *et al.* (1991). Pregnancy in persons with mild thyroid abnormalities: maternal and neonatal repercussions. *Journal of Clinical Endocrinology and Metabolism*, **73**, 421–7.

138. Mizejewski, C.J., Morris, J.E., Hauser, P., Weintraub, B.D., and Pass, K.A. (1995). A strategy for newborn screening for resistance to thyroid hormone: possible relevance to attention deficit hyperactivity disorder. *Screening*, **4**, 61–70.

16 *Congenital dislocation of the hip*

Ian Leck

INTRODUCTION

Strictly speaking, the term 'congenital dislocation of the hip' (CDH) means being born with the head of one femur outside the acetabulum (the socket in the bony pelvis in which the head of the femur is normally located). In this chapter, however, the term is reserved for persistent dislocation, since it is this that screening aims to prevent. Persistent dislocation is considered to be present when the head of the femur remains located either totally outside the acetabulum (luxation or complete dislocation) or only partially within it (subluxation or partial dislocation). The condition can arise before or after birth, and causes increasing disability once the child begins to walk.

In neonatal screening, the aim of preventing persistent dislocation is pursued by testing the hips for severe instability. In this condition, one or both hips are either already dislocated or temporarily become so when gently manipulated. Affected infants are generally treated by splinting, in order to promote stabilization by keeping each femoral head deep within the corresponding acetabulum.

The most commonly used primary screening test is the Ortolani–Barlow (O–B) manoeuvre. This is a manual test for which no instruments are needed, although ultrasound is sometimes used to observe the movement of the joint during the test, and/or to examine its anatomy for signs of imperfect development (dysplasia). At some centres (especially in Austria and Germany) this is done routinely; and even if the O–B test is negative, treatment is sometimes given when a hip is thought to be dysplastic.

The focus of this chapter is on screening for CDH rather than for dysplasia, and reflects the view that treating newborn infants for dysplasia not associated with severe instability is of doubtful benefit and would consume substantial resources. The proportion of infants in whom ultrasonic screening for dysplasia is positive varies very widely between observers and sometimes approaches 50 per cent;[1] and a positive finding in the newborn is not a strong predictor of hip problems later in infancy (whereas ultrasonic evidence of hip joint instability is).[2] In later life, there is evidence that dysplastic hips are at increased risk of becoming osteoarthritic;[3] but whether this risk is reduced by early detection and treatment of dysplasia cannot be proved without long-term follow-up data which are not available.

THE DISORDER

Natural history

CDH does not generally present clinically in unscreened children until they start walking. However, experience of neonatal screening, which is considered later in this chapter, indicates that most but not all potential cases of persistent CDH are born with severe instability, as are an even larger number of infants whose hips later stabilize spontaneously. The grounds for these conclusions are as follows:

1. The conclusion that *persistent CDH is usually preceded by severe instability in the newborn* rests on screening programmes in which the incidence of persistent CDH in infants whose hips had been stable at birth (and who therefore were not treated to prevent CDH) was only one-fifth or less of the incidence in complete populations which had no preventive treatment. Another reason for thinking that the neonatal and persistent conditions are related is that they share several risk factors—both are particularly common in the left hip, in females, in babies that have presented by the breech, and in firstborn infants.[4]

2. The conclusion that *severe instability of the newborn hip disappears spontaneously in a majority of cases* follows from the finding that when newborn infants are screened, the proportion in whom severe instability is detected is almost always several times as high as the prevalence of persistent dislocation in unscreened populations. Stabilization begins within a few days of birth: the majority of hips that are unstable according to the O–B test on the first day of birth appear to be stable when examined towards the end of the first week.[5,6]

3. The conclusion that *not all potential cases of persistent CDH are born with severe instability* is suggested by the finding that even in carefully screened populations, persistent dislocation in late infancy or early childhood is sometimes diagnosed in children whose hips were reported to be stable at birth. Some of these cases are no doubt missed at screening because of observer error or because they were born with irreducible dislocation (which the O–B test does not detect); but there are also well-documented cases on record in which increasingly obvious dysplasia was observed radiologically and dislocation eventually occurred after an experienced examiner had found the femoral head to be clinically stable within the acetabulum at birth.[7]

The natural history of CDH during the first year of life is therefore that severe instability of the hip in the newborn leads in a minority of cases to persistent CDH, and that less frequently CDH develops in hips which previously articulated normally. In the newborn the head of the femur can readily slip in and out of the acetabulum in most hips that are severely unstable; but when CDH persists, reduction becomes more difficult or impossible.

In persistent complete CDH, the head of the femur becomes displaced upwards in relation to the pelvis, especially when the child starts to walk. This makes the leg shorter, which causes limping and its complications (e.g. knee joint problems) except when the disorder is bilateral (which it is in about one-third of cases). Complete and incomplete CDH can both lead to pain, and to the degenerative changes of osteoarthrosis. In complete dislocation, a well-developed false acetabulum may form in the iliac wall adjacent to the dislocated femoral head, in which case the degenerative changes seem to be more severe than if there is little or no ilio-femoral articulation.[3]

Prevalence

Estimates of the natural prevalence of persistent CDH (i.e. its prevalence in the absence of screening and treatment) are given in Table 16.1. These figures relate to diagnoses made in young children born before the introduction of screening in places where the population is of predominantly northwest European ancestry—Australia, North America, Scandinavia, and the United Kingdom. CDH was ascertained in 0.84–1.5 per 1000 of these children, mainly from hospital records. Three other studies in England and Wales[16–18] yielded lower rates (0.66, 0.67, and 0.85/1000) than the English figures in the table (1.03 to 1.14/1000); but in calculating these three lower rates, no allowance was made for cases missed because of death or removal from the study area.

Natural prevalence rates below those shown in Table 16.1 have been reported for African, Chinese, and Inuit infants.[19] Elsewhere, e.g. in Amerindian, Czech, Japanese, Lapp, and Turkish communities, rates of 1 per cent-10 per cent (10 to 100 times as high as those in Table 16.1) have been described.[13,20–24] These differences are thought to reflect different nursing practices: high rates occur mainly in communities with traditions of nursing infants with their thighs extended and adducted, whereas in the low-prevalence communities it has been customary to carry infants on the backs of their mothers with their thighs flexed and abducted.[19] Abduction stabilizes the joint by 'screwing home' the femoral head deep within the acetabulum.[25] A sharp reduction in the prevalence of CDH was observed when a method of swaddling which maintained the thighs in extension was abandoned in a Japanese community.[22]

When the prevalence of persistent CDH is elevated by practices which limit abduction and flexion, the additional cases may often not arise until after birth, unlike most

Table 16.1 Reported prevalence of dislocation of one or both hips, in communities of mainly northwestern European ancestry in which screening was not carried out

Location	Prevalence per 1000 (95% CI if population size given)
Aberdeen, UK[8]	1.5
Vancouver, Canada[9]	1.31 (0.98–1.64)[a]
New York City, USA[10]	1.24 (0.32–2.16)
South Australia[11]	1.2
Newcastle-on-Tyne, UK[b]	1.14 (0.58–1.70)
Northern England[b]	1.12 (0.86–1.38)
Birmingham, UK[12]	1.03 (0.80–1.24)[c]
Norway (excluding Lapland)[13]	1.02 (0.90–1.14)[a]
Sweden[14]	0.86 (0.77–0.95)[d]
Rochester, Minn., USA[15]	0.84 (0.10–1.58)

[a] Figures revised using additional data supplied by E. Hey (personal communication).
[b] Prevalence/1000 children alive 1 year after birth, based on unpublised data supplied by E. Hey (personal communication).
[c] Prevalence rate revised from that given in the original report, by subtracting from the denominator the number of children estimated to have had insufficient follow-up for persistent dislocation to be ascertained.
[d] Prevalence rate not given in the original report, but estimated by relating the number of cases reported to have been ascertained in Sweden in 1948–50 to the number of surviving children who were estimated to have been born in Sweden 1½ years earlier (i.e. in July 1946–June 1949).

other cases of persistent CDH (p. 399): less than one-fifth of infants with persistent CDH in a Japanese population in which the prevalence of this condition was high (2.7 per cent) had shown signs of instability at birth.[26]

SCREENING TESTS

Routine neonatal screening for CDH was first introduced in 1952 in Malmö, Sweden, by von Rosen and his colleagues.[27] The screening procedure they used was Ortolani's test, a manual method of assessing whether the head of each femur is within the corresponding acetabulum.[28] The Ortolani–Barlow (O–B) test which is now the most widely used primary screening test for CDH was developed from the Ortolani test by Barlow in the late 1950s, in order to enable dislocatable as well as dislocated hips to be detected.[5]

In the O–B test, the knee and hip are held in 90° of flexion, with the upper thigh between the examiner's fingers and thumb so that the greater trochanter of the femur lies under the middle finger, the lesser trochanter under the thumb, and the flexed lower leg in the palm; and the thigh is abducted through about 45°. With the thighs in this position, forward pressure is applied behind the greater trochanter with the middle finger, and reducible luxation is diagnosed if this pressure is felt to cause the femoral head to slip forward into the acetabulum. If this does not happen, outward and backward pressure is applied with the thumb on the inner side of the thigh, and dislocatability is diagnosed if this pressure is felt to cause the femoral head to slip backwards out of the acetabulum. The femoral head should slip forward again into a reduced position either immediately the pressure by the thumb is released or when this release of pressure is accompanied by pressure on the greater trochanter by the middle finger. Movement of the femoral head into or out of the acetabulum is often but not always accompanied by a palpable and/or audible 'clunk'.

The test may be carried out on each hip simultaneously or on each in turn (Fig. 16.1). In the latter case, the examiner puts each hip through the above movements with one hand while steadying the infant's pelvis with the other hand, the thumb of which is placed on the symphysis pubis and the fingers under the sacrum.

In infants whose hips are not dislocated or dislocatable, the test may detect unusual mobility of the femoral head within the acetabulum (interpreted as mild joint laxity) or give rise to clicks and grating sensations. These infants are not generally regarded as screen-positive. They are kept under review in some screening programmes; and a few studies suggest that they are more likely than other screen-negative children to develop persistent dislocation, although the excess risks appear to be small (1.5 per cent or less).[29,30] The evidence for regarding clicks or grating as a risk factor has been contested.[31–33]

The O–B test is very often performed as part of the routine neonatal clinical examination. Other signs of CDH which may be sought at the same time include a reduction in the angle through which the affected thigh can be abducted, and asymmetry affecting the skin creases and length of the thighs and the position in which they are held when unrestricted. However, these signs do not usually develop until after the neonatal period,[5,34] unlike positive O–B results.

In the UK, there are national guidelines on screening for CDH which recommend

Examination of both hips simultaneously   Examination of each hip separately

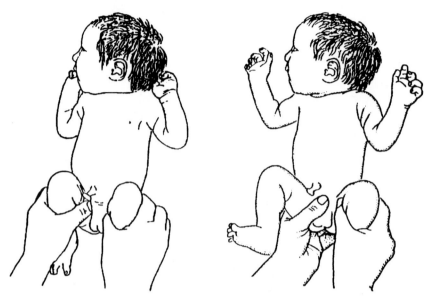

Fig. 16.1   Position of examiner's hands and infant for: (left) the Ortolani–Barlow test as carried out on both hips together; (right) the Ortolani–Barlow test as carried out when one hip (in this illustration the left) is examined separately from the other. (Reproduced from *Screening for the detection of congenital dislocation of the hip* (revised 1986), Standing Medical Advisory Committee and Standard Nursing Advisory Committee, 1986, pp. A2 and A4, by permission of the Controller of Her Majesty's Stationery Office.)

that the O–B test should be carried out twice before the newborn is discharged from the obstetric hospital, and for a third time at six weeks of age.[34] In fact, nearly 70 per cent of obstetric units in the UK test infants within 24 hours of birth and the rest within 48 hours, but only 8 per cent aim to test all infants twice before discharge.[35] A recent randomized controlled trial comparing policies of testing once and twice before discharge suggests that once is sufficient: retesting did not increase the number of infants thought to need treatment when seen at an orthopaedic clinic.[36]

It is not known how many infants are tested at six weeks. A single examination at this time would be preferable to earlier testing if all infants could be examined then, since it would result in fewer false-positives being splinted: most hips that are unstable at birth stabilize by six weeks even if untreated (p. 399). Splinting has not been shown to lose in effectiveness when delayed until six weeks, although there is a strong consensus among paediatric orthopaedic surgeons that delays longer than this lead to poorer results.[37,38] The main reason for not abandoning screening at birth in favour of testing at six weeks only is that 100 per cent coverage is easier to achieve in the obstetric hospital than in the community.

Most neonatal screening in hospital is carried out by junior paediatric staff, and especially in the UK by those in their first year of postgraduate paediatric training;[35] and child health centres staffed by community medical and nursing staff provide screening for infants not in hospital.[39] The person carrying out primary screening is expected to refer infants in whom the O–B test is positive to an experienced orthopaedic surgeon or paediatrician,[34] who will generally repeat the test and decide on management if the result is again positive. In the UK this decision is generally taken by an orthopaedic surgeon.[35] Among infants who tested positive at primary screening, the proportions in different studies who remained positive when retested in orthopaedic clinics varied from two-fifths[40] to four-fifths.[41]

At some units, primary screening includes not only O–B testing but also enquiry about certain other risk factors for CDH: infants are referred for secondary screening if any of these factors is present. The factors considered vary between units: apart from a positive O–B test, the most widely used are a family history of CDH and a personal history of breech presentation.[35]

Among the screening programmes for which it is possible to estimate effectiveness in discriminating between affected and unaffected, some have classified infants as O–B positive and negative on the basis of primary O–B screening by a junior examiner combined with secondary O–B screening by a senior, as described above; a few seem to have relied exclusively on primary screening by experienced observers (e.g. orthopaedic surgeons[6,9,42–45] and specially trained physiotherapists[30,46]); and there are a few for which the available reports do not state which approach was used. This diversity must be borne in mind through the review of screening statistics which follows.

Discrimination between affected and unaffected subjects

Direct estimates of detection and false-positive rates for the O–B test are not available. To determine these rates, one would need to withhold treatment from infants in whom the O–B test was positive. Indirect estimates can, however, be made from the proportion who test positive, the proportion who present with CDH after testing negative, and the natural prevalence of CDH (i.e. the proportion of infants who would present with CDH if there was no screening).

The *proportion of infants who tested positive* ranged from 1.6 to 28.5/1000, with a median of 7.6/1000, in 44 populations of predominantly northwestern European ancestry which were screened by the O–B test.[6,8,9,29,30,32,39–77] One reason for the wide variation in these rates is probably that some examiners classified O–B test findings as positive when they showed only minor laxity of the joint—i.e. not enough laxity to allow the femoral head to be moved beyond the rim of the acetabulum. This could substantially inflate the positive rate, since minor laxity is much commoner than severe instability.[71]

In efficiently screened populations, the *proportion of infants who present with CDH after testing negative* is similar to the proportion who present with CDH without having been treated for neonatal instability. The latter was reported for 30 of the above 44 populations, and ranged from 0.07 to 1.79/1000 infants screened, with a median of 0.45/1000. The figure for the UK as a whole (where O–B testing is routine) may be higher than this median according to a recent nationwide survey:[78] it was estimated from this that operative procedures for CDH were carried out in 0.78/1000 liveborn children, and the disorder was diagnosed after age three months in 70 per cent of those affected (i.e. in $0.70 \times 0.78/1000$, which is 0.55/1000).

The reported *natural prevalence of CDH* in populations of predominantly north-western European ancestry has already been shown to range from 0.84 to 1.5/1000, with a median value of 1.1/1000 (Table 16.1). The true range is probably rather higher, since complete ascertainment is difficult to achieve. For the purpose of estimating detection and false-positive rates, it is assumed here that the true natural prevalence is 1.3/1000.

Table 16.2 shows what the rates would in this case be for a hypothetical population of 100 000 infants in which the number who were O–B positive (760) and the number who presented with CDH after an O–B negative test (45) matched the median values for these outcomes in populations of mainly northwestern European ancestry. One hundred and thirty infants would present with CDH in the absence of screening. Eighty-five of these 130 infants would be 'true-positives', since 85 is the difference between 130 and 45 (the number affected by persistent CDH after testing negative— i.e. the 'false-negatives'). Subtraction of 85 from the total number who tested positive (760) gives the number of false-positives, i.e. 675. The estimated detection rate is therefore 65 per cent (85/130) and the false-positive rate is 0.7 per cent (675/ (100 000–130)).

Given the variation between studies in the proportions of infants who test positive and who present with dislocation after testing negative, it is predictable that the detection and false-positive rates will also vary widely. Estimates of these rates are plotted in Fig. 16.2 for 26 of the 30 populations of northwestern European origin for which data on the frequency of positive and false-negative results were available. In the four populations for which estimates are not given, estimation was impossible because the false-negative cases of CDH observed after screening equalled or outnumbered the total cases of CDH to be expected in the absence of screening if the natural preva-lence was 1.3/1000. Two of these four populations were from Aberdeen,[8,77] where CDH was reported in 1.5/1000 unscreened infants (Table 16.1). Data on natural prevalence are not available for the other two populations (from Southampton[57] and five counties in Norway[60]). It is possible that some of the 'false-negatives' in these populations (and indeed in others) were only ascertained as cases of CDH because of there being a screening programme. This would happen if O–B testing increased the risk of CDH (see below), or if the surveillance throughout infancy which some

Table 16.2   100 000 infants with median values for the proportions with positive and false-negative results: distribution by screening test result and outcome if not treated, assuming that the natural prevalence of CDH is 1.3/1000

	Screening test result		Total
	Positive	Negative	
Outcome if not treated:			
CDH	85	45	130
No CDH	675	99 195	99 870
Total	760	99 240	100 000

Detection rate = 85/130 = 65.4%.
False-positive rate = 675/99 870 = 0.7%

screening programmes include led to abnormalities which would resolve spontaneously being detected and counted as 'false-negatives'.

The detection rates shown in Fig. 16.2 range from 25 per cent to 94 per cent (median
72 per cent), and the false-positive rates from 0.1 per cent to 1.9 per cent (median 0.58
per cent). These ranges are so wide as to raise serious doubts about the value of the
O–B test, as does the lack of a positive correlation between the two rates. In any
screening test, when some examiners observe many more positives than others, the
assumption is that the threshold beyond which the former examiners regard results as
positive is relatively low. In this case, their detection and false-positive rates will both
be higher than those obtained by examiners whose threshold of abnormality is higher,
i.e. the different examiners' detection and false-positive rates will be positively correlated. With the O–B test, however, the examiners at some centres seem to obtain
positive results in ≥ 90 per cent of cases of CDH and ≤ 0.4 per cent of non-cases,
whereas others do so in ≤ 30 per cent of cases and ≥ 1.6 per cent of non-cases. There
must be fundamental differences between centres in the performance or interpretation
of the test; but what these differences are is not evident from the reports compared.
For example, the few centres where primary screening was done by orthopaedic surgeons [6,9,42–45] or specially trained physiotherapists [30,46] did not have consistently better
or worse rates than the other centres (Fig. 16.2).

Interobserver differences in O–B test results occur within as well as between centres.
Studies have been reported in which two observers differed as to whether the O–B test
was positive in between half and twice as many cases as were agreed to be abnormal;[79,80] and in a study in which infants were tested by up to four paediatricians, cases

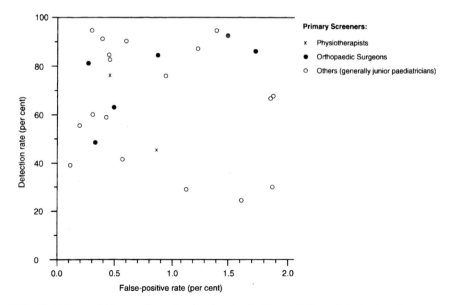

Fig. 16.2 Detection and false-positive rates of screening in 26 populations of predominantly
northwestern European ancestry,[6,9,30,32,40–46,50,52–54,56,58,61–68,73,76] estimated on the assumption that the
natural prevalence of CDH is 1.3/1000. The type of point plotted for each centre shows who carried out
primary screening there. (Data from reference 67 corrected by E Hey (personal communication).)

which were agreed to be abnormal were outnumbered much more heavily by cases of disagreement.[81]

Variations in technique which may lead to discordant findings have been demonstrated using videotapes of various categories of physicians and nurses carrying out the O–B test. When their performance was marked by experts, senior orthopaedic surgeons scored 95 per cent on average, senior paediatricians 64 per cent, community medical and nursing staff 59 per cent, and junior paediatric staff 52 per cent.[82] Given these findings and the fact that senior orthopaedic surgeons do not generally carry out primary screening, it is not surprising that the results of screening for CDH are poor overall. What is surprising is that the results from the centres where orthopaedic surgeons were the primary screeners did not compare more favourably with the results of the other centres analysed.

Odds of being affected given a positive result (OAPR)

For a population with the median total positive and false negative rates reported for populations of northwestern European ancestry (Table 16.2), the OAPR would be 1:8 (85:675) if the natural prevalence of CDH was 1.3/1000. The OAPRs yielded by the detection and false-positive rates for the populations shown in Fig. 16.2 range from 1:2 to 1:50, with a median of 1:7.

Safety of screening

Except in osteogenesis imperfecta (in which O–B testing can fracture the femur[83]), it is not certain whether CDH screening is completely safe. There is no conclusive evidence that it is not; but the possibility that it can reduce the stability of the hip joints has been raised, partly in order to account for certain changes in the prevalence of late cases of dislocation (i.e. cases presenting in infants who were O–B negative at birth) that have been observed following changes in screening practice. For example, prevalence increased at one unit when it introduced the O–B test in place of the simple Ortolani test (which tests for reducible dislocation as the O–B test does, but differs by not testing whether dislocation can be induced if it is not already present).[84] At another unit, an increase in the prevalence of late cases was succeeded by a decrease when the amount of repeat O–B testing was reduced.[85] It has also been reported that lax hip joints become more so when repeatedly examined in life[86] or at necropsy.[87] Post-mortem studies in the neonate suggest that the O–B test can cause even stable hips to become lax, although only if the O–B test is done frequently or harshly enough to break the vacuum seal in the joint space by producing an effusion or forcing gas out of solution.[88] These findings do not prove that the O–B test is unsafe as a screening procedure, but the possibility should be taken seriously, especially since even a low risk of damage could be substantial in relation to the natural risk of CDH.

Ancillary or alternative tests: ultrasound

The techniques other than physical examination which have been used in the detection of CDH include imaging with X-rays, magnetic resonance imaging, audible sound transmission, vibration arthrography, and ultrasound. Imaging with X-rays is unsuitable for neonatal screening because of the hazards of exposure to radiation and because the structures around the joint are not yet ossified enough to show up adequately. Magnetic resonance imaging is too time-consuming and costly and scarce a resource to use for screening. Audible sound transmission between the patella and the pubic symphysis, which was suggested as a screening test because it tends to be reduced when the femoral head and acetabulum are not closely apposed, has only been reported from one centre,[89,90] and the available data are far too limited to assess its performance. The same is true for vibration arthrometry (the use of instruments to record and analyse the vibrations that occur when joints are examined clinically) as a technique in CDH screening. This was introduced in the hope of identifying severe instability by analysing the vibrations which the O–B test produces.[91,92]

Ultrasound examination of the hips is much more widespread: in early 1994, 69 per cent of maternity units in the UK and the Irish Republic were using it and a further 4 per cent planned to introduce it over the next 12 months.[35] It is generally performed with the infant lying in a supine or lateral position, using a real-time linear-array transducer. The standard practice is for the test to be carried out between 10 days and six weeks after birth[38,93] and to include two procedures: (1) a *dynamic examination* in which the movement of the femoral head during the O–B test is viewed in a transverse plane whilst the hip is in 90° of flexion; (2) a *static or morphological examination* in which a view in the coronal plane passing through the centre of the acetabulum is obtained while the hip is slightly flexed or in 90° of flexion.[94] The purpose of the static examination is to detect signs of dysplasia of the hip, including complete or partial dislocation when at rest. Among the units using ultrasound in the UK and the Irish Republic in 1994 for which data were available, the dynamic method alone was used by 36 per cent, the static method alone by 24 per cent, and both methods by 40 per cent.[35]

The British and Irish units where ultrasound was used also varied in the contexts in which they reported using it. Forty-five per cent did so only in infants with clinically abnormal hips, 6 per cent only in infants at high risk of CDH, and 48 per cent in both these groups. Only one unit (out of 176 where some use was made of ultrasound) had a policy of screening every infant by ultrasound.[35] Data on the performance of ultrasound as a screening procedure are available for a few centres which use it in all infants and a few which do so only in infants who have clinically abnormal hips or other risk factors for CDH.

Results of ultrasound as a primary screening test
Results from four centres where all infants were screened by ultrasound are summarized in Table 16.3. There were considerable differences in practice between the first three of these centres and the fourth.

At the first three centres,[1,95–97] all infants with dysplasia on ultrasound and/or clinical instability were classified as positive, but immediate treatment was largely or entirely restricted to those with clinically detected severe instability. The remaining infants who were classified as positive had regular follow-up examinations and only received treatment if this was indicated then. The estimated detection rates of these three centres (69 per cent–100 per cent) were close to or above the median for the 26 centres using the O–B test alone on which Fig. 16.2 is based, but their false-positive rates (3.8–5.9 per cent) were much higher than those for the 26.

At the fourth centre,[98] infants were only classified as positive if severe instability was

Table 16.3 Discrimination between affected and unaffected infants reported with ultrasound as a primary screening test

Location of study	Definition of a positive result	Number of infants screened	Prevalence (per 1000 infants)		Screening parameters (assuming a natural prevalence of 1.3/1000)		
			Positive results (a)	Late diagnoses (b)	Detection rate (%), [(1.3 − b)/1.3]	False-positive rate (%), {[a − (1.3 −b)]/(1000−1.3)}	OAPR {(1.3 − b):[a − (1.3 − b)]}
Trondheim, Norway[1,95]	Reducible dislocation on clinical examination, and/or instability on dynamic ultrasound examination, and/or dysplasia on static ultrasound examination[a]	5457	52.0	0.4	69	5.1	1:57
Coventry, England[96]	Positive O–B test on clinical examination, and/or dysplasia on static ultrasound examination[a]	14 050	60.3	0.0	100	5.9	1:45
Bergen, Norway[97]	Positive O–B test on clinical examination, and/or dysplasia on static ultrasound examination[b]	3613	38.5	0.3	77	3.8	1:38
Trollhätten, Sweden[98]	Severe instability on dynamic ultrasound examination	4430	10.8	0.0	100	1.0	1:7

[a] Dysplasia here denotes low femoral head coverage (i.e. an abnormally small percentage of the head of the femur is located within the ossified part of the acetabulum).
[b] Dysplasia here denotes underdevelopment of the acetabular roof, and includes partial and total dislocation.

observed by ultrasound. These infants were treated immediately if their hips were dislocated, and otherwise followed up after three weeks and treated if their hips were still unstable then. The study size was too small for much reliance to be placed on the detection rate (100 per cent). The false-positive rate (1.0 per cent) was not much higher than the median for the 26 centres that did not use ultrasound (0.6 per cent), but this false-positive rate may not be typical: in another careful study,[80] severe instability was observed by ultrasound in 2.3 per cent of hips, which is equivalent to 3.5 per cent of infants (since CDH is bilateral in one-third of those affected) and therefore implies a false-positive rate of 3.4 per cent if the true-positive rate is 0.1 per cent as suggested.

Results of ultrasound as a secondary screening test

Results for five centres where ultrasound has been used as a secondary test in infants with risk factors for CDH (including clinically abnormal hips) are summarized in Table 16.4. The criteria for classifying infants as positive included dysplasia at three of these centres[97,99,100] but were limited to displacement of the head of the femur at the other two.[73,93] At all five centres, those classified as positive were treated immediately by splinting if the abnormality was severe. Otherwise they were followed up, and only splinted if they remained abnormal. As one would expect, the estimated detection rates and false-positive rates for these centres (46 per cent–92 per cent and 0.8 per cent–2.4 per cent respectively) both tended to be lower than those for the four centres where all infants were screened by ultrasound, although the ranges for the two groups of centres overlapped.

   Data on the performance of ultrasound are not available for any centres where it is used *only* in infants with clinically positive O–B tests. It would be valuable to know whether its use in this way can exclude false-positives and so reduce unnecessary splinting without impairing the detection of subjects at risk of persistent CDH, but this question has not yet been answered, although a trial by the UK Medical Research Council is currently addressing it.[106] A previous trial in which ultrasound was used in one of two groups of infants whose hips were clinically O–B positive[75] failed as a test of the use of ultrasound because the management of the two groups also differed in other respects.

Conclusions regarding ultrasound

The value of ultrasound in screening for CDH remains uncertain. As a method of distinguishing between true- and false-positives in infants whose hips are clinically O–B positive, its value may be clarified by the Medical Research Council's current trial. Its value in primary screening or as a secondary test in infants at high risk of CDH is not established by the analyses of performance shown in Tables 16.3 and 16.4. The estimated detection rates at the centres using ultrasound in these ways were not consistently higher than those obtained at some centres by clinical O–B testing alone, and the false-positive rates were relatively high (especially with primary screening by ultrasound). Consequently, most OAPRs were low. The most favourable OAPRs (1:7) came from two of the three centres where dysplasia without femoral displacement or instability was not regarded as a positive finding, which supports the view that this should be disregarded when screening for CDH (see p. 398).

Table 16.4 Discrimination between affected and unaffected infants reported with ultrasound as a secondary screening test

Location of study	Ultrasound findings defined as positive	Number of infants screened by physical examination	Percentage of infants selected for ultrasound as a secondary screening test[a]	Prevalence (per 1000 infants screened by physical examination)		Screening parameters (assuming a natural prevalence of 1.3/1000)		
				Positive results (a)	Late diagnoses (b)	Detection rate (%), $[(1.3 - b)/1.3]$	False positive rate (%), $\{[a - (1.3 - b)]/(1000 - 1.3)\}$	OAPR $\{(1.3 - b): [a - (1.3 - b)]\}$
Coventry, England[73]	Displacement on static or dynamic examination	4617	9.7	21.2	0.6	54	2.1	1:29
Swansea, Wales[99]	Severe instability on dynamic examination, and/or dysplasia or immaturity (Graf's criteria[2,3]) on static examination	3879	10.5	25.3	0.1[b]	92	2.4	1:20
Southampton, England[93]	Displacement on static or dynamic examination	26 952	7.0	8.6	0.2	85	0.8	1:7
Bergen, Norway[97]	Dysplasia (Graf's criteria[101,102]) on static examination	4388	11.8	21.2	0.7	46	2.1	1:34
Blackburn, England[100]	Severe instability on dynamic examination, and/or dysplasia (Zieger's criteria[103,104]) on static examination	4300 (estimate)	4.8	11.2	0.5	62	1.0	1:13

[a] Selection criteria included clinical instability, family history of CDH, and breech presentation in all studies, and also clicking hip and positional foot deformity in all studies except that from Bergen, and limited abduction in the studies from Coventry and Blackburn.
[b] Prevalence according to Jones.[105]

One three-way trial has been reported in which the policies compared were primary screening by physical examination alone; primary screening by both physical examination and ultrasound; and primary screening by physical examination followed by secondary screening by ultrasound if risk factors for CDH were reported.[97] The allocation of infants to the three arms was not formally randomized, but severe bias was unlikely. The trial was located in Bergen, and is the source of the Bergen data in Tables 16.3 and 16.4. The prevalence of late-diagnosed cases of CDH ('false negatives') was 1.3/1000 after screening by physical examination alone, and 0.7/1000 and 0.3/1000 when physical examination was combined with secondary and primary ultrasound screening respectively. As the trial was not large enough for this trend to be statistically significant ($P = 0.11$),[97] it leaves the value of ultrasound screening in doubt and demonstrates the need for a trial based on larger numbers.

NEONATAL TREATMENT

In screening for most conditions, a positive screening test is an indication for a diagnostic test, and treatment is only given if the latter test is positive. In screening for CDH, by contrast, diagnostic testing is impossible, since the objective of screening is to detect those at risk of a condition that is still in the future, and decisions to treat (which are generally made by orthopaedic surgeons) are taken mainly in response to positive O–B and ultrasound findings.

The objective in treatment is to keep the thighs flexed and partly abducted so that the head of each femur remains deep within the acetabulum during the first few weeks or months after birth. In these circumstances the acetabulum comes to encompass an increasing proportion of the femoral head, which grows more slowly than the acetabular cartilage during the early postnatal period,[107] and the joint thus becomes more stable.

A variety of methods of splinting the thighs in flexion and partial abduction have been devised, of which two are widely used—the Pavlik harness (the more popular in Britain and Ireland) and the von Rosen splint.[35] The Pavlik harness is made of soft material, and maintains the thighs in position by holding the feet in stirrups attached to a belt, which is worn under the arms and secured by straps around the shoulders. The von Rosen splint is a flat, padded piece of malleable metal, shaped rather like a capital H but with the horizontal line extending laterally beyond the vertical ones. This splint is anchored by moulding the lateral and upper projections around the trunk and shoulders respectively, and the thighs are held in position by moulding the two lower projections under them.

There have been no randomized trials to compare the merits of these methods or to assess how long splinting should continue. Durations of splinting varying from two to 52 weeks were reported by the British and Irish units surveyed. Seven-tenths of them splinted for less than 12 weeks.[35]

Safety of neonatal treatment

The main hazard of treatment of CDH is ischaemic or avascular necrosis. This is characterized by delayed and commonly multifocal ossification of the femoral head, often accompanied by reduced femoral growth. It is thought to be due to compression of the femoral head and impairment of its blood supply by stresses in the tissues of the joint when the hip is held in abduction and medial rotation.[108] Ischaemic necrosis can lead to deformity of the acetabulum, coxa vara, shortening of the leg and osteoarthrosis, although many cases become normal.

The incidence of ischaemic necrosis is highest after surgery for established dislocation, when it has exceeded one-third in some series.[109] The incidence rates reported after splinting for neonatal instability or dysplasia have ranged from 2 per cent to zero with the von Rosen splint and from 20 per cent to zero with the Pavlik harness.[30,110–112] Experience suggests that the rate of ischaemic necrosis following splinting is lowest when the hips are maintained in moderate as opposed to extreme abduction.[6,113] The importance of minimizing this rate is heightened by the large numbers at risk—0.8 per cent of all infants on average if each with a positive O–B test is splinted (p. 403). Among these infants who may be put at risk of ischaemic necrosis, an estimated seven-eighths or more are not prospective cases of CDH (p. 404) and therefore cannot be expected to benefit from splinting.

EFFECTIVENESS OF SCREENING AND NEONATAL TREATMENT

The value of neonatal screening and treatment programmes in preventing persistent CDH cannot be estimated accurately, since there have been no randomized clinical trials. We can, however, make some assessment of the effectiveness of these programmes from the proportions of infants within them who were eventually treated surgically for persistent CDH. There would be no such infants if screening and neonatal treatment were totally effective. If, on the other hand, these procedures had no effect, it is reasonable to suppose that the proportion of infants who would be treated surgically in a population of northwestern European descent would be close to the figure of 1.3/1000 which was adopted above as an overall estimate of the natural prevalence of persistent CDH in such populations. Hospital referrals were the main source of ascertainment for the estimates of prevalence in Table 16.1 on which this figure of 1.3/1000 is based.

Table 16.5 lists 16 centres with screening programmes (including three where ultrasound was used) from which data including the numbers of infants receiving surgical treatment for persistent CDH have been published for populations of more than 10 000. At all but one of these 16 centres, fewer children underwent surgery than the 1.3/1000 who might be expected to have done so in the absence of neonatal treatment. At 11 of the 16 centres, a majority of the children undergoing surgery had not previously been splinted as a result of screening: they were failures of screening rather than failures of splinting. Failures of screening also outnumber failures of splinting in the UK as a whole, where a recent survey of cases reported by orthopaedic surgeons[78] suggests that 0.78/1000 children (95 per cent CI 0.72–0.84) undergo surgery for CDH, of whom less than one-quarter are detected by screening (which is routine in the UK).

There are several reasons for being cautious when interpreting the findings when the surgical treatment rates in Table 16.5 are compared with one another and with the rate

Table 16.5 Frequency of surgery for CDH in screened populations

Place and date	Population size	Proportion (per 1000 total population)				
		Total splinted neonatally	Underwent surgery			Percentage of all recipients of surgery who underwent open surgery
			After splinting neonatally	Not splinted neonatally	Total	
Screening by clinical examination without ultrasound						
Aberdeen, UK						
1960–9[41]	71 169[a]	16.31	0.11	1.10	1.21	–
1970–9[8,77]	53 033	28.45	0.30	1.53	1.83	–
1980–9[77]	67 093	10.00[a]	0.31	1.79	2.10	21%[a]
Total	191 295	17.46	0.23	1.46	1.69	–
Leiden and Haarlem, Netherlands,1971–9[74]	14 264	9.81	0.28	1.12[a]	1.40[a]	90%[a]
Northern England, 1972–82[b]	348 304	6.04[a]	0.43	0.68	1.11	–
Uusimaa, Finland, 1966–75[68,114,115]	151 924	6.06	0.41	0.68	1.09	11%
Uppsala, Sweden, 1962–5[52]	11 868	19.55	0.25	0.42	0.67	25%
Bristol, UK, 1970–9[32]	23 002	19.35	0.22	0.43	0.65	47%
Newcastle-on-Tyne,UK, 1964–73[67]	25 921	10.45	0.31	0.27[b]	0.58	67%[b]
Solihull, UK, 1980–90[116]	37 511	12.48	0.37	0.08	0.45	100%
Western Australia, 1981–3[117]	66 822	5.70[c]	0.31[c]	0.09[d]	0.40	59%
East Dorset, UK, 1982–92[46]	42 421	6.01	0.14	0.21	0.35	27%
Edinburgh, UK, 1962–8[56]	31 961	4.44[a]	0.22	0.13	0.34	36%
Vancouver, Canada, 1967–76[45]	32 480	9.88	0.15	0.18	0.34	0%
New Plymouth, New Zealand, 1964–85[6]	20 657	16.02	0.05	0.10	0.15	100%
Primary screening by clinical examination and secondary ultrasound[e]						
Southampton, UK, 1988–92[93]	26 952	4.19[c]	0.19[c]	0.22[d]	0.41	82%
Blackburn, UK, 1992–4[118]	10 757	6.04[c]	0.00[c]	0.28[d]	0.28	–
Primary screening by clinical examination and ultrasound						
Coventry, UK, 1989–92[96]	14 050	2.42[c]	0.14[c]	0.00[d]	0.14	0%

a Estimated.
b Unpublished data supplied by E. Hey (personal communication).
c Figures relate to all cases diagnosed by screening (some more than four weeks after birth) and treated.
d Figures relate to cases not diagnosed by screening.
e Indications for ultrasound at Southampton were clinical hip instability, clicking hip, family history of CDH, breech delivery, and foot deformity; at Blackburn, clinical hip instability, any congenital abnormality (including talipes equinovarus, metatarsus adductus or torticollis) or condition causing diffuse ligamentous laxity, family history of CDH, and breech delivery.

to be expected in the absence of screening. Firstly, there may be a problem of defini-tion: some reports did not give enough details of the treatment which each child underwent for one to be sure that all the rates were based on the same range of sur-gical procedures. Secondly, it is clear from the percentages of recipients of surgery who were treated by open as opposed to closed surgery (Table 16.5) that treatment policies varied between centres. These variations may have extended to what were accepted as the indications for surgery of any kind, in which case treatment rates would vary between centres even if the prevalence of persistent CDH did not. Thirdly, the extent of underascertainment of episodes of treatment at the different centres is unknown, although the fact that treatment rates were high for the centres with the largest populations (where one would expect underascertainment to be most severe) suggests that this may not have been a serious problem. Fourthly, many of the reports on which the data were based were written because the clinicians involved in screen-ing and treatment at the centres concerned had a particular interest in this work, which is likely to have been reflected in better results than those to be expected gener-ally. This is supported by the fact that the surgical treatment rates for three-quarters of the centres in Table 16.6 are lower than the estimated rate for the UK (0.78/1000).[78]

Bearing in mind these limitations of the data, it is not surprising that not every series points to the same conclusion about the effectiveness of screening. Given that the rates of surgery observed after screening only exceeded 1.3/1000 (the expected rate without screening) at two centres, and were close to half this figure or less at three-quarters of centres, it seems on balance likely that there is benefit in screening for per-sistent CDH, although the magnitude of this benefit cannot be quantified.

FINANCIAL COSTS AND SAVINGS OF NEONATAL SCREENING AND TREATMENT

Costings of screening and treatment for CDH have been published for Vancouver, Canada,[119,120] and more recently for Bergen, Norway.[121] In Table 16.6, the Bergen cost-

Table 16.6   Estimated health care costs (using costings in US$ from Bergen, Norway[121]) of screening and not screening a population of 10 000 in which (a) 1.3/1000 infants would develop persistent CDH if not screened, and (b) 1 per cent of infants would be splinted and 0.5/1000 treated surgically for CDH if screening were practised

Type of care	Unit cost of care[121]	Number of recipients of care	Cost for total population
Requirements if screening is omitted:			
Surgical treatment	$400 per day in hospital	13 (in hospital for 40 days on average[122])	$208 000
Requirements if screening is practised:			
Screening	$6 per child	10 000	$60 000
Splinting	$150 per child	100	$15 000
Surgical treatment	$400 per day in hospital	5 (in hospital for 40 days on average[122])	$80 000
Total	–	–	$155 000

Ratio of costs with screening to costs without screening = 155:208 = 0.75:1.

ings are used to compare the costs of screening (by clinical examination without ultra-sound) and not screening in a population for which the natural prevalence of persist-ent CDH is 1.3/1000, and in which the proportions splinted and receiving surgery after ultrasound are 1 per cent and 0.5/1000 respectively (as in the median population screened without ultrasound in Table 16.5). Table 16.6 suggests that screening such a population would cost about three-quarters as much as not screening. The corre-sponding ratios for the other populations in Table 16.5 which were screened without ultrasound range from 1.5:1 (Aberdeen) to 0.5:1 (New Plymouth). It seems therefore that although programmes of screening for CDH by clinical examination can reduce health care costs, their effects on these costs are generally modest.

The financial implications of using ultrasound in screening were also examined in the Bergen study,[121] using the results of the trial described earlier (p. 311) which com-pared primary screening by physical examination alone, primary screening by physi-cal examination followed by secondary screening by ultrasound, and primary screening by both methods. The combined costs of screening, splinting, and surgical treatment incurred by these three approaches were too close together to judge whether using ultrasound in either of the ways described can reduce health care costs. To enable this question to be answered, a trial based on larger numbers is needed. The question cannot be answered from the data in Table 16.5 on centres using ultrasound, since the splinting and surgical treatment rates which would have occurred at these centres with screening by clinical examination alone are unknown.

CONCLUSION

A flow diagram of screening for CDH as it has been most widely practised is shown in Fig. 16.3. Primary screening by the O–B test without ultrasound is carried out during the early neonatal period by junior paediatricians. Infants in whom this test is positive for severe instability are retested by orthopaedic surgeons, and splinted if the test is again positive or if the surgeon finds other evidence of severe instability. The estimates of the results of this procedure in Fig. 16.3 are based on median values for the 13 centres in Table 16.5 where infants were screened by clinical examination with-out ultrasound. According to these estimates, approximately three-quarters of the infants who would develop persistent CDH in the absence of screening would be detected and half would be prevented from developing the condition by the screening programme. Among those splinted, 10 per cent would be true positives (i.e. the OAPR is 1:9), but only in 7 per cent would the splinting prevent persistent CDH.

Screening for CDH is considerably more successful at some centres and less so at others than in the example shown in Fig. 16.3, because of the variations in detection and false-positive rates described in this review. Although it has not been possible to pinpoint the sources of this variability, its occurrence seems less surprising when one considers the many differences in methodology between centres. These differences include variations in:

(1) the qualifications and experience of the primary screeners;

(2) the use of ultrasound;

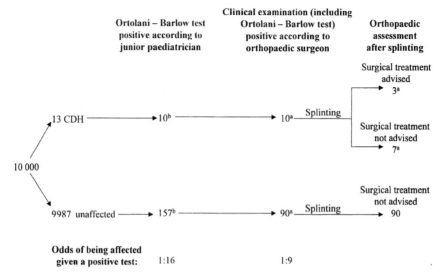

Fig. 16. 3 Flow diagram of screening for CDH. Key: [a]Based on median values for infants who were screened by clinical examination without ultrasound at centres in Table 16.5 (of whom approximately 0.3/1000 underwent surgery without having been splinted (i.e. were false-negatives), 10/1000 were splinted, and 0.3/1000 underwent surgery after splinting). [b]Estimated from proportion of infants classified as positive by orthopaedic surgeons (i.e. proportion splinted—1 per cent), on the assumptions (1) that these infants account for 60 per cent of infants classified as positive by junior paediatricians (different estimates put this proportion at 40–80 per cent, see p. 403) and (2) that far more cases of CDH would be missed by junior paediatricians screening all infants than by orthopaedic surgeons examining the 1.67 per cent of infants classified as positive by junior paediatricians.

(3) the extent to which findings at primary screening other than severe instability (e.g. positive family history, minor instability) are regarded as positive results;

(4) the procedure followed (neonatal splinting in all cases or secondary screening) if the result of primary screening is positive;

(5) the criteria for a positive result (and therefore for splinting) at secondary screening;

(6) the age at which any secondary screening is carried out and splinting initiated;

(7) the method and duration of splinting.

Randomized trials of adequate size have not been undertaken to assess whether and how variations in any of these features of screening affect its outcome, with one exception: as already noted (p. 409), the possible effects of not splinting clinically O–B positive infants if an ultrasound examination is normal are currently under investigation.[106] Large randomized trials of dynamic ultrasound examination as a primary screening test, and as a secondary test in infants identified as at high risk of persistent CDH by primary screening, are particularly needed, for three reasons. Firstly, encouraging results (Tables 16.3 and 16.4) have been reported from centres using dynamic ultrasound in these ways.[93,98] Secondly, lower false-negative rates were reported when ultrasound was used in screening, especially primary screening, in one small trial in which these procedures were compared with screening by physical examination alone[97] (p. 411); and the overall costs of screening and treatment in this trial were similar regardless of the method of screening [121] (p. 415). Thirdly, secondary ultrasound is already becoming widely accepted in clinical practice,[35] with significant implications for the cost of screening, which makes the need for randomized trials more urgent. It is much more difficult to mount a randomized trial of a procedure once it has becomes a part of routine clinical practice.

Screening by the O–B test was itself introduced into clinical practice without its value being assessed by randomized trial; and without data from such a trial, even the benefits of this test as a screening procedure cannot be quantified satisfactorily, given the widely varying results obtained from different centres (Table 16.5). There would be ethical objections to mounting such a trial in an area where there is evidence that the number of children who benefit from screening is as great as the 7 in 10 000 shown in Fig. 16.3. However, these objections could not apply were a trial to be mounted in areas where the prevalence of persistent CDH after screening is comparable to its prevalence in unscreened populations, as was the case in Aberdeen during the period when the data in Table 16.5 were collected. In the UK, such areas could probably be identified from routine hospital data, from which 77 per cent of infants commencing surgical treatment for CDH can be ascertained according to a recent survey.[78] It is therefore proposed that areas where at least 1/1000 children undergo surgical treatment for CDH according to hospital records should be identified, and that a randomized trial to compare the outcome of neonatal screening by the O–B test with no screening be undertaken in these areas.

In other areas, screening by physical examination should be continued, and kept under review by a designated health worker in each district as proposed in national guidelines for the UK.[34] Only a minority of British Health Districts seem to have such an arrangement.[35,123] One task of the designated worker should be to ensure that new screeners undergo formal training—an important requrement given the poor performance of the O–B test reported for junior doctors[82] (p. 406). To minimize the risk of infants' hips being made less stable by inexperienced handling (p. 406), it may be best if trainees are introduced to the signs of instability not by examining patients but by the use of a hip simulator model,[34] although this practice too has not been validated by randomized trial.

REFERENCES

1. Holen, K. J., Terjesen, T., Tegnander, A., Bredland, T., Saether, O. D., and Eik-Nes S. H. (1994). Ultrasound screening for hip dysplasia in newborns. *Journal of Pediatric Orthopaedics* **14**, 667–73.
2. Engesaeter, L. B., Wilson, D. J., Nag, D., and Benson, M. K. D. (1990). Ultrasound and congenital dislocation of the hip: the importance of dynamic assessment. *Journal of Bone and Joint Surgery* **72-B**, 197–201.
3. Weinstein, S. L. (1987). Natural history of congenital hip dislocation (CDH) and hip dysplasia. *Clinical Orthopaedics and Related Research* **225**, 62–76.
4. Leck, I. (1977). Correlations of malformation frequency with environmental and genetic attributes in man. In *Handbook of teratology vol. 3: comparative, maternal and epidemiologic aspects* (ed. J. G. Wilson and F. C. Fraser), pp. 243–324. Plenum, New York.

5. Barlow, T. G. (1962). Early diagnosis and treatment of congenital dislocation of the hip. *Journal of Bone and Joint Surgery* **44-B**, 292–301.

6. Hadlow, V. (1988). Neonatal screening for congenital dislocation of the hip: a prospective 21-year survey. *Journal of Bone and Joint Surgery* **70-B**, 740–3.

7. Davies, S. J. M. and Walker, G. (1984). Problems in the early recognition of hip dysplasia. *Journal of Bone and Joint Surgery* **66-B**, 479–84.

8. MacKenzie, I. G. and Wilson, J. G. (1981). Problems encountered in the early diagnosis and management of congenital dislocation of the hip. *Journal of Bone and Joint Surgery* **63-B**, 38–42.

9. Lehmann, E. C. H. and Street, D. G. (1981). Neonatal screening in Vancouver for congenital dislocation of the hip. *Canadian Medical Association Journal* **124**, 1003–8.

10. McIntosh, R., Merritt, K. K., Richards, M. R., Samuels, M. H., and Bellows, M. T. (1954). The incidence of congenital malformations: a study of 5,964 pregnancies. *Pediatrics* **14**, 505–21.

11. Paterson, D. (1982). The early diagnosis and screening of congenital dislocation of the hip. In *Congenital dislocation of the hip* (ed. M. O. Tachdjian), pp. 145–57. Churchill Livingstone, New York.

12. Leck, I., Record, R. G., McKeown, T., and Edwards, J. H. (1968). The incidence of malformations in Birmingham, England, 1950–59. *Teratology* **1**, 263–80.

13. Getz, B. (1955). The hip joint in Lapps and its bearing on the problem of congenital dislocation. *Acta Orthopaedica Scandinavica* **Suppl. 22** (misprinted as 18).

14. Palmén, K. (1961). Preluxation of the hip joint: diagnosis and treatment in the newborn and the diagnosis of congenital dislocation of the hip joint in Sweden during the years 1948–1960. *Acta Paediatrica* **50, Suppl. 129.**

15. Harris, L. E., Lipscomb, P. R., and Hodgson, J. R. (1960). Early diagnosis of congenital dysplasia and congenital dislocation of the hip. *Journal of the American Medical Association* **173**, 229–33.

16. Record, R. G. and Edwards, J. H. (1958). Environmental influences related to the aetiology of congenital dislocation of the hip. *British Journal of Preventive and Social Medicine* **12**, 8–22.

17. Smithells, R. W. (1968). Incidence of congenital abnormalities in Liverpool, 1960–64. *British Journal of Preventive and Social Medicine* **22**, 36–7.

18. Richards I. D. G. and Lowe C. R. (1971). Incidence of congenital defects in South Wales, 1964–66. *British Journal of Preventive and Social Medicine* **25**, 59–64.

19. Salter, R. B. (1968). Etiology, pathogenesis and possible prevention of congenital dislocation of the hip. *Canadian Medical Association Journal* **98**, 933–45.

20. Rabin, D. L., Barnett, C. R., Arnold, W. D., Freiberger, R. H., and Brooks, G. (1965). Untreated congenital hip disease. A study of the epidemiology, natural history, and social aspects of the disease in a Navajo population. *American Journal of Public Health* **55**, no.2, Suppl.

21. Walker, J. M. (1977). Congenital hip disease in a Cree-Ojibwa population: a retrospective study. *Canadian Medical Association Journal* **116**, 501–4.

22. Yamamuro, T. and Ishida, K. (1984). Recent advances in the prevention, early diagnosis, and treatment of congenital dislocation of the hip in Japan. *Clinical Orthopaedics and Related Research* **184**, 34–40.

23. Kutlu, A., Memik, R., Mutu, M., Kutlu, R., and Arslan, A. (1992). Congenital dislocation

of the hip and its relation to swaddling used in Turkey. *Journal of Pediatric Orthopaedics* **12**, 598–602.

24. Poul, J., Bajerova, J., Sommernitz, M., Straka, M., Pokorny, M., and Wong, F. H. Y. (1992). Early diagnosis of congenital dislocation of the hip. *Journal of Bone and Joint Surgery* **74-B**, 695–700.

25. Edelson, J. G., Hirsch, M., Weinberg, H., Attar, D., and Barmeir, E. (1984). Congenital dislocation of the hip and computerised axial tomography. *Journal of Bone and Joint Surgery* **66-B**, 472–8.

26. Tanabe, G., Kotakemori, K., Miyake, Y., and Mohri, M. (1972). Early diagnosis of congenital dislocation of the hip. *Acta Orthopaedica Scandinavica* **43**, 511–22.

27. von Rosen, S. (1962). Diagnosis and treatment of congenital dislocation of the hip in the new-born. *Journal of Bone and Joint Surgery* **44-B**, 284–91.

28. Ortolani, M. (1937). Un segno poco noto e sua importanza per la diagnosi precoce di prelussazione congenita dell'anca. *Pediatria* **45**, 129–36.

29. Cunningham, K. T., Moulton, A., Beningfield, S. A., and Maddock, C. R. (1984). A clicking hip in a newborn baby should never be ignored. *Lancet* **i**, 668–70.

30. Bernard, A.A., O'Hara, J. N., Bazin, S., Humby, B., Jarrett, R., and Dwyer, N. St.J. P. (1987). An improved screening system for the early detection of congenital dislocation of the hip. *Journal of Pediatric Orthopaedics* **7**, 277–82.

31. Dunn, P. M. (1984). Clicking hips should be ignored. *Lancet* **i**, 846.

32. Dunn, P. M., Evans, R. E., Thearle, M. J., Griffiths, H. E. D., and Witherow, P. J. (1985). Congenital dislocation of the hip: early and late diagnosis and management compared. *Archives of Disease in Childhood* **60**, 407–14.

33. Bond, C. D., Hennrikus, W. L., and Della Maggiore, E. D. (1997). Prospective evaluation of newborn soft-tissue hip 'clicks' with ultrasound. *Journal of Pediatric Orthopaedics* **17**, 199–201.

34. Standing Medical Advisory Committee and Standard Nursing Advisory Committee (1986). *Screening for the detection of congenital dislocation of the hip* (revised 1986). Department of Health and Social Security, London.

35. Dezateux, C. and Godward, S. (1996). A national survey of screening for congenital dislocation of the hip. *Archives of Disease in Childhood* **74**, 445–8.

36. Glazener, C. M. A., Ramsay, C. R., Campbell, M. K., Booth, P., Duffty, P., Lloyd, D. J., *et al.* (1999). Neonatal examination and screening trial (NEST): a randomised, controlled, switchback trial of alternative policies for low risk infants. *British Medical Journal* **318**, 627–31.

37. Clarke, N. M. P. (1994). Role of ultrasound in congenital dislocation of the hip. *Archives of Disease in Childhood* **70**, 362–3.

38. Harcke, H. T. (1994). Screening newborns for developmental dysplasia of the hip: the role of sonography. *American Journal of Roentgenology* **162**, 395–7.

39. Bower, C., Stanley, F. J., and Kricker, A. (1987). Congenital dislocation of the hip in Western Australia: a comparison of neonatally and postneonatally diagnosed cases. *Clinical Orthopaedics and Related Research* **224**, 37–44.

40. Almby, B. and Rehnberg, L. (1977). Neonatal hip instability: incidence, diagnosis and treatment at the University Hospital of Uppsala 1960–64 and 1970–74. *Acta Orthopaedica Scandinavica* **48**, 642–9.

41. MacKenzie, I. G. (1972). Congenital dislocation of the hip: the development of a regional service. *Journal of Bone and Joint Surgery* **54-B**, 18–39.
42. Barlow, T. G. (1966). Congenital dislocation of the hip in the newborn. *Proceedings of the Royal Society of Medicine* **59**, 1103–6.
43. Smaill, G. B. (1968). Congenital dislocation of the hip in the newborn. *Journal of Bone and Joint Surgery* **50-B**, 524–36.
44. Goodrich, E. R. (1973). Routine examination of newborn infants for congenital dislocated hips. *Journal of the American Medical Association* **226**, 1119–20.
45. Tredwell, S. J. and Bell, H. M. (1981).Efficacy of neonatal hip examination. *Journal of Pediatric Orthopaedics* **1**, 61–5.
46. Fiddian, N. J. and Gardiner, J. C. (1994). Screening for congenital dislocation of the hip by physiotherapists. *Journal of Bone and Joint Surgery* **76-B**, 458–9.
47. Coleman, S. S. (1956). Diagnosis of congenital dysplasia of the hip in the newborn infant. *Journal of the American Medical Association* **162**, 548–54.
48. Medbø, I. U. (1961). Early diagnosis and treatment of the hip joint dysplasia. *Acta Orthopaedica Scandinavica* **31**, 282–315.
49. Stanisavljevic, S. (1964). *Diagnosis and Treatment of Congenital Hip Pathology in the Newborn*. Baltimore: Williams and Wilkins.
50. Finlay, H. V. L., Maudsley, R. H., and Busfield, P. I. (1967). Dislocatable hip and dislocated hip in the newborn infant. *British Medical Journal* **iv**, 377–81.
51. Hirsch, C. and Scheller, S. (1970). Result of treatment from birth of unstable hips: a 5-year follow-up. *Acta Orthopaedica Scandinavica* **Suppl. 130**, 25–9.
52. James, U. and Sevastikoglou, J. A. (1970). Analysis of a material of congenital dislocation of the hip. *Acta Orthopaedica Scandinavica* **Suppl. 130**, 30–5.
53. Palmén, K. (1970). Preluxation of the hip in the newborn: the diagnostic work in Sweden during the years 1953–1966. *Acta Orthopaedica Scandinavica* **Suppl. 130**, 8–12.
54. von Rosen, S. (1970). Instability of the hip in the newborn. Fifteen years experience in Malmö. *Acta Orthopaedica Scandinavica* **Suppl. 130**, 13–24.
55. Sommer, J. (1971). Atypical click in the newborn. *Acta Orthopaedica Scandinavica* **42**, 353–6.
56. Mitchell, G. P. (1972). Problems in the early diagnosis and management of congenital dislocation of the hip. *Journal of Bone and Joint Surgery* **54-B**, 4–12.
57. Wilkinson, J. A. (1972). A post-natal survey for congenital displacement of the hip. *Journal of Bone and Joint Surgery* **54-B**, 40–9.
58. Williamson, J. (1972). Difficulties of early diagnosis and treatment of congenital dislocation of the hip in Northern Ireland. *Journal of Bone and Joint Surgery* **54-B**, 13–17.
59. Ritter, M. A. (1973). Congenital dislocation of the hip in the newborn. *American Journal of Diseases of Children* **125**, 30–2.
60. Bjerkrein, I. (1974). Congenital dislocation of the hip joint in Norway. *Acta Orthopaedica Scandinavica* **Suppl. 157**.
61. Artz, T. D., Lim W.N., Wilson, P. D. Levine, D.B., and Salvati, E.A. (1975). Neonatal diagnosis, treatment and related factors of congenital dislocation of the hip. *Clinical Orthopaedics and Related Research* **110**, 112–36.
62. Fredensborg, N. (1976). The effect of early diagnosis of congenital dislocation of the hip. *Acta Paediatrica Scandinavica* **65**, 323–8.

63. Fredensborg, N. (1976). The results of early treatment of typical congenital dislocation of the hip in Malmö. *Journal of Bone and Joint Surgery* **58-B**, 272–8.

64. Paterson, D. C. (1976). The early diagnosis and treatment of congenital dislocation of the hip. *Clinical Orthopaedics and Related Research* **119**, 28–38.

65. Cyvin, K. B. (1977). Congenital dislocation of the hip joint: clinical studies with special reference to the pathogenesis. *Acta Paediatrica Scandinavica* **Suppl. 263.**

66. Jones, D. (1977). An assessment of the value of examination of the hip in the newborn. *Journal of Bone and Joint Surgery* **59-B**, 318–22.

67. Noble, T. C., Pullan, C. R., Craft, A. W., and Leonard, M. A. (1978). Difficulties in diagnosing and managing congenital dislocation of the hip. *British Medical Journal* **ii**, 620–3.

68. Heikkilä, E. (1984). Congenital dislocation of the hip in Finland: an epidemiologic analysis of 1035 cases. *Acta Orthopaedica Scandinavica* **55**, 125–9.

69. Palmén, K. (1984). Prevention of congenital dislocation of the hip: the Swedish experience of neonatal treatment of hip joint instability. *Acta Orthopaedica Scandinavica* **55, Suppl. 208.**

70. Rao, S. and Thurston, A. J. (1986). Congenital dislocation of hip in the newborn: a postnatal survey. *New Zealand Medical Journal* **99**, 752.

71. Mubarak, S. J., Leach, J., and Wenger, D. R. (1987). Management of congenital dislocation of the hip in the infant. *Contemporary Orthopedics* **15**, 29–44.

72. Clausen, I. and Nielsen, K. T. (1988). Breech position, delivery route and congenital hip dislocation. *Acta Obstetrica et Gynaecologica Scandinavica* **67**, 595–7.

73. Clarke, N. M. P., Clegg, J., and Al-Chalabi, A. N. (1989). Ultrasound screening of hips at risk for CDH: failure to reduce the incidence of late cases. *Journal of Bone and Joint Surgery* **71-B**, 9–12.

74. Burger, B. J., Burger, J. D., Bos, C. F. A., Obermann, W. R., Rozing, P. M., and Vandenbroucke, J. P. (1990). Neonatal screening and staggered early treatment for congenital dislocation or dysplasia of the hip. *Lancet* **336**, 1549–53.

75. Gardiner, H. M. and Dunn, P. M. (1990). Controlled trial of immediate splinting versus ultrasonographic surveillance in congenitally dislocatable hips. *Lancet* **336**, 1553–6.

76. McNicol, M. F. (1990). Results of a 25-year screening programme for neonatal hip instability. *Journal of Bone and Joint Surgery* **72-B**, 1057–60.

77. Lennox, I. A. C., McLauchlin, J., and Murali, R. (1993). Failures of screening and management of congenital dislocation of the hip. *Journal of Bone and Joint Surgery* **75-B**, 72–5.

78. Godward, S. and Dezateux, C. (1998). Surgery for congenital dislocation of the hip in the UK as a measure of the outcome of screening. *Lancet* **351**, 1149–52.

79. Bialik, V., Fishman, J., Katzir, J., and Zeltzer, M. (1986). Clinical assessment of hip instability in the newborn by an orthopedic surgeon and a pediatrician. *Journal of Pediatric Orthopaedics* **6**, 703–5.

80. Rosendahl, K., Markestad, T., and Lie, R. T. (1996). Developmental dysplasia of the hip. A population-based comparison of ultrasound and clinical findings. *Acta Paediatrica* **85**, 64–9.

81. Baronciani, D., Atti, G., Andiloro, F., Bartesaghi, A., Gagliardi, L., Passamonti, C., *et al.* (1997). Screening for developmental dysplasia of the hip: from theory to practice. *Pediatrics* **99**, E5.

82. El-Shazly, M., Trainor, B., Kernohan, W. G., Turner, I., Haugh, P. E., Johnston, A. F.,

et al. (1994). Reliability of the Barlow and Ortolani tests for neonatal hip instability. *Journal of Medical Screening* **1**, 165–8.

83. Paterson, C. R., Beal, R. J., and Dent, J. A. (1992). Osteogenesis imperfecta: fractures of the femur when testing for congenital dislocation of the hip. *British Medical Journal* **305**, 464–6.

84. Sanfridson, J., Redlund-Johnell, I., and Udén, A. (1991). Why is congenital dislocation of the hip still missed? Analysis of 96,891 infants screened in Malmö 1956–1987. *Acta Orthopaedica Scandinavica* **62**, 87–91.

85. Moore, F. H. (1989). Examining infants' hips—can it do harm? *Journal of Bone and Joint Surgery* **71-B**, 4–8.

86. Cheetham, C. H. and Garrow, D. H. (1987). Screening for the detection of congenital dislocation of the hip. *Archives of Disease in Childhood* **62**, 315.

87. Dunn, P. M. (1987). Screening for the detection of congenital dislocation of the hip. *Archives of Disease in Childhood* **62**, 315–16.

88. Jones, D. A. (1991). Neonatal hip stability and the Barlow test: a study in stillborn babies. *Journal of Bone and Joint Surgery* **73-B**, 216–18.

89. Stone, M. H., Richardson, J. B., and Bennet, G. C. (1987). Another clinical test for dislocation of the hip. *Lancet* **i**, 954–5.

90. Stone, M. H., Clarke, N. M. P., Campbell, M. J., Richardson, J. B., and Johnson, P. A. (1990). Comparison of audible sound transmission with ultrasound in screening for congenital dislocation of the hip. *Lancet* **336**, 421–2.

91. Kernohan, W. G., Beverland, D. E., McCoy, G. F., Hamilton, A., Watson, P., and Mollan, R. (1990). Vibration arthrometry: a preview. *Acta Orthopaedica Scandinavica* **61**, 70–9.

92. Kernohan, W. G., Trainor, B., Nugent, G., Walker, P., Timoney, M., and Mollan, R. (1993). Low-frequency vibration emitted from unstable hip in human neonate. *Clinical Orthopaedics and Related Research* **288**, 214–18.

93. Boeree, N. R. and Clarke, N. M. P. (1994). Ultrasound imaging and secondary screening for congenital dislocation of the hip. *Journal of Bone and Joint Surgery* **76-B**, 525–33.

94. Harcke, H. T., Graf, R., and Clarke, N. M. P. (1993) at Symposium on Infant Hip Sonography, Alfred I du Pont Institute, Wilmington, Delaware; cited by Harcke, H. T., 1994, in 'Screening newborns for developmental dysplasia of the hip: the role of sonography', *American Journal of Roentgenology* **162**, 395–7.

95. Terjesen, T., Bredland, T., and Berg, V. (1989). Ultrasound for hip assessment in the newborn. *Journal of Bone and Joint Surgery* **71-B**, 767–73.

96. Marks D. S., Clegg, J., and Al-Chalabi, A. N. (1994). Routine ultrasound screening for neonatal hip instability. *Journal of Bone and Joint Surgery* **76-B**, 534–8.

97. Rosendahl, K., Markestad, T., and Lie, R. T. (1994). Ultrasound screening for developmental dysplasia of the hip in the neonate: the effect on treatment rate and prevalence of late cases. *Pediatrics* **94**, 47–52.

98. Andersson, J. E. and Funnemark, P.-O. (1995). Neonatal hip instability: screening with anterior-dynamic method. *Journal of Pediatric Orthopaedics* **15**, 322–4.

99. Jones, D. A. and Powell, N. (1990). Ultrasound and neonatal hip screening: a prospective study of 'high risk' babies. *Journal of Bone and Joint Surgery* **72-B**, 457–9.

100. Teanby, D. N. and Paton, R. W. (1997). Ultrasound screening for congenital dislocation of the hip: a limited targeted programme. *Journal of Pediatric Orthopaedics* **17**, 202–4.

101. Graf, R. (1984). Classification of hip joint dysplasias by means of ultrasonography. *Archives of Orthopaedic and Traumatic Surgery* **102**, 248–55.

102. Graf, R. (1987). The ultrasound examination of the hip. In *Congenital dysplasia and dislocation of the hip in children and adults* (ed. D. Tönnis), pp.172–212. Springer, Berlin.

103. Zieger, M., Hilpert, S., and Schulz, R. D. (1986). Ultrasound of the infant hip. Part 1, basic principles. *Pediatric Radiology* **16**, 483–7.

104. Zieger, M. and Schulz, R. D. (1987). Ultrasound of the infant hip. Part 3, clinical application. *Pediatric Radiology* **17**, 226–32.

105. Jones, D. A. (1994). Principles of screening and congenital dislocation of the hip. *Annals of the Royal College of Surgeons of England* **76**, 245–50.

106. Dezateux, C. and Godward, G. (1995). Evaluating the national screening programme for congenital dislocation of the hip. *Journal of Medical Screening* **2**, 200–6.

107. Ralis, Z. and McKibbin, B. (1973). Changes in shape of the human hip joint during its development and their relationship to its stability. *Journal of Bone and Joint Surgery* **55-B**, 780–5.

108. Pous, J. G., Camous, J.-Y., and El Blidi, S. (1992). Cause and prevention of osteochondritis in congenital dislocation of the hip. *Clinical Orthopaedics and Related Research* **281**, 56–62.

109. Brougham, D. I., Broughton, N. S., Cole, W. G., and Menelaus, M. B. (1990). Avascular necrosis following closed reduction of congenital dislocation of the hip. *Journal of Bone and Joint Surgery* **72-B**, 557–62.

110. Bradley, J., Wetherill, M., and Benson, M. K. D. (1987). Splintage for congenital dislocation of the hip: is it safe and reliable? *Journal of Bone and Joint Surgery* **69-B**, 257–63.

111. Bennett, J. T. and MacEwen, G. D. (1989). Congenital dislocation of the hip: recent advances and current problems. *Clinical Orthopaedics and Related Research* **247**, 15–21.

112. Langkamer, V. G., Clarke, N. M. P., and Witherow, P. (1991). Complications of splintage in congenital dislocation of the hip. *Archives of Disease in Childhood* **66**, 1322–5.

113. Hensinger, R. N. (1982). Treatment in early infancy: birth to two months. In *Congenital dislocation of the hip* (ed. M. O. Tachdjian), pp.159–71. Churchill Livingstone, New York.

114. Heikkilä, E. and Ryöppy, S. (1984). Treatment of congenital dislocation of hip after neonatal diagnosis. *Acta Orthopaedica Scandinavica* **55**, 130–4.

115. Heikkilä, E., Ryöppy, S., and Louhimo, I. (1984). Late diagnosis in congenital dislocation of the hip. *Acta Orthopaedica Scandinavica* **55**, 256–60.

116. Krikler, S. J. and Dwyer, N. St.J. P. (1992). Comparison of results of two approaches to hip screening in infants. *Journal of Bone and Joint Surgery* **74-B**, 701–3.

117. Bower, C., Stanley, F. J., Morgan, B., Slattery, H., and Stanton, C. (1989). Screening for congenital dislocation of the hip by child-health nurses in Western Australia. *Medical Journal of Australia*, **150**, 61–5.

118. Sochart, D. H. and Paton, R. W. (1996). Role of ultrasound assessment and harness treatment in the management of developmental dysplasia of the hip. *Journal of the Royal College of Surgeons of England* **78**, 505–8.

119. Fulton, M. J. and Barer, M. L. (1984). Screening for congenital dislocation of the hip: an economic appraisal. *Canadian Medical Association Journal* **130**, 1149–56.

120. Tredwell, S. J. (1990). Economic evaluation of neonatal screening for congenital dislocation of the hip. *Journal of Pediatric Orthopaedics* **10**, 327–30.

121. Rosendahl, K., Markestad, T., Lie, R. T., Sudmann, E., and Geitung, J. T. (1995). Cost-effectiveness of alternative screening strategies for developmental dysplasia of the hip. *Archives of Pediatrics and Adolescent Medicine* **149**, 643–8.
122. Kernohan, G., Trainor, B., Mollan, R., and Normand, C. (1991). Cost of treatment of congenital dislocation of the hip. *International Journal of Health Planning and Management* **6**, 229–33.
123. Jones, D. A., Beynon, D., and Littlepage, B. N. C. (1991). Audit of an official recommendation on screening for congenital dislocation of the hip. *British Medical Journal* **302**, 1435–6.

III

Certain procedures used in screening programmes

17 *Ultrasound as an ancillary investigation in the management of pregnancy*

Amy B. Levine and Charles J. Lockwood

INTRODUCTION

Over the past decade, there has been a dramatic increase in the use of ultrasound in obstetrics. Proponents of universal ultrasound screening in pregnancy cite benefits which include accurate assignment of gestational age, early detection of multiple gestation and placenta praevia, and identification of intrauterine growth retardation. It is assumed that this knowledge would result in decreases in perinatal morbidity and mortality and decreases in inductions for postdate pregnancies. However, before widespread adoption of a policy of routine ultrasound screening in pregnancy can be justified, the efficacy of this technology should be subjected to scientific evaluation. To date, there have been 13 randomized clinical trials (RCT) which have evaluated the efficacy of routine ultrasound screening in pregnancy.

The purpose of this chapter will be to review the role of ultrasound as an ancillary technique in the management of pregnancy. Specifically, it will focus on the following issues:

(1) establishment of gestational age;

(2) diagnosis of placenta praevia;

(3) identification of intrauterine growth retardation;

(4) detection and surveillance of multiple gestation.

Each of these topics will be discussed with references being made to any RCTs which have addressed the efficacy of ultrasound diagnosis in improving pregnancy outcome.

The role of ultrasound in the detection of malformations is considered in Chapter 18.

ESTABLISHMENT OF GESTATIONAL AGE

The accurate determination of gestational age is an essential element of obstetric care. Knowledge of fetal age enables the obstetrician to (1) avoid elective iatrogenic prematurity, (2) institute surveillance/delivery in post term cases, (3) identify growth disorders, and (4) properly interpret results from maternal serum screening for Down's syndrome and neural tube defects.

Traditionally, obstetricians use the length of time since the first day of the patient's last menstrual period ('menstrual age') as a proxy for gestational age. This historic method is of limited accuracy due to the potential for faulty recall, as well as to the erroneous dating that can arise from other sources including variation in the length of the follicular phase, hormonal therapy, and implantation bleeding. Clinical methods of dating a pregnancy, such as assessment of uterine size, auscultation of fetal heart tones, and patients' perception of fetal movements have proved inadequate for gestational age assignment.

The first structure that can be identified and measured ultrasonically is the gestational sac, which is visible as early as 4.5 weeks using transvaginal sonography. Gestational sac size correlates with menstrual age in a linear relationship in the first trimester.[1,2] However, the relationship to menstrual age is not as accurate during the latter part of the first trimester; for example, at 12 weeks menstrual age, 5 per cent of sacs appear from their size to be at least nine days younger or older than this.[3] The reliability of the measurement is decreased in the presence of an irregularly shaped sac, myometrial contractions, and bladder distention. Hence, gestational sac size is of limited value. It is probably best used to assign gestational age only in the absence of a measurable fetal pole.

Measurement of the fetus itself early in pregnancy should provide an accurate assessment of gestational age, as this is a time of rapid curvilinear growth with little biologic variation. Robinson and Fleming[4] performed 334 crown rump length (CRL) measurements between six and 14 weeks and found that menstrual age could be predicted to within 2.7 days in 95 per cent of cases if three independent measurements were utilized. Several other investigators have demonstrated the high degree of accuracy of the first trimester CRL measurements in assigning gestational age. Drumm et al.[5] and Pedersen[6] studied patients with known ovulation data and found a good correlation between age from ovulation and CRL measurements, with 95 per cent confidence limits of 2.6 and 3.2 days respectively. Most recently, Daya[7] created a CRL table in IVF pregnancies (known conception date) and compared these data with pre-existing CRL tables based on menstrual and ovulating dating. He found that menstrual data under-estimated gestational age by a mean of 1.9 days, while ovulation-based data over-estimated gestational age by means varying from 2.4 to 3.9 days depending on the pre-existing table used.

After 12 weeks of gestation, the biparietal diameter (BPD) is the measure most often used in the assignment of gestational age. The relative accuracy of CRL versus BPD measurements in predicting gestational age has been debated in the literature. In small series of patients, Kopta et al.[8] and Selbing[9] found BPD and CRL to be equally predictive in establishing an estimated date of confinement. Drumm,[10] however, found CRL to be a better predictor than BPD measurement, while Campbell et al.[11] found that BPD measurements prior to 18 weeks of gestation were significantly more accurate than CRL predictions.

Some have advocated the use of multiple measurements (BPD, head circumference, abdominal diameter or circumference, and femur length) to provide a composite fetal age assessment. While this method is acceptable when all biometric parameters are similar, it presents a problem when these sonographically derived gestational age estimates differ. In the latter situation, averaging the measurements will produce a less accurate assessment than the best predictor. Furthermore, as described by Wald *et al.*,[12] averaging measurements could result in a decreased detection of fetuses with Down's syndrome, as these fetuses tend to have shortened long bones and averaging would result in an under-estimation of gestational age.

The fundamental issues concerning the use of sonography in predicting gestational age are (1) whether sonographic estimations of fetometry are more accurate than menstrual dates in predicting gestational age and (2) whether accurate knowledge of gestational age results in improved obstetric care. Two large studies have addressed the first issue by comparing the accuracy of certain last menstrual period (LMP) and ultrasound in predicting the date of delivery in women with spontaneous onset of labor. Campbell *et al.*[11] found that of the 1317 patients with optimal menstrual histories and the 876 patients with suspect menstrual histories, 84.7 per cent and 69.7 per cent respectively delivered within two weeks of their due date. Of the 744 pregnancies dated by CRL, 84.6 per cent delivered within two weeks of the due date, not statistically different from those with optimal menstrual histories, but more accurate ($p<0.001$) than those with suspect menstrual histories. In contrast, of the 1678 pregnancies dated by BPD prior to 18 weeks, 89.4 per cent delivered within two weeks of the due date, a statistically significant improvement compared with those dated by both optimal and suspect menstrual histories. In another study,[13] 2289 women had dating by LMP and 2320 women had dating by both LMP and BPD estimates. Of those who went into spontaneous labor at term, 89.4 per cent of those dated by ultrasound delivered within two weeks of the due date compared with 85.5 per cent of those dated by menstrual history, a statistically significant difference. In addition, of the 2320 women with both optimal LMP and BPD estimates of due date, in 20 per cent of cases the two differed by more than one week and the BPD was a better predictor. Hence, there is evidence to support the assertion that sonographic estimates of gestational age are more accurate than menstrual dating.

Whether accurate knowledge of gestational age improves obstetric care is a more difficult question to answer. Several randomized clinical trials have addressed the issue of whether routine ultrasound screening can decrease the rate of postdate inductions. As shown in Table 17.1, four of five studies found that ultrasound screening did result in a significantly decreased rate of postdate inductions. While this did not result in any changes in perinatal outcome, it does decrease the need for unnecessary maternal intervention, which is potentially deleterious if it results in an increased rate of cesarean delivery for failed inductions.

Another aspect of obstetric care for which accurate assignment of gestational age is crucial is in the interpretation of maternal serum marker screening. In the large study of 'triple' marker (i.e. AFP, E, hCG) screening for Down's syndrome, Haddow *et al.*[19] found that the percentage of women who initially screened positive was higher in those dated by last menstrual period compared with those dated by ultrasonography (8.7 versus 3.7 per cent). In another study, Wald *et al.*[12] demonstrated that the routine use of ultrasonography to estimate gestational age could improve the performance of serum screening for Down's syndrome. Specifically, they found that routine use of

Table 17.1   Summary of randomized controlled trials assessing efficacy of routine ultrasound in decreasing rate of postdate inductions

Author	Inductions for post dates (%)		Significance of difference between screened and control groups
	Screened	Control	
Eik-Nes et al. (1984)[14]	1.9%	7.8%	*
Bakketeig et al. (1984)[15]	1.6%	4.0%	*
Waldenstrom et al. (1988)[16]	1.7%	3.7%	*
Ewigman et al. (1990)[17]	7.0%	7.5%	N.S.
LeFevre et al. (1993)[18]	1.6%	2.1%	*

* = statistically significant.
N.S. = not significant.

ultrasound to date pregnancies increased the detection rate from 58 per cent to 67 per cent while maintaining the false-positive rate at 5 per cent.

The issue of accurate assignment of gestational age in diagnosing fetal growth disorders will be discussed in the section on intrauterine growth retardation.

PLACENTA PRAEVIA

Placenta praevia is defined as the implantation of the placenta in the lower uterine segment and overlying the cervix. Depending on the degree of abnormal placentation, there are three types of placenta praevia: complete, partial, and marginal. Placenta praevia is an obstetric condition which predisposes both the mother and fetus to increased morbidity and mortality, as a result of maternal hemorrhage and preterm delivery respectively.

The prevalence of placenta praevia varies with gestational age, ranging from 5 to 10 per cent at mid gestation to less than 1 per cent at term.[20] Clinical risk factors for placenta praevia include history of previous placenta praevia, prior cesarean delivery or other uterine surgery, smoking, multiparity, increased maternal age, and multiple gestations. It is believed that defective vascularization of the endometrium may predispose to trophoblast nidation and/or migration in the relatively unscarred lower uterine segment.

Accurate diagnosis of placenta praevia is important in that profuse hemorrhage can occur if labor is allowed to proceed or as a result of trauma (e.g. by digital vaginal examination). Prior to delivery, the diagnosis of placenta praevia is suspected in cases of vaginal bleeding and confirmed with sonography. The ultrasound diagnosis of placenta praevia is based on noting the relation of the placenta to the internal cervical os. Using transabdominal sonography, placental localization can be accurately ascertained in the majority of cases. However, technical factors may create situations in which either the cervix cannot be adequately visualized or false results are obtained. Visualization of the cervix may be limited by maternal obesity as well as acoustic shadowing from the fetal presenting part residing in the pelvis. False-negative diagnosis may also occur in cases of lateral wall implantation. In contrast, false-positive diagnosis may occur in the following situations: (1) overdistention of the maternal bladder, (2) uterine contraction, (3) hematoma in the lower uterine segment. Reported false-positive and detection rates of transabdominal sonography in diagnosing placenta praevia in selected patients are 2 per cent to 6 per cent and 93 per cent to over 98 per cent respectively [21,22].

Transvaginal sonography has become an increasingly popular means of imaging the pelvis. Placement of the probe in the vagina allows it to be in close proximity to the internal os of the cervix, resulting in enhanced resolution, and avoiding technical problems such as maternal obesity, fetal presenting part, and bladder overdistention. The safety of using the vaginal approach in cases with placenta praevia has been demonstrated.[23] Several authors have evaluated the accuracy of transvaginal sonography in the diagnosis of placenta praevia.[24,25] Table 17.2 summarizes their data.

These studies suggest that transvaginal sonography is superior to transabdominal sonography in the diagnosis of placenta praevia. The role of transperineal sonography in assessing placental localization requires investigation.

To date, there are no studies available which have evaluated the role of routine ultrasound screening in decreasing the potential maternal and fetal morbidities and mortalities associated with placenta praevia.

INTRAUTERINE GROWTH RETARDATION (IUGR)

The antenatal detection of the growth retarded fetus is important for the obstetrician as this condition is associated with increased perinatal morbidity and mortality. Early identification of IUGR enables the initiation of further diagnostic testing, including evaluation of structural anomalies, karyotypic abnormalities, and congenital infections. Moreover, early recognition of affected pregnancies enables these fetuses to be monitored using a variety of antenatal surveillance techniques, so that timely interventions are facilitated.

The diagnosis of IUGR is not standardized, though most commonly a birthweight of less than the tenth, fifth, or third percentile for gestational age has been employed in the literature. One of the concerns in using an absolute birthweight percentile as the diagnostic criterion is that it cannot discriminate between a constitutionally small, but healthy, fetus and the fetus that is growth retarded due to a pathologic process. Additionally, this criterion will be insensitive to the fetus whose weight is greater than the tenth percentile, but who is underweight compared with height.

Prior to the widespread availability of ultrasound, fetal growth was assessed using serial fundal height measurements. However, this technique is inappropriate as either

Table 17.2 Predictive value of transvaginal sonography in diagnosing placenta praevia in selected cases

Author	Ultrasound method	Detection rate (%)	False-positive rate (%)	Odds of being affected given a positive result
Farine et al.[24] (N = 45)	TA	80	66	1:2.9
	TV	100	17	1:0.6
Leerentveld et al.[25] (N = 100)	TV	88	1	1:0.07

TA = transabdominal ultrasound.
TV = transvaginal ultrasound.

a screening or diagnostic tool in the identification of IUGR, since it has a low detection rate (56 per cent in a study in which fetal growth and fundal growth respectively were defined as low when birthweight and fundal height were below the 10 per cent percentile for gestation length[26]). Sonographic measurements of various fetal biometric parameters including biparietal diameter, head circumference, abdominal circumference, and femur length, isolated and in combination, have been proposed as a means of detecting the growth retarded fetus. Studies evaluating biparietal diameter measurements demonstrate a wide range of detection rates (44–90 per cent).[27] This probably reflects the heterogeneous nature of the populations studied, the use of different cut-off points to define low biparietal diameter, and the fact that brain-sparing IUGR accounts for a major proportion of all cases of IUGR. Therefore, cephalometry alone is not a sensitive tool for the detection of IUGR. The fetal abdominal circumference (AC) has also been investigated as a means of detecting the growth retarded fetus. Affected fetuses have a decrease in hepatic glycogen stores and liver mass.[28] Hence, the abdominal circumference, which is largely a measure of the fetal liver, reflects this visceral wasting.[29] In most reports, the detection rate of abdominal circumference measurements in detecting IUGR has been found to exceed 80 per cent, greater than most of the detection rates observed with cephalometry.[30,31]

Since the most common definition of IUGR is birthweight below the tenth percentile for gestational age, investigators have examined the role of sonographic-estimated fetal weight (EFW) in predicting birthweight. Various combinations of sonographic measures of head size, body girth, and length have been incorporated into computer-derived regression equations that estimate weight. Several of these formulae estimate fetal weight to within 15 per cent in 95 per cent of cases.[32] EFW formulas that use BPD, AC, and femur length (FL) have the highest correlation with actual birthweight in IUGR fetuses.[33]

The primary limitation of fetal biometry in the diagnosis of IUGR is that correct interpretation of measurements is dependent upon accurate assignment of gestational age. In clinical practice, however, uncertainty about dating frequently occurs. Thus, a common problem is to distinguish between a growth retarded fetus and a pregnancy with incorrect dating. The use of indices other than menstrual age to assess gestational age has therefore been suggested. One such index is the true transverse cerebellar diameter. Reece *et al.*[34] found that in nineteen cases of IUGR, this index was unaffected by fetal growth retardation, i.e. was appropriate for gestational age . However, Hill *et al.*[35] reported conflicting data in their series of 44 cases of IUGR where in 26 cases (59 per cent) the transcerebellar diameter was two standard deviations below the mean. Hence, further investigation regarding this index is needed. The use of body proportionality indices instead of menstrual age in detecting the fetus with IUGR has also been proposed. Specifically, the head to abdominal circumference ratio[36] and the femur length to abdominal circumference ratio[37] have been evaluated. While these indices may be helpful in identifying cases of asymmetric IUGR, they are unable to detect symmetric IUGR where all biometric parameters are reduced. As an alternative to a single set of measurements obtained at one point in time, serial measurements to assess interval growth have also been proposed as a means of identifying the growth retarded fetus, especially in cases where menstrual age assignment is uncertain. Divon found that an abnormal rate of growth of the abdominal circumference (<10 mm in 14 days) had a detection rate of 85 per cent in identifying infants with birthweights below the 10th centile, and a false-positive rate of 74 per cent.[38] The odds of being affected given a positive result were therefore 1:2.75.

Doppler velocimetry has also been studied in the detection of the growth retarded fetus. Current technology permits interrogation of numerous fetal blood vessels. The most commonly studied vessels in the detection of IUGR have been the uterine and umbilical arteries, though the middle cerebral artery, the descending aorta, and the inferior vena cava have also been evaluated. Investigations of uterine and umbilical artery doppler ultrasonography[39-43] have found this modality to be a poor screening tool in the prediction of IUGR in the general population.

Several randomized clinical trials have evaluated the critical question of whether routine ultrasound screening for the detection of IUGR can decrease perinatal morbidity and mortality. As shown in Table 17.3, these studies revealed no improvement in perinatal outcome following the use of ultrasound.

MULTIPLE GESTATION

Sonography plays a major role in the diagnosis and management of multiple gestations. Early diagnosis enables optimization of antenatal care. This includes serial ultrasound examinations to detect those obstetric complications unique to multiple gestations which require specialized plans of management.

Using transabdominal sonography, separate gestational sacs can be discriminated by six weeks from the last menstrual period, and by seven to eight weeks, multiple

Table 17. 3 Summary of randomized controlled trials assessing efficiency of routine ultrasound in decreasing perinatal morbidity and mortality

Author	Timing of ultrasound	Perinatal deaths/pregnancies		Other findings
		Screened	Control	
Eik-Nes *et al.*[14]	18th and 32nd weeks	3/809	8/819	Decreased maternal hospital admissions; decreased perinatal morbidity
Neilson *et al.*[44]	34–37 weeks	0/433	1/444	No significant difference in obstetric management or perinatal morbidity
Bakketeig *et al.*[15]	19th and 32nd weeks	5/496	3/478	No significant difference in perinatal morbidity
Secher et al.[45]	32nd and 37th weeks	8/1570	7/1741	No significant difference in perinatal morbidity
Larsen *et al.*[46]	28th week and every 3 weeks thereafter	5/484	3/481	Increased rate of induction for IUGR; increased number of hospital admissions; no significant difference in perinatal morbidity
Ewigman et al.,[47] LeFevre *et al.*[18]	15–22 weeks and 31–35 weeks	52/7685	41/7596	Increased rate of induction for IUGR; no significant difference in perinatal morbidity
Total (95% confidence intervals)		73/11 477 = 6.4/1000 (4.9, 7.9)	63/11 559 = 5.5/1000 (4.2, 6.8)	

fetal poles with cardiac activity are detectable. Transvaginal sonography permits diagnosis approximately one to two weeks earlier than the transabdominal technique. With the increased use of early sonography, it has become apparent that the number of twins observed at delivery is significantly less than the number of twins identified by ultrasound during the first trimester. Explanations for this phenomenon of twin disappearance with resultant singleton pregnancy include both inaccurate ultrasound diagnosis (false-positive diagnoses in the presence of hematomas, decidual reaction in a bicornuate uterus, and other ultrasound artifacts), and early pregnancy wastage with resorption of the sac and embryo. The exact prevalence of this vanishing twin phenomenon is unknown. In a prospective study, Landy *et al.*[48] found that 21 per cent of multiple gestations in which both fetuses were viable at the time of first trimester ultrasound examination resulted in the birth of a singleton. The only clinical complication associated with the disappearance of one twin was vaginal bleeding, though the majority of patients were asymptomatic.

Placentation is one of the most important factors related to the increased perinatal morbidity and mortality rate seen in twin pregnancies. Adverse outcomes result from the higher incidence of preterm labor, intrauterine growth retardation, and fetal death seen in monochorionic compared wtih dichorionic twin gestations. Monoamniotic twinning is associated with the highest perinatal morbidity and mortality rates due to cord entanglement. The sonographic evaluation of placentation should be approached in a systematic manner. If separate placentas are identified or if the fetuses are of different genders, the pregnancy must be dichorionic. When a single placenta is present and the twins are the same sex, the characteristics of the dividing membrane must be evaluated. In dichorionic placentations, the membrane is thick and either three or four layers can usually be seen.[49] A thin membrane is most likely consistent with a monochorionic placentation. The absence of a dividing membrane signifies the rare monoamniotic placentation. The presence of a single amniotic cavity can be confirmed by demonstrating entanglement of the two umbilical cords[50,51] or by injection of bubbles into the sac.[52]

The overall frequency of congenital anomalies is increased in monozygotic twins,[53] perhaps reflective of the teratogenic insult which caused the twinning, or due to a malformed fetus being less likely to miscarry when accompanied by a healthy twin. The latter phenomenon is illustrated by acardiac fetuses (only seen in pregnancies in which there is another fetus to maintain the circulation). Anomalies in twins are often discordant, that is, affecting only one twin. Detailed sonographic evaluation of all twins provides the opportunity to diagnose many congenital anomalies. In addition to fetal anomalies, placental abnormalities such as vasa praevia and velamentous cord insertion occur more often in multiple gestations. These conditions are detectable with ultrasound examination, especially now that color flow doppler sonography is available.[54]

Serial ultrasound examinations are the only means of assessing individual fetal growth in a multiple gestation. The most accurate means of assessing growth in each individual fetus and comparing growth between fetuses is to obtain an estimated fetal weight based on multiple parameters which include the abdominal circumference.[55,56] Fetal growth in a multiple gestation can be discordant between fetuses. This discordance can result from individual biological variation, unfavorable implantation site, discordance for a chromosomal abnormality, or twin to twin transfusion syndrome. Discordance may arise in situations where neither, one, or both twins are growth retarded. The most useful definition of growth discordance is a birthweight discrepancy of >25 per cent when the difference in birthweights is expressed as a percentage of the birthweight of the larger twin. This definition was originally derived from the knowledge that when the birthweight difference was greater than 25 per cent, the smaller twin was at increased risk of impaired growth and intellectual development compared with the larger twin.[57] More recent studies have confirmed that the presence of growth discordance places the smaller twin at significantly increased risk of low Apgar scores, intrauterine growth retardation, prolonged hospitalization, and perinatal death.[58,59] Knowledge that discordance is present enables the obstetrician to increase fetal surveillance and choose the optimal time for delivery.

Perhaps the most extreme complication observed in monochorionic twins is the twin to twin transfusion syndrome. This arises when the circulation of one twin is in contact with that of the co-twin through a shared placental cotyledon. The extent, direction, and size of the anastomoses determine the severity of the syndrome. Typically, the donor is growth retarded and develops oligohydramnios and anemia, while the recipient develops polyhydramnios and polycythemia. The diagnosis should be suspected when the following sonographic criteria are present:

(1) twin gestation with a single placenta and a thin dividing membrane;

(2) discordant fetal growth;

(3) discordant amniotic fluid volumes, including the 'stuck twin' appearance secondary to severe oligohydramnios in the smaller twin's sac.

In severe cases, hydrops may develop in either or both twins and one or both fetuses may expire. Active intervention appears to improve outcome compared with expectant management.[60] Treatments for this syndrome have included serial amniocenteses,[61] laser ablation of vascular anastomoses,[62] umbilical cord ligation of one twin,[63] and fetal reduction.[64]

The increased use of ovulation-inducing agents and assisted reproductive techniques has resulted in an increased incidence of multiple gestations with three or more fetuses. These can be diagnosed on ultrasound in the first trimester. It is known that as the number of fetuses in a pregnancy increases, the gestational age at delivery and the birthweight will decrease. In an effort to decrease the high morbidity and mortality resulting from premature delivery in these higher-order multiple gestations, first trimester fetal reduction using ultrasound guidance has been employed. While not an optimal solution to the problems associated with higher-order multiple gestations, it appears to be a relatively safe option for reducing the consequences associated with severe prematurity of multiple fetuses.[65]

Routine ultrasound screening during pregnancy would result in the early diagnosis of approximately 98 per cent of all multiple gestations.[66] Such detection has been presumed to be important in reducing the perinatal morbidity and mortality associated with multiple fetuses.[66,67] A review of the randomized controlled trials assessing the efficacy of routine ultrasound in pregnancy reveals that five studies have evaluated twins as a separate subset of the total population. Table 17.4 summarizes the data from these studies.

Table 17.4   Summary of randomized controlled trials assessing efficacy of routine ultrasound in decreasing perinatal morbidity and mortality associated with twins

Author	Number of pregnancies	Outcome(s) assessed	Study	Control	Significance
Eik-Nes *et al.*[14]	Not stated	Mean birthweight (g)	2600	2180	N.S.
Bakketeig *et al.*[15]	6 study, 4 control	Mean birthweight (g)	2268	1662	N.S.
		Mean gestational age at delivery (days)	252	227	N.S.
		Perinatal deaths	0	2	N.S.
Waldenström *et al.*[16]	24 study, 20 control	Mean birthweight (g)	2486	2539	N.S.
		Mean gestational age at delivery (days)	258	262	N.S.
		Perinatal deaths	4	0	N.S.
Saari-Kemppainen *et al.*[68]	36 study, 38 control	Perinatal deaths	2	5	N.S.
Ewigman *et al.*[47]	68 study, 61 control	Mean birthweight (g)	2461	2411	N.S.
		Perinatal deaths	4	4	N.S.

N.S. = not significant.

None of the studies was able to demonstrate a statistically significant improvement in the outcome of twins when routine ultrasound screening had been employed. However, it should be noted that in two of the four studies evaluating birthweight, mean birthweight was higher by more than 400 g in the screened group. One limitation of all of these studies is the small number of multiple gestations available for analysis. For example, in the four studies in which perinatal deaths were reported there were totals of only 170 pregnancies and 10 perinatal deaths in the screened groups, and 161 pregnancies and 11 deaths in the controls. Further investigation with larger sample size is necessary before one can assess the utility of routine ultrasound screening in improving the outcomes of multiple gestations.

CONCLUSIONS

Ultrasound is widely thought to play an important role in the management of pregnancies complicated by uncertain dates, vaginal bleeding, multiple gestations, and growth disorders. This conclusion is not supported by the randomized controlled trials of routine ultrasound screening in pregnancy, which have failed to demonstrate a significant improvement in perinatal outcomes. However the measures of outcome used (e.g. perinatal mortality) are non-specific, and would not be expected to show a significant difference in trials of the sizes described. Our conclusion therefore is that there is no firm evidence of benefit with respect to these outcomes, but there is insufficient evidence available to exclude a medically useful effect.

REFERENCES

1. Nyberg D A, Mack L A, Laing F C, and Patten R M (1987). Distinguishing normal from abnormal gestational sac growth in early pregnancy. *J Ultrasound Med*, **6**, 23–7.

2. Hellman L M, Kobayashi M, Fillisti L, and Lavenhar M (1969). Growth and development of the human fetus prior to the 20th week of gestation. *Am J Obstet Gynecol*, **103**, 789–800.

3. Robinson H P (1975). Gestational sac volumes as determined by sonar in the first trimester of pregnancy. *Br J Obstet Gynecol*, **82**, 100–7.

4. Robinson H P and Fleming J E E (1975). A critical evaluation of sonar crown-rump length measurements. *Br J Obstet Gynecol*, **82**, 702–10.

5. Drumm J E, Coinch J, and MacKenzie S (1976). The ultrasonic measurement of fetal crown-rump length as a means of assessing gestational age. *Br J Obstet Gynecol*, **83**, 417–21.

6. Pedersen J F (1982). Fetal crown-rump length measurement by ultrasound in normal pregnancy. *Br J Obstet Gynecol*, **89**, 926–30.

7. Daya S (1993). Accuracy of gestational age estimation by means of fetal crown-rump length measurement. *Am J Obstet Gynecol*, **168**, 903–8.

8. Kopta M M, May R R, and Crane J P (1983). A comparison of the reliability of the estimated date of confinement predicted by crown-rump length and biparietal diameter. *Am J Obstet Gynecol*, **145**, 562–5.

9. Selbing A (1982). Gestational age and ultrasonic measurement of gestational sac, crown-rump length, and biparietal diameter during first 15 weeks of pregnancy. *Acta Obstet Gynecol Scand*, **61**, 233–5.

10. Drumm J E (1977). The prediction of delivery date by ultrasonic measurement of fetal crown rump length. *Br J Obstet Gynecol*, **84**, 1–5.

11. Campbell S, Warsof S L, Little D, and Cooper D J (1985). Routine ultrasound screening for the prediction of gestational age. *Obstet Gynecol*, **65**, 613–19.

12. Wald N J, Cuckle H S, Densem J W, Kennard A, and Smith D (1992). Maternal serum screening for Down's syndrome: the effect of routine ultrasound scan determination of gestational age and adjustment for maternal weight. *Br J Obstet Gynecol*, **99**, 144–9.

13. Waldenström U, Axelsson O, and Nilsson S A (1990). Comparison of the ability of a sonographically measured biparietal diameter and the last menstrual period to predict the spontaneous onset of labor. *Obstet Gynecol*, **76**, 336–8.

14. Eik-Nes S H, Okland O, Aure J C, and Ulstein M (1984). Ultrasound screening in pregnancy: a randomized controlled trial. *Lancet*, **1**, 1347.

15. Bakketeig L S, Jacobsen G, Brodtkorb C J, Eriksen B C, Eik-Nes S H, Ulstein M K, *et al.* (1984). Randomized controlled trial of ultrasonographic screening in pregnancy. *Lancet*, **2**, 207–10.

16. Waldenström U, Nilsson S, Fall O, Axelsson O, Eklund G, Lindeberg S, *et al.* (1988). Effects of routine one-stage ultrasound screening in pregnancy: a randomized controlled trial. *Lancet*, **2**, 585–8.

17. Ewigman B, LeFevre M, and Hesser J A (1990). Randomised trial of routine prenatal ultrasound. *Obstet Gynecol*, **76**, 189–194.

18. LeFevre M D, Bain R P, Ewingman B G, Frigoletto F D, Crane J P, and McNellis D A (1993). Randomized trial of prenatal utrasonographic screening: impact on maternal management and outcome. *Am J Obstet Gynecol*, **169**, 483–9.

19. Haddow J E, Palomaki G E, Knight G J, Williams J, Pulkkinen A, Canick J A, *et al.* (1992). Prenatal screening for Down's syndrome with use of maternal serum markers *New Engl J Med*, **327**, 588–93.
20. Rizos N, Doran T A, Miskin M, Benzie R J, and Ford J A (1979). Natural history of placenta praevia ascertained by diagnostic ultrasound. *Am J Obstet Gynecol*, **133**, 287–91.
21. Laing F C (1981). Placenta previa: Avoiding false negative diagnoses. *J Clin Ultrasound*, **9**, 109–13.
22. Cotton D B, Read J A, Paul R H, and Quilligan E J (1980). The conservative aggressive management of placenta previa. *Am J Obstet Gynecol*, **137**, 687–95.
23. Farine D, Peisner D B, and Timor Trisch I E (1990). Placenta previa-Is the traditional diagnostic approach satisfactory? *JCU*, **18**, 328–30.
24. Farine D, Fox H E, Jakobson S, and Timor Trisch I E (1989). Is it really placenta previa? *Eur J Obstet Gynecol*, **31**, 103–108.
25. Leerentveld R A, Gilberts E, Arnold M, and Waldimiroff, J W (1990). Accuracy and safety of transvaginal sonographic placental localization. *Obstet Gynecol*, **76**, 759–62.
26. Rosenberg K, Grant J M, and Aitchison T (1982). Measurement of fundal height as a screening test for fetal growth retardation. *Br J Obstet Gynecol*, **89**, 447–50.
27. Guidetti D A and Divon M Y (1991). Sonographic detection of the IUGR fetus In *Abnormal Fetal Growth* (ed. M Y Divon), pp. 129–146. Elsevier Science, Amsterdam.
28. Evans M I, Mukherjee A B, and Schulman J D (1983). Animal models of intrauterine growth retardation. *Obstet Gynecol Surv*, **38**, 183–92.
29. Lockwood C J and Weiner S (1986). Assessment of fetal growth. *Clin. Perinatol*, **13**, 3–35.
30. Kurjak A, Kirkinen P, and Latin V (1980). Biometric and dynamic ultrasound assessment of small for dates infants: report of 260 cases. *Obstet Gynecol*, **56**, 281–4.
31. Geirsson R T and Persson P (1984). Diagnosis of intrauterine growth retardation using ultrasound. *Clin Obstet Gynecol*, **11**, 457–80.
32. Hadlock F P, Harrist R B, Sharman R S, Deter R L, and Park S K (1985). Estimation of fetal weight with the use of head, body, and femur measurements-a prospective study. *Am J Obstet Gynecol*, **151**, 333–7.
33. Guidetti D, Divon M Y, Braverman J J, Langer O, and Merkatz I R (1990). Sonographic estimates of fetal weight in the intrauterine growth retarded population. *Am J Perinatol*, **7**, 5–7.
34. Reece E A, Goldstein I, Pilu G, and Hobbins J C (1987). Fetal cerebellar growth unaffected by intrauterine growth retardation: a new parameter for prenatal diagnosis. *Am J Obstet Gynecol*, **157**, 632–8.
35. Hill L M, Guzick D, Rivello D, Hixson J, and Peterson C (1990). The transverse cerebellar diameter cannot be used to assess gestational age in the small for gestational age fetus. *Obstet Gynecol*, **75**, 329–33.
36. Crane J P and Kopta M M (1979). Prediction of intrauterine growth retardation via ultrasonically measured head/abdominal circumference ratios. *Obstet Gynecol*, **54**, 597–601.
37. Hadlock F P, Deter R L, Harrit R B, Roecker E, and Park S K (1983). A date-independent predictor of intrauterine growth retardation: femur length: abdominal circumference ratio. *Am J Roentgenol*, **141**, 979–84.
38. Divon M Y, Chamberlain P F, Sipos L, Manning F A, and Platt L D (1986). Identification of the small for gestational age fetus with the use of gestational age-independent indices of fetal growth. *Am J Obstet Gynecol*, **115**, 1197–1201.

39. North R A, Ferrier C, Long D, Townend K, and Kincaid-Smith P (1994). Uterine artery doppler flow velocity waveforms in the second trimester for the prediction of preeclampsia and fetal growth retardation. *Obstet Gynecol*, **83**, 378–86.

40. Todros T, Ferrazzi E, Arduini D, Bastonero S, Bezzeccheri V, and Biolcati M (1995). Performance of doppler ultrasonography as a screening test in low risk pregnancies: Results of a multicentric study. *J Ultrasound Med*, **14**, 343–8.

41. Atkinson M W, Maher J E, Owen J, Hauth J, Goldenberg R L, and Copper R L (1994). The predictive value of umbilical artery doppler studies for preeclampsia or fetal growth retardation in a preeclampsia prevention trial. *Obstet Gynecol*, **83**, 609–12.

42. Bruinse H W, Sijmons E A, and Reawer P (1989). Clinical value of screening for fetal growth retardation by doppler ultrasound. *J Ultrasound Med*, **8**, 207–9.

43. Beattie R B and Dornan J C (1989). Antenatal screening of intrauterine growth retardation with umbilical artery doppler ultrasonography. *Br Med J*, **298**, 631–5.

44. Neilson J, Munjanja S P, and Whitfield C R (1984). Screening for small for dates fetuses: a controlled trial. *Br Med J*, **289**, 1179–82.

45. Secher N J, Hansen P K, Lenstrup C, and Eriksen P S (1986). Controlled trial of ultrasound screening for light for gestational age infants in late pregnancy. *Eur J Obstet Gynecol Reprod Biol*, **23**, 307–13.

46. Larsen T, Larsen J F, Petersen S, and Greisen G (1992). Detection of small-for-gestational-age fetuses by ultrasound screening in a high risk population: a randomized controlled study. *Br J Obstet Gynecol*, **99**, 467–74.

47. Ewigman B G, Crane J P, Frigoletto F D, LeFevre M L, Bain R P, and McNellis D (1993). Effect of prenatal ultrasound screening on perinatal outcome. *New Engl J Med*, **329**, 821–7.

48. Landy H J, Weiner S, Corson S L, Batzer F R, and Bolognese R J (1986). The 'Vanishing twin': Ultrasonographic assessment of fetal disappearance in the first trimester. *Am J Obstet Gynecol*, **155**, 14–19.

49. D'Alton M E and Mercer B M (1990). Antepartum management of twin gestation: ultrasound. *Clin Obstet Gynecol*, **33**, 42–51.

50. Nyberg D A, Filly R A, Golbus M S, and Stephens J D (1984). Entangled umbilical cords: A sign of monoamniotic twins. *J Ultrasound Med*, **3**, 29–32.

51. Aisenbrey G A, Catanzarite U A, Hurley T J, Spiegel J H, Schrimmer D B, and Mendoza A (1995). Monoamniotic and pseudoamniotic twins: Sonographic diagnosis, detection of cord entanglement and obstetric management. *Obstet Gynecol*, **8**, 218–22.

52. Tabsh K (1990). Genetic amniocentesis in multiple gestation: a new technique to diagnose monoamniotic twins. *Obstet Gynecol*, **75**, 296–8.

53. Schinzel A, Smith D W, and Miller J R (1979). Monozygotic twinning and structural defects. *J Pediatr*, **95**, 921–30.

54. Pretorius D H, Chau C, Poeltler D M, Mendoza A, Catanzarite V A, and Hollenbach K A (1996). Placental cord insertion visualization with prenatal ultrasonography. *J Ultrasound Med*, **15**, 585–93.

55. Chitkara U, Berkowitz G S, Levine R, Riden D J, Fagerstrom R M, Chervenak F A, *et al.* (1985). Twin pregnancy: routine use of ultrasound examinations in the prenatal diagnosis of intrauterine growth retardation and discordant growth. *Am J Perinatol*, **2**, 49–54.

56. Storlazzi E, Vintzileos A M, Campbell W A, Nochimson D J, and Weinbaum P J (1987). Ultrasound diagnosis of discordant fetal growth in twin gestations. *Obstet Gynecol*, **69**, 363–7.

57. Babson S G and Phillips D S (1973). Growth and development of twins dissimilar in size at birth. *New Engl J Med*, **289**, 937–40.
58. Erkkola R, Ala-Mello S, Piiroinen O, Kero P, and Sillanpaa M (1985). Growth discordancy in twin pregnancies: A risk factor not detected by measurements of biparietal diameter. *Obstet Gynecol*, **66**, 203–6.
59. Blickstein I, Shoham-Schwartz Z, Lancet M, and Borenstein R (1987). Characterization of the growth discordant twin. *Obstet Gynecol*, **70**, 11–15.
60. Reisner D P, Mahony B S, Petty C N, Nyberg D A, Porter T F, Zingheim R W, *et al.* (1993). Stuck twin syndrome: outcome in 37 consecutive cases. *Am J Obstet Gynecol*, **169**, 991–5.
61. Elliott J P, Urig M A, and Clewell W H (1991). Aggressive therapeutic amniocentesis for treatment of twin–twin transfusion syndrome. *Obstet Gynecol*, **77**, 537–40.
62. Ville Y, Hyett J, Hecher K, and Nicolaides K (1995). Preliminary experience with endoscopic laser surgery for severe twin-twin transfusion syndrome. *New Engl J Med*, **332**, 224–7.
63. Quintero R A, Reich H, Puder K S, Bardicef M, Evans M, Cotton D B, and Romero R (1994). Brief report: umbilical cord ligation of an acardiac twin by fetoscopy at 19 weeks of gestation. *New Engl J Med*, **330**, 469–71.
64. Bebbington M W, Wilson R D, Machan L, and Wittmann B K (1995). Selective feticide in twin transfusion syndrome using ultrasound-guided insertion of thrombogenic coils. *Fetal Diagn Ther*, **10**, 32–6.
65. Berkowitz R L, Lynch L, Stone J, and Alvarez M (1996). The current status of multifetal pregnancy reduction. *Am J Obstet Gynecol*, **174**, 1265–72.
66. Persson P H and Kullander S (1983). Longterm experience of general ultrasound screening in pregnancy. *Am J Obstet Gynecol*, **146**, 942–7.
67. Persson P H, Grennert L, Gennser G, and Kullander S (1979). On improved outcome of twin pregnancies. *Acta Obstet Gynecol Scand*, **58**, 3–7.
68. Saari-Kemppainen A, Karjalainen O, Ylostalo P, and Heinonen O P (1990). Ultrasound screening and perinatal mortality: controlled trial of systematic one-stage screening in pregnancy. *Lancet*, **336**, 387–91.

18 *Ultrasound scanning for congenital abnormalities*

Nicholas Wald, Anne Kennard, Alan Donnenfeld, and Ian Leck

INTRODUCTION

Routine antenatal ultrasound anomaly scanning is now widely practised. A 1996 United Kingdom survey[1] reported that 82 per cent of maternity units now offer such a scan, usually at about 18 weeks of pregnancy. There is a firm belief by many that such scanning is useful while others remain unconvinced. The Radius study[2] concluded that routine ultrasound did not improve perinatal outcome compared with ultrasound performed on a clinically selected population. A review of published studies by Romero,[3] however, concluded that routine ultrasound scanning is worthwhile, if the standard of scanning is sufficiently high. Scanning can identify abnormalities in certain pregnancies, but it can also cause harm by prompting unnecessary medical intervention. There is a common assumption that the detection of an abnormality *per se* is worthwhile. This chapter assesses the value of ultrasound scanning both as a diagnostic and a screening test for fetal abnormalities, considering published evidence of ultrasound scanning performance, natural history, and birth prevalence of the disorders. On the basis of this evidence we then draw up a list of abnormalities for which ultrasound scanning and subsequent action can lead to a clear benefit.

Problems in assessing screening performance

There are practical problems in assessing ultrasound scanning for fetal abnormalities.

1. As currently offered, it is a non-specific investigation in which the ultrasound examiner looks for a wide range of structural abnormalities and other findings that might be markers of a medical disorder. Over 100 different abnormalities can be identified using ultrasound, which explains both the attraction of the procedure and the problems in its evaluation. Few tests in medicine examine everything that can be seen or measured. For example, a blood sample is not tested for everything that can be measured, even though the cost of extra tests may be small. It is recognized that, when performed without a prior indication, abnormal values can occur more often by chance than because of genuine disease, and many diseases identified have no effective treatment.

2. Many studies publish estimates of detection rates without giving the corresponding false-positive rates, or present only an odds of being affected given a positive result (OAPR). This arises because in clinical practice a population is scanned but only women with positive ultrasound findings are followed up. This yields the OAPR which, by itself, is insufficient to evaluate the test.

3. Most of the important disorders are rare, so the numbers in any particular study are small and estimates of detection rates are correspondingly unreliable.

4. A positive result is often followed by medical intervention such as termination of pregnancy. Including such cases in estimates of detection rates, even though many affected pregnancies would end naturally in a miscarriage, makes these estimates too high.

Need to define purpose

The approach to ultrasound screening for fetal abnormalities that we advocate is 'Specified Abnormality Scanning', i.e. not scanning for all abnormalities but only for those for which antenatal screening confers benefits which outweigh harm and cost. There are four groups of congenital abnormalities in which there is benefit from antenatal ultrasound scanning. Our definitions of these groups, in terms of the clinical action that may be taken, (based partly on those specified by the working party of the Royal College of Obstetricians[1]) are:

A. Abnormalities associated with serious disability for which termination of pregnancy is justifiable*.

B. Fatal abnormalities for which a termination of pregnancy avoids continuing with an unproductive pregnancy.

C. Abnormalities for which *in utero* treatment reduces morbidity.

D. Abnormalities for which immediate post-natal treatment reduces morbidity.

The other abnormalities which are sometimes detected by scanning can be classified under two headings:

P. Those for which there is a *possible* benefit in antenatal identification but no clear evidence whether this is so.

O. Those for which there is *no* benefit in antenatal identification.

We refer to the six groups as 'categories of benefit'.

Screening or diagnosis

Abnormalities can be identified directly or indirectly from an ultrasound scan. In the first case, scanning detects structural defects which directly identify the disorder. Ultrasound is then a *diagnostic test*, because the examination makes the diagnosis. In the second case, ultrasound identifies defects or markers that indicate an increased risk of a disorder but not the abnormality requiring action; used in this way, ultrasound is a *screening test*. For example, using ultrasound to identify the cra-

---

* We recognize the difficulty in defining 'justifiable' in this context, but take it to cover abnormalities for which there is a consensus that termination is a justified action.

nial signs associated with spina bifida is screening; confirming that there is spina bifida present is diagnosis. Using ultrasound to identify markers of Down's syndrome is also screening.

This chapter is divided into two parts: one on ultrasound *diagnosis* and the other on ultrasound *screening*. Certain defects such as cystic hygroma are sometimes classified as a disorder and sometimes as a marker for a disorder. Where there is doubt, we classify such defects as markers and include them under ultrasound screening.

ULTRASOUND AS A DIAGNOSTIC TEST

We have limited our review of the published literature on ultrasound as a diagnostic test to cohort studies of routine ultrasound anomaly scanning around 16–24 weeks of pregnancy, based on data collected in or after 1986. Table 18.1 summarizes the 19 studies included.[4–22] Our review covers over 180 000 scanned pregnancies, and about 2400 reported abnormalities, a rate of about 1.3 per cent. Most studies reported on all major fetal abnormalities detectable on ultrasound, although four reported on heart defects only. Individual fetal abnormalities are only considered if they were reported in at least three studies.

Ultrasound detection of fetal disorders

Table 18.2 gives, for each disorder, summary estimates of the ultrasound detection rate together with the approximate birth prevalence[23,24] and the category of benefit

Table 18.1   Cohort studies of routine ultrasound scanning (excluding data obtained before 1986)

Study	Gestation	Total pregnancies scanned	Fetal abnormalities scanned	Period studied
Achiron et al. 1992[4]	18–24 weeks	5347	23†	1988–90
Anderson et al. 1995[5]	16–20 weeks	7880	144	1991–3
Buskens et al. 1996[6]	16–24 weeks	5319	80‡	1991–3
Chitty et al. 1991[7]	18–20 weeks	8342	125	1988–9
Constantine and McCormack 1991[8]	16–18 weeks	4984	49	1988–9
Crane et al. 1994[9]	15–23 weeks	7327	118	1987–91
Eurenius et al. 1999[10]	15–22 weeks	8228	145	1990–2
Gonçalves et al. 1994[11]*	> 16 weeks	574	287	1987–91
Jorgensen et al. 1999[12]	17–19 weeks	27 844	73#	1989–91
Levi et al. 1995[13]	80% <20 weeks	9392	235	1990–2
Luck 1992[14]	19 weeks	8523	166	1988–91
Ott 1995[15]	Not reported	1136	14†	1991–3
Papp et al. 1995[16]	18–20 weeks	51 675	496	1988–90
Roberts et al. 1993[17]	16–24 weeks	11 360**	114	1988–9
Rustico et al. 1990[18]	mean 23 weeks	1841	18†	1986–7
Shirley et al. 1992[19]	19–22 weeks	6183	84	1989–90
Stefos et al. 1999[20]	18–22 weeks	7236	162	1990–6
Van Dorsten et al. 1998[21]	15–22 weeks	1611	21	1993–6
Vergani et al. 1992[22]	18–20 weeks	5336	32†	1987–9

* Nested case-control study in a cohort.
** Estimate based on cohort of 12 909, adjusted by 88 per cent rate of scanning in abnormality group (12 909 × 0.88=11 360).
† Only heart defects reported.
‡ Abnormalities reported as either 'heart defects' or 'other defects'.
# Only neural tube defects, abdominal wall defects and Down's syndrome reported.

Table 18.2 Category of benefit, birth prevalence and summary estimates of reported detection rate for individual fetal abnormalities

Main disorder	Category of benefit‡	Approximate birth prevalence (per 1000)*	Number reported	Number detected	Detection rate (%) (range)	Additional details of abnormalities included in estimates	Number of studies on which detection rates are based
Central nervous system:							
Spina bifida/encephalocele	A	1.0	173	146	84 (65–100)		14[5,7–14,16,17,19–21]
Holoprosencephaly	A	0.1	13	12	92 (67–100)		4[7,14,16,17]
Microcephaly	A	1.0	26	9	35 (0–100)	Occipitofrontal circumference >2.5 or 3 sds below mean	6[10,11,13,16,17,21]
Dandy-Walker syndrome	A	≤0.1	12	10	83 (0–100)		6[7,9,11,16,20,21]
Anencephaly	B	0.5	134	133	99 (80–100)		13[5,7–14,16,17,19,20]
Iniencephaly	B	≤0.1	7	7	100 (all 100)		3[7,11,16]
Hydrocephaly	P^M	1.0	112	102	91 (40–100)	Excludes cases also affected by spina bifida	10[7,8,10,11,13,16,17,19–21]
Agenesis of corpus callosum	P^M	0.1	10	5	50 (0–75)		4[5,9,11,16]
Respiratory tract:							
Diaphragmatic hernia	P^M	0.5	49	30	61 (0–100)		14[5,7–14,16,17,19–21]
Congenital cystic adenomatoid malformation	O	0.1	23	22	96 (0–100)		8[5,7,11,14,16,17,19,20]
Digestive tract:							
Cleft lip/palate	P^M	1.5	49	13	27 (13–75)		7[5,7,9,11,17,19,20]
Exomphalos	P^M	0.5	38	33	87 (73–100)		10[5,7,9,11,14,16,17,19–21]
Gastroschisis	P	0.1	30	27	90 (0–100)		8[5,7,11,14,16,17,19,20]
Intestinal atresia	P^M	0.2	61	38	62 (0–100)		12[5,7–11,13,14,16,17,19,20]
Oesophageal atresia/tracheo-oesophageal fistula	P	0.2	27	5	19 (0–100)	Excludes rectal and anal atresia	9[5,7,9–11,14,16,17,21]
Genito-urinary tract:							
Bilateral renal agenesis	B	0.1	38	33	87 (0–100)		9[5,7,9,11,13,14,16,17,20]
Hydronephrosis/multicystic dysplastic kidneys/obstructive uropathy	P^M	1.0	246	195	79 (21–100)		12[5,7,9–11,13,14,16,17,19–21]

Cardiac:

	‡						
Severe	A/B/D	2.0	149	69	46 (0–100)	Hypoplastic left/right heart, Ebstein's anomaly, single atrium, truncus arteriosus, total anomalous pulmonary drainage, ectopia cordis, complex heart disease, atrio-ventricular defect, transposition of great vessels	17[4–11,13–15,17–22]
Moderate	P[M]	2.0	89	18	20 (0–78)	Fallot's tetralogy, coarctation of aorta, pulmonary stenosis, cardiomyopathy, cardiohypertrophy, double outlet ventricle	16[4–11,13–15,17–20,22]
Mild	P[M]	3.5	211	33	16 (0–100)	Ventricular septal defect, atrial septal defect, aortic stenosis	17[4–11,13–15,17–22]
Combined	A/B/D/P[M]	7.5	449	120	27 (0–64)	See severe/moderate/mild above	17[4–11,13–15,17–22]
Hypoplastic left heart	A/B	0.5	31	16	52 (0–100)		11[4–8,10,11,14,17,20,22]
Atrio-ventricular septal defect	A/B	0.5	25	16	64 (0–100)		10[4–7,13,15,17,18,20,22]
Double outlet ventricle	P[M]	0.1	5	2	40 (0–100)		5[4,6,11,14,19]
Ventricular septal defect	P[M]	3.5	173	28	16 (0–67)		16[4–11,13–15,17,18,20–22]
Skeletal:							
Osteogenesis imperfecta	B/O	≤0.1	6	6	100 (all 100)		4[5,11,16,17]
Thanatophoric dysplasia	B	≤0.1	8	8	100 (all 100)		3[7,13,16]
Achondrogenesis	B	≤0.1	4	4	100 (all 100)		3[11,14,19]
Limb reduction defect	P[M]	0.5	28	12	43 (20–100)		4[9,11,16,17]
Other:							
Meckel-Gruber syndrome	B	≤0.1	7	7	100 (all 100)	Encephalocele, polydactyly and renal cystic dysplasia	4[7,11,16,20]
Sacrococcygeal tumour	P	≤0.1	5	3	60 (0–100)		3[7,16,19]

* Birth prevalences rounded and based on Heinonen et al.[23] where figures available, otherwise estimates from Rimoin et al.[24] where available, otherwise prevalence derived from number of reported abnormalities in reviewed studies.

‡ Definition of categories on page 442; M signifies that the disorder is also a marker for another condition.

arising from detection (A, B, C, D, P, or O). The estimates of detection rate are based on a simple summation, across the studies, of the number of each disorder detected, divided by the total number of each disorder reported. They therefore ignore possible heterogeneity between studies. Disorders for which there may be an indirect benefit because the ultrasound finding is a marker for another disorder are annotated with a superscript M and any indirect benefit is discussed under screening.

Disorders of the central nervous system

Four disorders (spina bifida, holoprosencephaly, microcephaly, and Dandy–Walker syndrome) are associated with serious disability for which termination of pregnancy is justifiable (category A). *Spina bifida* is the most common with a natural birth prevalence over 1 per 1000, and ultrasound detected 84 per cent of reported cases (see Table 18.2). Because of the importance of ultrasound in the diagnosis of spina bifida a summary of the individual studies is given in Table 18.3. *Holoprosencephaly* has a birth prevalence of about 0.1 per 1000. The most severe forms result in a short life expectancy, and although others may survive several years, they show little, if any, developmental progress. Most cases are associated with other abnormalities, mainly trisomy 13 (see screening section below). Most cases were detected. *Microcephaly* is not straightforward, its definition sometimes being taken to be an occipitofrontal circumference measurement further than 2 standard deviations below the mean and sometimes further than 2.5 or 3 standard deviations below the mean. The cut-off has significant implications for prognosis and only one reviewed study specified a

Table 18.3   Summary of routine ultrasound anomaly scanning as a method of diagnosing spina bifida and encephalocele* (excluding data collected before 1986)

| Study | Study period | Spina bifida pregnancies (including encephalocoele) | | False-positives | No of pregnancies scanned |
		No. detected	Total no.		
Anderson et al 1995[5]	1991–3	7	7	0	7880
Chitty *et al*.1991[7]	1988–9	7	7	0	8342
Constantine and McCormack 1991[8]	1988–9	5	6	0	4984
Crane *et al*. 1994[9]	1987–91	3	4	0	7327
Eurenius *et al*. 1999[10]	1990–2	4	6	Not given	8228
Gonçalves *et al*.* 1994[11]	1987–91	20	24	0	574
Jorgensen *et al*. 1999[12]	1989–91	13	20	4	27 844
Levi *et al*. 1995[13]	1990–92	9	11	0	9392
Luck 1992[14]	1988–91	3	3	0	8523
Papp *et al*.† 1995[16]	1988–9	47	53	0	51 675
Roberts *et al*. 1993[17]	1988–9	14	17	Not given	11 360
Shirley *et al*. 1992[19]	1989–90	4	4	0	6183
Stefos *et al*. 1999[20]	1990–6	8	9	1	7236
Van Dorsten *et al*. 1998[21]	1993–6	2	2	0	1611
All		146 (detection rate = 84%)	173	5 (false-positive rate = 0.004%)	141 571‡

* In at least one of these studies,[12] screening tests (lemon and banana signs) as well as visualization of a spinal lesion were used in diagnosis of spina bifida.
† Includes cases referred due to raised level of serum alphafetoprotein.
‡ Excludes studies 10 and 17 where description of false-positives not given.

definition.[13] For the purposes of this chapter, we assume an occipitofrontal circumference measurement of ≥3 standard deviations below the mean because this is indicative of severe mental handicap and because the proportion of microcephaly found in the studies was less than 0.1 per cent (over 2 per cent would be expected with an occipitofrontal circumference measurement further than 2 standard deviations below the mean). About 40 per cent of reported cases of microcephaly were detected. *Dandy–Walker syndrome*, with a birth prevalence of ≤0.1 per 1000, is usually fatal *in utero* or shortly after birth, and in survivors there is an extremely high mortality rate and significant morbidity. Ten out of twelve reported cases were detected.

Anencephaly is the most common of the fatal disorders (category of benefit B) and 133 out of 134 cases reported were detected. The other fatal disorder considered is *iniencephaly* and all seven cases reported were detected.

Hydrocephaly in the absence of spina bifida is a common disorder with a birth prevalence of over 1 per 1000. There is some uncertainty over the benefit arising from antenatal detection, which depends on the severity of the defect. Over 90 per cent of cases were detected.

Agenesis of the corpus callosum has a birth prevalence of about 0.1 per 1000 and over half of cases are associated with chromosomal abnormalities or with other abnormalities of the central nervous system, when mental retardation usually occurs. In cases of agenesis of the corpus callosum alone, however, development is usually normal. Half of the reported cases were detected. But for its value in screening for autosomal abnormalities (see below) it would not be worth including in a scan examination unless other central nervous system abnormalities were present.

Disorders of the respiratory system

Congenital diaphragmatic hernia, with a birth prevalence of about 0.5 per 1000, is a serious and often fatal disorder when the defect is large, but smaller defects may be reparable. The major cause of death is pulmonary hypoplasia and pulmonary hypertension. Antenatal identification, prompting appropriate planned care at the time of delivery, may reduce morbidity. About 60 per cent of cases were detected. It should be included in an ultrasound scan examination as a marker for trisomy 18.

Congenital cystic adenomatoid malformation is a solid and/or cystic mass in the lung. Antenatal diagnosis and increased ultrasound surveillance to determine if fetal deterioration is occurring may be beneficial. However, prognosis is variable. This malformation may lead to hydrops and fetal death, and nearly all reported cases were detected, but with a birth prevalence of 0.1 per 1000 the disorder is uncommon, and the natural history insufficiently well known to warrant inclusion in an ultrasound scan examination.

Disorders of the digestive system

The most common disorders in this group are *cleft lip and palate*. As they are present in most cases of trisomy 13, antenatal diagnosis may be advocated. Otherwise there is no advantage in detecting these defects *in utero*. About a quarter of cases were detected.

The *abdominal wall defects* are *exomphalos* (also called omphalocoele) and *gastroschisis*. Exomphalos can be fatal and about half of cases are associated with other anomalies, particularly trisomy 18 and trisomy 13 (see screening section below). Nearly 90 per cent of abdominal wall defects were detected (87 per cent of exomphalos and 90 per cent of gastroschisis). Both exomphalos and gastroschisis are often reparable, but survival at one year is more favourable for gastroschisis (92 per cent) than for exomphalos (60 per cent). Caesarean section appears not to reduce morbidity or mortality. When exomphalos is identified in the second trimester, ultrasonography can help determine odds for survival by characterizing the size of the defect and identifying other malformations. Rarely, gastroschisis present early in pregnancy may subsequently disappear; bowel atresia then occurs, presumably due to a compromised blood supply which leads to autolysis.[25-31]

Intestinal (mainly duodenal) atresia is associated with an increased risk of Down's syndrome (see screening section below), but otherwise prognosis is good. Antenatal diagnosis with immediate surgical correction in the neonatal period may prevent complications such as aspiration of gastric contents, perforation, or electrolyte imbalance.[32] *Oesophageal atresia with tracheoesophageal fistula* has a good prognosis if the abnormality is isolated. Over half of the cases of intestinal atresia were detected, which is surprising because the sonographic signs are often not apparent until after 24 weeks. Oesophageal atresia and tracheoesophageal fistula were detected in about one-fifth of the reported cases.

The atresias and abdominal wall defects considered here may benefit from antenatal identification with subsequent planned delivery and neonatal care, but there is no conclusive evidence for this. Examination for exomphalos and intestinal atresia is justified in screening for autosomal anomalies.

Disorders of the genito-urinary system

Disorders of the genito-urinary tract are associated in 2–33 per cent of cases with chromosomal abnormalities.[33] *Bilateral renal agenesis*, the most serious disorder considered in this group, is fatal, with a birth prevalence of about 0.1 per 1000. Nearly 90 per cent of cases were detected.

The other major genito-urinary disorders reported were *hydronephrosis* and *multicystic dysplastic kidneys*, with a total birth prevalence of about 1 per 1000. *Obstructions of the genito-urinary tract* may result in hydronephrosis, multicystic dysplastic kidneys, or both.[34] In bilateral early onset obstruction, *in utero* surgery to salvage renal function and avoid pulmonary hypoplasia is of possible benefit (category of benefit P). In some cases of bilateral abnormalities (for example, infantile polycystic kidneys with a birth prevalence of about 1 in 50 000), the disorder will be fatal (category of benefit B). For unilateral lesions, the benefit of surgery is uncertain. If hydronephrosis is confirmed after delivery, prophylactic antibiotics may reduce the possibility of urinary tract infections and renal scarring.[14] The combined detection rate for hydronephrosis, multicystic dysplastic kidneys, and obstructions of the genito-urinary tract was 79 per cent. Adult onset polycystic disease is rarely detected on ultrasound (late age of presentation, birth prevalence of about 1 in 1000) and has been excluded from this category.

Disorders of the heart

Cardiac abnormalities are the most frequent birth defects, with a birth prevalence of about 7.5 per 1000 when patent ductus arteriosus (which is not a prenatal malformation) is excluded. We have divided them into three groups: *severe* (birth prevalence about 2/1000), *moderate* (2/1000), and *mild* (3.5/1000). Rare cardiac abnormalities and those not specified in detail were excluded from detection rates. About half of the severe heart defects were detected, among which the most common was hypoplastic left heart with a mortality rate of over 70 per cent. One-fifth of moderate heart defects were detected; some of these *may* benefit from antenatal identification although the evidence is conflicting.[35,36] For example, if an infant is born with aortic atresia, a prostaglandin infusion may be given to keep open the ductus arteriosus to allow blood perfusion to the systematic circulation. Antenatal diagnosis will probably avoid delay in initiating the treatment. Mild cardiac defects, usually ventricular septal defects, were detected in only 16 per cent of cases, and there is no clear benefit in diagnosing mild heart defects antenatally except, as with other heart defects, in screening for chromosomal abnormalities (see screening section). The heart defects mainly associated with chromosomal abnormalities are hypoplastic left heart, atrioventricular and ventricular septal defects, and double outlet right ventricle,[37] which are listed separately in Table 18.2. The risk of other structural abnormalities, such as diaphragmatic hernia, is increased in the presence of heart defects.

Disorders of the skeletal system

Ultrasound diagnosis of *osteogenesis imperfecta* is based on undermineralized bones, often with evidence of intrauterine fractures. Some forms of the disease are lethal in the immediate perinatal period (type II cases), and warrant the offer of a termination of pregnancy. Others are relatively mild and consistent with normal life expectancy. In the studies reviewed, all six cases reported were detected.

Thanatophoric dysplasia and *achondrogenesis*, both fatal disorders each with a birth prevalence of ≤0.1 per 1000, were detected in all 12 reported cases.

There were 28 reported cases of *limb reduction defects*, of which 12 (43 per cent) were detected. Most limb reduction defects affect only the hands or feet, and do not warrant termination of pregnancy, though reduction defects of the thumbs and radii are sometimes markers for trisomy 18.

Meckel-Gruber syndrome

Meckel-Gruber syndrome comprises encephalocele, polydactyly, and cystic dysplasia of the kidneys. It is lethal at or before birth and has a birth prevalence of ≤0.1 per 1000. All reported cases were detected.

Sacrococcygeal tumour

Prognosis varies with tumour size. Three of the five reported cases were detected. There may be a benefit in antenatal identification, because very large lesions may lead to fetal cardiac failure, and early delivery or *in utero* surgery may be appropriate when the failure is evident.

False-positive results following routine ultrasound

Table 18.4 summarizes the false-positive results that were reported in the studies. All but one of these studies yielded a false-positive rate, based on the authors' definition of false-positive, ranging from 0 per cent to 0.7 per cent. The combined rate across the studies was 0.06 per cent, primarily including suspected renal, cardiac,

Table 18.4   Reported false-positives in studies of routine ultrasound screening. (The false-positive rates may be too low; see text.)

Study	False-positive rate (%)	Details of reported false-positives
Achiron *et al.* 1992[4]	0.02% [1/5324]	1 coarctation of aorta
Anderson *et al.* 1995[5]	0.1% [10/7736]	7 mild ventriculomegaly, 1 lung cyst, 1 microcephaly, 1 renal dilation
Buskens *et al.* 1996[6]	0.1% [7/5239]	5 cardiac defects, 2 other defects
Chitty *et al.* 1991[7]	0.02% [2/8217]	1 tracheo-oesophageal fistula, 1 cystic adenomatoid malformation
Constantine and McCormack 1991[8]	0 % [0/4935]	
Crane *et al.* 1994[9]	0.1 % [7/7209]	2 hydronephrosis, 1 unilateral multicystic renal dysplasia, 3 cerebral ventriculomegaly, 1 sacrococcygeal teratoma
Eurenius *et al.* 1999[10]	0.2% [20/8083]	Not specified
Gonçalves *et al.* 1994[11]	0.7 % [2/287]	1 bilateral mild pyelectasis, 1 unilateral renal agenesis
Jorgensen *et al.* 1999[12]	0.02% [5/27 771]	4 spina bifida, 1 abdominal wall defect
Levi *et al.* 1995[13]	0.1 % [9/9157]	3 microcephaly, 4 dilated renal pelvis, 1 talipes, 1 megacystis
Luck 1992[14]	0.05% [4/8357]	1 oesophageal atresia, 1 diaphragmatic hernia, 2 cardiac defects
Ott 1995[15]	1.1% [12/1122]	12 cardiac defects initially but normal on rescan
Papp *et al.* 1995[16]	0% [0/51 179]	
Roberts *et al.* 1993[17]	Not given	Not given
Rustico *et al.* 1990[18]	0% [0/1823]	
Shirley *et al.* 1992[19]	0.02% [1/6099]	1 omphalocele
Stefos *et al.* 1999[20]	0.1% [9/7074]	1 meningomyelocele, 1 atrial septal defect, 1 transposition of great arteries, 1 cleft lip, 2 multicystic dysplastic kidney, 2 limb/skeletal abnormality, 1 achondroplasia
Van Dorsten *et al.* 1998[21]	0.1% [1/1590]	1 non-immune hydrops
Vergani *et al.* 1992[22]	0.04% [2/5304]	1 hypoplastic left heart, 1 abnormal tricuspid valve
Combined false-positive rate (all abnormalities)†	0.06% [72/125 162]	
Combined false-positive rate (known heart defects only)‡	0.02% [24/130 652]	

† Excludes studies 4, 15, 18, 22 (heart defects only), 17 (false-positive rate not given), and 12 (spina bifida, abdominal wall defects, Down's syndrome only).
‡ Excludes studies 10 and 17 (false-positives not specified) and 12 (heart defects not reported).

and gastrointestinal defects. The combined false-positive rate for cardiac defects alone, again based on the authors' definition of false-positive, was 0.02 per cent.

Discrimination between affected and unaffected fetuses

The detection and false-positive rates in Tables 18.2 and 18.4 are unlikely to be accurate; the detection rates are likely to be over-estimated and the false-positive rates under-estimated. One reason for this is that when a pregnancy is terminated as a result of a positive finding, there is often no necropsy to determine whether the fetus is affected, in which case it may be counted as a true-positive when it is in reality a false-positive. From follow-up studies of pregnancies terminated because fetal abnormalities had been diagnosed by an ultrasound examination, it seems likely that the frequency of diagnostic errors in these cases varies widely between centres: the ultrasound diagnosis was incorrect in 9 per cent of 357 fetuses from terminated pregnancies in one such study,[38] and in 40 per cent of 133 in another.[39] The former of these studies also included follow-up data on 1139 fetuses in which an ultrasound diagnosis of abnormality was not followed by termination, and 1 per cent of these fetuses was unaffected at birth.

A second reason why false-positive rates may be under-estimated is that a second scan may be carried out if the first suggests that an abnormality is present; and if the second scan does not confirm this suggestion, the case may not be counted as a false-positive, although it should be.

A further reason why the detection and false-positive rates in Tables 18.2 and 18.4 must be viewed with caution is that all cases in which malformations were diagnosed by ultrasound were classified as positive. The only cases that should be so classified ('genuine' true- and false-positives) are those in which the antenatal diagnosis can if correct lead to a benefit (termination of pregnancy, intra-uterine surgery, or effective treatment immediately after birth) which is not available or more difficult to provide if diagnosis is delayed until birth. In other words, we suggest that the correct definitions of true- and false-positives to use in the context of ultrasound screening and diagnosis are:

1. True-positive: an affected pregnancy with a positive result, defining an affected pregnancy as one with a disorder for which antenatal detection has a clear benefit (termination, intrauterine surgery, or effective treatment immediately after birth), and defining a positive result as an ultrasound report that the pregnancy is affected.

2. False-positive: an unaffected pregnancy with a positive result, defining an unaffected pregnancy as one without a disorder for which antenatal detection has a clear benefit (termination, intra-uterine surgery, or effective treatment immediately after birth), and defining a positive result as an ultrasound report that the pregnancy is affected by such a disorder.

The numbers of 'genuine' true-positives can be estimated by taking the numbers terminated because of ultrasound diagnosis of malformation and adjusting them to allow for cases in which an offer of termination was declined or in which treatment before or immediately after birth was carried out. The latter cases are estimated to be far fewer than those terminated: Down's syndrome screening experience[40] and a British study in which cases diagnosed by ultrasound were analysed by outcome[14] indicate that 90 per cent of offers of termination are accepted, and in the latter study only 3 per cent of cases that were not terminated were treated by neonatal surgery and none by surgery before birth.

Ultrasound screening performance using specified definitions for true and false-positives

Table 18.5 includes estimates of the numbers of 'genuine' true-positives in those of the studies reviewed which gave the numbers of pregnancies terminated after an ultrasound diagnosis of fetal abnormality.[4,5,7,9,10,12,14,16,19–22] These numbers were calculated using the above estimate for the proportion of offers of termination that are accepted (90 per cent) and assuming that 5 per cent of cases not offered termination received treatment or surgery before or immediately after birth. Table 18.5 also shows the numbers of true- and false-positives originally reported, and the numbers of 'genuine' false-positives.

Table 18.5 True- and false-positives in studies of routine ultrasound scanning where numbers of terminations are given: all cases reported and 'genuine' cases (cases in which the antenatal diagnosis can if correct lead to benefit)

Study	Rate of termination following ultrasound diagnosis of abnormality	True positives		False-positives[e]		Odds of being affected given a positive result[g]	
		Reported (I)	Genuine(II)[d]	Reported (III)	Genuine (IV)[f]	Reported (I:III)	Adjusted (II:IV)
Achiron et al. 1992[4] (heart defects study)	28% (5/18[b])	11	6	1	1	11:1	6:1
Anderson et al. 1995[5]	45% (42/93)	93	49	10	2	46:1	24:1
Chitty et al. 1991[7]	56% (52/93)	93	60	2	2	46:1	30:1
Crane et al. 1994[9]	29% (9/31[c])	27	11	7	6	4:1	2:1
Eurenius et al. 1999[10]	50% (16/32)	32	18	20	Not available	2:1	–
Jorgensen et al. 1999[12] (selected defects study[a])	48% (35/73)	73	41	33	33	2:1	1.2:1
Luck 1992[14]	17% (25/147)	147	34	4	4	37:1	8:1
Papp et al. 1995[16]	86% (273/317)	317	304	0	0	–	–
Shirley et al. 1992[19]	50% (29/58)	58	34	1	1	58:1	34:1
Stefos et al. 1999[20]	31% (40/130)	130	49	8	8	16:1	6:1
Van Dorsten et al. 1998[21]	36% (4/11)	11	5	1	1	11:1	5:1
Vergani et al. 1992[22] (heart defects study)	31% (8/26)	26	10	2	2	13:1	5:1

[a] Neural tube defects, abdominal wall defects and Down's syndrome.
[b] Denominator includes those detected by extended ultrasonography.
[c] Denominator includes some scans performed on clinical indication.
[d] $(T/0.9) + \{0.05 \times [N - (T/0.9)]\}$, where T = terminations of pregnancy and N = true-positives reported.
[e] These numbers may be too low; see text.
[f] Assessed directly from studies.
[g] These OAPRs may be too favourable; see text.

In one of the 12 studies (the largest, which took place in Hungary[16]) no false-positives were identified. Two sets of OAPRs for the other 11 studies are given in Table 18.5. The first set is based on the reported positives. These OAPRs lie between 2:1 and 58:1, a misleading overestimate of screening performance because many of the true-positives have no clear benefit associated with their detection. The OAPRs in the second set are restricted to diagnoses of disorders that benefit from antenatal detection, and range from 1.2:1 to 34:1.

Despite the differences between studies, it seems from this limited analysis that in each study there were more true-positives than false-positives, and in most studies many more. However, this would not necessarily be so if some terminated cases were false-positives. For example, if 20 per cent of the terminated cases in each study had been false-positives, the adjusted OAPRs for all 12 studies would lie between 0.8:1 and 4:1.

ULTRASOUND AS A SCREENING TEST

Ultrasound screening for fetal abnormalities identifies markers that indicate an increased risk of a disorder; they do not directly indicate the presence of the disorder. Depending on the disorder, identification of a marker is usually followed by a more detailed ultrasound scan and/or an invasive diagnostic procedure such as amniocentesis or chorionic villus sampling. There are two categories of ultrasound markers, (1) major structural abnormalities associated with an increased risk of a disorder that may require action in their own right (holoprosencephaly associated with trisomy 13 for example) and (2) fetal ultrasound measurements that differ between affected and unaffected pregnancies (reduced femur length associated with Down's syndrome, for example).

We deal only with reasonably common abnormalities that benefit from antenatal identification. There are four such disorders: trisomy 21 (Down's syndrome), trisomy 18 (Edwards' syndrome), trisomy 13 (Patau's syndrome), and spina bifida. In all four, detection justifies the offer of a termination of pregnancy, either because of serious disability (Down's syndrome, spina bifida) or because the disorder is usually fatal at or soon after birth (trisomies 18 and 13).

An invasive procedure is sometimes needed to confirm a diagnosis, and the associated risk of miscarriage of an unaffected fetus may outweigh the benefit of detection. For example, a choroid plexus cyst is associated with increased risk of trisomy 18, a fatal condition, but usually the fetus is unaffected. A judgment is needed on whether unaffected fetuses should be put at risk from an invasive procedure to detect a non-viable fetus. It would be reasonable to restrict the markers considered of benefit to those with a high OAPR (higher than 1:20 for example).

As in the diagnosis section above, we have limited our review of the published literature on ultrasound screening to studies of ultrasound performed around 16–24 weeks of pregnancy, based on data collected in 1986 or later. In contrast to what we have done in the diagnosis section, we have included studies of high-risk pregnancies when assessing the performance of markers that are not serious disorders in their own right (increased nuchal thickness, for example). Data are not routinely collected on such markers unless the information is used for other obstetric purposes, for example, femur length for estimating gestational age. The main reservation is that a higher index of suspicion exists in scanning a high-risk population than in a general population, which may lead to over-estimates of the general population detection and false-positive rates.

There are insufficient published data to estimate the ultrasound performance of major structural abnormalities as markers for a disorder. We have therefore estimated the *detection rate* by multiplying the proportion of affected pregnancies with the marker present at birth (from the published literature) by the ultrasound detection rate of the marker (from Table 18.2). The *false-positive rate* of the marker is calculated by adding the proportion of unaffected fetuses in whom the marker is not present but incorrectly identified (ultrasound false-positive rate of the marker) to the proportion of unaffected fetuses in whom the marker is detected (birth prevalence of the marker in unaffected pregnancies × ultrasound detection rate of the marker). This is illustrated below, using intestinal atresia as a marker for Down's syndrome as an example:

Detection rate = detection rate of intestinal atresia using routine ultrasound × proportion of Down's syndrome births with intestinal atresia

$$= 62\% \times 5\% = 3\%.$$

(62% comes from Table 18.2 and 5% is the proportion of Down's syndrome births with intestinal atresia according to Twining[37].)

False-positive rate = false-positive rate for intestinal atresia using routine ultrasound + [detection rate of intestinal atresia using routine ultrasound × proportion of all non-Down's syndrome births with intestinal atresia]

$$= 0\% + \{62\% \times [0.02 - (0.17 \times 0.05)]\%\} = 0.007\%.$$

(0% comes from Table 18.4, and 62% and 0.02% (the proportion of all births with intestinal atresia) from Table 18.2. 0.17% is the birth prevalence of Down's syndrome and 0.05 (that is, 5%) is the proportion of Down's syndrome births with intestinal atresia.[37])

The ultrasound screening performance of the markers that are not major structural abnormalities has been estimated using a summation of the true- and false-positives across the relevant studies, divided by the total number of affected and unaffected cases respectively.

Down's syndrome
Second trimester

Table 18.6 gives summary estimates of the screening performance of the two types of early second trimester ultrasound markers—the major structural abnormalities (cardiac defects, intestinal atresia, and exomphalos) and fetal ultrasound measurements (nuchal fold thickness, femur and humerus length, pyelectasis, and hyperechogenic bowel). The screening performance of the ultrasound measurements has been estimated using a summation of true- and false-positives across the relevant studies[41–71] divided by the total numbers of affected and unaffected pregnancies respectively. This method was previously used in the review commissioned by the NHS Technology Assessment Programme.[40] Nuchal fold thickness using a cut-off level of 6 mm yields the

Table 18.6 Summary estimate of performance of second trimester ultrasound screening for Down's syndrome

Ultrasound markers	Detection rate (%) (range if applicable)	False-positive rate (%) (range if applicable)	Odds of being affected given a positive result	Number of studies used to derive estimates
Major structural abnormalities:				
Atrioventricular septal defect	11	0.014	1:0.8	See footnotes 1–3
Ventricular septal defect	2	0.052	1:13	See footnotes 1–3
Intestinal atresia	3	0.007	1:1.3	See footnote 1
Exomphalos	2	0.042	1:14	See footnote 1
Other markers:				
Nuchal fold thickness ≥6 mm	39 (8–75)	1.3 (0–8.5)	1:26	17[41–57]
Femur length (comparing observed with expected)	28 (13–48)	5.8 (3–16)	1:159	13[41,43,48,49,58–66]
Femur length (ratio of BPD to femur length)	26 (10–55)	5.1 (1.1–9)	1:151	6[42,57,59,64,67,68]
Humerus length (comparing observed with expected)	29 (24–64)	4.6 (1–15)	1:122	8[43,48,57,59,62–65,68]
Femur length and humerus length combined (comparing observed with expected)	36 (18–53)	3.7 (1.6–7.6)	1:79	3[45,62,63]
Pyelectasis	18 (6–46)	2.5 (1.6–4.0)	1:107	7[54,57,65,66,68–70]
Hyperechogenic bowel	16 (6–20)	0.7 (0.6–2.2)	1:34	5[54,65,66,68,71]

1. Detection rate = ab and false-positive rate = $c + b(d - ae)$, where a = proportion of Down's syndrome fetuses with specified anomaly (from Twining 1995);[37] b = overall detection rate for anomaly (Table 18.2); c = false-positive rate for anomaly (Table 18.4); d = overall prevalence of anomaly (Table 18.2); e = overall prevalence of Down's syndrome (0.17%).
2. Twining[37] did not give the proportion of Down's syndrome fetuses with specific heart defects (a in footnote 1), but listed atrioventricular and ventricular septal defects as those most often found antenatally in Down's syndrome. From his figure for the total prevalence of heart defects in Down's syndrome (40%), and from the series of heart defects in trisomic fetuses that he cited[72–75] and the detection rates shown in Table 18.2, we estimate that a (the proportion of Down's syndrome fetuses with anomalies) is 17% for atrioventricular septal defect and 15% for ventricular septal defect.
3. For each heart defect, the false-positive rate (c in footnote 1) was estimated on the assumption that the false-positive rate for all congenital heart disease is 0.02% (Table 18.4) and that these false-positive cases are distributed by reported diagnosis in the same proportions as the 95 cases of congenital heart disease detected by ultrasound that are listed in Table 18.2.

highest detection rate (39 per cent), for a 1.3 per cent false-positive rate. Detection rates varied from 8–75 per cent and false-positive rates from 0–8.5 per cent. Other useful markers with very low false-positive rates include atrioventricular and ventricular septal defects, intestinal atresia, exomphalos, and hyperechogenic bowel. For each of these markers the odds of being affected by Down's syndrome given a positive result are greater than 1:60, which are the odds accepted with current serum screening methods. Less commonly described markers include cerebral ventricular dilation, choroid plexus cysts, ear length, fifth-digit midphalanx hypoplasia, increased ilial length, short frontal lobe, sandal gap, and enlargement of the iliac wing. There are insufficient data on these markers to estimate screening performance.

The performance of ultrasound screening for Down's syndrome could be improved by producing a risk estimate based on the presence or absence of a combination of ultrasound markers. This was the subject of a review by Vintzileos *et al*,[76] but information on the extent to which these markers are independent of each other in both affected and unaffected pregnancies, needed to do this reliably, is not currently available.

Five studies that examined the effectiveness of routine ultrasound screening for Down's syndrome, but did not specify the markers used, collectively identified only 15 out of 66 (23 per cent) affected pregnancies.[5,7,11,17,19] No false-positive rates were given. The Multiscan study in Scandinavia[12] obtained a detection rate of only 6 per cent (2 out of 32 affected pregnancies) and a false-positive rate of 0.1 per cent using femur length and biparietal diameter, increased nuchal skin fold (although this was not routinely measured), cardiac and abdominal wall defects, and duodenal atresia/ stenosis as markers for Down's syndrome.

First trimester

Nuchal translucency measurement, which is the maximum depth of a fluid-filled space at the back of the fetal neck, is a useful ultrasound marker for Down's syndrome between 10 and 14 weeks of pregnancy. This measurement increases with gestational age. There are significant unexplained study-to-study differences in the estimates of screening performance using this marker. In one intervention study in which nuchal translucency was adjusted for gestational age and used together with maternal age, the reported detection rate was 84 per cent for a 6 per cent false-positive rate.[77] This estimate does not allow for detected pregnancies that would have miscarried in the absence of screening and termination of pregnancy. One study that allowed for this bias estimated that the detection rate using nuchal translucency measurement with maternal age was 63 per cent for a 5 per cent false-positive rate[78] and a more recent analysis estimated that it was 73 per cent.[79]

Spina bifida

Spina bifida affects the cerebellum and frontal bones. The cerebellum is drawn into the foramen magnum and produces a 'banana sign', sometimes measured as a reduced transverse cerebellar diameter. The frontal bones are pinched in laterally, producing a 'lemon' sign instead of the usual ovoid shape. Table 18.7 summarizes the data on cerebellar abnormalities and spina bifida. Table 18.8 does so for cranial abnormalities. If the birth prevalence of spina bifida without intervention was 1 per 1000, the odds of being affected given a positive result would be 1:0.5 for the qualitative banana sign and 1:3 for the lemon sign according to the combined figures. The true odds are probably considerably lower, for reasons discussed in Chapter 3 (p. 65).

Trisomy 18

Table 18.9 summarizes data on markers for trisomy 18. No single marker has a high detection rate. Among the major structural anomalies, exomphalos has the highest rate (17 per cent). All have a low false-positive rate so the OAPR for some markers is acceptable.

Table 18.7 Ultrasound and neural tube defects: screening performance of the cerebellar ('banana') sign. Except where indicated, the women screened were known to be at high risk of a neural tube defect pregnancy.

Study (first author and publication date)	Period	Detection rate % (n)[a] (spina bifida)	False-positive rate % (n) (all non-NTD pregnancies)
Qualitative assessments:			
Nicolaides[80] 1986	1983–5	95 (20/21)	0.0 (0/100)[b]
Campbell[81] 1987	1985–6	96 (25/26)	0.0 (0/410)
Pilu[82] 1988	Pre 1988	100 (19/19)	0.0 (0/17)[c]
Goldstein[83] 1989	Pre 1989	100 (19/19)	10.6 (5/47)[d]
Thiagarajah[84] 1990	1986–9	92 (22/24)	–
Van den Hof[85] 1990	1986–8	95 (124/130)	0.0 (0/1388)
Petrikovsky[86] 1990	Pre 1990	53 (8/15)	0.0 (0/313)
Blumenfeld[87] 1993	1987–92	100 (6/6)[b]	0.0 (0/7180)[b]
Combined		93 (243/260)	0.05 (5/9455)
Quantitative assessment:			
de Courcy-Wheeler[88] 1994	1986–93	68 (141/208)[e]	1.4 (6/440)[e]

[a] The denominator is those cases for which the appropriate view of the fetus was available.
[b] These were women who presented for routine ultrasound scans.
[c] All 17 cases had isolated hydrocephalus.
[d] All 5 false-positives had isolated ventriculomegaly.
[e] Test regarded as positive when the transverse cerebellar diameter was ≤85 per cent of the median.

Table 18.8 Ultrasound and neural tube defects: screening performance of the cranial ('lemon') sign. Except where indicated, the women screened were known to be at high risk of a neural tube defect pregnancy.

Study (first author and publication date)	Period	Detection rate % (n)[a] (spina bifida)	False-positive rate % (n) (all non-NTD pregnancies)
Nicolaides[80] 1986	1983–5	100 (54/54)	0.0 (0/100)[b]
Campbell[81] 1987	1985–6	100 (26/26)	1.2 (5/410)
Penso[89] 1987	1983–6	67 (16/24)	0.0 (0/12)[c]
Chambers[90] 1988	Pre 1988	75 (9/12)	0.0 (0/169)
Gabbe[91] 1988	Pre 1988	75 (6/8)	–
Nyberg[92] 1988 (i)	Pre 1988	55 (17/31)	0.0 (0/30)[d]
Nyberg[92] 1988 (ii)	Pre 1988	79 (15/19)	1.3 (3/230)
Goldstein[83] 1989	Pre 1989	70 (14/20)	2.1 (1/47)
Thiagarajah[84] 1990	1986–9	75 (18/24)	–
Van den Hof[85] 1990	1986–8	83 (108/130)	0.6 (9/1388)
Petrikovsky[86] 1990	Pre 1990	67 (10/15)	1.6 (5/313)
Blumenfeld[87] 1993	1987–92	67 (4/6)[b]	0.0 (0/7180)[b]
de Courcy-Wheeler[88] 1994	1986–93	96 (200/208)	–
Combined		86 (497/577)	0.23 (23/9879)

[a] The denominator is those cases for which the appropriate view of the fetus was available.
[b] These were women who presented for routine ultrasound scans.
[c] The spina bifida and non-NTD pregnancies were all associated with hydrocephalus.
[d] All 30 cases had isolated hydrocephalus.

Table 18.9 Summary estimates of performance of second trimester ultrasound screening for trisomy 18 (Edwards' syndrome) using anomalies listed in Table 18.2 as markers. The birth prevalence of trisomy 18 is taken to be 0.2/1000.

Ultrasound marker	Prevalence of marker in trisomy 18 according to Twining 1995[37] (%) (a)	Detection rate for the marker (%) (from Table 18.2) (b)	Detection rate for trisomy 18 (%) ($0.01 \times a \times b$)	False-positive rate for the marker (%) (from Table 18.4) (c)	Proportion of all births with the marker (%) (from Table 18.2) (d)	False-positive rate for trisomy 18 (%) ($e = c + b \{[0.01 \times d] - [0.01 \times a \times 0.0002]\}$)	Odds of being affected given a positive result ($1{:}e/[0.01 \times a \times b \times 0.0002]$)
Major structural abnormalities							
Neural tube defects	<10	89	≤9	0.004	0.15	≈0.14	1: ≥80
Holoprosencephaly	≤10 (i)	92	≤9	0	0.01	≈0.008	1: ≥4
Dandy–Walker syndrome	≤10 (i)	83	≤8	0	≤0.01	≈0.003 (viii)	1: ≥1.8 (viii)
Hydrocephaly	≤10 (i)	91	≤9	0.009	0.15	≈0.14	1: ≥77
Agenesis of corpus callosum	≤10 (i)	50	≤5	0	0.01	≈0.005	1: ≥5
Diaphragmatic hernia	20	61	12	0.0009	0.05	0.029	1:12
Cleft lip and/or palate	15	27	4	0.0009	0.15	0.041	1:51
Exomphalos	20	87	17	0.002	0.05	0.042	1:12
Double outlet right ventricle	5 (ii)	40	2	0.0003 (iii)	0.01	0.004	1:10
Hypoplastic left heart	1 (ii)	52	1	0.003 (iii)	0.05	0.029	1:145

Ultrasound marker	Prevalence of marker in trisomy 18 according to Twining 1995[37] (%) (a)	Detection rate for the marker (%) (from Table 18.2) (b)	Detection rate for trisomy 18 (%) (0.01 × a × b)	False-positive rate for the marker (%) (from Table 18.4) (c)	Proportion of all births with the marker (%) (from Table 18.2) (d)	False-positive rate for trisomy 18 (%) (e = c + b {[0.01 × d] − [0.01 × a × 0.0002]})	Odds of being affected given a positive result (1:e/[0.01 × a × b × 0.0002])
Atrioventricular septal defect	3 (ii)	64	2	0.003 (iii)	0.05	0.035	1:88
Ventricular septal defect	55 (ii)	16	9	0.005 (iii)	0.35	0.059	1:33
Hydronephrosis etc	15 (iv)	79	12	0.012	0.1	0.089	1:37
Limb reduction defects	15 (v)	43	6	0	0.05	0.020	1:17
Other Markers							
Choroid plexus cysts	42 (vi)	90 (vi) (est.)	38	0	1 (vii)	0.892	1:118

(i) Assumed to be ≤10 per cent in the absence of any estimate by Twining 1995.[37]

(ii) Twining did not give the proportions of trisomy 18 fetuses with specific heart defects, but listed double outlet right ventricle, hypoplastic left heart, and atrioventricular and ventricular septal defects as those most often found antenatally in trisomy 18 and/or trisomy 13. The prevalence of these defects in trisomy 18 was estimated for the above table from Twining's figure for the total prevalence of heart defects in trisomy 18 (80 per cent), from the results of the series of heart defects in trisomic fetuses that he cited,[72–75] and from the detection rates shown in Table 18.2.

(iii) The false-positive rate for each heart defect was estimated on the assumption that the false-positive rate for all congenital heart disease is 0.02 per cent (Table 18.4) and that these false-positive cases are distributed by reported diagnosis in the same proportions as the 120 cases of congenital heart disease detected by ultrasound that are listed in Table 18.2.

(iv) Twining's[37] figure includes horseshoe kidney.

(v) Radial aplasia, absent or hypoplastic thumb. Twining gives a figure of 10 per cent for radial aplasia, and says that hypoplasia and absence of thumb occur 'less commonly'.

(vi) From Donnenfeld 1995.[93]

(vii) Proportion of all *fetuses* with the marker.

(viii) Estimated on the assumption that the population prevalence of Dandy-Walker syndrome is 0.005%.

Table 18.10 Summary estimates of performance of second trimester ultrasound screening for trisomy 13 (Patau's syndrome) using anomalies listed in Table 18.2 as markers. The birth prevalence of trisomy 13 is taken to be 0.1/1000.

Ultrasound marker	Prevalence of marker in trisomy 13 according to Twining 1995[37] (%) (a)	Detection rate for the marker (%) (from Table 18.2) (b)	Detection rate for trisomy 13 (%) (0.01 × a × b)	False-positive rate for the marker (%) (from Table 18.4) (c)	Proportion of all births with the marker (%) (from Table 18.2) (d)	False-positive rate for trisomy 13 (%) (e = c + b {[0.01 × d] − [0.01 × a × 0.0001]})	Odds of being affected given a positive result (1:e/[0.01 × a × b × 0.0001])
Holoprosencephaly	75	92	69	0	0.01	0.002	1:0.3
Dandy–Walker syndrome	20	83	17	0	≤0.01	0.002 (iv)	1:1.2 (iv)
Hydrocephaly	13	91	12	0.009	0.15	0.144	1:120
Agenesis of corpus callosum	22	50	11	0	0.01	0.004	1:4
Diaphragmatic hernia	≤10 (i)	61	≤6	0.0009	0.05	0.031	1:≥51
Cleft lip and/or palate	75	27	20	0.0009	0.15	0.039	1:20
Exomphalos	30	87	26	0.002	0.05	0.043	1:17
Double outlet right ventricle	9	40	4	0.0003 (iii)	0.01	0.004	1:11
Hypoplastic left heart	10 (ii)	52	5	0.003 (iii)	0.05	0.028	1:56
Atrioventricular septal defect	6 (ii)	64	4	0.003 (iii)	0.05	0.035	1:88
Ventricular septal defect	33 (ii)	16	5	0.005 (iii)	0.35	0.060	1:120
Hydronephrosis etc.	30	79	24	0.012	0.1	0.089	1:37

(i) Assumed to be ≤10 per cent in the absence of any estimate by Twining 1995.[37]

(ii) Twining did not give the proportions of trisomy 13 fetuses with specific heart defects, but listed double outlet right ventricle, hypoplastic left heart, and atrioventricular and ventricular septal defects as those most often found antenatally in trisomy 13 and/or trisomy 18. The prevalence of these defects in trisomy 13 was estimated for the above table from Twining's figure for the total prevalence of heart defects in trisomy 13 (80 per cent), from the results of the series of heart defects in trisomic fetuses that he cited,[72–75] and from the detection rates shown in Table 18.2.

(iii) The false-positive rate for each heart defect was estimated on the assumption that the false-positive rate for all congenital heart disease is 0.02 per cent (Table 18.4) and that these false-positive cases are distributed by reported diagnosis in the same proportions as the 120 cases of congenital heart disease detected by ultrasound that are listed in Table 18.2.

(iv) Estimated on the assumption that the population prevalence of Dandy–Walker syndrome is 0.005%.

Trisomy 13

Table 18.10 summarizes data on markers for trisomy 13. Holoprosencephaly is the best marker.

Odds of being affected with trisomy 18 or 13 given the presence of an ultrasound marker

Some markers are associated with both trisomy 18 and 13. Table 18.11 summarizes the OAPRs for either abnormality. They range from greater than 1:1 (holoprosencephaly) to less than 1:75 (neural tube defect).

ABNORMALITIES TO BE INCLUDED IN AN ULTRASOUND ANOMALY SCAN

Table 18.12 lists abnormalities worth identifying in a routine ultrasound anomaly scan, on the basis of the studies reviewed and the natural history of the disorders. Disorders classified as having a 'possible' benefit in antenatal detection are excluded (P in Table 18.2). This list could form the basis of an information leaflet in which the defects being sought are made explicit when women are asked if they wish to have the ultrasound examination. It would clarify the purpose of the examination, and avoid subsequent complaints that an abnormality not specified had been missed.

Limitations of our approach

We recognize that Specified Abnormality Scanning is a new approach to ultrasound screening. It focuses on detecting serious abnormalities for which a remedy, usually termination of pregnancy, is available. We have not considered the extent to which variation in the severity of each disorder may influence detection rates. Some abnormalities of little consequence if seen in isolation may be suggestive of a more severe

Table 18.11 Approximate odds of being affected by trisomy 13 or 18 if one of the major anomalies listed in Tables 18.9 and 18.10 is detected by ultrasound screening

Ultrasound marker	Odds of being affected by trisomy 13 or 18 given a positive test	Prevalence per 1000 births
Neural tube defects	1:≥ 80	1.5
Holoprosencephaly	1:≥ 0.03	0.1
Dandy–Walker syndrome	1:≥ 0.17*	≤0.1
Hydrocephaly	1:≥ 46	1
Agenesis of corpus callosum	1:≥ 1.7	0.1
Diaphragmatic hernia	1:≥ 9	0.5
Cleft lip and/or palate	1:14	1.5
Exomphalos	1:7	0.5
Double outlet right ventricle	1:5	0.1
Hypoplastic left heart	1:40	0.5
Atrioventricular septal defect	1:43	0.5
Ventricular septal defect	1:26	3.5
Hydronephrosis etc.	1:18	1
Limb reduction defects	1:17	0.5
Total		11

* Estimated on the assumption that the population prevalence of Dandy-Walker syndrome is 0.005%.

prognosis if associated with other abnormalities. Allowing for these effects would be difficult, and would be unlikely to make a material difference to our practical conclusion that ultrasound screening for congenital abnormalities should focus on those listed in Table 18.12. Of course, this list is only a start and is likely to be modified in the light of discussion and any new data.

Our review is confined to studies of routine ultrasound scanning for screening. Ultrasound scanning for a particular clinical purpose, for example because of a condition for which there is a family history, falls outside the approach we propose. The specificity of the examination would be determined by the history and the clinical need.

It is likely that a more detailed ultrasound scan than we propose—for example lasting 45 minutes and using sophisticated technology such as Doppler imaging—would have higher detection and lower false-positive rates. This would be unlikely to alter our conclusions on which abnormalities are worth detecting by ultrasound, because these conclusions were based mainly on the benefits of detection rather than on ultrasound performance.

CONCLUSION

Ultrasound scanning in pregnancy should aim to identify and report only disorders for which there is an effective intervention. Women should be given information leaflets listing the disorders, and explaining for each the implications of a positive screening test, the further tests and intervention which might be offered, and the possible consequences of not intervening. In this way, genuine consent would be obtained. Patients could also indicate particular abnormalities of concern to them, including any not on the list (for example, those in their family), and the ultrasonographer could consider these as well as the listed abnormalities. A broad non-specific examination including abnormalities in which nothing is gained by diagnosis before birth could thus be avoided without omitting anything of special concern to a couple. Patients who would not consider termination of pregnancy for conditions on the list could choose not to be told the findings for these conditions, or decline to have an ultrasound scan examination for fetal abnormalities.

Screening for abnormalities for which no intervention can be offered is unjustified. Doing so simply to prepare parents before the birth is not helpful. If no intervention is to be offered, the psychological cost of an uncertain prognosis, or in the case of minor abnormalities an excessive preoccupation with the condition, can easily outweigh any benefits of being prepared, and this is not a sound basis for a screening investigation.

The application of this approach, Specified Abnormality Scanning, will require discussion, education, and examination of data to determine the specified disorders. We have attempted to do this, though our list (Table 18.12) is unlikely to be the last word. Having specified what should be sought and reported, there would no longer be a need to report abnormalities for which there is no effective intervention. Indeed, to do so is unjustified because it causes needless distress and the temptation to carry out further unnecessary medical investigations. We acknowledge that there may be a reluctance to withhold apparently positive findings for which there is no effective remedy, but the

Table 18.12 Possible checklist of specific ultrasound abnormalities which would benefit from antenatal identification (that is, those specifically covered by specified abnormality scanning)*

Ultrasound finding	Diagnostic/ screening	Abnormality at increased risk (screening only)	Action to be offered
Central nervous system:			
Lemon sign	Screening	Spina bifida	Diagnostic ultrasound and/or amniocentesis
Banana sign	Screening	Spina bifida	Diagnostic ultrasound and/or amniocentesis
Spina bifida	Diagnostic		Amniocentesis to confirm diagnosis or termination of pregnancy
Holoprosencephaly	Diagnostic		Termination of pregnancy
Severe microcephaly	Diagnostic		Termination of pregnancy
Anencephaly	Diagnostic		Termination of pregnancy
Iniencephaly	Diagnostic		Termination of pregnancy
Dandy–Walker syndrome	Diagnostic		Termination of pregnancy
Agenesis of corpus callosum	Screening	trisomy 13, 18	Amniocentesis
Respiratory tract/neck:			
Diaphragmatic hernia	Screening	trisomy 13, 18	Amniocentesis
Nuchal fold thickness (≥6 mm)	Screening	Down's syndrome	Amniocentesis
Digestive tract:			
Cleft lip/palate	Screening	trisomy 13, 18	Amniocentesis
Exomphalos	Screening	trisomy 13, 18, Down's syndrome	Amniocentesis
Duodenal atresia	Screening	Down's syndrome	Amniocentesis
Hyperechogenic bowel	Screening	Down's syndrome	Amniocentesis
Genito-urinary tract:			
Bilateral renal agenesis	Diagnostic		Termination of pregnancy
Hydronephrosis/multicystic dysplastic kidneys/	Diagnostic		*In utero* treatment if bilateral
obstructive uropathy	Screening	trisomy 13, 18	Amniocentesis
Cardiac:			
Severe†	Diagnostic		Termination of pregnancy Immediate postnatal treatment
Double outlet right ventricle	Screening	trisomy 18, 13	Amniocentesis
Ventricular septal defect	Screening	Down's syndrome	Amniocentesis
Skeletal:			
Osteogenesis imperfecta (severe)	Diagnostic		Termination of pregnancy
Thanatophoric dysplasia	Diagnostic		Termination of pregnancy
Achondrogenesis	Diagnostic		Termination of pregnancy
Limb reduction defects	Screening	trisomy 18	Amniocentesis
Other:			
Meckel's syndrome	Diagnostic		Termination of pregnancy
Cystic hygroma	Screening	Down's syndrome	Amniocentesis

* Conditions are listed as benefiting from diagnostic ultrasound if in category of benefit A, B, C or D, and as benefiting from screening ultrasound if in category of benefit A or B and OAPR ≥1:60 for Down's syndrome or ≥1:20 for spina bifida or for one of the other common autosomal trisomies (13 or 18). The reasons for specifying these cut-off thresholds are that those for Down's syndrome and spina bifida match those accepted with present serum screening methods, and that the OAPR must be high to justify an invasive procedure where fatal chromosomal abnormalities (trisomies 13 and 18) are concerned.

† As in Table 18.2: Hypoplastic left/right heart, Ebstein's anomaly, single atrium, truncus arteriosus, total anomalous pulmonary drainage, ectopia cordis, complex heart disease, atrio-ventricular defect, transposition of great vessels.

new approach aims to improve the benefit of the anomaly scan, to simplify the examination by only seeking specified abnormalities instead of all possible abnormalities, and to better quantify its value.

REFERENCES

1. RCOG/RCR (1996). Survey on the use of obstetric ultrasound in the UK, cited in the *Report of the RCOG Working Party on Ultrasound Screening for Fetal Abnormalities—Consultation Document.*(Submitted.)
2. Ewigman BG, Crane JP, Frigoletto FD, LeFevre ML, Bain RP, McNellis D, and the RADIUS study group (1993). Effect of prenatal ultrasound screening on perinatal outcome. *New Engl J Med*, **329**, 821–7.
3. Romero R (1993). Routine obstetric ultrasound. *Ultrasound Obstet Gynecol*, **3**, 303–7.
4. Achiron R, Glaser J, Gelernter I, Hegesh J, and Yagel S (1992). Extended fetal echocardiographic examination for detecting cardiac malformations in low risk pregnancies. *Br Med J*, **304**, 671–4.
5. Anderson N, Boswell O, and Duff G (1995). Prenatal sonography for the detection of fetal anomalies: results of a prospective study and comparison with prior series. *Am. J. Roentgenol.*, **155**, 943–50.
6. Buskens E, Grobbe DE, Frohn-Mulder JME, Stewart PA, Juttmann RE, Wladimiroff JW, and Hess J (1996). Efficacy of routine fetal ultrasound screening for congenital heart disease in normal pregnancy *Circulation*, **94**, 67–72.
7. Chitty LS, Hunt GH, Moore J, and Lobb MO (1991). Effectiveness of routine ultrasonography in detecting fetal structural abnormalities in a low risk population. *Br Med J*, **93**, 1165–9.
8. Constantine G and McCormack J (1991). Comparative audit of booking and mid-trimester ultrasound scans in the prenatal diagnosis of congenital anomalies. *Prenat Diagn*, **11**, 909–14.
9. Crane JP, LeFevre ML, Winborn RC, Evans JK, Ewigman BG, Bain RP, Frigoletto FD, McNellis D, and the RADIUS Study Group (1994). A randomised trial of prenatal ultrasonographic screening: Impact on the detection, management and outcome of anomalous fetuses. *Am J Obstet Gynecol*, **71**, 392–9.
10. Eurenius K, Axelsson O, Cnattingius S, Eriksson L, and Norsted T (1999). Second trimester ultrasound screening performed by midwives; sensitivity for detection of fetal anomalies. *Acta Obstet Gynecol Scand*, **78**, 98–104.
11. Gonçalves LF, Jeanty P, and Piper JM (1994). The accuracy of prenatal ultrasonography in detecting congenital anomalies. *Am J Obstet Gynecol*, **71**, 1606–12.
12. Jorgensen FS, Valentin L, Salvesen KA, Jorgensen C, Jensen FR, Bang J, Eik-Nes SH, Madsen M, Marsal K, Persson PH, Philip J, Bogstad JW, and Norgaard-Pedersen B (1999). MULTISCAN-α Scandinavian multicenter second trimester obstetric ultrasound and serum screening study. *Acta Obstet Gynecol Scand*, **78**, 501–10.
13. Levi S, Schaaaps JP, De Havay P, Coulon R, and Defoor P (1995). End-result of routine ultrasound screening for congenital anomalies: The Belgian Multicentric Study 1984–92. *Ultrasound Obstet Gynecol*, **5**, 366–71.
14. Luck CA (1992). Value of routine ultrasound scanning at 19 weeks: a four year study of 8849 deliveries. *Br Med J*, **304**, 1474–8.

15. Ott WJ (1995). The accuracy of antenatal fetal echocardiography screening in high and low risk patients. *Am J Obstet Gynecol*, **172**, 1741–9.
16. Papp Z, Tóth-Pál E, Papp Cs, Tóth Z, Szabó M, Veress L, and Török O (1995). Impact of prental mid-trimester screening on the prevalence of fetal structure anomalies: a prospective epidemiological study. *Ultrasound Obstet Gynecol*, **6**, 320–6.
17. Roberts AB, Hampton E, and Wilson N (1993). Ultrasound detection of fetal structural abnormalities in Auckland 1988–9. *NZ Med J*, **106**, 441–3.
18. Rustico MA, Bennettoni A, D'Ottario G, Bogatti P, Fontana A, Pecite V, and Mandrizzeto GP (1990). Fetal echocardiography: the role of the screening procedure. *Europ J Obstet Gynecol Reprod Biol*, **36**, 19–25.
19. Shirley IM, Bottomley F, and Robinson VP (1992). Routine radiographer screening for fetal abnormalities by ultrasound in an unselected low risk population. *Br J Radiol*, **65**, 5649.
20. Stefos T, Plachouras N *et al.* (1999). Routine obstetrical ultrasound at 18–22 weeks: our experience of 7236 fetuses. *J Matern Fetal Med*, **8**, 64–9.
21. Van Dorsten JP, Husley TC, Newman RB, and Menard MK (1998). Fetal anomaly detection by second-trimester ultrasonography in a tertiary center. *Am J Obstet Gynecol*, **178**, 742–9.
22. Vergani P, Mariani S, Ghidini A, Schiavina R, Cavallone M, Locatelli, Strobelt N, and Cerruti P (1992). Screening for congenital heart disease with the four-chamber view of the heart. *Am J Obstet Gynecol*, **167**, 1000–3.
23. Heinonen OP, Slone D, and Shapiro S (1977). *Birth defects and drugs in pregnancy*. Publishing Sciences Group, Massachusetts.
24. Rimoin DL, Connor JM, and Pyeritz RE (ed) (1996). *Emery and Rimoin's Principles and Practice of Medical Genetics*, 3rd edn. Churchill Livingstone, Edinburgh.
25. Quirk JG, Fortney J, Collins HB, West J, Hassad SJ, and Wagner C (1996). Outcomes of newborns with gastroschisis: The effects of mode of delivery, site of delivery, and interval from birth to surgery. *Am J Obstet Gynecol*, **174**, 1134–40.
26. Lewis DF, Towers CV, Garite TJ, Jackson DN, Nageotte MP, and Major SA (1990). Fetal gastroschisis and omphalocele: Is cesarian section the best mode of delivery? *Am J Obstet Gynecol*, **163**, 773–5.
27. Lenke R and Hatch EI (1986). Fetal gastroschisis: A preliminary report advocating the use of Cesarian section. *Obstet Gynecol*, **67**, 395.
28. Carpenter MW, Curci MR, Dibbins AW, and Haddow JE (1984). Perinatal management of ventral wall defects. *Obstet Gynecol*, **64**, 646.
29. Johnson N, Lilford RJ, Irving H, Crabbe D, and Cartmill R (1991). The vanishing bowel. Case report of bowel atresia following gastroschisis. *Br J Obstet Gynaecol*, **98**, 214–15.
30. Benacerraf BR, Saltzman DH, Estroff JA, and Frigoletto FD (1990). Abnormal karyotype of fetuses with omphalocele: Prediction based on omphalocele contents. *Obstet Gynecol*, **75**, 317.
31. Tucci M and Bard H (1990). The associated anomalies that determine prognosis in congenital omphaloceles. *Am J Obstet Gynecol*, **163**, 1646–9.
32. Romero R, Ghidini A, Costigan K, Touloukian R, and Hobbins JC (1988). Prenatal diagnosis of duodenal atresia: does it make any difference? *Obstet Gynecol*, **71**, 739–41.
33. Nicolaides K, Shawwa L, Brizot M, and Snijders R (1993). Ultrasonographically detectable markers of fetal chromosomal defects. *Ultrasound Obstet Gynecol*, **3**, 56–69.

34. Quinlan RW, Cruz AC, and Huddleston JF (1986). Sonographic detection of fetal urinary-tract anomalies. *Obstet Gynecol*, **67**, 558–65.
35. Copel JA, Tan ASA, and Kleinman CS (1997). Does prenatal diagnosis of congenital heart disease alter short term outcome? *Ultrasound Obstet Gynecol*, **10**, 237–41.
36. Chang AC, Huhta JC, Yoon GY, Wood DC, Tulzer G, Cohen A, Mennuti M, and Norwood WI (1991). Diagnosis, transport and outcome in fetuses with left ventricular outflow tract obstruction. *J Thorac Cardiovasc Surg*, **102**, 841–8.
37. Twining P (1995). Ultrasound diagnosis of chromosomal disease. In *Diseases of the fetus and newborn*, 2nd edn, (ed. GB Reed, AF Claireaux, and F Cockburn), pp. 934–953. Chapman and Hall, London.
38. Brand IR, Kaminopetros P, Cave M, Irving HC, and Lilford R (1994). Specificity of antenatal ultrasound in the Yorkshire Region: a prospective study of 2261 ultrasound detected anomalies. *Br J Obstet Gynaecol*, **101**, 392–7.
39. Clayton-Smith, Farndon PA, McKeown C, and Donnai D (1990). Examination of fetuses after induced abortion for fetal abnormality. *Br Med J*, **300**, 295–7.
40. Wald NJ, Kennard A, Hackshaw A, and McGuire A (1997). Antenatal screening for Down's syndrome. *J Med Screen*, **4**, 181–246.
41. Benacerraf BR, Cnann A, Gelman R, Laboda LA, and Frigoletto FD (1989). Can sonographers reliably identify anatomic features associated with Down syndrome in fetuses? *Radiology*, **173**, 377–80.
42. Ginsberg N, Cadkin A, Pergament E, and Verlinsky Y (1990). Ultrasonographic detection of the second-trimester fetus with trisomy 18 and trisomy 21. *Am J Obstet Gynecol*, **163**, 1186–90.
43. Benacerraf BR, Neuberg D, and Frigoletto FD (1991). Humeral shortening in second-trimester fetuses with Down syndrome. *Obstet Gynecol*, **77**, 223–7.
44. Crane JP and Gray DL (1991). Sonographically measured nuchal skinfold thickness as a screening tool for Down syndrome. results of a prospective clinical trial. *Obstet Gynecol*, **77**, 533–6.
45. Benacerraf BR, Neuberg D, Bromley B, and Frigoletto FD (1992). Sonographic scoring index for prenatal detection of chromosomal abnormalities. *J Ultrasound Med*, **11**, 449–58.
46. Kirk JS, Comstock CH, Fassnacht MA, Yang SS, and Lee W (1992). Routine measurement of nuchal thickness in the second trimester. *J Maternal Fetal Med*, **1**, 82–6.
47. De Vore GR and Alfi O (1993). The association between an abnormal nuchal skinfold, trisomy 21 and ultrasound abnormalities identified during the second trimester of pregnancy. *Ultrasound Obstet Gynecol*, **3**, 387–94.
48. Lockwood CJ, Lynch L , Ghidini QA, Lapinski R, Berkowitz G, Thayer B, and Miller WA (1993). The effect of fetal gender on the prediction of Down syndrome by means of maternal serum α-fetoprotein and ultrasonographic parameters. *Am J Obstet Gynecol*, **169**, 1190–7.
49. Benacerraf BR, ,Nadel A, and Bromley B (1994). Identification of second trimester fetuses with autosomal trisomy by the use of a sonographic scoring index. *Radiology*, **193**, 135–40.
50. Donnenfeld AE, Carlson DE, Palomaki GE, Librizzi RJ, Weiner S, and Platt LD (1994). Prospective multicenter study of second-trimester nuchal skinfold thickness in unaffected and Down syndrome pregnancies. *Obstet Gynecol*, **84**, 844–7.
51. Gray DL and Crane JP (1994). Optimal nuchal skin-fold threshold based on gestational age for prenatal detection of Down syndrome. *Am J Obstet Gynecol*, **171**, 1282–6.

52. Watson WJ, Miller RC, Menard K, Chescheir NC, Katz VL, Hansen WF, and Wolf EJ (1994). Ultrasonographic measurement of fetal nuchal skin to screen for chromosomal abnormalities. *Am J Obstet Gynecol*, **170**, 583–6.

53. Bahado-Singh RO, Goldstein I, Uerpairojkit B, Copel JA, Mahoney MJ, and Baumgarten A (1995). Normal nuchal thickness in the midtrimester indicates reduced risk of Down syndrome in pregnancies with abnormal triple-screen results. *Am J Obstet Gynecol*, **173**, 1106–10.

54. DeVore GR and Alfi O (1995). The use of color doppler ultrasound to identify fetuses at increased risk of trisomy 21. An alternative for high risk patients who decline genetic amniocentesis. *Obstet Gynecol*, **85**, 378–86.

55. Grandjean H, Sarramon MF, and AFDPHE Study Group (1995). Sonographic measurement of nuchal skinfold thickness for determination of Down syndrome in the second trimester fetus: A multicenter prosepective study. *Obstet Gynecol*, **85**, 103–6.

56. Borrell A, Costa D, Martinez JM, Delgado RD, Forguell T, and Fortuny A (1997). Criteria for fetal nuchal thickness cut-off: a re-evaluation. *Prenat Diag*, **17**, 23–9.

57. Vintzileos AM, Campbell WA, *et al.* (1997). Second trimester ultrasound markers for detection of Trisomy 21: which markers are best? *Obstet Gynecol*, **89**, 941–4.

58. Cuckle H, Wald N, Quinn J, Royston P, and Butler L (1989). Ultrasound fetal femur length measurement in the screening for Down syndrome. *Br J Obstet Gynaecol*, **96**, 1373–8.

59. Rodis JF, Vintzileos AM, Fleming AD, Ciarleglio L, Nardi D, Feeney L, Scorza WE, Campbell WA, and Ingardia C (1991). Comparison of humerus length with femur length in fetuses with Down's syndrome. *Am J Obstet Gynecol*, **165**, 1051–6.

60. Biagiotti R, Periti E, Cariati E, and Nannini R (1992). Echogenic measuring of the length of the fetal femur length in the screening for Down syndrome. *Minerva Ginecol*, **44**, 609–12.

61. LaFollette L, Filly RA, Anderson R, and Golbus MS (1989). Fetal femur length to detect trisomy 21. A reappraisal. *J Ultrasound Med*, **8**, 657–60.

62. Nyberg DA, Resta RG, Luthy DA, Hickok DE, and Williams MA (1993). Humerus and femur length shortening in the detection of Down's syndrome. *Am J Obstet Gynecol*, **168**, 534–8.

63. Biagiotti R, Periti E, and Cariati E (1994). Humerus and femur length in fetuses with Down syndrome. *Prenat Diagn*, **14**, 429–34.

64. Johnson MP, Michaelson JE, Barr M, Treadwell MC, Hume RF, Dombrowski MP, and Evans MI (1995). Combining humerus and femur length for improved ultrasonographic identification of pregnancies at increased risk for trisomy 21. *Am J Obstet Gynecol*, **172**, 1229–35.

65. Nyberg DA, Luthy DA, Cheng EY, Sheley RC, Resta RG, and Williams MA (1995). Role of prenatal ultrasonography in women with positive screen for Down syndrome on the basis of maternal serum markers. *Am J Obstet Gynecol*, **173**, 1030–5.

66. Verdin SM and Economides DL (1998). The role of ultrasonagraphic markers for Trisomy 21 in women with positive serum biochemistry. *Br J Obstet Gynaecol*, **105**, 63–7.

67. Marquette GP, Boucher M, Desrochers M, and Dellaire L (1990). Screening for trisomy 21 with ultrasonographic determination of biparietal diameter/femur length ratio. *Am J Obstet Gynecol*, **163**, 1604–5.

68. Nyberg DA, Luthy DA, *et al.* (1998). Age-adjusted ultrasound risk assessment for fetal Down's syndrome during the second trimester: description of the method and analysis of 142 cases. *Ultrasound Obstet Gynecol*, **12**, 8–14.

69. Benacerraf BR, Mandell J, Estroff JA, Harlow BL, and Frigoletto FD (1990). Fetal pyelectasis: A possible association with Down syndrome. *Obstet Gynecol*, **76**, 58–60.
70. Corteville JE, Dicke JM, and Crane JP (1992). Fetal pyelectasis and Down syndrome: Is genetic amniocentesis warranted? *Obstet Gynecol*, **79**, 770–2.
71. Bromley B, Doubilet P, Frigoletto FD, Krauss C, Estroff JA, and Benacerraf BR (1994). Is fetal hyperechoic bowel on second trimester sonogram an indication for amniocentesis? *Obstet Gynecol*, **83**, 647–51.
72. Copel J, Cullen M, Green JS, *et al.* (1988). The frequency of aneuploidy in prenatally diagnosed congenital heart disease: an indication for fetal karyotype. *Am J Obstet Gynecol*, **158**, 409–13.
73. Allen LD, Sharland GK, and Chita SK (1991). Chromosomal abnormalities in fetal congenital heart disease. *Ultrasound Obstet Gynecol*, **1**, 8–11.
74. Brown DL, Emerson DS, Schulman LP, *et al.* (1993). Predicting aneuploidy in fetuses with cardiac anomalies. *J Ultrasound Med*, **3**, 153–61.
75. Paladini D, Calabro R, Palmieri S, and D'Andrea T (1993). Prenatal diagnosis of congenital heart disease and fetal karyotyping. *Obstet Gynecol*, **81**, 679–82.
76. Vintzileos AM and Egan JFX (1995). Adjusting the risk for Trisomy 21 on the basis of second-trimester ultrasonography. *Am J Obstet Gynecol*, **172**, 837–44.
77. Nicolaides KH, Sebire NJ, Snijders RJM, and Johnson S (1996). Down's syndrome screening in the UK. *Lancet*, **347**, 906–7.
78. Wald NJ and Hackshaw AK (1997). Combining ultrasound and biochemistry in first-trimester screening for Down's syndrome. *Prenat Diagn*, **17**, 821–9.
79. Nicolaides KH, Snijders RJM, and Cuckle HS (1998). Correct estimation of parameters for ultrasound nuchal translucency screening. *Prenat Diagn*, **18**, 519–20.
80. Nicolaides KH, Campbell S, Gabbe SG, and Guidetti R (1986). Ultrasound screening for spina bifida: cranial and cerebellar signs. *Lancet*, **ii**, 72–4.
81. Campbell J, Gilbert WM, Nicolaides KH, and Campbell S (1987). Ultrasound screening for spina bifida: cranial and cerebellar signs in a high risk population. *Obstet Gynecol*, **70**, 247–50.
82. Pilu G, Romero R, Reece EA, Goldstein I, Hobbins JC, and Bovicelli L. (1988). Subnormal cerebellum in fetuses with spina bifida. *Am J Obstet Gynecol*, **158**, 1052–6.
83. Goldstein RB, Podrasky AE, Filly RA, and Callen PW (1989). Effacement of the fetal cisterna magna in association with myelomeningocele. *Radiology*, **172**, 409–13.
84. Thiagarajah S, Henke J, Hogge WA, Abbitt PL, Breeden N, and Ferguson JE (1990). Early diagnosis of spina bifida: the value of cranial ultrasound markers. *Obstet Gynecol*, **76**, 54–7.
85. Van den Hof MC, Nicolaides KH, Campbell J, and Campbell S (1990). Evaluation of the lemon and banana signs in one hundred thiry fetuses with open spina bifida. *Am J Obstet Gynecol*, **162**, 322–7.
86. Petrikovsky BM (1990). Fruit signs and neural tube defects. *Prenat Diagn*, **10**, 134.
87. Blumenfeld Z, Siegler E, and Bronshtein M (1993). The early diagnosis of neural tube defects. *Prenat Diagn*, **13**, 863–71.
88. de Courcy-Wheeler RHB, Pomeranz MM, Wald NJ, and Nicolaides KH (1994). Small fetal transverse cerebellar diameter: a screening test for spina bifida. *Br J Obstet Gynaecol*, **101**, 904–5.
89. Penso C, Redline RW, and Benacerraf BR (1987). A sonographic sign which predicts which fetuses with hydrocephalus have an associated neural tube defect. *J Ultrasound Med*, **6**, 307–11.

90. Chambers SE, Muir BB, and Bell JE (1988). Bullet-shaped head in fetuses with spina bifida: a pointer to the spinal lesion. *J Clin Ultrasound*, **16**, 25–8.

91. Gabbe SG, Mintz MC, Mennuti MT, and McDonnell AE (1998). Detection of open spina bifida by the lemon sign: pathologic correlation *J Clin Ultrasound*, **16**, 399–402.

92. Nyberg DA, Mack LA, Hirsch J, and Mahony BS (1988). Abnormalities of fetal cranial contour in sonographic detection of spina bifida: evaluation of the 'lemon' sign. *Radiology*, **167**, 387–92.

93. Donnenfeld AE (1995). Prenatal sonographic detection of isolated fetal choroid plexus cysts: should we screen for trisomy 18? *J Med Screen*, **2**, 18–21.

19 *Amniocentesis and chorionic villus sampling*

Christine Gosden, Ann Tabor, Ian Leck, Adrian Grant, Zarko Alfirevic, and Nicholas Wald

INTRODUCTION

Amniocentesis and chorionic villus sampling (CVS) are methods which have the aim of obtaining tissue of the same genetic origin as the fetus for diagnostic purposes without removing any tissue from the fetus itself. These purposes include the diagnosis of chromosomal anomalies (most often Down's syndrome) and Mendelian genetic disorders (e.g. inborn errors of metabolism). Amniocentesis is also performed to allow for the measurement of amniotic fluid bilirubin in Rh-incompatible pregnancies (Chapter 12) and of amniotic alpha fetoprotein and acetylcholinesterase in the diagnosis of open neural tube defects (Chapter 3). Amniocentesis can be used therapeutically to induce abortion or to relieve a uterus distended by hydramnios, but these are not relevant to our subject.

Amniocentesis has been used for longer than CVS in diagnosing fetal disorders. The karyotyping of cultured amniotic fluid cells was reported in 1966.[1] The first examples of antenatal detection of severe inherited metabolic disorders were described in 1968.[2] In 1972 Brock and Sutcliffe reported that open neural tube defects could be detected by amniotic fluid alphafetoprotein analysis.[3] First-trimester CVS emerged in the early 1980s as an alternative to second-trimester amniocentesis for obtaining tissue of the same genetic origin as the fetus. CVS had the obvious attraction of allowing an earlier diagnosis and therefore an earlier termination of pregnancy if indicated.

SAMPLING AND CULTURING PROCEDURES

Amniocentesis

Features of amniotic fluid and amniotic fluid cells

Amniotic fluid production begins in the sixth week of pregnancy and continues until term. Fetal urine is its major source in the latter half of pregnancy, but first enters the amniotic space at 8–11 weeks gestation. The most likely source of amniotic fluid very early in pregnancy is an inward transfer of solute across the amnion with water following passively.

Amniotic fluid cells are derived from the fetal skin, the urogenital tract, respiratory tract, gastrointestinal tract, umbilical cord, epithelium of the amniotic membrane, and cells from the upper layer of trophoblast which migrate through pores in the amniotic membrane.[4-6] Cells derived from extraembryonic membranes, cord and trophoblast predominate until nearly half-way through pregnancy. After this time, the change from fetal periderm to epidermis together with the increased circulation of amniotic fluid accompanied by much greater fetal swallowing, production of fetal urine, and flow through the fetal urinary tract causes the number of cells derived from the fetus itself to increase.[6,7]

The cell content of amniotic fluid samples increases steadily with gestation. The proportion of viable cells among the total decreases from about 20 per cent at 14 weeks to less than 5 per cent in the third trimester.

Sampling procedure

Amniocentesis is now always performed by the abdominal route. In early pregnancy, the vaginal route has been used, but it is unsatisfactory, with a high culture failure rate (17 per cent in one study[8]) because of bacterial or fungal overgrowth.

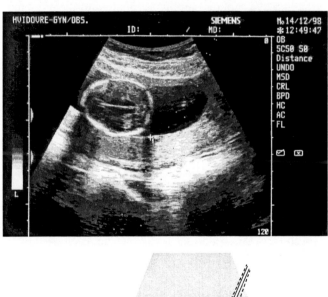

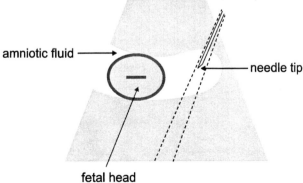

Fig. 19.1 Second-trimester amniocentesis under ultrasound-guidance, as seen on the ultrasound display and in a line drawing. The punctured line represents the needle guide.

The use of *ultrasound* (Fig. 19.1) to guide needle insertion reduces the failure rate of amniocentesis.[9,10] A correlation between the use of ultrasound (before or during amniocentesis) and the post-amniocentesis rate of miscarriage has never been demonstrated, but it is generally agreed that amniocentesis should be performed with the help of real-time ultrasound scanning, preferably under direct ultrasound guidance.[11]

The *experience* of the operator has been shown to be of importance. The failure rate of amniocentesis,[10] the rate of feto-maternal haemorrhage during amniocentesis,[12] and the miscarriage rate[13] are reduced with greater operator experience. In Denmark, the National Board of Health recommends that a gynaecologist should learn the technique by doing 100 amniocenteses under supervision, and then keep up the routine by doing 200 amniocenteses per year.[14]

The miscarriage rate increases when the *size of needle* used exceeds 18[15] or 20[9] Gauge. Most centres now employ the narrower Gauge 20–22 needle, corresponding to an external diameter between approximately 0.9 and 0.7 mm.

The risk of fetal loss increases with the *number of needle insertions*.[9,15] Current practice is therefore to perform only two attempts at amniocentesis on the same day. If unsuccessful, the procedure should be postponed for a week. Failure to retrieve fluid suggests that the pregnancy is not developing normally, and therefore may *per se* have an increased risk of miscarriage.

Perforation of the placenta by the needle was followed by a substantially increased risk of miscarriage in two large studies, although not in two rather smaller ones in which all amniocenteses were performed by a single physician (Table 19.1). Despite the latter finding, it is widely agreed that, whenever possible, placental perforation should be avoided. If the placenta covers the whole anterior uterine wall and therefore cannot be bypassed, many centres postpone amniocentesis for one to two weeks.

In summary, amniocentesis should be performed with standard aseptic precautions, under ultrasound guidance, by a trained operator regularly performing the procedure, taking care to avoid placental perforation, and with no more than two insertions per patient on the same day, using needles no larger than 20-Gauge.

In twin pregnancies, retrieval of amniotic fluid from both sacs used to be secured by injecting a marker (dye or chemically recognizable substance) into the first sac. Fluid subsequently removed from the second sac could then be recognized by the absence of the marker. The advent of real-time ultrasound has made dye-injection obsolete, since it allows visually guided amniotic fluid sampling from both sacs.[20]

Table 19.1   Spontaneous abortion rate following amniocentesis in singleton pregnancies according to whether the test was done transplacentally

Study	*n*	Rate of placental perforation (%)	Abortion rate (%)	
			Transplacental amniocentesis	No placental perforation
Crane and Kopta 1984[16]	998	35	0.9	0.9
Hanson *et al.* 1985[17]	2136	29	1.8	1.6
Tabor *et al.* 1986[18]	2302	15	2.9	1.2
Kappel *et al.* 1987[19]	7181	15	2.7	1.7

Timing in pregnancy

Although removal of amniotic fluid is possible from the seventh week of pregnancy, the usual time for carrying out amniocentesis has been the 14th–16th week of pregnancy. Success rates for fetal karyotyping at this time now exceed 99 per cent in most centres. Results are usually available between 16 and 19 weeks of gestation. If the pregnancy is to be terminated, the woman has to go through a late abortion. This may cause greater physical and emotional distress than a first-trimester termination. The risks of complications are also greater. While the risk of maternal death from termination is low (14 per million at 11–12 weeks of gestation in the United States) it increases nearly seven-fold from about 11 weeks to 18 weeks of gestation; and the incidence of other major complications increases nearly three-fold.[21,22] There are therefore advantages in performing antenatal diagnosis earlier.

Until recently, early amniocentesis (before 15 weeks) was thought to be contraindicated because during this period the volume of amniotic fluid is small (so that the proportion of fluid that is removed at amniocentesis is greater) and cell numbers are low. Improved ultrasound in the first trimester and the development of new sampling and culture techniques have combined to make early amniocentesis possible, but the number of cases reported is still small.[23–30] The technique is similar to amniocentesis performed at later gestational ages, but in up to 5 per cent of procedures aspiration of fluid may be hampered due to tenting of membranes.[31] Most authors recommend the removal of approximately 1 ml of amniotic fluid per week of gestation.[24–26] This volume has been chosen as a balance between the number of living cells present in the amniotic fluid and the volume of amniotic fluid which may be removed without increasing the risk of miscarriage.

There are still difficulties with early amniocentesis. Because the cells sampled are predominantly of extra-embryonic origin, they come from cell lines which diverged from the fetus very early in embryonic life. They may therefore differ in karyotype from the fetus itself.

During the first trimester, unlike the second, two sacs are present—the amniotic cavity and the extra-embryonic coelom. The fluid in the latter is jelly-like and difficult to aspirate, and has a different alphafetoprotein concentration to amniotic fluid.[32]

The greatest difficulty with early amniocentesis is that the success rate of karyotyping amniotic fluid cells in the first trimester is low. It used only to be between 60 and 75 per cent,[33] although after 11 completed weeks the success rate approaches that in the second trimester.[30] The karyotyping success rate may be increased by using a new filter technique,[34] in which the amniotic fluid is aspirated into a syringe as is normally done, but the cells are retained on a filter, while most of the amniotic fluid is reinjected into the uterus. This technique has been shown to reduce the reporting time, but the possible complications of this method still have to be evaluated.

Amniotic fluid alphafetoprotein and acetylcholinesterase measurements that are of use in the diagnosis of neural tube defects can be obtained from 12 weeks of gestation.[35] This is a benefit of amniocentesis at this time which chorionic villus sampling does not offer.

Cell culture and the use of uncultured cells

It is tempting to use uncultured cells for antenatal diagnosis because of the advantages of obtaining a rapid result (the cells are available for immediate analysis) and because it avoids cell culture which is complicated, expensive, liable to problems of slow cell growth or infection and, above all, time-consuming. Uncultured amniotic fluid cells have been used for a number of different diagnoses and Huisjes[4] has reviewed their uses. In the second trimester, the three principal uses are for the detection of biochemical abnormalities,[36] for the isolation of DNA for recombinant DNA analysis, and for rapid fetal sexing using X and Y chromatin.

The use of uncultured cells is hindered by three related problems—maternal blood cell contamination, a preponderance (usually more than 80 per cent) of dead or dying cells in the sample, and a frequency of cell division so low that uncultured cell studies result in successful cytogenetic analysis in 1 per cent of cases or less. The dead cells release proteolytic and lysosomal enzymes as well as DNAase and RNAase, and the resulting degradation products sometimes cause diagnostic problems, especially for metabolic disorders and some DNA analyses.

Determination of sex chromatin status (either X chromatin (Barr bodies) or Y bodies) may also be difficult in dead cells, which have pyknotic nuclei.[37] Although the scope for using uncultured cells is increasing as chromosome-specific probes and fluorescent *in situ* hybridization open up the prospects of detecting chromosomal abnormalities on interphase cells,[38] dead cells cause problems even with these methods, and usually less than 60–70 per cent of the cells examined show the appropriate number of signals, e.g. three fluorescent signals in trisomy 21 with a chromosome 21 specific probe.[39]

Because of the difficulties in using uncultured cells, amniotic fluid cells are generally cultured for about two weeks. The cultured cells can be used to test for metabolic or biochemical disorders caused by many genetic diseases; and mitotic figures can be observed in dividing cells so that chromosomal abnormalities can be detected. Cell culture has the advantage that it separates viable cells (which adhere to the surface of the culture vessels) from dead or dying amniotic fluid cells and maternal blood cells.

Chorionic villus sampling

Features of chorionic villi

Divergence between the embryological cell line that gives rise to the chorionic villi (the placenta) and the line that forms the fetus occurs at a very early stage of gestation, probably prior to the 64 cell blastocyst. At about six days after conception, cells of the trophoblast (which will form much of the chorion and placenta) penetrate the endometrial mucosa and begin to grow deep into the endometrium. The trophoblast then differentiates into two layers, the cytotrophoblast which remains mitotically active and the syncytiotrophoblast which is in direct contact with the maternal endometrium. The syncytiotrophoblast develops fluid-filled spaces and forms, as its name implies, a multinucleated syncytium. The spaces in the syncytiotrophoblast later become continuous with the maternal blood vessels and form the utero-placental circulation. At about 14 days from conception, proliferations of the cytotrophoblast into the fluid-filled cavities in the syncytiotrophoblast form 'primary' chorionic villi. At about 15–20 days from conception, mesenchymal cells invade the villi, where some of them differentiate to form blood vessels; the villi are called 'secondary' while they have a mesenchymal core but no blood vessels, and 'tertiary' when vascularized. Growth occurs at the tips of the tertiary villi until they reach the maternal endometrium. There is rapid development of side branches of these anchoring villi between 21 and 28 days after conception; and from this time until the end of the second month of pregnancy the entire surface of the gestational sac is covered with villi, thus increasing the surface area for maternal–fetal exchange. During and beyond the third month the villi continue to develop in the placental area; but over the rest of the chorion they atrophy and disappear by about 14 weeks of gestation.

Sampling procedures

Chorionic villi may be sampled through the uterine cervix (transcervical) or through the maternal abdomen (transabdominal).

In transcervical CVS, a flexible cannula is passed through the uterine cervix, usually under ultrasound guidance.[40,41] Villi can be removed using biopsy forceps, or more commonly by aspiration through the cannula.[42]

In transabdominal CVS, a two-stage approach is widely used. A hollow needle with a stylette is first introduced under ultrasound guidance through the abdominal wall and myometrium to a point near the placental edge. A finer needle is then passed down inside the introducer until it protrudes slightly beyond the tip of the introducer, deeper into the chorionic villi but not beyond the fused chorionic and amniotic membranes which form the edge of the gestation sac. Villi are then removed by aspiration. The technique may be carried out 'free-hand' with the introducer separate from the ultrasound transducer, or with the needle attached to the transducer.[43]

Cell culture and the use of uncultured cells

During CVS, villi are removed together with maternal blood clot and maternal decidua. The maternal tissues are usually intimately associated with the fetal tissues and their removal necessitates dissection of all the visible adherent maternal tissue under a dissecting microscope. Failure to remove decidua and blood clot from the sample may result in maternal cell contamination—a source of misdiagnosis if the maternal cells are karyotyped. No ways of removing contaminating maternal cells by mechanical methods, enzymatic digestion, or cell lysis methods have yet been devised. For this reason, processing is more labour-intensive and demands more specialist expertise for CVS than for amniocentesis.

Two methods of processing are used: direct preparation (implying examination after no more than 48 hours of incubation) and long-term culture. These methods use different tissue layers and cell lineages, yield results over different periods, and are therefore associated with different error rates. The mitotic divisions studied in direct preparations are those occurring in the chorionic villus cells at the time of sampling. It is possible to obtain a karyotype within 3–4 hours, although this may be extended to 24–48 hours by subjecting the villi to short-term culture to provide better-quality divisions. The advantage of this method is the speed of diagnosis. Its principal disadvantage is that direct preparations are prone to false-positive results because the mitotic figures obtained from direct preparations or from short-term cultures are derived from the cytotrophoblastic layer of the chorionic villi; these cells diverge from the fetus at an earlier stage in embryological development than the mesenchyme from which the long-term cultures are derived, and are more likely to acquire a different karyotype. This can lead to findings such as uniparental disomy (a karyotype in which both chromosomes of a pair are inherited from the same parent) and mosaicism. Another disadvantage of direct preparations is that they may be of poor quality and so lead to false-negative results.

The cells from the mesenchymal layer of the villi which give rise to long-term cultures are derived from the embryonic epiblast. As well as these mesenchymal cells being less likely to differ in karyotype from the fetus than the cells examined by the direct method, the technical quality (including banding) of the cultured preparations is superior to that of the direct preparations, reducing the risk of false-negative results.

These advantages of long-term culture are offset by some disadvantages. The cultures take some 5 to 14 days to grow and karyotype, so there is a longer wait for results. Sometimes the cells may fail to grow, or become infected, necessitating another test. Antibiotics—commonly penicillin, streptomycin, and a fungicide—are included in the culture medium to reduce the risk of infection. Another source of difficulty in long-term culturing is that abnormal or contaminating maternal cells sometimes achieve a higher mitotic rate than the normal cells of the conceptus, and so become predominant. This may accentuate confined placental mosaicism or maternal cell contamination. Maternal cell contamination may be minimized by dissection of the maternal tissue from the villi prior to culture, but it remains a problem.

EXAMINATION OF CELLS

Chromosome analysis

Indications

The principal indication for cytogenetic analysis of amniotic fluid cells or chorionic villi is increased risk for trisomy 21. Serum screening for Down's syndrome is now widely available and can detect over 85 per cent of affected pregnancies with a 0.9 per cent false-positive rate (see Chapter 4). Sometimes karyotyping is indicated because a specific condition other than Down's syndrome is suspected, for example when there is a family history of pregnancy or child with a chromosome disorder, or a balanced chromosomal abnormality in one of the parents, or an abnormal ultrasonogram of the fetus.[2,44] Certain fetal structural malformations, e.g. of the skeleton, kidneys and heart, carry risks of chromosome disorder which may be as high as 10–20 per cent. Less frequent indications for chromosome analysis in pregnancy are maternal anxiety, exposure to radiation or radioisotopes, risk of chromosomal instability syndromes, and parental treatment for cancer.

CVS and amniocentesis data have been used to examine the extent to which Down's syndrome and other trisomies decline in prevalence through mid and late pregnancy as a result of the high natural fetal loss rates in these disorders. It is estimated that in the absence of intervention, 31 per cent of fetuses with Down's syndrome who are alive at the time when CVS is performed (about 11 weeks) are lost by the time when amniocentesis is performed (about 16 weeks), and a further 17 per cent are lost before term.[45,46]

This implies the loss of about 48 per cent of affected fetuses who are alive at 11 weeks and 25 per cent who are alive at 16 weeks. Greater losses occur in other trisomies: in one study[47] the frequency of trisomy 13 and 18 fell from 30 per cent of all trisomic fetuses at 9–14 weeks to 22 per cent at 15–20 weeks, and 14 per cent at birth.

Procedure

At present, it is customary to look for chromosomal abnormalities by undertaking full karyotyping of the CVS or amniotic fluid cell preparation, and to offer termination if a serious abnormal karyotype is found (usually Down's syndrome). When mosaicism or certain other anomalies are observed, it may be necessary to take a further sample for karyotyping (an amniotic fluid sample if the sample already karyotyped was a CVS, or even a fetal blood sample if amniotic fluid cells have already been karyotyped[48]), mainly to determine whether the abnormality is present in the fetus itself as opposed to being confined to extra-embryonic tissue.

Increasingly, methods other than karyotyping are also being used to examine CVS or amniotic fluid cells for chromosomal anomalies in pregnancies in which the results of serum screening are positive. One such method is fluorescence *in situ* hybridization (FISH) using chromosome-specific DNA probes. This technique is applicable to uncultured interphase cells from chorionic villi or amniotic fluid, in which it can detect 13, 18 and 21 trisomies, X and Y abnormalities, and other anomalies for which probes are available.[49,50]

Another technique based on DNA analysis of uncultured amniotic fluid cells is the amplification of polymorphic chromosome-specific DNA markers by polymerase chain reaction (PCR). This test relies on the fetus being heterozygous for one or more of the marker genes, in which case the number of chromosomes of the type under consideration (e.g. chromosome 21) can be determined by analysing the products of the PCR on a DNA sequencer.

The tests based on FISH and PCR share the advantage of giving results more quickly than cell culture followed by karyotyping, since they use freshly sampled cells; but their performance has not yet been quantified sufficiently to indicate whether they should replace karyotyping in the diagnosis of Down's syndrome and other aneuploidies.

Sources of error

Attempts to determine the karyotype may fail or give false-positive or false-negative results. Culture failure can occur after amniocentesis or CVS when there are too few viable cells in the sample. Amniocentesis can also be followed by culture failure (1) when the amniotic fluid is heavily contaminated by blood or its breakdown products, and (2) when (as occasionally happens) the predominant cells are of a large flat type in which few, if any, mitoses are seen. After CVS, a direct preparation or culture may be recognized to have failed even when cells in metaphase are present, if these cells (1) are obviously of maternal origin or of poor quality (e.g. hypodiploid), or (2) exhibit variations in karyotype which are thought to be artifacts and not signs that two or more cell lines with different karyotypes have arisen during the development of the fetus and placenta. Another cause of failure in long-term cultures after CVS is overwhelming contamination by micro-organisms.

When a culture is obtained, it may yield false-positive or false-negative results as a consequence of mosaicism, death of an unrecognized twin, maternal cell contamination, and laboratory and technical errors.

Mosaicism

Mosaicism is the term used to describe the presence of two (or more) different cell lines which have diverged after their derivation from a single conceptus. (The situation when two different cell lines are present but these are derived from two different conceptuses is described as chimaerism; the chimaera of Greek mythology was part lion, part goat, and part serpent.)

Usually in chromosomal mosaicism, there is one normal cell line which retains the original karyotype, and one line in which the karyotype is abnormal because of a somatic mutation in the cell from which this line has arisen. If the mutation occurred very early in development, both lines may be present throughout the fetus and placenta. With mutations occurring later, after the embryo and placenta have become distinct, the fetal cells may be normal and the extra-embryonic ones mosaic, or vice versa. Conversely, if the original karyotype is trisomic, one of the three chromosomes may later be lost in some or all the cells of the fetus or in the placenta. When this occurs in a fetus and the lost chromosome is paternal, the fetus is left with maternal uniparental disomy, which can lead to antenatal loss, intra-uterine growth retardation, and other disorders (e.g. Prader–Willi syndrome if there is uniparental disomy for chromosome 15[52]).

Even cases in which mosaicism is present throughout the fetus and placenta can be missed by CVS or amniocentesis, since normal and abnormal cells may not both be represented in the particular sample examined. When the fetus and some extra-embryonic tissues differ in karyotype, the results of CVS are much more likely to be false-positive or false-negative so far as the fetus is concerned, especially if karyotyping is carried out on a direct preparation: the cells seen in direct preparations are from the cytotrophoblastic cell line, which diverges from the fetal line at an earlier stage in development than the mesenchymal line from which CVS cultures derive (see pp. 475–6). Differences in karyotype between the fetus and extra-embryonic tissues may also lead to false-positive and false-negative results with amniocentesis, especially at 16 weeks or earlier (when a majority of amniotic fluid cells are extraembryonic in origin).[53]

There are a few conditions, not generally regarded as forms of mosaicism, in which chromosomal abnormalities are found in some cells but not others. These are syndromes caused by karyotypic abnormalities which do not express themselves in every tissue. For example, in the Pallister Killian syndrome the chromosomal abnormality is expressed in fibroblasts but cannot usually be detected in cultured blood cells. In these syndromes, karyotyping will give a false-negative result if carried out on tissues in which the abnormality is not expressed.

Death of an unrecognized twin

After a karyotypically abnormal twin has died, abnormal cells derived from its chorion may persist, and be sampled if an attempt is made to carry out CVS or amniocentesis on the surviving fetus. If this sample is karyotyped, it will give a false-positive result for the surviving twin, if this is normal. This is a form of chimaerism rather than of mosaicism, but without full genetic analysis it is difficult to recognize that this is the case. It is particularly likely to occur in pregnancies of older women, because both the risk of multiple pregnancy and the risk of chromosomal abnormality rise as maternal age increases.

Maternal cell contamination

In amniocentesis, the specimen may be contaminated by maternal blood cells following haemorrhage from the perforation caused by the needle, or by a plug of other cells which may enter the needle as it penetrates the maternal tissues. To avoid the latter complication, the operator may use a stylet or discard the first 1–2 ml of the aspirated sample.

In CVS, contamination may occur if the maternal decidua and blood clot that are often firmly attached to the villous sample are not removed. Any maternal cells that remain in this sample may grow more rapidly in culture than cells from the mesenchymal core of the villi. This is because they have better access to the surface of the culture vessel and culture medium (the mesenchymal villous core may be covered in layers of syncytiotrophoblast, cytotrophoblast, and basement membrane) and because they have a higher cellular proliferation rate. This means that the proportion of maternal cells may increase with time in culture.[54]

The most common presentation of maternal cell contamination is a 46,XX/46,XY karyotype. Genuine mosaicism of this type (which may lead to true hermaphroditism or intersexuality) is rare (about 1 in 10 000 births), so the likelihood when an XX/XY karyotype is found in cells from CVS or amniocentesis is that the fetus is male and maternal contamination has occurred. To determine whether this is the case, it is necessary to determine whether the XX cell line is of maternal origin by testing it for maternal cell markers (i.e. comparing chromosomal heteromorphisms in metaphases from this line and from a cultured maternal blood sample).

Extreme levels of maternal cell contamination will give rise to a 46,XX karyotype. If the fetus has a trisomy or other karyotypic error, this diagnosis will be missed. In the case of a normal male fetus, the fetal gender will be misdiagnosed. However, if the fetus is a normal female, no diagnostic error will be made despite the fact that the wrong cells have been karyotyped. Testing for maternal cell markers may therefore also be indicated if a 46,XX karyotype is found in cells from amniocentesis or CVS where heavy maternal cell contamination is suspected.

Laboratory and technical errors

There is always a risk that samples from different pregnancies or the reports on them may become mixed up so that normal fetuses are reported to be abnormal and vice versa. Such laboratory errors can be expected to happen mainly in the processes involved in CVS, which are more labour-intensive and have more stages than the procedures associated with amniocentesis.

Technical errors—those due to chromosomal changes during processing, and observer error—can also lead to both false-positive and false-negative reports. False-positive findings include apparent aneuploidy, usually due to loss of a chromosome; sex chromosome loss leading to a false diagnosis of Turner's syndrome (45,X) is particularly common. Prolonged culture may induce tetraploidy (92,XXXX or 92,XXYY) or tetraploid mosaicism. High levels of antibiotics or hormonal supplementation of culture media[55] may give rise to structural rearrangements such as translocations. Single cell aberrations may occur, and be confused with mosaicism if cell numbers are low. False-positives for technical reasons are more common with CVS than with amniocentesis, because the preparative methods applied to CVS samples lead to more chromosome loss and breakage than occur in the processing of amniotic fluid and cells. This can falsely yield an aneuploid result.

False-negative results for technical reasons most often happen in direct CVS preparations. These are more likely to be of poor quality than are preparations of amniotic fluid cells and long-term CVS cultures; but even with these other methods small chromosomal deletions and rearrangements which are clinically significant may be overlooked, because either the quality of the preparations or the standard of the analysis is unsatisfactory.

Detection of single gene disorders

The single gene disorders which can be diagnosed using amniocentesis or CVS include some for which these tests are indicated only when the family history is positive, and others for which there is also a laboratory-based population screening test.

The conditions for which diagnostic testing is indicated only when there is a positive family history include Duchenne muscular dystrophy, X-linked retinitis pigmentosa (Chapter 5), and most of the inborn errors of metabolism that can be detected in cells of chorionic or amniotic origin (e.g. Hurler and Hunter syndromes, metachromatic leukodystrophy, Pompe's disease, Fabry's disease, congenital adrenal hypoplasia, and ornithine carbamyltransferase deficiency). Most of these disorders are very rare: in Britain, only about 120 antenatal diagnoses of inborn errors of metabolism are made each year.[56] These include cases of at least 20 disorders which can be detected using amniocentesis or CVS.

The conditions for which it is appropriate to offer diagnostic testing when a laboratory-based population screening test is positive include cystic fibrosis, β thalassaemia, sickle-cell disease, and Tay–Sachs disease. These conditions include some (e.g. cystic fibrosis) where the laboratory-based screening test can be offered to the whole population, and others (e.g. Tay–Sachs disease) where this offer should be restricted to a high-risk group (in this case people who are Jewish or have a Jewish parent).

Various procedures are used to test for single gene disorders in cells of chorionic or amniotic origin, including DNA analysis (e.g. for cystic fibrosis) and specific enzyme analysis (e.g. for Tay–Sachs disease). The technology used in these analyses has developed greatly over the past 10 years. Identification of the genes responsible for certain conditions has led to the ability to diagnose these disorders using direct gene analysis, rather than the error-prone techniques of gene tracking using polymorphic markers near to the genes involved but not necessarily very close to them. The introduction of the polymerase chain reaction (PCR) for DNA analysis as an alternative to conventional Southern blotting has reduced the amount of tissue required from sampling, which has improved success rates and safety. The diagnosis of metabolic disorders has benefitted from more sophisticated assay techniques and more complete information about enzyme levels.

As in chromosomal analysis, maternal cell contamination is a problem which can lead to errors when long-term cell culture or PCR DNA analysis is undertaken. Another difficulty is a shortage of data on the performance of testing for most of these disorders. This shortage of data exists partly because positive results may not be confirmed in the fetus if a termination is carried out, and partly because a large number of individually rare disorders are involved, each with its own problems and error rates. To add to this diversity, some conditions occur in different forms (e.g. methylmalonicaciduria) or involve a number of different mutations which give the same phenotype but raise different diagnostic problems (e.g. the mutations leading to β thalassaemia or haemophilia A).

PERFORMANCE

This section will focus mainly on the performance of amniocentesis and CVS in the context of chromosome analysis. This was the context in which most of the available data on performance were gathered. These data came principally from comparisons of the following:

1. *Second-trimester amniocentesis versus neither procedure*—compared in a randomized clinical trial in Danish women aged 25–34,[18] and in four non-randomized studies in centres where amniocentesis was offered mainly to women with fetuses at high risk of chromosomal or neural tube defect (three prospective studies with non-randomized controls in multiple centres in Canada,[9] the United Kingdom,[10] and the United States,[15,57] and one retrospective observational study at a single centre in Los Angeles[58]).

2. *Second-trimester amniocentesis versus early amniocentesis*—compared in two randomized clinical trials in Canadian women who were being tested either on grounds of age or because of other indications involving a genetic risk of less than 0.5 per cent.[59,60]

3. *Second-trimester amniocentesis versus CVS*—compared in randomized clinical trials in Canada,[61] Denmark,[62] and several European countries (the MRC European Study[63]), which were based on women who were mainly seeking antenatal diagnosis because their age put them at increased risk of a trisomy 21 fetus.

4. *Early amniocentesis versus CVS*—compared in a randomized clinical trial in Denmark,[64] and in two trials, one in Britain[30] and one in the Netherlands,[65] in which women could either make their own choice between these two procedures (both done transabdominally) or opt for random allocation.

5. *Transcervical versus transabdominal CVS*—compared in two randomized clinical trials in Italy[66,67] and one each in Denmark[62] and the United States.[68]

The Danish randomized trial of second-trimester amniocentesis and CVS[62] is mentioned twice because it was designed as a three-way comparison (amniocentesis versus transabdominal CVS versus transcervical CVS) amongst women classified as at low genetic risk. All high-risk women in this trial were allocated to one of the two CVS groups. The transcervical approach was used in most of the women investigated by CVS in the other trials of second-trimester amniocentesis versus CVS.

Table 19.2 Failure rates with amniocentesis and CVS

Study	Second-trimester amniocentesis			Early amniocentesis			CVS			Odds ratio (odds of failure for sample failures and laboratory failures) (95% CI)
	Number studied[a]	Sample failure rate[b]	Laboratory failure rate	Number studied[a]	Sample failure rate[b]	Laboratory failure rate	Number studied[a]	Sample failure rate[b]	Laboratory failure rate	
Studies of second-trimester amniocentesis alone										
United States[15]	1040[c]	5.9%[d]	5.6%							
Canada[9]	1020[c]	7.4%[d]	7.0%							
Los Angeles, USA[58]	2000[c]	0.5%	2.2%							
Denmark[18]	2264[c]	0.0%	0.6%							
Studies of second-trimester amniocentesis versus early amniocentesis										
Canada (pilot study)[59]	299[c]	0.3%	0.0%	330[c]	2.4%	0.6%				9.3 (1.2 to 73.1)[e]
Canada (full-scale trial)[60]	1775[c]		0.4%[f]	1916[c]		3.1%[f]				8.0 (3.6 to 17.6)[e]
Studies of second-trimester amniocentesis versus CVS										
Canada[61]	862	2.1%[g]	0.0%				998	9.5%[h]	1.3%	5.7 (3.4 to 9.5)[i]
MRC EuropeanTrial[63]	1464	1.7%[g]	0.6%				1527	5.1%[g]	0.5%	2.5 (1.7 to 3.7)[i]
Denmark[62]	1042	0.0%	0.3%				2037	2.1%	0.6%	9.6 (3.0 to 30.8)[i]
Studies of early amniocentesis versus CVS										
London, UK[30]				731	0.0%	2.3%	570	0.7%	0.5%	0.52 (0.21 to 1.26)[j]
Copenhagen, Denmark[64]				548	0.4%[d]	0.2%	559	1.4%[d]	1.3%	5.0 (1.4 to 17.4)[j]
Leiden, Netherlands[65]				130[k]	1.5%[l]	0.8%	74[k]	4.1%[l]	2.7%	3.1 (0.7 to 13.4)[j]

[a] Number allocated specified procedure (excluding those who did not receive either procedure) except where stated.
[b] Acceptable sample not obtained at first or second attempt, except where stated.
[c] Number in which allocated procedure was carried out.
[d] Acceptable sample not obtained at first attendance for amniocentesis (results not analysed by number of samples).
[e] Odds of failure with early amniocentesis/odds with second-trimester amniocentesis.
[f] Sample failures and laboratory failures.
[g] Number of attempts to obtain an acceptable sample not stated.
[h] Acceptable sample not obtained in up to three attempts.
[i] Odds of failure with CVS/odds with amniocentesis.
[j] Cases at low genetic risk (percentages for CVS estimated by interpolation).
[k] Number in which specified procedure was carried out.
[l] Acceptable sample not obtained at all.

Data on the reliability of cytogenetic diagnosis based on CVS are also available from large observational studies in Italy,[69] the United Kingdom,[70] and the United States.[71]

The above data are our main sources for studying the completeness, reliability, and safety of antenatal diagnosis based on amniocentesis and CVS.

Completeness

The term 'completeness' is here used to denote the proportion of procedures (amniocentesis or CVS) which yield a result (generally a karyotype, sometimes biochemical or DNA data). In most reports that give data on incompleteness, failure to obtain an adequate sample is distinguished from failure at a later stage (laboratory or culture failure). Failure rates of these kinds are given in Table 19.2 for studies in which amniocentesis was studied either alone or alongside CVS. Table 19.3 gives corresponding figures for studies comparing transabdominal and transcervical CVS.

In second-trimester amniocentesis, the average sampling failure rate after two attempts was 0.2 per cent. The average laboratory failure rate was 0.4 per cent in trials of second-trimester amniocentesis carried out since 1980, although it was considerably higher in earlier trials. In the trials of first-trimester amniocentesis, the sampling failure and laboratory failure rates each varied from less than 0.3 per cent to more than 2 per cent. The overall risk of failure after early amniocentesis was significantly higher than after second-trimester amniocentesis in the two trials in which these two methods were directly compared.

The sample failure rate for CVS was consistently and substantially higher than for early or second-trimester amniocentesis, with an average value of 1.8 per cent after two attempts. The average laboratory failure rate with CVS was 0.8 per cent, again higher (although less so) than the rate after second-trimester amniocentesis. The laboratory failure rate was considerably lower after CVS than after early amniocentesis in one of the three trials comparing these procedures, but the reverse was true in the other two.

The overall risk of failure in CVS (i.e. the sum of sampling and laboratory failure

Table 19.3   Failure rates with transabdominal and transcervical CVS

Study	Transabdominal CVS			Transcervical CVS			Odds ratio*
	Number studied[a]	Sample failure rate[b]	Laboratory failure rate	Number studied[a]	Sample failure rate[b]	Laboratory failure rate	
Bologna, Italy[66]	60	13%	0.0%	60	23%	0.0%	2.0 (0.77 to 5.2)
Milan, Italy[67]	575	0.2%	0.7%	581	0.2%	1.5%	2.0 (0.68 to 5.9)
Denmark[62]	1443	1.2%	0.5%	1419	3.1%	0.8%	2.3 (1.4 to 3.7)
United States[68]	1860[c]	1.4%[d]		1879[c]	2.5%[d]		1.8 (1.1 to 2.9)[e]

* Odds of failure with transcervical CVS/odds with transabdominal CVS, for sample failures and laboratory failures except where stated (95% CI).
[a] Number allocated specified procedure (excluding those who did not receive either procedure) except where stated.
[b] Acceptable sample not obtained at first or second attempt, except where stated.
[c] Number in whom allocated procedure was carried out.
[d] Acceptable sample not obtained after one to three attempts (at one attendence).
[e] Ratio based on sample failures alone.

rates) was about twice as high with the transcervical approach as with the trans-abdominal, and this trend was statistically significant in the larger trials (Table 19.3).

Accuracy
Data used in estimating detection and false-positive rates
The estimation of detection and false-positive rates poses a problem because often there is no confirmation of the karyotype in the neonate or terminated fetus, especially when the findings at amniocentesis or CVS are negative. The anomalies of affected fetuses with negative results who die before or soon after birth are not likely to be diagnosed unless fetal karyotyping is undertaken in all cases of miscarriage, still-birth, or neonatal death following amniocentesis or CVS. Even in surviving infants in whom false-negative results have occurred, although important anomalies (mainly Down's syndrome) are likely to be diagnosed eventually, such diagnoses may not be entered in the records of the screening programme.

When CVS or amniocentesis yields a positive result, it is relatively easy to determine whether this is correct by tests on the fetus or newborn; but often this is not done, even when the pregnancy is terminated. For example, 55 per cent of the pregnancies terminated in the MRC European Trial[63] had no confirmatory testing. In support of omitting this, it is argued that the initial tests are reliable on their own, fetal parts are difficult to find after suction termination of pregnancy, and parental stress should not be prolonged.

Data which can be used to estimate false-positive rates and detection rates for specific disorders were only available in six of the reports listed above (p. 481): those dealing with the non-randomized Canadian study in which second-trimester amnio-centesis but not CVS was used,[9] the randomized trials in Canada[61] and Europe[63] in which the two tests were compared, and the observational studies of CVS in Italy,[69] the United Kingdom,[70] and the United States.[71] Comparable data for early amniocen-tesis are not available.

In these studies, some CVS specimens were examined only as direct preparations, others were used only to grow long-term cultures, and others were tested using both methods. The methods of examination used in individual cases were never specified in the trial reports. However, in the reports of the observational studies of CVS, par-ticulars were given of the karyotype seen in the direct preparation and of the kary-otype seen after long-term culture in each case in which these methods were both used and gave discordant findings (except when the discordance was likely to be due only to maternal contamination of one preparation). A discordant pair analysis was undertaken on the pregnancies for which discordant CVS results were reported and for which there was also information on whether the fetus was affected. Table 19.4 gives the results of this analysis for pregnancies in which the karyotype was affected according to one method of examining CVS specimens and unaffected according to the other ($n = 148$), and Table 19.5 gives the results for pregnancies in which there was mosaicism according to one method and a non-mosaic chromosomal anomaly according to the other ($n = 13$).

The fetal findings matched those in the long-term cultures (and not those in the direct preparations) in 101 of the 148 pregnancies in Table 19.4—13 (93 per cent) of 14 in which the fetus was affected and 88 (66 per cent) of 134 in which it was not. The

Table 19.4   Numbers of cases examined by CVS[69-71] in which one type of preparation (direct or long-term culture) contained cells with abnormal karyotypes and the other did not (discordant pair analysis)

Karyotype in positive test	Fetus affected		Fetus unaffected	
	Direct preparation +ve, culture −ve	Direct preparation −ve, culture +ve	Direct preparation +ve, culture −ve	Direct preparation −ve, culture +ve
Trisomy 18[a]	0	2	0	0
Other autosomal aneuploidies	0	1[b]	11	4
Sex chromosome aneuploidies	1[b]	1[b]	10	1
Polyploidy	0	0	3	2
Balanced rearrangements	0	0	2	0
Unbalanced rearrangements	0	0	3	0
Mosaicism	0	9[c]	59	39
Total	1	13	88	46

[a] There were no cases of discordance for trisomy 21 or 13.
[b] The fetus (unlike the abnormal CVS preparation) was mosaic in these cases.
[c] Including one case in which the abnormality was present in all cells of the fetus.

Table 19.5   Numbers of cases examined by CVS[69-71] in which direct preparations and long-term cultures both contained cells with abnormal karyotypes but where the anomaly was mosaic in one type of preparation and homogeneous in the other

Type of anomaly		Fetal karyotype abnormal		Fetal karyotype normal
In direct preparation	In long-term culture	Homogeneous	Mosaic	
Homogenous	Mosaic	0	3[a]	7[b]
Mosaic	Homogeneous	2	0	1

[a] Includes one case in which the direct preparation was 47,XXX, the culture was 45,X/46,XX, and the fetus was 45,X/46,XX/47,XXX.
[b] Includes one case in which the direct preparation was 92,XXYY and the culture was 47,+8/46.

differences between these percentages and 50 per cent (the figure to be expected if both methods were equally accurate) are both highly statistically significant. The 13 pregnancies in Table 19.5 included three cases of concordance for mosaicism and two of concordance for non-mosaic anomalies between fetus and long-term culture, with discordance between these and the direct preparations. The fetus was normal in the remaining eight pregnancies in Table 19.5; and in seven of these pregnancies the long-term cultures were mosaic, and therefore resembled the fetuses more closely than did the matching direct preparations (in which no normal cells were seen). Because of this evidence that long-term cultures are more accurate than direct preparations in diagnosing the karyotype of the fetus, the analyses of detection rates and false-positive rates that follow make use of long-term culture findings in cases where the results obtained with both methods were available. These analyses do not include errors due to maternal contamination, which are discussed later.

Detection rates

Table 19.6 gives the detection rates of chromosomal anomalies from amniocentesis and CVS in the six studies listed in the preceding section as sources of data on

Table 19.6   Detection of chromosomal anomalies: confirmed cases (true-positives and false-negatives) examined by second-trimester amniocentesis or chorionic villus sampling. Results of long-term cultures were used in this analysis in CVS cases where different karyotypes had been reported in cultures and in direct preparations.

	Amniocentesis	Chorionic villus sampling				
	(Canada,[9,61] Europe[63]) n (detection rate %)	Canada,[61] Europe[63] n	United States[71] n	United Kingdom[70] n	Italy[69] n	Total n (detection rate %)
Column no.	(1)	(2)	(3)	(4)	(5)	(6)
All pregnancies	2938	2105	11 436	7415	4787	25 743
Pregnancies with anomalies:						
Trisomy 21	20 (100%)	13	38	65	34	150 (100%)
Trisomy 13 or 18	6 (100%)	5	12	38	17	72 (100%)
Other autosomal aneuploidies	0 (–)	0	1	2	2	5 (100%)
Sex chromosome aneuploidies	3 (100%)	5	17	21	13	56 (100%)
Polyploidy	0 (–)	0	3	3	4	10 (100%)
Balanced rearrangements	20 (100%)	19	–	5[a]	33	52 100%)[b,c]
Unbalanced rearrangements	9 (100%)	1*	11	6***[a]	6*	18** (89%)[b]
Mosaicism	4 (100%)	1	10	9*	8	28* (96%)
Total with anomalies	62 (100%)	44*	92	149****	117*	321* (99.7%)[d]

[a] Non-inherited rearrangements only.
[b] Data from United Kingdom[70] not included.
[c] Data from United States[71] not included.
[d] Rearrangements not included.
* Including one false-negative.
** Including two false-negatives.
*** Including three false-negatives.
**** Including four false-negatives.

detection and false-positive rates. The absolute numbers of confirmed cases are also shown, and each of these numbers that includes one or more missed (i.e. false-negative) cases is accompanied by an asterisk for each missed case.

Columns (1) and (2) of Table 19.6 are based on the randomized Canadian and European trials of amniocentesis and CVS and the non-randomized Canadian study in which amniocentesis but not CVS was used. The data from these studies are pooled because the numbers are relatively small. All three studies were designed mainly to explore the possibility that amniocentesis or CVS was harmful to the fetus, whereas the CVS studies on which columns (3), (4), and (5) are based lacked this incentive to detect anomalies in infants whose CVS results had been negative.

In the three studies shown in columns (1) and (2), no confirmed case was missed by amniocentesis (*n* = 62), and only one (an unbalanced rearrangement) by CVS (*n* = 44). Two confirmed cases (both of Down's syndrome) were, however, missed in the United States' study in which second-trimester amniocentesis but not CVS was used (*n* = 26).[15] This study, like those on which columns (1) and (2) are based, was concerned with the possible hazards of amniocentesis. Its results could not be included in column (1) because no breakdown of the 26 confirmed cases by type of anomaly was published. If these cases had been included in column (1), the detection rate for the anomalies listed would have been 97.7 per cent for amniocentesis (two missed cases in

88) as well as for CVS (one missed case in 44 in the clinical trials). The detection rates for all anomalies combined which were yielded by the two largest observational studies of CVS (columns (3) and (4)) are not directly comparable with these figures, since the observational studies did not cover all rearrangements. Excluding rearrangements, Table 19.6 includes 33 confirmed cases of anomalies tested by amniocentesis, none of which was missed, and 321 tested by CVS, of which one (0.3 per cent) was missed.

CVS would have missed fewer cases if long-term culture had been carried out in all instances instead of direct preparations alone sometimes being used. This is illustrated in the Italian study, in which both methods were used throughout; the detection rate was 99.1 per cent for long-term cultures and only 95.7 per cent for direct preparations.[69]

In summary, high detection rates can be achieved both with amniocentesis and with CVS, and long-term CVS cultures are more sensitive than direct CVS preparations. For Down's syndrome, the detection of which is usually the main aim of antenatal karyotyping, this conclusion about CVS is consistent with the small number of reports in the world literature of cases of Down's syndrome that were missed with CVS. Reports of five affected pregnancies in which direct preparations of CVS tissue were negative have been published,[72–76] and Lilford *et al.*[76] estimated that if half of all such cases had been reported (which seems optimistic) the detection rate of Down's syndrome in direct preparations might be 99.6 per cent. Down's syndrome was correctly identified in long-term culture in three of the five reported cases with false-negative direct preparations, and no cases with false-negative results in both procedures have been reported. Trisomy 18 is another autosomal trisomy that is sometimes missed in direct preparations (Table 19.4).

False-positive rates

Table 19.7 gives false-positive rates based on the same sources as the figures for confirmed cases in Table 19.6. Use of the term 'false-positive' here does not imply that those who reported on the CVS or amniotic fluid cells were mistaken in thinking that these cells were abnormal. All that is implied is that the *fetus* was unaffected.

In Table 19.7 as in Table 19.6, CVS cases in which discrepancies between the findings in direct preparations and long-term cultures were reported were classified according to the findings in long-term cultures. In the Italian study (the only one in which both direct preparations and long-term cultures were examined in all cases), the overall false-positive rate for direct preparations was 10.5/1000—twice as high as the rate for long-term cultures (5.2/1000).[69]

Table 19.7 contains three columns of figures for the pregnancies tested by amniocentesis, three for those tested by CVS in clinical trials, and three for those in each CVS observational study. The first column of each set of three gives the numbers of false-positive results observed (O), the second gives adjusted numbers (A), and the third gives false-positive rates per cent (FPR%) based on the adjusted numbers. The need to adjust the numbers of false-positive results arose because there were many instances where an anomalous karyotype at amniocentesis or CVS was neither confirmed nor excluded at follow up. For example, in the United States study, this was true of 17 out of 60 pregnancies in which the final CVS finding was mosaicism. Among the remaining 43 pregnancies in this group, follow-up was negative in 33 and positive in 10. It seems likely that many of the 17 cases not followed up were also false-positive, in which case the false-positive rate would be under-estimated if calculated

Table 19.7 False-positive results: observed numbers (O) obtained by karyotyping cells derived from amniotic fluid and chorionic villi, adjusted numbers (A) which take account of the lack of follow-up data on some fetuses reported to be positive, and estimated false-positive rates per 100 fetuses (FPR%). Adjusted numbers and false-positive rates were calculated on the assumption that for each anomaly the ratio of true- to false-positives was the same for the total reported to be positive (t) as for the number reported to be positive who were followed up (f). In this case, A = Ot/f, and FPR% = 100A/[n-(ct/f)] where n is the total number of fetuses karyotyped and c is the number with chromosomal anomalies at follow-up. Results of long-term cultures were used in this analysis in CVS cases where different karyotypes had been reported in cultures and in direct preparations.

| | Second-trimester amniocentesis | | | Chorionic villus sampling | | | | | | | | | | | | | | | |
	(Canada,[9,61] Europe[65]) (n = 2938)			Canada,[61] Europe[63] (n = 2105)			United States[71] (n = 11 436)			United Kingdom[70] (n = 7415)			Italy[69] (n = 4787)			Total (n = 25 743)		
	O	A	FPR%	O	A	FPR%	O	A	FPR%	O	A	FPR%	O	A	FPR%	O	A	FPR%
Trisomy 13, 18, or 21	0	0	0	0	0	0	0	0	0	0	0	0	0	0	0	0	0	0
Other autosomal aneuploidies	0	0	0	2	4.0	0.19	6	9.4	0.08	4	11.3	0.15	3	4.8	0.10	15	29.5	0.11
Sex chromosome aneuploidies	0	0	0	1	1.7	0.08	0	0	0	0	0	0	2	2.3	0.05	3	4.0	0.02
Polyploidy	0	0	0	0	0	0	1	2.5	0.02	3	5.0	0.07	1	1.0	0.02	5	8.5	0.03
Balanced rearrangements	0	0	0	0	0	0	–	–	–	1[c]	1.8[c]	0.02[c]	1	1.1	0.02	1[e]	1.1[e]	0.02[e]
Unbalanced rearrangements	0	0	0	0	0	0	0	0	0	0[c]	0[c]	0[c]	0	0	0	0	0	0
Mosaicism[a]	9[b]	13.2	0.45	28[b]	38.6	1.83	33	46.0	0.40	41	62.8	0.85	16[d]	16.0	0.33	118	163.4	0.64
Total[f]	9	13.2	0.45	31	44.3	2.10	40	57.9	0.50	48	79.1	1.07	22	24.1	0.50	141	205.4	0.80

[a] Level II or III mosaicism (i.e. cases in which two or more karyotypes were seen, each in at least two cells) except where stated.
[b] Criteria for diagnosing mosaicism not specified (except in Canadian trial[61] where Levels II and III were accepted).
[c] Non-inherited rearrangements only.
[d] Level III mosaicism (i.e. cases in which two or more karyotypes were seen, each in at least two cells, in multiple colonies or flask cultures of mesenchyme).
[e] Data from United Kingdom[70] and United States[71] not included.
[f] Rearrangements not included.

by dividing 33 by the number of unaffected pregnancies. A more accurate estimate can be obtained by assuming that the 17 cases not followed up were divided betweeen true- and false-positives in the same proportions as the other 43. On this assumption, four of the 17 (i.e. $17 \times 10/43$) would be true-positive and 13 (i.e. $17 \times 33/43$) would be false-positive; there would be a total of 14 true positives (i.e. $4 + 10$) and 46 false-positives (i.e. $13 + 33$); and the false-positive rate would be 0.40 per cent [i.e. $46/(11\,436 - 14)$]. The adjusted numbers of false-positive results and the false-positive rates in Table 19.7 were estimated in this way.

False-positive results occurred in an estimated 0.45 per cent of pregnancies tested by amniocentesis, 2.10 per cent tested by CVS in clinical trials, and 0.50 to 1.07 per cent in the three observational studies of CVS results. Chromosomal rearrangements are excluded from these totals, because the data for them were not comparable between series.

In all the studies listed, most of the false-positive reports were of mosaicism, and most of the variation between the total false-positive rates was due to these cases. Among the pregnancies tabulated in Tables 19.6 and 19.7 for which the condition of the fetus was known, false-positive cases of mosaicism exceeded true mosaics by two to one among the 3000 tested by amniocentesis, and by four to one among the 25 000 tested by CVS. Autosomal aneuploidies other than trisomies 13, 18, and 21 were the only other anomalies listed for which false-positives exceeded true-positives, in this instance by three to one among those tested by CVS. Neither amniocentesis nor CVS yielded any false-positive reports of trisomy 13, 18, or 21 in the studies listed.

Maternal contamination rates

Table 19.8 shows the frequency of 46,XX/46,XY and 46,XX karyotypes in material obtained by amniocentesis or CVS in pregnancies with a male fetus. If the fetus is male, a 46,XX karyotype can be regarded as a false-negative result (since the main purpose of sexing in early pregnancy is to identify males at risk of X-linked disease), whereas 46,XX/46,XY is a mosaic diagnosis and the great majority of reports of it are false-positive (p. 479). The two findings are discussed together here (rather than with other false-negative and false-positive results respectively) because they are both indicative of maternal contamination.

Table 19.8 Frequency of karyotypes generally due to maternal contamination in preparations of amniotic fluid cells or chorionic villi from pregnancies with male fetuses

Procedure	Number of male fetuses			Percentage with XX/XY or XX karyotype
	Estimated total*	XX/XY karyotype	XX karyotype	
Second-trimester amniocentesis				
Canada[9]	504	3	2	1.0
Canada[61]	503	3	0	0.6
Europe[63]	521	3	2	1.0
CVS (direct preparation)				
Canada[61]	455	3	1	0.9
United States[71]	3437	4	0	0.1
CVS (long-term culture)				
Canada[61]	301	18	20	12.6
United States[71]	4378	77	1	1.8

* Taken as 52 per cent of all pregnancies.

The amniocentesis data in Table 19.8 are derived from the trials used in Tables 19.6 and 19.7. The CVS data are taken from only two of the studies in Tables 19.6 and 19.7 (the second Canadian clinical trial[61] and the American observational study[71]), since the other reports did not provide all the data needed to calculate separate rates for direct preparations and long-term cultures. Separate rates are needed because the speed at which maternal cells multiply in long-term cultures may make their prevalence in these cultures higher than in direct preparations (p. 479).

To estimate the percentages of male fetuses for whom 46,XX/46,XY and 46,XX karyotypes were reported, it was assumed that males accounted for 52 per cent of each related population. Unlike in Table 19.7, no adjustment was made for cases not followed up, since 46,XX/46,XY and 46,XX karyotypes in preparations of amniotic fluid cells or chorionic villi are not indications for termination or precursors of spontaneous abortion (the main sources of failure to follow up the karyotypes listed in Table 19.7)—except that as a XX/XY karyotype usually means that the fetus is male, it may lead to termination in the rare event of the mother carrying an X-linked recessive mutation.

Table 19.8 shows that in the three trials, 46,XX/46,XY or 46,XX was reported in about 1 per cent of male pregnancies tested by amniocentesis. The findings for CVS are more heterogeneous. Both in the direct preparations and in the long-term cultures, contamination was several times more common in the Canadian trial[61] than in the United States study.[71] Also, the contamination was extensive enough to produce an XX karyotype as opposed to a mosaic one in many more of the contaminated Canadian cases than of the United States ones. These differences are presumably technical, and make it inappropriate to compare the results of different procedures across studies. It seems more reasonable to compare within studies. When this is done, no significant difference is found between the contamination rates for amniocentesis and CVS direct preparations (0.6 per cent and 0.9 per cent respectively in the Canadian trial) but the rates for long-term cultures are more than 10 times higher than for direct preparations (12.6 per cent versus 0.9 per cent in the Canadian trial and 1.8 per cent versus 0.1 per cent in the United States study).

It therefore seems that although long-term cultures are more accurate than direct preparations for detecting the anomalies considered in Tables 19.4–19.7, they are also much more prone to maternal contamination.

Safety

The main focus of concern about the safety of amniocentesis and CVS is their effects on the risks of miscarriage and perinatal death. There have also been reports of an excess risk of limb deficiencies (i.e. absence of all or part of one or more limbs) in infants born after CVS, and of congenital dislocation of the hip, talipes equinovarus, and neonatal respiratory distress in those born after amniocentesis. Maternal effects include feto-maternal haemorrhage during amniocentesis, vaginal bleeding and spotting after CVS, and amniotic fluid leakage after both tests. More serious maternal effects have not been detected in large-scale studies, although there are case reports of amniotic fluid embolism following amniocentesis and of serious, even fatal, infection following transcervical CVS.[77,78]

Assessing safety is not straightforward. This can be illustrated by consideration of the risk of miscarriage. Any increase will occur against the background of a pre-existing risk of spontaneous miscarriage. It is, however, impossible to predict the background risk of spontaneous miscarriage with any accuracy because this is dependent on other factors. One factor is whether the fetuses under study have been shown by ultrasound examination to be alive at the time in pregnancy from which their survival is being monitored. Also, increased maternal age is associated with increased risk of miscarriage, and the miscarriage rate will necessarily appear higher after earlier testing. For these reasons, it is impossible to judge the extent to which miscarriages observed following amniocentesis or CVS are causally linked to the test by comparing figures from case series or other observational studies. The only way of ensuring that selection bias is avoided is by random allocation of women to alternative policies for antenatal diagnosis. This discussion of safety will therefore focus, when possible, on the few studies of amniocentesis and/or CVS that have been randomized controlled trials.

In all but one of the randomized trials (p. 481), alternative diagnostic procedures were compared. The interpretation of the results of these trials therefore needs to take into account that even the procedure with the lower complication rate may be more hazardous than no procedure at all.

To minimize selection bias in studies of safety based on randomized trials, the denominator used in calculating the risk of adverse outcome in any trial arm should be the total number of pregnancies randomized to that arm (or this number less any pregnancies lost to follow up), and the numerator should be the sum of the following three figures for the arm:

1. *All spontaneous fetal losses from the time of randomization.* This is straightforward if the procedures being compared are performed at the same time of pregnancy; but if, for example, CVS at 11 weeks is being compared with amniocentesis at 16 weeks, it is important to include the fetal losses in the amniocentesis group that occur after randomization but before the procedure is performed. Of course, the amniocentesis could not have caused these fetal losses; but if they are not included the results will be biased in favour of 16-week amniocentesis.

2. *All terminations of pregnancy from the time of randomization.* It is recognized that pregnancies in which the fetus is chromosomally abnormal are at increased risk of spontaneous fetal loss. It follows that CVS at 11 weeks will detect fetal abnormalities (and so lead to termination) in some pregnancies which would have ended in spontaneous fetal loss at 11–16 weeks if they had been randomized to amniocentesis at 16 weeks. If this effect were ignored and only spontaneous fetal deaths in the arms of a trial of these procedures were compared, it would bias the results in favour of CVS. Similarly, if one attempted to assess the safety of amniocentesis by comparing only spontaneous fetal mortality in pregnancies investigated by amniocentesis and in pregnancies in which neither amniocentesis nor CVS was carried out, the results would be biased in favour of amniocentesis.

3. *All infants born alive who are affected by disorders such as Down's syndrome which the procedures under study are designed to diagnose.* If two programmes were being compared and one of them prevented more affected births than the other, ignoring the cases whose birth was not prevented would bias the results against the

more successful programme. For example, if one programme offered amniocentesis and the other did not, and if the only difference in outcome was that termination of pregnancy was carried out in all cases of Down's syndrome in the first programme and none in the second, the risk of adverse outcome would appear to be higher in the first programme than in the second if only spontaneous fetal losses and terminations of pregnancy were counted.

The sum of these three figures gives the total number of fetal losses (from the time in pregnancy beyond which data have been gathered) if all affected pregnancies were terminated, and is hereafter referred to as 'total' fetal losses. Clearly the 'total' fetal loss rate occurring in any arm of a study is not the same as the fetal loss rate caused by the procedure to which the pregnancies in that arm were allocated; but the difference between the 'total' fetal loss rates in two arms will be an unbiased estimate of the excess fetal loss rate (excluding fetuses with defects for which termination of pregnancy was performed) due to the more hazardous of the two procedures being compared.

Using mainly data from the studies listed on p. 481, this review examines the safety of (1) second-trimester amniocentesis (compared with non-intervention); (2) CVS (drawing on the comparisons with second-trimester amniocentesis, comparisons between transabdominal and transcervical CVS, and comparisons of the risk of limb deficiences after CVS and in the general population of births); (3) early amniocentesis (compared with CVS and second-trimester amniocentesis).

Second-trimester amniocentesis

The risk of fetal loss following amniocentesis will be considered first, followed by possible complications of pregnancy and complications in the infants.

Risks of fetal loss

The results of the Danish randomized trial and of the four non-randomized studies of amniocentesis are summarized in Tables 19.9 and 19.10 respectively. In the Danish trial[18] women allocated to the control group had an ultrasound scan to assess fetal viability at the gestational age at which the study group had amniocentesis. To make this design ethically acceptable, the trial was restricted to women aged 25–34 years, who would not otherwise have been offered genetic amniocentesis. Amniocentesis was followed by an excess 'total' fetal loss rate of 0.9 per cent (95 per cent CI = 0.0 to 1.9 per cent). Another procedure for estimating the excess fetal loss rate after amniocentesis yielded a similar result for this study (0.9 per cent; 95 per cent CI = 0.1 to 1.6 per cent).[79] This procedure made use of the excess number of pregnancies terminated for abnormal fetuses in the amniocentesis arm of the trial compared with the number in the control arm. One-third of the excess was added to the number of spontaneous losses in the amniocentesis arm before converting the number to a rate. This was to allow for those of the abnormal pregnancies terminated as a result of amniocentesis that would have miscarried if they had been in the control arm of the trial.

Most of the excess of fetal losses in the amniocentesis arm of the Danish trial was attributed to miscarriages occurring in the first three to four weeks after amniocentesis (Fig. 19.2).

As the study group and control group in the Danish trial seem to be comparable

Table 19.9 Fetal loss in Danish randomized trial comparing low-risk women aged 25–34 who were allocated ultrasound and second-trimester amniocentesis (study group) or ultrasound alone (control group)[18]

	No. of pregnancies studied	Miscarriages and stillbirths			No. of terminations of pregnancy (b)	No of infants born alive with anomalies that were tested for (c)	'Total' fetal losses[b]		
		No. (a)	%	Difference[a] (95% CI)			No. (a + b + c)	%	Difference[a] (95% CI)
Study group	2302	58	2.5%	} 0.7% (−0.1 to 1.5%)	15	0	73	3.2%	} 0.9% (0.0 to 1.9%)
Control group	2304	42	1.8%		6	4	52	2.3%	

[a] Percentage for study group minus percentage for control group.
[b] Total fetal losses if all affected pregnancies were terminated.

Table 19.10 Fetal loss after second-trimester amniocentesis (non-randomized studies)

Source		Percentage of study group having ultrasound before amniocentesis	No. of pregnancies studied	Miscarriages and stillbirths			No of terminations of pregnancy	No. of infants born alive with anomalies that were tested for	'Total' fetal losses[c]		
				No.	%	Difference[b] (95% CI)			No.	%	Difference[b] (95% CI)
				(a)			(b)	(c)	(a + b + c)		
Canada[9]	Study group	98%	447[d,e]	21	4.7%	0.0% (−2.6 to 2.5%)	−[f]	–	–	–	3.4% (1.4 to 5.5%)
	Control group	–	718[e]	34	4.7%		–	–	–	–	
United States[15,57]	Study group	29%	1034	36	3.5%	0.2% (−1.4 to 1.8%)	39	4	79	7.6%	
	Control group	–	978	32	3.3%		1	8	41	4.2%	
United Kingdom[10] (supplementary study)	Study group	68%	1026[e]	38	3.7%	1.6% (0.1 to 3.0%)	63	–	–	–	
	Control group	–	1026[e]	22	2.1%		–	–	–	–	
Los Angeles[58]	Study group	90%	1943	52[g]	2.7%	0.4% (−0.6 to 1.4%)	51	–	–	–	
	Control group	–	2000	46[g]	2.3%		–	–	–	–	

a Excluding losses to follow-up.
b Percentage for study group minus percentage for control group.
c Total fetal losses if all affected pregnancies were terminated.
d Women selected for amniocentesis because they were aged 35 years or more. (The study group also included 518 other pregnancies which were not terminated, of which 12 ended in spontaneous abortions or stillbirth.)
e Denominators do not include terminated pregnancies.
f The whole study group included 1020 pregnancies, of which 55 were terminated.
g Including neonatal deaths.

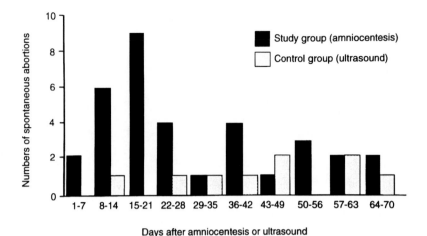

Fig. 19.2 Numbers of spontaneous abortions at different periods after amniocentesis (study group) or ultrasound scan (control group).[18]

with each other and representative of the Danish population,[18] the findings may be generalized to other groups of younger women at low genetic risk. In older women, the miscarriage rate *per se* increases,[80] and there is no reason to believe that the amniocentesis-related miscarriage rate should be any smaller in those women.

In the four non-randomized studies (Table 19.10), the indications for inclusion (especially being at high risk of having a trisomic fetus) meant that the participants tended to be older than most pregnant women. Caution is needed in interpreting these studies, not only because of the risks of selection bias that are common to most comparisons of non-randomized groups, but also because fetal viability was not assessed in the control groups at entry to the studies. As a result the fetal loss rate among controls can be expected to be higher than in the women having an amniocentesis, and this will tend to conceal any fetal losses due to amniocentesis. Another source of bias in this direction in three of the four studies in Table 19.9 is that only their spontaneous fetal loss rates (as opposed to their 'total' fetal loss rates) can be compared. As already indicated (p. 491) comparisons of this kind tend to be biased in favour of amniocentesis when this is compared with a no-procedure control group.

Although biases of these kinds may conceal risks due to amniocentesis, the spontaneous fetal loss rate in each group examined by amniocentesis was at least as high as in the corresponding control group; and in the United Kingdom study,[10] with well over 2000 cases and 2000 controls, there were significantly more fetal losses in the study group. The main part of the United Kingdom study may have been subject to ascertainment bias, mainly because many of the controls were selected later in gestation than the times when amniocentesis was carried out on their matches (so that some potentially acceptable controls might have experienced fetal loss before they had had the opportunity to be selected). However, this was avoided in a supplementary enquiry, from which the data for this study in Table 19.10 are taken. These data confirm the finding of an increased fetal loss rate following amniocentesis: the excess over the rate for the control group was 1.6 per cent (95 per cent CI = 0.1 to 3.0 per cent).

In the United States study, the only non-randomized one for which 'total' fetal loss rates could be compared, Table 19.10 suggests that the excess fetal loss rate following amniocentesis (excluding fetuses with defects for which termination of pregnancy was performed) was 3.4 per cent (95 per cent CI = 1.4 to 5.5 per cent).

The risk of fetal loss due to amniocentesis in twins has not been reliably documented. Among studies of all fetal losses after amniocentesis in twins, much the largest (based on 339 twins) was that of Anderson *et al.*,[81] who reported that 3.6 per cent miscarried before 28 weeks of gestation. This figure does not suggest that amniocentesis is an important cause of fetal loss in twins, given their relatively high background miscarriage rate.

Feto-maternal haemorrhage

This condition tends to raise the level of maternal serum AFP, and has been studied in a randomized trial[12] in which the distribution of changes in AFP in a control group having ultrasonography (*n* = 268) and a study group having amniocentesis (*n* = 283) was compared. This comparison suggested that a feto-maternal haemorrhage had occurred in 17 per cent of the study group during amniocentesis. The rate of feto-maternal haemorrhage was higher after transplacental amniocentesis (26 per cent) than in other cases (15 per cent). When analysed by fetal birthweight, the data gave no support to a previous suggestion[82] that feto-maternal haemorrhage during amniocentesis decreases mean birthweight, but the number of women was too small to draw any conclusion on whether it increases the miscarriage rate, as has also been suggested.[83]

The risk of feto-maternal haemorrhage during amniocentesis causing Rhesus iso-immunization is small—2–3 per cent according to two retrospective studies.[84,85] In a prospective cohort study[86] three women (0.8 per cent) had anti-D in their serum by the time of delivery, and two more by six months later, giving an immunization rate of 1.4 per cent (95 per cent CI = 0.2 to 2.6), which does not differ to a statistically significant extent from the spontaneous immunization rate. The studies are, however, consistent with a 1–2 per cent risk of Rh immunization following amniocentesis. Because of this possibility, and because of the *a priori* grounds for judging that there is a risk, the World Health Organization recommends that a small dose of anti-D be given at the time of amniocentesis to D-negative women.[87] The effectiveness of this procedure has not been proven in a controlled study. A protective effect was, however, suggested by the results of a retrospective study of 300 pregnancies, in which anti-D was given at the time of amniocentesis, and only one woman was immunized.[88] Likewise, the MRC study[10] reported that none of 59 women who had been given anti-D was iso-immunized, as compared with three cases among untreated women.

Other complications of pregnancy

In the Canadian study[9] and the NICHD study,[15] the incidences of maternal complications reported within 72 hours of or in the first week after amniocentesis were 3.6 per cent and 2.4 per cent. The complication rate in the control group was not studied. In the Danish randomized trial,[18] complications were recorded approximately four weeks after amniocentesis or ultrasonography in the study and in the control group, respectively. The women were specifically asked about bleeding, abdominal pain, and amniotic fluid leakage. The complication rate was higher after amniocentesis (12.1 per cent) than after ultrasonography (5.8 per cent). While vaginal bleeding occurred equally often in the two groups, amniotic fluid leakage was reported four times more often in the study group (39 versus 10 women).

Neonatal respiratory difficulties

These were associated with a history of amniocentesis in the randomized Danish trial[18] and the non-randomized MRC trial.[10] The three other studies that compared pregnancies in which amniocentesis was used and non-randomized controls[9,15,58] found no increased incidence of neonatal respiratory difficulties following amniocentesis.

In the MRC study[10] severe unexplained respiratory difficulties at birth were reported significantly more often in babies born to subjects (1.3 per cent) than in controls (0.4 per cent). This increase was most marked in those infants born between 34 and 37 weeks of gestation (8.2 per cent in subjects and 0.9 per cent in controls). The mortality attributable to respiratory distress syndrome was also higher among subjects than controls (0.26 per cent compared with 0.13 per cent). It has, however, been suggested that the experience of the control group was unusually favourable.

In the Danish randomized trial,[18] 1.1 per cent of infants in the study group and 0.5 per cent in the control group developed respiratory distress syndrome. The difference (0.6 per cent) is statistically significant (95 per cent CI = 0.1 to 1.1 per cent). Pneumonia was also diagnosed more often in the study group (15 infants versus 6). The association between amniocentesis and respiratory distress syndrome was independent of birthweight and gestational age.

Several other findings also suggest that amniocentesis affects lung function. Firstly, structural changes were observed in the lungs of baby monkeys after amniocentesis compared with control monkeys.[89] Secondly, in a randomized trial of first-trimester amniocentesis versus CVS,[90] both tests were found to be associated with an increase in the newborn in the proportions of functional residual capacity values below the 2.5 centile of the normal range. Thirdly, a lower ratio of crying vital capacity to birthweight was found in 10 newborns whose mothers had amniocentesis, than in 10 infants born after uneventful pregnancies[91] (although this last difference may have arisen because of the conditions in the first group that led to amniocentesis, rather than because of the test itself).

The association of amniocentesis with respiratory distress syndrome in the only randomized study[18] was not significant enough to prove beyond reasonable doubt that it increases the rate of respiratory difficulties in the newborn. If it does, the reason may be that altered amniotic fluid volume after amniocentesis or subsequent chronic amniotic fluid leakage interferes with normal lung development and lung structure at term, thus giving rise to pulmonary hypoplasia and consequently to respiratory distress syndrome in the newborn.[90] Whether these antenatal and neonatal changes have any long-term impact on lung development remains to be shown.

Other complications in infants

In the main part of the United Kingdom study,[10] the proportion of live births after amniocentesis that occurred before 39 weeks (25 per cent, including 5 per cent before 36 weeks of gestation) was significantly higher ($p < 0.05$) than the corresponding percentage for controls (22 per cent, including 3 per cent before 36 weeks). In the other two trials for which data on gestation length were reported,[18,57] the proportion of infants born before 37 weeks was slightly but not significantly higher after amnio- centesis than in the controls, and mean birthweight was not significantly related to amniocentesis. However, the number of very low birthweight infants, i.e. ≤1500 g, was significantly higher after amniocentesis (21 (0.9 per cent) in the study group versus 9 (0.4 per cent) in the control group) in the randomized controlled trial of amnio- centesis.[18] The rate of low birthweight infants (i.e. 1501–2500 g) was similar in the study and control groups of this trial (89 (4.0 per cent) and 92 (4.0 per cent)).

Injury to the infant may evidently be caused by the needle during amniocentesis. Before the introduction of simultaneous ultrasonography during amniocentesis, severe fetal complications were sporadically reported. Since then Verjaal *et al.*[92] reported needle injury marks on eight out of 1500 babies, while the NICHD study[15] and Tabor *et al.*[18] found no signs of injury attributable to the amniocentesis. Although it has been suggested that only a minority of needle marks are apparent in the neo- natal period,[93] the risk of direct injury to the fetus seems very small. Real-time ultrasonography guidance of the needle tip may further reduce this risk.

Congenital dislocation of the hip and talipes equinovarus were found more often among infants born after amniocentesis in the main part of the MRC study.[10] This finding could not be confirmed in the methodologically more correct supplementary part of the MRC study[10] or the other three trials.[9,15,18] Furthermore a case-control study[94] of 257 cases of talipes and/or hip malformation and 1075 control infants found no association between amniocentesis and talipes or hip malformations. Studies of children to age one year or more have identified no associations between amnio- centesis and physical growth or neurological or mental development.[15,93,95,96] It may be concluded that second-trimester amniocentesis has no proved ill effects on offspring who survive until late pregnancy, although there is some evidence that it increases the risk of respiratory problems.

A procedure more likely than amniocentesis to damage the fetus is the injection of methylene blue into the amniotic sac. This used to be undertaken during amnio- centesis in twin pregnancies to avoid sampling from the same sac twice (p. 472), and appears to cause jejunal atresia: this defect occurred in 17 (10 per cent) of 172 twins in a retrospective study[97] of 86 twin pairs following amniocentesis with injection of 1–2 ml of 1 per cent methylene blue into the first sac, and in 15 of these pregnancies the twin with the atresia could be identified as the one who received the methylene blue. As other dyes have not been evaluated as regards the safety of intrauterine injection, the use of dye injection into the uterus should be avoided as far as possible.

First-trimester chorionic villus sampling

Comparisons with second-trimester amniocentesis

The frequency of spontaneous and 'total' fetal losses in the three large randomized trials[61-63] is compared in Table 19.11. The Canadian and Danish trials of CVS and amniocentesis are each represented by two sets of figures. Amniocentesis is compared with transcervical CVS in the first set of figures for the Danish CVS trial and with transabdominal CVS in the second. For the Canadian trial, two sets of figures are given because some women were allocated to one or other arm before being scanned by ultrasound to exclude 'ineligible' pregnancies (i.e. multiple pregnancies, pregnancies

Table 19.11 Fetal loss in randomized trials comparing first-trimester chorionic villus sampling and second-trimester amniocentesis

Source/test allocated	No. of pregnancies studied	Miscarriages and stillbirths			No. of terminations of pregnancy	No. of infants born alive with anomalies that were tested for (c)	'Total' fetal losses[a]		
		No. (a)	%	Difference[b] (95% CI)	(b)		No. (a + b + c)	%	Difference[b] (95% CI)
Canada[61] (all pregnancies randomized and followed up):									
Transcervical CVS	1363	196	14.4%	2.2% (−0.4 to 4.7%)	34	0	230	16.9%	1.6% (−1.2 to 4.4%)
Amniocentesis	1361	166	12.2%		41	1	208	15.3%	
Canada[61] (pregnancies eligible at first ultrasound and followed up):									
Transcervical CVS	1164	63	5.4%	1.0% (−0.7 to 2.8%)	26	0	89	7.6%	0.5% (−1.6 to 2.7%)
Amniocentesis	1169	51	4.4%		31	1	83	7.1%	
Europe[63]:									
CVS[c]	1609	152	9.4%	3.2% (1.4 to 5.1%)	59	−	211[d]	13.1%	4.3% (2.2 to 6.5%)
Amniocentesis	1592	99	6.2%		41	−	140[d]	8.8%	
Denmark[62][e]:									
Transcervical CVS	1010	86[f]	8.5%	4.0% (1.9 to 6.1%)	24	0	110	10.9%	4.5% (2.0 to 6.9%)
Amniocentesis	1042	47[f]	4.5%		20	0	67	6.4%	
Denmark[62][e]:									
Transabdominal CVS	1027	38[f]	3.7%	−0.8% (−2.5 to 0.9%)	27	0	65[f]	6.3%	−0.1% (−2.2 to 2.0%)
Amniocentesis	1042	47[f]	4.5%		20	0	67[f]	6.4%	

[a] Total fetal losses if all affected pregnancies were terminated.

[b] Percentage for CVS group minus percentage for amniocentesis group.

[c] 72% had transcervical and 28% transabdominal CVS.

[d] Not including infants born alive with anomalies that were tested for.

[e] Excluding women who refused to participate or were found to be ineligible and those with a history of translocation or late termination or a fetus at risk of metabolic disease.

[f] Including neonatal deaths.

beyond 12 weeks of gestation, and those in which the fetus was already dead). These cases are included in the first set of figures and excluded from the second. The first set of Canadian figures is the less likely to be biased; but the second is more comparable to the results of the other trials, since in these all pregnancies were scanned and ineligible ones excluded before allocation.

In the CVS arms of the trials, the transcervical approach was used exclusively in the Canadian study and in nearly three-quarters of pregnancies in the European trial. In these trials and in the transcervical CVS and amniocentesis arms of the Danish trial, CVS was associated with the higher fetal loss rate, the excess being statistically significant in the European and Danish trials. Combining these figures (including those for the eligible pregnancies in the Canadian study) gives an excess 'total' fetal loss rate of 3.2 per cent (95 per cent CI 1.9 to 4.5 per cent) following transcervical CVS. Most of the excess was attributable to spontaneous fetal loss.

This difference in fetal loss rates is greater than those reported in non-randomized cohort studies, particularly the large study sponsored by the US National Institutes of Child Health and Human Development.[98] This study showed a crude excess pregnancy loss associated with CVS of 1.5 per cent, which was reduced to 0.8 per cent (95 per cent CI −1.3 to 2.9) after statistical adjustment for differences between the groups in gestational and maternal age. On the basis of these findings or personal case series, some commentators have argued that the excess risks associated with transcervical CVS were higher in the randomized trials because some of the operators in these trials were too inexperienced to perform CVS properly. Had this been so, performance would be expected to have improved over the recruitment period. However, secondary analyses of the European trial in which the data were stratified into three time periods and by the size of a centre's contribution failed to identify any improvement over the course of the trial or any clear differences between centres according to whether they made larger or smaller contributions. Furthermore, the results of the three multicentre trials and the American non-randomized cohort study are statistically consistent with each other.

Events in late pregnancy do not appear to be influenced by transcervical CVS; for example, it was not related to admission to hospital, induction of labour, and Caesarean delivery.[99] In the randomized controlled trials, the differences in the number of pregnancies that failed to reach term or achieve a normal birthweight reflected the differences in fetal losses, rather than an effect in later pregnancy.

Transabdominal CVS seems to compare more favourably than transcervical CVS with amniocentesis: the total fetal loss rates in the transabdominal CVS and amniocentesis arms of the Danish study (shown on the last two rows of Table 19.11) were almost identical.

Comparisons between transabdominal and transcervical CVS

The four randomized trials comparing transabdominal and transcervical CVS[62,66–68] are compared in Table 19.12. In the Danish trial transcervical CVS was associated with an excess 'total' fetal loss rate of 4.6 per cent (95 per cent CI 2.1 to 7.0 per cent) which was due to a difference in the risk of spontaneous fetal loss. In the Italian and United States trials, by contrast, there were no significant differences betweeen the two approaches. In the bigger of the two Italian trials, a larger proportion of the

Table 19.12 Fetal loss in randomized trials comparing transcervical and transabdominal chorionic villus sampling

Source/test allocated	No. of pregnancies studied	Miscarriages and stillbirths No. (a)	%	Difference[b] (95% CI)	No. of terminations of pregnancy (b)	No. of infants born alive with anomalies that were tested for (c)	'Total' fetal losses[a] No. (a + b + c)	%	Difference[b] (95% CI)
Bologna, Italy[66]									
Transcervical CVS	60	2[c]	3.3%	} 0.0% (−6.4% to 6.4%)	3	—	5[c,d]	8.3%	} 0.0% (−9.9 to 9.9%)
Transabdominal CVS	60	2[c]	3.3%		3	—	5[c,d]	8.3%	
Milan, Italy[67]									
Transcervical CVS	592	51[f]	8.6%	} 1.0% (−2.1 to 4.1%)	40	—	91[d]	15.4%	} −0.5% (−4.7 to 3.6%)
Transabdominal CVS	591	45	7.6%		49	—	94[d]	15.9%	
United States[100][e]									
Transcervical CVS	2001	91[f]	4.5%	} −0.2% (−1.4 to 1.2%)	66	—	157[d,f]	7.8%	} −0.3% (−1.9 to 1.4%)
Transabdominal CVS	1978	92[f]	4.7%		68	—	160[d,f]	8.1%	
Denmark[62][g]									
Transcervical CVS	1010	86[f]	8.5%	} 4.8% (2.7 to 6.9%)	24	0	110[f]	10.9%	} 4.6% (2.1 to 7.0%)
Transabdominal CVS	1027	38[f]	3.7%		27	0	65[f]	6.3%	

[a] Total fetal losses if all affected pregnancies were terminated.
[b] Percentage for transcervical CVS group minus percentage for transabdominal CVS group.
[c] Not including stillbirths.
[d] Not including infants born alive with anomalies that were tested for.
[e] Data are as recorded in the Cochrane database,[100] since the published figures[68] excluded 'genetically abnormal' pregnancies.
[f] Including neonatal deaths.
[g] Excluding women who after randomization refused to participate or were found to be ineligible, and those with a history of translocation or late termination or a fetus at risk of metabolic disease.

women allocated transcervical CVS received transabdominal CVS, which could have diluted a difference; but the heterogeneity between the Danish and United States trials cannot have arisen in this way, and remains unexplained. The Danish workers suggested that the difference between their study and others might indicate that the Danish obstetricians had received less training in transcervical CVS.[62]

In each series the numbers of terminations of pregnancy associated with the two procedures were similar, suggesting that laboratory performance was unaffected by the method of sampling. Judged on induction of labour and Caesarean delivery, there was no evidence of a differential effect on obstetric management in late pregnancy.[100] The pattern of short-term complications, however, did differ; spotting and bleeding were more common after transcervical CVS. No life-threatening maternal complications were reported amongst the 8000 participants in these randomized studies.

Association with fetal limb deficiencies

In 1991, severe limb deficiencies (most of them combined with oromandibular abnormalities) were reported in 5 out of 289 cases examined by CVS at 56–66 days of gestation.[101] Subsequent cohort and case-control studies have provided further evidence of a causal relationship between CVS and deficiencies in which the distal part of one or more limbs or digits is missing across its entire width ('transverse terminal deficiencies'). The odds of being affected by these deficiencies were 12.6 times as high for infants born after CVS as for other infants in an Italian case-control study.[102] Birth prevalence in 12 cohort studies involving nearly 40 000 CVS pregnancies (7.4/10 000) was three to five times as high as in the general populations with which the studies were compared (1.5–2.3/10 000).[103] The association was not supported by a study based on notifications to a voluntary international registry of malformations occurring after CVS;[104] but the birth prevalence of major limb deficiencies was much lower according to these data than in the general population with which they were compared, suggesting that notification had been incomplete.[105]

Table 19.13 **Frequency of transverse limb deficiencies after CVS, according to two case-control studies and one cohort study**

Study		Gestational age at which CVS was carried out			
		Any age	≤9 weeks	10 weeks	≥11 weeks
Case-control studies[103]					
United States	Number of transverse digital deficiencies in exposed fetuses	7	2	4	1
	Odds ratio (95% CI)	6.4 (1.1–38.6)	11.3 (1.0–131.6)	7.5 (1.5–36.7)	5.6 (0.3–94.7)
Italy	Number of transverse limb deficiencies in exposed fetuses	11	8	3	0
	Odds ratio (95% CI)	12.6 (6.2–23.9)	21.6 (9.0–47.7)	14.3 (3.2–47.2)	–
Cohort study[106]					
Germany	Number of limb deficiencies in exposed fetuses	10	5	4	1
	Rate/10 000	8	24	11	1

Studies of the relationship of gestational age at CVS to the risk of limb deficiencies have provided further evidence of a relationship. In two case-control studies, the odds ratios decreased with increasing duration until at 11 or more weeks they did not differ significantly from unity.[103] A consistent trend was observed in a German cohort study.[106] These trends with gestation length at CVS are shown in Table 19.13.

Another study has provided strong evidence that the time at which CVS is performed is closely related to the severity as well as the risk of limb deficiency. In this study[107] post-CVS limb reduction defects were classified into five groups according to whether the defect was proximal (upper arm) or distal (fingers). Within each group the median gestational age at which the CVS was performed was determined; and it was found that the more distal the defect the more advanced was the median age at CVS. These median gestations ranked perfectly in relation to the location of the limb reduction defect (Fig. 19.3). The probability of correctly ranking five ordered categories by chance if there were no underlying difference would be $1/5 \times 1/4 \times 1/3 \times 1/2 \times 1$ or 0.008. The result of this study is therefore statistically highly significant.

It must therefore be concluded that CVS in early pregnancy carries a risk of damage to the fetal limbs. Given the figures in Table 19.13 and the reported birth prevalence of transverse terminal limb deficiencies in the general population (1.5–3.5/10 000[103,108]), it seems likely that CVS leads to an extra risk of these defects of between 20 and 70/10 000 in fetuses exposed at or before nine weeks of gestation. The risk decreases as pregnancy advances and there is no evidence that it is present beyond 10 weeks of gestation.

Early amniocentesis

Comparisons with second-trimester amniocentesis

The frequency of spontaneous and 'total' fetal losses in the two randomized trials (both Canadian) is compared in Table 19.14. These trials were carried out by the same

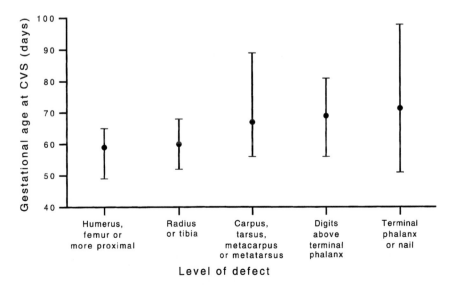

Fig. 19.3 Median and range of gestational ages at CVS according to level of defect in most severely affected limb. (HV Firth, personal communication).

Table 19.14 Fetal loss in Canadian randomized trials directly comparing early and second-trimester amniocentesis[59,60]

Source/test allocated	Number of pregnancies studied	Miscarriages, stillbirths and neonatal deaths			No. of terminations of pregnancy	No. of infants born alive with anomalies that were tested for[a]	'Total' fetal losses[b]		
		No. (a)	%	Difference[c] (95% CI)	(b)	(c)	No. (a + b + c)	%	Difference[c] (95% CI)
Pilot study[59]									
Early amniocentesis	344	13	3.8%	−1.8% (−5.0 to 1.4%)	14	1	28	8.1%	0.7% (−3.3 to 4.7%)
Second-trimester amniocentesis	339	19	5.6%		6	0	25	7.4%	
Full-scale study[60]									
Early amniocentesis	2183	94	4.3%	1.1% (0.0 to 2.2%)	72	1	167	7.7%	1.8% (0.3 to 3.3%)
Second-trimester amniocentesis	2185	71	3.2%		57	1	129	5.9%	

a Assuming that infants born alive with anomalies tested for accounted for half of all births in which 'central nervous system' anomalies were reported.
b Total fetal losses if all affected pregnancies were terminated.
c Percentage for early amniocentesis group minus percentage for mid-trimester amniocentesis group.

team, but there was no overlap of data between them.[59,60] In each trial, the 'total' fetal loss rate in pregnancies assigned to early amniocentesis was higher than in those assigned to second-trimester amniocentesis, significantly so in the larger trial. In the combined trials, the difference in 'total' fetal loss rate between the two groups was 1.6 per cent (95 per cent CI 0.2–3.0), of which 0.6 per cent (95 per cent CI −0.5–1.7) was attributable to the difference in spontaneous losses.

In the larger trial, the birth prevalence of talipes equinovarus was 1.3 per cent in pregnancies assigned to early amniocentesis and 0.1 per cent in those assigned second-trimester amniocentesis. Also, among the women in this trial who had received their allotted treatment, amniotic fluid leakage was observed in 4.6 per cent of those receiving early amniocentesis and in 2.4 per cent of those receiving second-trimester amnio-centesis. For both these outcomes, the excesses associated with early amniocentesis were statistically significant (for the 1.2 per cent excess of talipes, 95 per cent CI = 0.7–1.7; for the 2.2 per cent excess of amniotic fluid leakage, 95 per cent CI = 1.0–3.4). After amniotic fluid leakage, the risk of talipes was increased.[60]

Comparisons with transabdominal CVS

Table 19.15 shows the frequency of spontaneous and 'total' fetal losses in the pregnancies that were randomly allocated early amniocentesis or transabdominal CVS in the trials in Denmark,[64] Britain,[30] and the Netherlands.[65] In each trial, the 'total' fetal loss rate in pregnancies allocated early amniocentesis exceeded the rate in those allocated CVS, but not to a statistically significant extent, and the excess was confined to spontaneous fetal deaths. Combining the figures for the three trials gives excess rates in pregnancies assigned to early amniocentesis which are significant for spontaneous losses (2.2 per cent; 95 per cent CI 0.6–3.8) but not for 'total' losses (1.5 per cent; 95 per cent CI −0.6–3.6).

Talipes equinovarus was unusually common after early amniocentesis in the three trials comparing early amniocentesis and CVS, as well as in the larger of the two trials comparing early and second-trimester amniocentesis. In the trials of early amniocentesis and CVS, the birth prevalence of talipes among the infants whose mothers accepted random allocation was 1.9 per cent in those born after early amniocentesis and 0.1 per cent in those born after CVS. The difference of 1.8 per cent between these percentages is statistically significant (95 per cent CI 0.8–2.8). Within the early amniocentesis arm of the Danish study, the frequency of talipes was found to increase with decreasing gestational age at amniocentesis.[64]

Summary of variations in 'total' fetal losses

There is insufficient evidence available to say conclusively which is the safest of the methods of antenatal diagnosis compared above. The differences in 'total' fetal mortality observed in the randomized trials are summarized in Fig. 19.4. Transabdominal CVS and second-trimester amniocentesis appear to be of comparable safety. Transcervical CVS seems to be less safe than second-trimester amniocentesis, and was also associated with a higher risk than transabdominal CVS in one trial. Early amniocentesis was followed by higher total fetal loss rates than second-trimester amniocentesis and transabdominal CVS, although the comparison between early amniocentesis and CVS was not based on enough pregnancies for firm conclusions to be drawn from this.

Table 19.15 Fetal loss in randomized trials comparing early amniocentesis and transabdominal chorionic villus sampling

Source/ test allocated	Number of pregnancies studied	Miscarriages and stillbirths			No. of terminations of pregnancy	No. of infants born alive with anomalies that were tested for	'Total' fetal losses[b]		
		No. (a)	%	Difference[b] (95% CI)	(b)	(c)	No. (a + b + c)	%	Difference[b] (95% CI)
London[30]									
Early amniocentesis	238	14[c]	5.9%	4.7% (1.4 to 8.0%)	6	0	20	8.4%	3.6% (−0.8 to 8.0%)
Transabdominal CVS	250	3[c]	1.2%		9	0	12	4.8%	
Copenhagen[64]									
Early amniocentesis	579	20	3.5%	1.2% (−0.7 to 3.1%)	9	0	29	5.0%	0.5% (−2.0 to 3.0%)
Transabdominal CVS	575[d]	13	2.3%		13	0	26	4.5%	
Leiden[65]									
Early amniocentesis	55	3	5.5%	2.2% (−5.3 to 9.7%)	0	0	3	5.5%	2.2% (−5.3 to 9.7%)
Transabdominal CVS	60	2	3.3%		0	0	2	3.3%	

[a] Total fetal losses if all affected pregnancies were terminated.
[b] Percentage for early amniocentesis group minus percentage for transabdominal CVS group.
[c] Including neonatal deaths.
[d] Excluding four women switched from CVS to amniocentesis after randomization, for whom outcome was not reported.

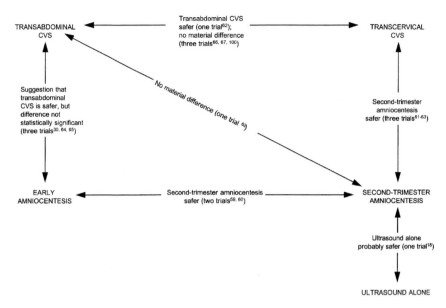

Fig. 19.4 Summary of differences in 'total' fetal loss rates observed in randomized clinical trials of amniocentesis and/or CVS.

POLICY IMPLICATIONS

The above analyses support the view that unless it is important to diagnose chromosomal abnormalities before 14 weeks of gestation, second-trimester amniocentesis is preferable to first-trimester CVS. Although the detection rates for both methods were close to 100 per cent in the trials reviewed (Table 19.6 and pp. 487–8), failure rates (Table 19.2) and false-positive rates (Table 19.7) tended to be lower with second-trimester amniocentesis than with early CVS, and the same was true of the risk of maternal contamination in the Canadian trial[61] (the only trial for which adequate data on this problem were published—Table 19.8). There is also evidence that CVS can lead to limb deficiencies in the fetus when performed before 11 weeks of gestation (Table 19.13), and that the risk of fetal loss is higher after transcervical CVS than after second-trimester amniocentesis (Table 19.11). According to the Danish trial of CVS and amniocentesis,[62] the fetal loss rate after transabdominal (unlike transcervical) CVS is as low as after amniocentesis (Table 19.11), but other trials suggest that transabdominal and transcervical CVS carry similar risks of fetal loss (Table 19.12). Finally, second-trimester amniocentesis costs less than CVS.

Second-trimester amniocentesis compares favourably with early amniocentesis as well as with CVS. Early amniocentesis has a much higher failure rate than second-trimester amniocentesis (Table 19.2) and is associated with more fetal losses (Table 19.14) and a higher birth prevalence of talipes equinovarus.

Among the procedures that may be used if it is important to make a diagnosis before 14 weeks of gestation, transabdominal CVS is less likely than early amniocentesis to lead to fetal loss (Table 19.15) or talipes equinovarus according to the limited trial data that are available, and the Danish trial suggests that it is associated with fewer fetal deaths than transcervical CVS (Table 19.12). Failure rates are lower with transabdominal than with transcervical CVS (Table 19.3), although the evidence as to whether they are lower with transabdominal CVS than with early amniocentesis is conflicting (Table 19.2).

If CVS is used, the data indicate that the best policy is to examine direct CVS preparations first, and to follow this by long-term culture *unless* one of the following two criteria applies:

1. *The direct preparation exhibits trisomy 21, 18, or 13* (referred to below as the 'common' autosomal trisomies, since they are the ones most often seen in infants). An immediate termination of pregnancy can reasonably be offered when one of these trisomies is reported in a direct preparation, since there were no false-positive reports of this kind in the CVS data analysed (Tables 19.4 and 19.7). Following this course would mean that rapid action could be taken in most pregnancies in which a termination of pregnancy for a chromosomal anomaly was appropriate: according to Table 19.6, the 'common' autosomal trisomies account for about 70 per cent of confirmed cases of chromosomal anomalies (excluding rearrangements, which are under-represented in Table 19.6, but most of which are balanced and therefore not associated with disability).

2. *The indication for determining the karyotype is a high risk of X-linked recessive disorder*. In these circumstances, the aim is to determine whether the fetus is male, which can be done more accurately in a direct preparation than in a long-term culture (Table 19.8).

If neither of these criteria is met, a decision on whether to offer a termination of pregnancy should not be taken until long-term cultures have been examined. This is because CVS direct preparations sometimes give false-negative and false-positive results which can be corrected using long-term cultures (Table 19.4). False-positive results of this kind have included reports of abnormal karyotypes of most types, although not of the three 'common' autosomal trisomies. There are fewer reports of false-negative results in direct preparations being corrected with long-term cultures, but these include cases of trisomies 18 and 21 (p. 487).

Should the long-term CVS culture results be negative, the discordant pair analysis (Table 19.4) shows that no further action is indicated, even after a positive direct preparation report: among 89 positive findings in direct preparations that were combined with negative long-term culture results, the results of follow-up were negative in 88 and positive in only one, and in the latter instance the final diagnosis was 45,X/46,XX mosaicism,[70] which is arguably not a firm indication for termination of pregnancy.

If the long-term CVS culture is positive for a sex-chromosome aneuploidy some would offer a termination of pregnancy without further testing, since Tables 19.6 and 19.7 suggest that the odds on being affected are very high (14:1). Others would take the view that the common sex chromosome aneuploidies (X0, XXX, XXY, XYY) do not have severe enough effects to justify termination.

If the long-term CVS culture result is positive for mosaicism, polyploidy, or an autosomal aneuploidy other than one of the 'common' trisomies, a termination of pregnancy should not be offered without further confirmation from an amniocentesis or fetal blood test. In the Italian observational study[69] (the only one in which long-term cultures were used throughout), mosaicism, polyploidy, and autosomal aneuploidies

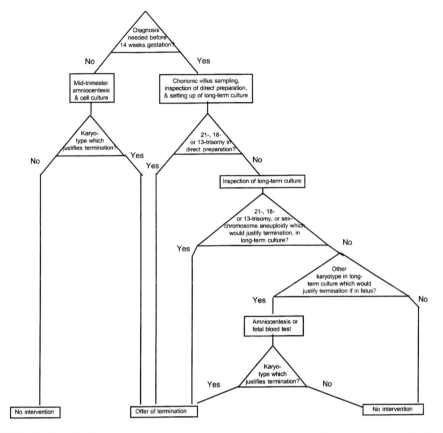

Fig. 19.5 Algorithm for diagnosis and management of chromosomal anomalies using amniocentesis or CVS.

other than the common trisomies were all reported falsely in long-term cultures (Table 19.7). There were 20 such false-positives, more than the 14 confirmed cases in the same categories which were identified in the Italian study (Table 19.6).

Further testing may not always be indicated when a CVS culture is positive for mosaicism, polyploidy, or an uncommon autosomal aneuploidy. Some may feel that a form of mosaicism that will have little effect on the phenotype does not justify termination, in which case confirmation by amniocentesis or fetal blood test is unwarranted. If polyploidy, or an autosomal aneuploidy other than the 'common' ones, is reported in a CVS culture, some parents may prefer the pregnancy to continue without further testing in order to avoid putting at risk a possibly normal fetus, given that if the abnormal finding is correct the fetus will almost certainly miscarry spontaneously.

An algorithm summarizing the diagnosis and management of chromosomal anomalies by the above policy is given in Fig. 19.5.

CONCLUSION

Both second-trimester amniocentesis and early CVS have very high detection rates as tests for significant chromosomal abnormalities (their main function).

Second-trimester amniocentesis is associated with the lower failure rates and false-positive rates, and does not increase the risk of limb deficiencies as CVS before 11 weeks of gestation does. Also, second-trimester amniocentesis is followed by lower fetal death rates than those seen after transcervical CVS; and the risk of fetal death after transabdominal CVS is as high as after transcervical CVS according to most clinical trials of these alternatives. Second-trimester amniocentesis is therefore preferable to CVS, except when first-trimester testing is strongly indicated for maternal reasons—e.g. if concern about the state of the fetus is causing the mother severe stress which needs urgent relief, or if a late termination would carry a significant risk of complications (which are less common after early termination).

When first-trimester testing is strongly indicated, the method of choice appears to be transabdominal CVS, given that this yields lower failure rates than transcervical CVS and that lower fetal loss rates have been reported after transabdominal CVS than after early amniocentesis or transcervical CVS.

In CVS testing, direct preparations should be inspected first. If trisomy 21, 18, or 13 is found, termination of pregnancy can be offered immediately. Otherwise, unless the only aim is to sex the fetus, long-term cultures should be examined. After this, an offer of immediate termination is again appropriate if trisomy 21, 18, or 13 or a serious sex-chromosome aneuploidy is found; but if a culture reveals other anomalies for which termination might be considered, the obstetrician should arrange an amniocentesis or fetal blood test to confirm that the fetus is affected before offering to terminate the pregnancy.

REFERENCES

1. Steele, M.W. and Breg Jr, W.R. (1966). Chromosome analysis of human amniotic fluid cells. *Lancet*, **i**, 383–5.
2. Nadler, H.L. (1968). Antenatal detection of hereditary disorders. *Pediatrics*, **42**, 912–8.
3. Brock, D.J.H. and Sutcliffe, R.G. (1972). Alpha-fetoprotein in the antenatal diagnosis of anencephaly and spina bifida. *Lancet*, **ii**, 197–9.
4. Huisjes, H.J. (1978). Cytology of amniotic fluid and its clinical application. In *Amniotic Fluid: Research and clinical Application*. (eds. D.W. Fairweather and E. Eskes). pp. 93–129. Excerpta Medica, Amsterdam.
5. Gosden, C.M. (1983). Amniotic fluid cell types and culture. *British Medical Bulletin*, **39**, 348–54.
6. Chen, W.W. (1982). Studies on the origin of human amniotic fluid cells by immunofluorescent staining of keratin filaments. *Journal of Medical Genetics*, **19**, 433–6.
7. Von Koskull, H., Aula, P., Trejdosiwicz, L.K., and Virtanen, I. (1984). Identification of cells from fetal bladder epithelium in human amniotic fluid. *Human Genetics*, **65**, 262–7.
8. Jørgensen, F.S., Bang, J., Lind, A.-M., Christensen, B., Lundsteen, C., and Philip, J. (1992). Genetic amniocentesis at 7–14 weeks of gestation. *Prenatal Diagnosis*, **12**, 277–83.
9. Simpson, N.E., Dallaire, L., Miller, J.R., Siminovich, L., Hamerton, J.L., Miller, J., and McKeen, C. (1976). Prenatal diagnosis of genetic disease in Canada: Report of a collaborative study. *Canadian Medical Association Journal*, **115**, 739–46.
10. MRC Working Party on Amniocentesis. (1978). An assessment of the hazards of amniocentesis. *British Journal of Obstetrics and Gynaecology*, **85**, suppl. 2, 1–41.

11. Turnbull, A.C. and MacKenzie, I.Z. (1983). Second-trimester amniocentesis and termination of pregnancy. *British Medical Bulletin*, **4**, 315–21.

12. Tabor, A., Bang, J., and Nørgaard-Pedersen, B. (1987). Feto-maternal haemorrhage associated with genetic amniocentesis: results of a randomized trial. *British Journal of Obstetrics and Gynaecology*, **94**, 528–35.

13. Leschot, N.J., Verjaal, M., and Treffers, P.E. (1985). Risks of midtrimester amniocentesis: assessment in 3,000 pregnancies. *British Journal of Obstetrics and Gynaecology*, **92**, 804–7.

14. Knudsen, J.L. and de Neergaard, L. (1994). *Prenatal Genetic Information, Counselling and Testing*. National Board of Health, Copenhagen, Denmark.

15. NICHD National Registry for Amniocentesis Study Group. (1977). Midtrimester amniocentesis for prenatal diagnosis. Safety and accuracy. *Journal of the American Medical Association*, **236**, 1471–6.

16. Crane, J.P. and Kopta, M.M. (1984). Genetic amniocentesis: Impact of placental position upon the risk of pregnancy loss. *American Journal of Obstetrics and Gynecology*, **150**, 813–6.

17. Hanson, F.W., Tennant, F.R., Zorn, E.M., and Samuels, S. (1985). Analysis of 2,136 genetic amniocenteses: Experience of a single physician. *American Journal of Obstetrics and Gynecology*, **152**, 436–43.

18. Tabor, A., Philip, J., Madsen, M., Bang, J., Obel, E., and Nørgaard-Pedersen, B. (1986). Randomised controlled trial of genetic amniocentesis in 4606 low-risk women. *Lancet*, **i**, 1287–93.

19. Kappel, B., Nielsen, J., Hansen, K.B., Mikkelsen, M., and Therkelsen, A. J. (1987). Spontaneous abortion following mid-trimester amniocentesis. Clinical significance of placental perforation and blood-stained amniotic fluid. *British Journal of Obstetrics and Gynaecology*, **94**, 50–4.

20. Elias, S., Gerbie, A.B., Simpson, J.L., Nadler, H.L., Sabbagha, R.E., and Shkolnik, A. (1980). Genetic amniocentesis in twin gestations. *American Journal of Obstetrics and Gynecology*, **138**, 169–73.

21. Tietze, C. (1983). Induced abortion. In *Obstetrical Epidemiology*, (ed. S.L. Barron and A.M. Thomson), pp. 319–346. Academic Press, London.

22. Lawson, H.W., Frye, A., Atrash, H.K., Smith, J.C., Shulman, H.B., and Ranick, M. (1994). Abortion mortality, United States, 1972 through 1987. *American Journal of Obstetrics and Gynecology*, **171**, 1365–72.

23. Hanson, F.W., Zorn, E.M., Tennant, F.R., Marianos, S., and Samuels, S. (1987). Amniocentesis before 15 weeks' gestation: Outcome, risks and technical problems. *American Journal of Obstetrics and Gynecology*, **156**, 1524–31.

24. Hanson, F.W., Happ, R.L., Tennant, F.R., Hune, S., and Peterson, A.G. (1990). Ultrasonography-guided early amniocentesis in singleton pregnancies. *American Journal of Obstetrics and Gynecology*, **162**, 1376–83.

25. Penso, C.A., Sandstrom, M.M., Garber, M.-F., Ladoulis, M., Stryker, J.M., and Benacerraf, B.B. (1990). Early amniocentesis: Report of 407 cases with neonatal follow-up. *Obstetrics and Gynecology*, **76**, 1032–6.

26. Stripparo, L., Buscaglia, M., Logatti, L., Ghisoni, L., Dambrosio, F., Guerneri, S., Rosella, F., Lituania, M., Cordone, M., de Biasio, P., Passamonti, U., Gimelli, G., and Cuoco, C. (1990). Genetic amniocentesis: 505 cases performed before the sixteenth week of gestation. *Prenatal Diagnosis*, **10**, 359–64.

27. Assel, B.G., Lewis, S.M., Dickerman, L.H., Park, V.M., and Jassani, M.N. (1992). Single-operator comparison of early and mid-second trimester amniocentesis. *Obstetrics and Gynecology*, **79**, 940–4.

28. Shulman, L.P., Elias, S., Phillips, O.P., Grevengood, C., Dungan, J.S., and Simpson, J.L. (1994). Amniocentesis performed at 14 weeks' gestation or earlier: Comparison with first-trimester transabdominal chorionic villus sampling. *Obstetrics and Gynecology*, **83**, 543–8.

29. Crandall, B.F., Kulch, P., and Tabsh, K. (1994). Risk assessment of amniocentesis between 11 and 15 weeks: Comparison to later amniocentesis controls. *Prenatal Diagnosis*, **14**, 913–9.

30. Nicolaides, K., Brizot, M. de L., Patel, F., and Snijders, R. (1994). Comparison of chorionic villus sampling and amniocentesis for fetal karyotyping at 10–13 weeks' gestation. *Lancet*, **344**, 435–9.

31. Evans, M.I., Drugan A., Koppitch III, F.C., Zador, I.E., Sacks, A.J., and Sokol, R.J. (1989). Genetic diagnosis in the first trimester: The norm for the 1990s. *American Journal of Obstetrics and Gynecology*, **160**, 1332–9.

32. Wathen, N.C., Cass, P.L., Campbell, D.J., Kitau, M.J., and Chard, T. (1991). Early amniocentesis: alphafetoprotein levels in amniotic fluid, extraembryonic coelomic fluid and maternal serum between 8 and 13 weeks. *British Journal of Obstetrics and Gynaecology*, **98**, 866–70.

33. Rooney, D.E., MacLachlan, N., Smith, J., Rebello, M.T., Loeffler, F.E., Beard, R.W., Rodeck, C., and Coleman, D.V. (1989). Early amniocentesis: a cytogenetic evaluation. *British Medical Journal*, **299**, 25.

34. Sundberg, K., Smidt-Jensen, S., and Philip, J. (1991). Amniocentesis with increased cell yield, obtained by filtration and reinjection of the amniotic fluid. *Ultrasound in Obstetrics and Gynecology*, **1**, 91–4.

35. Crandall, B.F., Hanson, F.W., Tennant, F., and Perdue, S.T. (1989). Alfa-fetoprotein levels in amniotic fluid between 11 and 15 weeks. *American Journal of Obstetrics and Gynecology*, **160**, 1204–6.

36. Patrick, A.D. (1983). Inherited metabolic disorders. *British Medical Bulletin*, **39**, 378–85.

37. Cederquist, L.L. and Fuchs, F. (1970). Antenatal sex determination. A historical review. *Clinical Obstetrics and Gynecology*, **13**, 159–77.

38. Cremer, T., Landegent, J., Brucker, A., Scholl, H.P., Schardin, M., Hager, H.D., *et al.* (1986) Detection of chromosome aberrations in the human interphase nucleus by visualisation of specific target DNAs with radioactive and non-radioactive in-situ hybridisation techniques: diagnosis of trisomy 18 with probe L1.84. *Human Genetics*, **74**, 346–52.

39. Bryndorf, T., Christensen, B., Philip, J., Hansen, W., Yokobata, K., Bui, N., and Gaiser, C. (1992). New rapid test for prenatal detection of trisomy 21 (Down's syndrome): preliminary report. *British Medical Journal*, **304**, 1536–9.

40. Brambati, B., Oldrini, A., Aladerun, S.A. (1983). Methods of chorionic villus sampling in first trimester fetal diagnosis. In *Progress in perinatal medicine: biochemical and biophysical diagnostic procedures*, (ed. A. Albertini and P.G. Crosignani), pp. 275–84. Excerpta Medica, Amsterdam.

41. Horwell, D.H., Loeffler, F.E., and Coleman, D.V. (1983). Assessment of a transcervical aspiration technique for chorionic villus biopsy in the first trimester of pregnancy. *British Journal of Obstetrics and Gynaecology*, **90**, 196–8.

42. Rodeck, C.H., Morsman, J.M., Gosden, C.M., and Gosden, J.R. (1983). Development of

an improved technique for first trimester microsampling of chorion. *British Journal of Obstetrics and Gynaecology*, **90**, 1113–8.

43. Brambati, B., Oldrini, A., and Lanzani, A. (1987). Transabdominal chorion villus sampling: a freehand ultrasound-guided technique. *American Journal of Obstetrics and Gynecology*, **157**, 134–7.

44. Benacerraf, B.R. and Frigoletto, F.D.J.R. (1987). Soft tissue nuchal fold in the second trimester fetus; standards for normal measurements compared with those in Down's syndrome. *American Journal of Obstetrics and Gynecology*, **157**, 1146–9.

45. Macintosh, M.C.M., Wald, N.J., Chard, T., Hansen, J., Mikkelsen, M., Therkelsen, A.J., *et al.* (1995). Selective miscarriage of Down's syndrome fetuses in women aged 35 years and over. *British Journal of Obstetrics and Gynaecology*, **102**, 798–801.

46. Macintosh, M.C.M., Wald, N.J., Chard, T., Hansen, J., Mikkelsen, M., Therkelsen, A.J., *et al.* (1996). The selective miscarriage of Down's syndrome from 10 weeks of pregnancy. *British Journal of Obstetrics and Gynaecology*, **103**, 1172–3.

47. Snijders, R.J.M., Holtgreve, W., Cuckle, H., and Nicolaides, K.H. (1994). Maternal age specific risks for trisomies at 9–14 weeks gestation. *Prenatal Diagnosis*, **14**, 543–52.

48. Gosden, C.M., Nicolaides, K.H., and Rodeck, C.H. (1988). Fetal blood sampling in investigation of chromosome mosaicism in amniotic fluid cell culture. *Lancet*, **i**, 613–7.

49. Philip, J., Bryndorf, T., and Christensen, B. (1994). Prenatal aneuploidy detection in interphase cells by fluorescence *in situ* hybridisation. *Prenatal Diagnosis*, **14**, 1203–15.

50. Van Opstal, D., Van Hemel, J.O., Eussen, B.H., Van Der Heide, A., Van den Berg, C., In't Veld, P.A., *et al.* (1995). A chromosome 21 specific cosmid cocktail for the detection of chromosome 21 aberration in interphase nuclei. *Prenatal Diagnosis*, **15**, 705–11.

51. Verma, L., Macdonald, F., Leedham, P., McConachie, M., Dhanjal, S., and Hultén, M. (1998). Rapid and simple prenatal DNA diagnosis of Down's syndrome. *Lancet*, **352**, 9–12.

52. Christian, S.L., Smith, A.C.M., Macha, M., Black, S.H., Elder, F.F.B., Johnson, J.M.P., *et al.* (1996). Prenatal diagnosis of uniparental disomy 15 following trisomy 15 mosaicism. *Prenatal Diagnosis*, **16**, 323–32.

53. Kalousek, D.K., Dill, F.J., Dantzar, T., McGillivray, B.C., Yong, S.L., and Wilson, R.D. (1987). Confined chorionic mosaicism in prenatal diagnosis. *Human Genetics*, **77**, 163–7.

54. Gosden, C. (1991). Fetal karyotyping using chorionic villus samples. In *Antenatal diagnosis of fetal abnormalities*, (ed. J.O. Drife and D. Donnai), pp.153–167. Springer, London.

55. Chang, H.-C., Jones, O.W., and Masui, H. (1982). Human amniotic fluid cells given in a hormone-supplemented medium – suitability for prenatal diagnosis. *Proceedings of the National Academy of Science, USA*, **79**, 4795–9.

56. Poenaru, L. (1987). First trimester diagnosis of metabolic diseases: a survey in countries from the European Community. *Prenatal Diagnosis*, **7**, 331–4.

57. Lowe C.U., Alexander, D., Bryla, D., and Seigel, D. (1978). *The Safety and Accuracy of Mid-trimester Amniocentesis*, DHEW Publication No (NIH) 78–190. US Department of Health, Education and Welfare, Washington, DC.

58. Crandall, B.F., Howard, J., Lebherz, T.B., Rubinstein, L., Sample, W.F., and Sarti, D. (1980). Follow-up of 2000 second-trimester amniocenteses. *Obstetrics and Gynecology*, **56**, 625–8.

59. Johnson, J-A.M., Wilson, R.D., Winsor, E.J.T., Singer, J., Dansereau, J., and Kalousek, D.K. (1996). The Early Amniocentesis Study: a randomised clinical trial of early amniocentesis versus midtrimester amniocentesis. *Fetal Diagnosis and Therapy*, **11**, 85–95.

60. Canadian Early and Mid-Trimester Amniocentesis Trial (CEMAT) Group (1998). Randomised trial to assess safety and fetal outcome of early and midtrimester amniocentesis. *Lancet*, **351**, 242–7.
61. Lippman, A., Tomkins, D.J., Shine, J., and Hamilton, J.L. (1992). Canadian multicentre randomised clinical trial of chorionic villus sampling and amniocentesis: final report. *Prenatal Diagnosis*, **12**, 385–476.
62. Smidt-Jensen, S., Permin, M., Philip, J., Lundsteen, C., Zachary, J.M., Fowler, S.E., *et al.* (1992). Randomised comparison of amniocentesis and transabdominal and transcervical chorionic villus sampling. *Lancet*, **340**, 1237–44.
63. MRC Working Party on the Evaluation of Chorionic Villus Sampling (1991). Medical Research Council European trial of chorion villus sampling. *Lancet*, **337**, 1491–9.
64. Sundberg, R., Bang, J., Smidt-Jensen, S., Brocks, V., Lundsteen, C., Permin, J., Keiding, N., and Philip, J. (1997). Randomised study of risk of fetal loss related to early amniocentesis versus chorionic villus sampling. *Lancet*, **350**, 697–703.
65. Nagel, H.T.C., Vandenbussche, F.P.H.K., Keirse, M.J.N.C., Oepkes, D., Oosterwijk, J.C., Beverstock, G. *et al.* (1998). Amniocentesis before 14 completed weeks as an alternative to transabdominal chorionic villus sampling: a controlled trial with infant follow-up. *Prenatal Diagnosis*, **18**, 465–75.
66. Bovicelli, L., Rizzo, N., Montacuti, V., and Morandi, R. (1986). Transabdominal vs transcervical routes for chorionic villus sampling. *Lancet*, **2**, 290.
67. Brambati, B., Terzian, E., and Tognoni, G. (1991). Randomized clinical trial of transabdominal vs transcervical chorionic villus sampling methods. *Prenatal Diagnosis*, **11**, 285–93.
68. Jackson, L.G., Zachary, J.M., Fowler, S.E., Desnick, R.J., Golbus, M.S., Ledbetter, D.H. *et al.* (1992). A randomised comparison of transcervical and transabdominal chorionic-villus sampling. *New England Journal of Medicine*, **327**, 594–8.
69. Pittalis, M.C., Dalpra, L., Torricelli, F., Rizzo, N., Noceras, G., Cariati, E., *et al.* (1994). The predictive value of cytogenetic diagnosis after CVS based on 4860 cases with both direct and culture methods. *Prenatal Diagnosis*, **14**, 267–78.
70. Association of Clinical Cytogeneticists Working Party on Chorionic Villi in Prenatal Diagnosis (1994). Cytogenetic analysis of chorionic villi for prenatal diagnosis: ACC collaborative study of UK data. *Prenatal Diagnosis*, **14**, 363–79.
71. Ledbetter, D.H., Zachary, J.M., Simpson, J.L., Golbus, M.S., Pergament, E., Jackson, L. *et al.* (1992). Cytogenetic results from the US Collaborative study on CVS. *Prenatal Diagnosis*, **12**, 317–45.
72. Miny, P., Basaran, S., Hozgreve, W., Horst, J., Pawlowitzki, I.H., and Ngo, T.K. (1988). False negative cytogenetic result in direct preparations after CVS. *Prenatal Diagnosis*, **8**, 633.
73. Bartels, I., Hansmann, I., Holland, U., Zoll, B., and Bauskolb, R. (1989). Down syndrome at birth not detected by first trimester chorionic villus sampling. *American Journal of Medical Genetics*, **34**, 606–7.
74. Simoni, G., Terzoli, G., and Rossella, F. (1990). Direct chromosome preparation and culture using chorionic villi: an evaluation of the two techniques. *American Journal of Medical Genetics*, **35**, 181–3.
75. Hammer, P., Holzgreve, W., Katabacak, Z., Horst, J., and Miny, P. (1991). False-negative and false-positive prenatal cytogenetic results due to true mosaicism. *Prenatal Diagnosis*, **11**, 133–6.

76. Lilford, R.J., Caine, A., Linton, F., and Mason, G. (1991). Short-term culture and false-negative results for Down's syndrome on chorionic villus sampling. *Lancet*, **337**, 861.

77. Blackmore, K.J., Mahoney, M.J., and Hobbins, J.C. (1985). Infection and chorionic villus sampling. *Lancet*, **ii**, 339.

78. Barela, A.I., Kleinman, G.E., Golbus, I.M., Menke, D.J., Hogge, W.A., and Golbus, M.S. (1986). Septic shock with renal failure after chorionic villus sampling. *American Journal of Obstetrics and Gynecology*, **154**, 1100–2.

79. Wald. N.J. (1995). Biochemical detection of neural tube defects and Down's syndrome. In *Turnbull's Obstetrics*, 2nd edn, (ed. G. Chamberlain), pp.195–209. Churchill Livingstone, Edinburgh.

80. Obel, E.B. (1980). Risk of spontaneous abortion following legally induced abortion. *Acta Obstetricia et Gynecologica Scandinavica*, **59**, 131–7.

81. Anderson, R.L., Goldberg, J.D., and Golbus, M.S. (1991). Prenatal diagnosis in multiple gestation: 20 years experience with amniocentesis. *Prenatal Diagnosis*, **11**, 263–70.

82. Thomsen, S.G., Isager-Sally, L., Lange, A.P., Saurbrey, N., Grønvall, S., and Schiøler, V. (1983). Elevated maternal serum alpha-fetoprotein caused by midtrimester amniocentesis: A prognostic factor. *Obstetrics and Gynecology*, **62**, 297–300.

83. Mennuti, M.T., DiGaetano, A., McDonnell, A., Cohen, A.W., and Liston, R.M. (1983). Fetal-maternal bleeding associated with genetic amniocentesis: real-time versus static ultrasound. *Obstetrics and Gynecology*, **62**, 26–30.

84. Golbus, M.S., Stephens, J.D., Cann, H.M., Mann, J., and Hensleigh, P.A. (1982). Rh iso-immunization following genetic amniocentesis. *Prenatal Diagnosis*, **2**, 149–56.

85. Murray, J.C., Karp, L.E., Williamson, R.A., Cheng, E.Y., and Luthy, D.A. (1983). Rh iso-immunization related to amniocentesis. *American Journal of Medical Genetics*, **16**, 527–34.

86. Tabor, A., Jerne, D., and Bock, J.E. (1987). Incidence of rhesus immunisation after genetic amniocentesis. *British Medical Journal*, **293**, 533–6.

87. WHO (World Health Organization) (1971). Prevention of Rh sensitization. *WHO Technical Report Series*, no. 468.

88. Tabsh, K.M.A., Lebherz, T.B., and Crandall, B.F. (1984). Risks of prophylactic anti-D immunoglobulin after second-trimester amniocentesis. *American Journal of Obstetrics and Gynecology*, **149**, 225–6.

89. Hislop, A. and Fairweather, D.V.I. (1982). Amniocentesis and lung growth: an animal experiment with clinical implications. *Lancet*, **ii**, 1271–2.

90. Thompson, P.J., Greenough, A., and Nicolaides, K.H. (1992). Lung volume measured by functional residual capacity in infants following first trimester amniocentesis or chorion villus sampling. *British Journal of Obstetrics and Gynaecology*, **99**, 479–82.

91. Vyas, H., Milner, A.D., and Hopkin, I.E. (1982). Amniocentesis and fetal lung development. *Archives of Disease in Childhood*, **57**, 627–8.

92. Verjaal, M., Leschot, N.J., and Treffers, P.E. (1981). Risk of amniocentesis and laboratory findings in a series of 1500 prenatal diagnoses. *Prenatal Diagnosis*, **1**, 173–81.

93. Finegan, J.-A.K., Quarrington, B.J., Hughes, H.E., Rudd, N.L., Stevens, L.J., Weeksberg, R., and Doran, T.A. (1985). Infant outcome following mid-trimester amniocentesis: development and physical status at age six months. *British Journal of Obstetrics and Gynaecology*, **92**, 1015–23.

94. Wald, N.J., Terzian, E., Vickers, P.A., and Weatherall, J.A.C. (1983). Congenital talipes and hip malformation in relation to amniocentesis: A case-control study. *Lancet*, **ii**, 246–9.

95. Finegan, J-A.K., Quarrington, B.J., Hughes, H.E., Mervyn, J.M., Hood, J.E., Zacher, J.E., *et al.* (1990). Child outcome following mid-trimester amniocentesis: development, behaviour and physical status at age 4 years. *British Journal of Obstetrics and Gynaecology*, **97**, 32–40.

96. Baird, P.A., Lee, I.M.L., and Sadovnik, A.D. (1994). Population-based study of long-term outcomes after amniocentesis. *Lancet*, **344**, 1134–6.

97. van der Pol, J.G., Wolf, H., Boer, K., Treffers, P.E., Leschot, N.J., Hey, H.A. *et al.* (1992). Jejunal atresia related to the use of methylene blue in genetic amniocentesis in twins. *British Journal of Obstetrics and Gynaecology*, **99**, 141–3.

98. Rhoads, G.G., Jackson, L.G., Schlesselman, S.E., de la Cruz, F.F., Desnick, R.J., Golbus, M.S. *et al.* (1989). The safety and efficacy of chorionic villus sampling for early prenatal diagnosis of cytogenetic abnormalities. *New England Journal of Medicine*, **320**, 609–617.

99. Grant, A.M. (1992). Chorionic villus sampling versus amniocentesis. In *Oxford Database of Perinatal Trials*, version 1.2, Disk issue 7, (ed. I. Chalmers), record no. 6007.

100. Grant, A.M. (1992). Transabdominal versus transcervical chorion villus sampling. In *Oxford Database of Perinatal Trials*, version 1.2, Disk issue 7, (ed. I Chalmers), record no. 6005.

101. Firth, H.V., Boyd, P.A., Chamberlain, P., MacKenzie, I.Z., Lindenbaum, R.H., and Huson, S.M. (1991). Severe limb abnormalities after chorion villus sampling at 56–66 days gestation. *Lancet*, **337**, 762–3.

102. Mastroiacovo, P. and Botto, L.D. (1994). Chorionic villus sampling and transverse limb deficiencies: maternal age is not a confounder. *American Journal of Medical Genetics*, **53**, 182–6.

103. Centers for Disease Control and Prevention (1995). Chorionic villus sampling and amniocentesis: recommendations for prenatal counseling, *MMWR*, **44**, (no. RR-9), 1–12.

104. Froster, U.G. and Jackson, L. (1996). Limb defects and chorion villus sampling: results from an international registry, 1992–4. *Lancet*, **347**, 489–94.

105. Evans, J.A. and Hamerton, J.L. (1996). Limb defects and chorionic villus sampling. *Lancet*, **347**, 484–5.

106. Stengel-Rutkowski, S. (ed.) (1993). *Pränatale Diagnostik an Chorionzotten: Abschlussbericht über die Dokumentation der Untersuchungen innerhalb der Gemeinschaftsstudie in der Bundesrepublik-Deutschland 1985–1991*. Munich.

107. Firth, H.V., Boyd, P.A., Chamberlain, P., MacKenzie, I.Z., Morris-Kay, G.M., and Huson, S.M. (1994). Analysis of limb reduction defects in babies exposed to chorion villus sampling. *Lancet*, **343**, 1069–71.

108. Leck, I. (1969). The incidence of limb deficiencies in recent years. In *Limb development and deformity: problems of evaluation and rehabilitation*, (ed. C.A. Swinyard), pp. 248–68. Thomas, Springfield, IL.

20 *Fetal blood and tissue sampling*

Pauline A. Hurley and Charles H. Rodeck

INTRODUCTION

Fetal tissue or body fluids are needed for many of the diagnostic tests that are indicated when antenatal screening tests are positive. This is, for example, often true when family history indicates that the fetus is at risk of a single gene disorder, or when testing for Down's syndrome is indicated by maternal age and biochemistry combined. Even if the disease is an anatomical defect which has been recognized by ultrasound, the diagnosis and prognosis can frequently only be completed when the fetal karyotype has been obtained from a fetal sample. The type of procedure performed will depend on the sample required for diagnosis, ranging from the simplest, amniocentesis, through the more invasive chorionic villus biopsy, to fetal blood or tissue sampling.

The indications for fetal tissue sampling fall broadly into three categories: firstly, where the diagnosis is currently not possible by karyotyping or DNA technology (e.g. some platelet and skin disorders); secondly, where a result from either chorionic villus sampling or amniocentesis needs to be checked (e.g. mosaicism); thirdly, where a rapid result is necessary if a patient at specific risk of an inborn error of metabolism or karyotypic abnormality presents late for antenatal care, or an anatomical marker of an aneuploidy has been identified by ultrasound.

Before embarking on fetal tissue sampling it is essential that: (1) the correct diagnosis has been made in the parents; (2) the fetus is at risk of the disease; (3) an accurate test is available to establish the diagnosis; and (4) the parents are fully informed of the risks and benefits of any planned procedure.

FETAL BLOOD SAMPLING

Indications

The main conditions which can be diagnosed by fetal blood sampling are listed in Table 20.1, as are the screening tests by which those in need of sampling may be identified. Antenatal diagnosis of the haemoglobinopathies and haemophilias prompted the introduction of fetal blood sampling techniques in the 1970s, but most of these diagnoses are now being performed by DNA analysis of chorionic villi.[1-3] Fetal blood sampling for other indications has therefore become more important.

Table 20.1 Indications for fetal blood sampling

Disorder		Screening test
Blood disorders:	Haemoglobinopathies	Genetic history
	Coagulation disorders	Carrier testing
	Factor VIII and IX deficiency	
Metabolic disorders		Genetic history
		Carrier testing
Fetal infections:	Rubella	History
	Toxoplasmosis	Maternal serology
	CMV	
	Parvovirus	
	Varicella	
Abnormal karyotype:	Trisomy	History
	Mosaicism	Maternal age
	Fragile-X	Serum screening
		Ultrasound
Immunodeficiencies		Genetic history
Intrauterine growth retardation (sample to measure blood gas and acid-base status)		Ultrasound
Unexplained fetal hydrops		Ultrasound
Red cell alloimmunization (sample to assess and treat fetal anaemia)		History
		Maternal serology
		Ultrasound
Platelet disorders:	Alloimmune thrombocytopenia	History
	Glanzmann's disease	Maternal serology

The list of metabolic disorders which are amenable to antenatal diagnosis either by enzyme or DNA analysis is continually being updated. They include the mucopolysaccharidoses, metachromatic leucodystrophy, homocystinuria, galactosaemia, and α1 antitrypsin deficiency. Although some of these may be diagnosed from fetal blood, in the majority chorionic villi are used.[4-6]

The investigation and antenatal management of other blood disorders such as alloimmune thrombocytopenia and, of course, Rhesus disease still require fetal blood sampling.[7,8]

Probably the major indication for fetal blood sampling in current clinical practice is the identification of a malformation at a routine ultrasound examination. Many of the defects detectable by ultrasound are associated with karyotypic abnormalities,[9-11] e.g. 16 per cent of fetuses with cardiac abnormalities.[12]

A number of fetal infections can also be diagnosed with fetal blood, such as rubella,[13,14] toxoplasmosis,[15,16] cytomegalovirus,[17] varicella-zoster,[18] and parvovirus.[19] But DNA techniques are increasingly being used on cells from chorionic villi or amniotic fluid.

An indication for fetal blood sampling that may increase is the assessment of small for gestational age fetuses or those suspected of being hypoxic.[20] The analysis of fetal blood gas and acid base status in clinical practice is far from established, however.[21]

Current techniques

Improvements in ultrasound technology led to the replacement of fetoscopic blood sampling[22] by sampling under ultrasound guidance. This technique was first introduced by Bang *et al.* in 1982 using the intrahepatic portion of the umbilical vein as a site for sampling.[23]

The original approach was to pass a guide needle (1.2 × 150 mm) down a puncture transducer through the maternal abdomen into the fetal abdomen 3–4 mm from the

Table 20.2 Sites for fetal blood sampling

Umbilical cord: artery or vein	Placental insertion
	Fetal insertion
	Free loop
Intra-hepatic portion of the umbilical vein	
Heart	

hepatic part of the umbilical vein. Through this, an inner needle (0.6 × 180 mm) was inserted into the lumen of the umbilical vein. The initial attempts were performed for intravascular transfusion in severe Rhesus disease. This technique was rapidly followed by a freehand ultrasound guided approach to the placental cord insertion[24] for the antenatal diagnosis of congenitally acquired infection (toxoplasmosis and rubella). It is this basic technique that is most extensively used today.

Using ultrasound guidance, fetal blood can now be obtained from a variety of sites (see Table 20.2). The preparation and technique for sampling is very similar whichever site is chosen. An initial ultrasound scan assessment is made of the fetal lie, placental location, amniotic fluid quantity and distribution, and umbilical cord insertion. At this assessment a decision is made about which site is best seen and of easiest access: a clear image is crucial. No pre-medication is necessary but local anaesthetic is usually infiltrated at the site of needle insertion.

In most centres full aseptic conditions are used throughout, including cleansing the skin, draping the abdomen and covering the ultrasound transducer. A single operator technique is usually used with the transducer held in one hand and the needle in the other. No special needle guide is necessary (although some prefer it) and a 20 or 22 gauge spinal needle is used depending on operator preference. The length of the needle is determined by the sonographically assessed depth of the target vessel (usually the umbilical vein at the placental cord insertion) from the maternal abdominal surface.

Once the sample is obtained it should be checked immediately to ensure that it is pure fetal blood. This may be achieved by assessment of the MCV (mean red cell volume) and Hct (haematocrit) using a Coulter counter. The MCV of fetal cells is 50 per cent greater than that of the maternal, although it falls with gestational age.[25]

At most sites the vein or artery may be entered. The vein is the preferred target, since it is the larger, less rigid of the vessels. Insertion of the needle into the artery may cause spasm of the vessel wall leading to alterations in blood flow and fetal heart rate that may necessitate delivery or preclude further sampling attempts; occasionally, fetal death may occur.

The vessel being sampled may be identified by injection of 1–2 ml of normal saline and sonographic observation of the turbulence and the direction of flow: in the artery towards the placenta and in the vein towards the fetus.

Sites for fetal blood sampling
Placental insertion of umbilical cord

The advantage of using the placental cord insertion is that it is a relatively fixed point which is affected only minimally by fetal movement. With an anterior placenta a transplacental approach avoids the introduction of the needle into the amniotic cavity

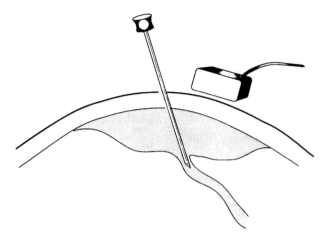

Fig. 20.1 Fetal blood sampling: approach to the anterior placenta.

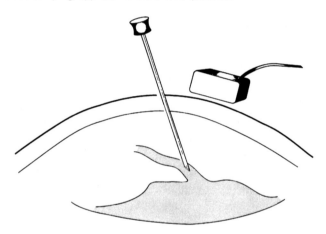

Fig. 20.2 Fetal blood sampling: approach to the posterior placenta.

(Fig. 20.1) therefore reducing the risk of amniotic fluid leak, but it has the disadvantage of producing feto-maternal haemorrhage which may cause sensitization of a Rhesus negative mother and will increase antibodies in an already alloimmunized woman. It is also possible erroneously to obtain a maternal sample from the intervillous space despite apparently correct placement of the needle.

If the placenta is posterior the amniotic cavity has to be traversed before the cord is entered at approximately 1 cm from the insertion site (Fig. 20.2), which can potentially lead to a persistent amniotic fluid leak. In the process of entering the cord it may be pinned against the placenta and the chorionic plate may be inadvertently punctured with consequent bleeding. Intra-amniotic bleeding from the cord is usually negligible or slight due to the haemostatic pressure of Wharton's jelly.

Fetal insertion of umbilical cord

The advantage of using the fetal insertion of the cord is that only fetal blood can be obtained from this point, and there is an increased quantity of Wharton's jelly so that haemostasis is in theory more effective and therefore blood loss is reduced.

However, in the presence of a normal amount of amniotic fluid, the fetus is mobile and if the initial attempt is unsuccessful a change in fetal position may make the target vessel more inaccessible.

Free loop of umbilical cord

In some circumstances, as with severe oligohydramnios, neither insertion of the cord may be visible or accessible to needling and the same may apply to the other sites, e.g. if the fetal spine is anterior. Most of the intrauterine sonolucencies seen with ultrasound are loops of cord, and this can be confirmed by colour Doppler. Such a loop can then be punctured. It is best to do this before infusion of any saline, so as to maintain the loop in a relatively fixed position. With normal amniotic fluid, or after amnioinfusion, loops of cord are very mobile and puncture is difficult.

Intrahepatic portion of the umbilical vein

Some groups now use the intrahepatic vein as a sampling site in preference to the cord.[26] However, in most centres the intrahepatic vein is selected if there is difficulty in visualizing or approaching the cord insertion, if there is concern regarding possible feto-maternal haemorrhage due to transplacental passage of the needle (i.e. when Rhesus alloimmunization can occur) or in twin pregnancies where allocation of the cord insertions to their respective fetuses may be difficult or impossible.

Under ultrasound guidance a 20 gauge spinal needle is introduced through the fetal abdominal wall either in the right or left hypochondrium or anteriorly in the midline. The needle can then be advanced through the substance of the liver in a horizontal plane and into the vein at an angle of about 60°.[27]

No alteration of the fetal liver enzymes has been reported with this technique.[26] The surrounding parenchyma reduces haemorrhage, and intraperitoneal bleeding was noted in only 2.3 per cent; this was shown to be reabsorbed over a few days with no serious complications.

Heart

The fetal heart has also been used in situations where no other sampling site is accessible.[28,29] The fetal heart is a large structure relative to the cord and lies in close proximity to the anterior chest wall. It is therefore easy to obtain blood from this site. However, movement of the needle within the myocardium is likely to produce rhythm disturbances which may be fatal. The technique is similar to all the other needling procedures but should be confined to cases where it is essential to obtain a blood sample that cannot be achieved safely from any other site.

Risks

The first large series of ultrasound guided fetal blood sampling was published in 1985 by Daffos *et al.*[30] They reported a fetal loss rate of 2 per cent . In this series of 606 samples the predominant indication for sampling was the investigation of possible toxoplasmosis infection and most of the fetuses were healthy. The main reasons for fetal loss are intrauterine death either at or near the time of sampling, spontaneous abortion as a result of chorioamnionitis, and premature delivery with consequent death from prematurity.

There is evidence that fetal loss is related to the gestational age at which sampling is performed. Orlandi *et al.*[31] showed a 5.2 per cent loss rate prior to 18 weeks of gestation compared with a 2.5 per cent loss rate between 19 and 21 weeks. Comparable fetal loss rates (2.5 per cent) have been found with intra-hepatic vein sampling.[26,27]

Maxwell *et al.*[32] showed that the loss rate is related to the indication for sampling, being 1.3 per cent for the diagnosis of the haemoglobinopathies (mean gestation 19 weeks), but 25 per cent where the indication is the investigation of non-immune hydrops. Clearly, a major factor in the fetal loss rate is the natural history of the disease process under investigation.

Pathological examination reveals macroscopic evidence of the needle entry in most instances of fetal blood sampling. In approximately 8 per cent there is evidence of haematoma encircling the vessel[33] but by the end of one week the vessel wall has healed. In this small series no thromboses were found in the umbilical vessels.

Acute fetal distress may be caused by reduction in blood flow due to haematoma formation at the site of needle insertion. It happens very rarely after fetal blood sampling, but occasionally after intravascular transfusion. Exsanguination only occurs in extremely thrombocytopenic fetuses. Weiner and Anderson[34] have shown that independent of the difficulty of the procedure there is a significant reduction in the Doppler waveform indices derived from the umbilical artery after fetal blood sampling from the cord. This suggests that puncture of the umbilical cord vessels leads to a release of vasoactive substances.

It is likely that premature delivery is a direct consequence of chorioamnionitis and therefore strict asepsis is of the utmost importance during any of these procedures.

SAMPLING FROM FETAL TISSUES OTHER THAN BLOOD

There are instances where fetal tissues other than blood are required for diagnostic purposes. These may include fetal liver, skin, muscle, tumour biopsy, or fluid aspiration from abnormal collections. The risks of these procedures appear to be similar to those of fetal blood sampling.

Fetal liver biopsy

The indications for fetal liver biopsy include high risk of the genetically inherited enzyme deficiencies of the urea cycle, including ornithine carbamyl transferase (OCT) and carbamyl phosphate synthetase deficiencies (see Table 20.3). First trimester diagnosis by DNA analysis is now usually possible.

Originally performed fetoscopically,[35] an ultrasound guided double-needle aspiration technique is now used.[36] An 18 gauge guide needle is inserted into the edge of the fetal liver and a 20 gauge needle is then advanced through this into the substance of the liver. Suction on a 10 ml syringe containing either culture medium or saline, and up and down movement of the needle within the liver substance yields a core of tissue that may be submitted to enzyme assay or microscopic examination. The procedure is usually done at 18–20 weeks of gestation.

Table 20.3 Indications for fetal liver biopsy.*
(Screening for these disorders is by family and past obstetric history)

Ornithine carbamyl transferase deficiency
Carbamyl phosphate synthetase deficiency
Primary hyperoxaluria type I
Aromatic aminoacid decarboxylase deficiency
Glucose-6-phosphate (G6P) deficiency
Glycogen storage disease type Ia and Ib

---

* Early diagnosis by chorion villus sampling and DNA analysis is possible in many cases.

Table 20.4 Genodermatoses in which antenatal diagnosis has been achieved by fetal skin biopsy. (Screening for these disorders is by family and past obstetric history)

Epidermolysis bullosa*: Junctional (letalis)
                        Dystrophic
Non-bullous ichthyosiform erythroderma
Bullous ichthyosiform erythroderma
Harlequin fetus
Lamellar ichthyosis
Sjögren–Larsson syndrome
Oculo-cutaneous albinism

---

* Early diagnosis by chorion villus sampling and DNA analysis is available in some cases.

Fetal tumour biopsy

Fetal tumours may be biopsied in a similar manner to that for fetal liver biopsy for identification of tumour type and prognosis. Tumours identified by this technique to date include congenital adenomatoid malformation of the lung and fetal teratomas.[37]

Fetal skin biopsy

Fetal skin was also biopsied initially by fetoscopy,[38] but ultrasound guided techniques using fine biopsy forceps[8] or Tru-cut needles[39] are now employed.

Skin sampling is used to make the antenatal diagnosis of some of the genodermatoses (see Table 20.4) in families with one affected child or a strong family history.

Some of these conditions may be associated with accelerated keratinization, which can cause diagnostic problems. Normal keratinization does not usually occur *in utero* until the 24th week and it may be uncertain when the abnormal gene is expressed, potentially making skin biopsy a late diagnostic test in some conditions, e.g. harlequin fetus, ichthyosis. Immunofluorescent antibodies to basement membrane antigens can be used as early as 15–16 weeks for junctional epidermolysis bullosa[40] and DNA techniques are also becoming applicable, particularly in some families with dystrophic epidemolysis bullosa.[41]

Multiple sampling sites may be required or a specific site may have to be targeted in some conditions, e.g. the sacral area in Hallopeau–Siemens dystrophic epidermolysis bullosa, and hair follicle (e.g. eyebrow or scalp) for oculocutaneous albinism.

The taking of the sample may produce biopsy artefact and disruption of the normal structures leading to difficulty and errors in diagnosis. Skin biopsy is therefore another antenatal diagnostic test which should only be performed in centres of expertise.

Fetal muscle biopsy

Fetal muscle biopsies can be tested for the presence of dystrophin to diagnose Duchenne muscular dystrophy.[42] This is only appropriate if the family are uninformative for DNA markers.

Fluid aspiration

A number of abnormal fetal fluid collections can be aspirated to provide diagnostic information. The fetal karyotype can be obtained by culturing cells present in ascites, pleural effusions,[43] cystic hygroma fluid, and fetal urine.[44]

The most useful application of fluid aspiration has been biochemical analysis of urine in the management of fetal obstructive uropathies detected by ultrasound, particularly the posterior urethral valve syndrome. Therapeutic results of vesico-amniotic shunting depend on the identification of those cases in which there is still good renal function and the kidneys are not dysplastic. Normal values are now available for fetal urinary electrolytes at various gestational ages, and sodium and calcium concentrations appear to be the most predictive.[45] Levels above the normal range suggest renal dysplasia and a poor prognosis. Repeat sampling after bladder emptying[46] and serial sampling[47] may be necessary to increase the reliability of the diagnosis of renal dysplasia.

CONCLUSION

In conclusion there are now many fetal tissues that can be sampled with relative safety for antenatal diagnosis of genetically inherited and structural abnormalities. The awareness that such an intervention is indicated most commonly arises as a result of the widespread use of ultrasound to screen for malformations. A familial or past obstetric history may bring to light the possibility of a genetic disorder. Usually, these are complex cases which should be managed in fetal medicine centres with the appropriate clinical, genetic counselling, and laboratory facilities.

REFERENCES

1. Williamson, R., Eskdale, J., Coleman, D.V., Niazi, M. *et al.* (1981). Direct gene analysis of chorionic villi: a possible technique for first trimester antenatal diagnosis of haemoglobinopathies. *Lancet*, **ii**, 1125–7.
2. Old, J.M., Ward, R.H.T., Modell, B. *et al.* (1982). First trimester diagnosis for haemoglobinopathies: 3 cases. *Lancet*, **ii**, 1413–16.
3. Old, J.M., Ward, R.H.T., Petrou, M. *et al.* (1986). First trimester diagnosis for haemoglobinopathies: report on 200 cases. *Lancet*, **ii**, 763–7.
4. Cooper, D.N. and Schmidtke, J. (1989). Diagnosis of genetic disease using recombinant DNA. *Human Genetics*, **83**, 307–34.

5. Poenarul, L. (1987). First trimester diagnosis of metabolic disease: a survey in countries from the European Community. *Prenatal Diagnosis*, **7**, 331–41.

6. Kleijer, W.J., Thoomes, R., Galjaard, H., Wendel, U., and Fowler, B. (1984). First trimester (chorion biopsy) diagnosis of Citrullinaemia and methyl aciduria. *Lancet*, **ii**, 1340.

7. Mibashan, R.S. and Rodeck, C.H. (1984). Haemophilia and other genetic defects of haemostasis. In *Prenatal Diagnosis*, (ed. C.H. Rodeck and K.H. Nicolaides), pp. 179–194. Wiley, Chichester.

8. Fisk, N.M. and Rodeck, C.H. (1996). Antenatal diagnosis and fetal medicine. In *Texbook of Neonatology* (ed. N. R. C. Roberton, J. M. Rennie), 3rd edn, pp. 199–233. Churchill Livingstone, Edinburgh.

9. Nicolaides, K.H., Rodeck, C.H., and Gosden, C.M. (1986). Rapid karyotyping in non-lethal fetal malformations. *Lancet*, **i**, 283–7.

10. Marchese, C.A., Garozzi, F., Mosso, R. *et al.* (1985). Fetal karyotype in malformations detected by ultrasound. *American Journal of Human Genetics*, **37**, A223.

11. Palmer, C.G., Miles, J.H., Howard-Peebles, P.N. *et al.* (1987). Fetal karyotype following ascertainment of fetal anomalies by ultrasound. *Prenatal Diagnosis*, **7**, 551–5.

12. Allan, L.D., Sharland, G.K., Chita, S.K. *et al.* (1991). Chromosomal abnormalities in fetal congenital heart disease. *Ultrasound in Obstetrics and Gynecology*, **1**, 8–11.

13. Daffos, F., Forestier, F., Grangeot-Keros, L. *et al.* (1984). Prenatal diagnosis of congenital rubella. *Lancet* **ii**, 1–3.

14. Morgan-Capner, P., Rodeck, C.H., Nicolaides, K.H. *et al.* (1985). Prenatal detection of rubella specific IgM in fetal sera. *Prenatal Diagnosis*, **5**, 21–3.

15. Desmonts, G., Daffos, F., Forestier, F. *et al.* (1985). Prenatal diagnosis of congenital toxoplasmosis. *Lancet* **i**, 500–3.

16. Daffos, F., Forestier, F., Capella-Pavlosky, M. *et al.* (1988). Prenatal management of 746 pregnancies at risk of congenital toxoplasmosis. *New England Journal of Medicine*, **318**, 271–5.

17. Lange, I., Rodeck, C.H., Morgan-Capner, P. *et al.* (1982). Prenatal serological diagnosis of intrauterine cytomegalovirus infection. *British Medical Journal*, **284**, 1673–4.

18. Cuthberson, G., Weiner, C.O., Giller, R.H. *et al.* (1987). Prenatal diagnosis of second trimester congenital varicella syndrome by virus specific IgM. *Journal of Paediatrics*, **11**, 592–5.

19. Peters, M.T. and Nicolaides, K.H. (1990). Cordocentesis for diagnosis and treatment of human parvovirus infection. *Obstetrics and Gynecology*, **75**, 501–4.

20. Soothill, P.W., Nicolaides, K.H., Bilardo, C. *et al.* (1987). Utero-placental blood velocity resistance index and umbilical venous p02, pC02, pH, lactate and erythroblast count in growth retarded fetuses. *Fetal Therapy*, **4**, 174–8.

21. Nicolini, U., Nicolaidis, P., Fisk, N.M., Vaughan, J., Fusi, L., Gleeson, R., and Rodeck, C.H. (1990). Limited role of fetal blood sampling in prediction of outcome in intrauterine growth retardation. *Lancet*, **336**, 768–71.

22. Rodeck, C.H. (1980). Fetoscopy guided by real-time ultrasound for pure fetal blood sampling, fetal skin samples and visualisation of the fetus *in utero*. *British Journal of Obstetrics and Gynaecology*, **87**, 449–56.

23. Bang, J., Bock, T.E., and Trolle, D. (1982). Ultrasound-guided fetal intravascular transfusion for severe Rhesus haemolytic disease. *British Medical Journal*, **284**, 373–4.

24. Daffos, F., Capella-Pavlovsky, M., and Forestier, F. (1983). Fetal blood sampling via the umbilical cord using needle guided by ultrasound. *Prenatal Diagnosis*, **3**, 271–7.

25. Fisk, N.M., Tannirandorn, Y., Santolaya, J., Nicolini, U., Letsky, E.A., and Rodeck, C.H. (1989). Fetal macrocytosis in association with chromosomal abnormalities. *Obstetrics and Gynecology*, **74**, 611–14.

26. Nicolini, U., Nicolaidis, P., Fisk, N.M., Tannirandorn, Y., and Rodeck, C.H. (1990). Fetal blood sampling from the intrahepatic vein: analysis of safety and clinical experience with 214 procedures. *Obstetrics and Gynecology*, **76**, 47.

27. Nicolini, U., Santolaya, J., Ojo, O.E. *et al.* (1988). The fetal intrahepatic vein as an alternative to cord needling for prenatal diagnosis and therapy. *Prenatal Diagnosis*, **8**, 665–71.

28. De Crespigny, L.C., Robinson, H.P., Quinn, M., Doyle, L. *et al.* (1985). Ultrasound guided fetal trasfusion for severe Rhesus isoimmunisation. *Obstetrics and Gynecology*, **66**, 529–32.

29. Westgren, M., Selbing, A., and Stangenberg, M. (1988). Fetal intracardiac transfusion in patients with severe Rhesus isoimmunisation. *British Medical Journal*, **295**, 885–6.

30. Daffos, F., Capella-Pavlovsky, M., and Forestier, F. (1985). Fetal blood sampling during pregnancy with use of needle guide by ultrasound: a study of 606 consecutive cases. *American Journal of Obstetrics and Gynecology*, **153**, 655–60.

31. Orlandi, F., Damiani, G., Jakil, C. *et al.* (1990). The risks of early cordocentesis (12–21 weeks): analysis of 500 procedures. *Prenatal Diagnosis*, **10**, 425–8.

32. Maxwell, D.J., Johnson, P., Hurley, P.A. *et al.* (1991). Fetal blood sampling and pregnancy loss in relation to indication. *British Journal of Obstetrics and Gynaecology*, **98**, 892–7.

33. Jauniaux, E., Donner, C., Simon, P. *et al.* (1989). Pathological aspects of umbilical cord after percutaneous umbilical blood sampling. *Obstetrics and Gynecology*, **73**, 215–18.

34. Weiner, C.P. and Anderson, T.L. (1989). The acute effect of cordocentesis with or without fetal curarization and intravascular transfusion upon umbilical waveform indices. *Obstetrics and Gynecology*, **73**, 219–23.

35. Rodeck, C.H., Patrick, A.D., Pembrey, M.E., Tzannatos, C., and Whitfield, A.E. (1982). Fetal liver biopsy for prenatal diagnosis of ornithine carbamyl transferase deficiency. *Lancet*, **ii**, 297–300.

36. Rodeck, C.H. and Fisk, N.M. (1993). Fetal liver biopsy. In *Ultrasound in Obstetrics and Gynaecology*, Vol. 2 (ed. F. Chervenk, G. Isacson, and S. Campbell), pp. 1267–72. Little Brown, Philadelphia.

37. Rodeck, C.H. and Nicolaides, K.H. (1986). Fetal tissue biopsy: techniques and indications. *Fetal Therapy*, **1**, 46–58.

38. Rodeck, C.H., Eady, R.A.J., and Gosden, C.M. (1980). Prenatal diagnosis of epidermolysis bullosa letalis. *Lancet* **i**, 949–52.

39. Bakharev, V.A., Aivazyan, A.A., Karentnikova, N.A. *et al.* (1990). Skin biopsy in prenatal diagnosis of some genodermatoses. *Prenatal Diagnosis*, **10**, 1–12.

40. Heagarty, A.H.M., Eady, R.A.J., Nicolaides, K.H., Rodeck, C.H., Hsi, B-L., and Ortonne, J.P. (1987). Rapid prenatal diagnosis of epidermolysis bullosa letalis using GB3 monoclonal antibody. *British Journal of Dermatology*, **117**, 271–5.

41. Dunnill, M.G.S., Rodeck, C.H., Richard, A.J., Atherton, D., Lake, B.D., Petrou, M. *et al.* (1995). Use of type VII collagen gene (COL 7A1) markers in prenatal diagnosis of recessive dystrophic epidermolysis bullosa. *Journal of Medical Genetics*, **32**, 749–50.

42. Evans, M.I., Greb, A., Kunkel, L.M., Sacks, A.J., Johnson, M.P., Boehm, M.S., Kazazian, Jr., H.H., and Hoffman, E.P. (1991). *In utero* fetal muscle biopsy for the diagnosis of Duchenne muscular dystrophy. *American Journal of Obstetrics and Gynecology*, **165**, 728–32.

43. Rodeck, C.H., Fisk, N.M., Fraser, D.I., and Nicolini, U. (1988). Long term drainage of fetal hydrothorax. *New England Journal of Medicine*, **391**, 1135–8.
44. Manning, F.A., Harrison, M.R., Rodeck, C.H. *et al.* (1986). Catheter shunts for hydronephrosis and hydrocephalus: report of the International Fetal Surgery Register. *New England Journal of Medicine*, **315**, 336–40.
45. Nicolini, U., Fisk, N.M., Beacham, J., and Rodeck, C.H. (1992). Fetal urine biochemistry: an index of renal maturation and dysfunction. *British Journal of Obstetrics and Gynaecology*, **99**, 46–50.
46. Nicolini, U., Tannirandorn, Y., Vaughan, J., Fisk, N.M., Nicolaidis, P, and Rodeck C.H. (1991). Further prediction of renal dysplasia in fetal obstructive uropathy: bladder pressusre and biochemistry of 'fresh' urine. *Prenatal Diagnosis*, **11**, 159–66.
47. Nicolini, U., Rodeck, C.H., and Fisk, N.M. (1987). Shunt treatment for fetal uropathy. *Lancet*, **ii**, 1338–9.

21 *Continuous electronic fetal monitoring during labour*

Ian Leck and Stephen B. Thacker

INTRODUCTION

Electronic fetal monitoring (EFM) during labour involves recording the fetal heart rate by means of an electrode on the fetal scalp or an ultrasound probe on the mother's abdomen. It was introduced during the 1960s, with the objective of recording fetal heart-rate patterns associated with hypoxia during labour. The aim is to identify fetal hypoxia at an early enough stage in labour to carry out a Caesarean or instrumental delivery before the hypoxia can lead to perinatal death or lasting neuropsychiatric disability.

ADVERSE OUTCOMES OF HYPOXIA DURING LABOUR

The use of EFM can be justified only if it is followed by a lower incidence of adverse effects of fetal hypoxia than is seen when less complex methods of detecting hypoxia (e.g. intermittent auscultation of the fetal heart) are used. Intrapartum hypoxia can lead to perinatal death or cerebral palsy (CP). The key question affecting the use of EFM is whether the fetuses selected for treatment by this method include some in which the treatment prevents death or CP.

The frequency of perinatal deaths, and of CP in survivors, is examined in Table 21.1. The perinatal death statistics are based on all births (including stillbirths from 24 weeks of gestation) in England and Wales in 1997, the most recent year for which data are available. The perinatal death rate from all causes was 8/1000 total births. Using both fetal and maternal certified causes of death, all deaths were assigned to Office of National Statistics' Cause Groups. This classification includes one group for anoxia, asphyxia, and trauma of intrapartum onset and one for those of antepartum onset. The perinatal death rate from intrapartum anoxia, asphyxia, and trauma was 0.6/1000 total births (7 per cent of all perinatal deaths).[1]

The figure given in Table 21.1 for the overall prevalence of CP in survivors (2/1000) is based on many population studies in industrialized countries.[2] Most of these studies yielded estimates of prevalence of between 1.6 and 2.5 per 1000 live births, although rates of nearly 6/1000 have been reported when complete birth cohorts have

Table 21.1 Estimated prevalence of perinatal death and cerebral palsy caused by hypoxia or trauma during labour

Outcome	Total prevalence per 1000 births	Proportion caused by hypoxia or trauma during labour	Prevalence of cases caused by hypoxia or trauma during labour, per 1000 births
Perinatal death	8[a]	7%	0.6[a]
Cerebral palsy in survivors	2[b]	9%[c]	0.2
Perinatal death or cerebral palsy	10	7–8%	0.8

[a] Office for National Statistics[1] (rate per 1000 total births).
[b] Stanley and Blair[2] (rate per 1000 live births).
[c] Nelson and Ellenberg;[3] Blair and Stanley.[4]

been followed up regularly and cases of motor impairment followed by early death or resolution have been included.

The estimate of 9 per cent for the proportion of cases of CP in survivors caused by hypoxia or trauma during labour (Table 21.1) is based on work by Nelson and Ellenberg[3] and Blair and Stanley.[4] Other current estimates of this percentage range from 3 per cent to 20 per cent.[5,6] Earlier estimates[7,8] were higher (approximately 50 per cent), reflecting the fact that up to half of all children with CP have a history of findings such as low Apgar scores, delayed breathing, seizures, and recurrent apnoea which can be brought about by intrapartum asphyxia.[3,4] However, recent population-based studies based on careful history-taking and multifactorial analysis suggest that these findings and the associated CP are both caused in a majority of cases by factors operating before the onset of labour.[3,4,9]

Given the estimates in Table 21.1 that intrapartum asphyxia leads to perinatal death in 0.6/1000 total births and survival with CP in 0.2/1000, and allowing for a margin of uncertainty around these estimates, 1/1000 total births is a reasonable estimate of the total prevalence of serious consequences of birth asphyxia. Separate figures for severe intellectual impairment and epilepsy are not included in this estimate, because birth asphyxia seldom seems to cause these conditions without causing CP also.[10]

THE SCREENING TEST

EFM (also known as cardiotocography) involves the production by a cardiotocograph of a continuous record (cardiotocogram) of the fetal heart rate and uterine contractions, and the interpretation of this record. The test has recently been described in detail by Parer.[11]

Procedure

Each fetal heartbeat is recorded either through an electrode placed on the presenting part of the fetus ('scalp electrode') or by means of an ultrasound Doppler transducer affixed (e.g. by a belt) to the mother's abdomen. The transducer works by directing an ultrasonic beam at the fetal heart, and detecting heartbeats by the changes in frequency of the reflected beam that occur whenever the heart moves. Unlike a scalp electrode, a Doppler transducer can be used before the membranes rupture. Whichever method is used, the cardiotocograph converts the interval between each pair of heartbeats to the pulse rate in beats per minute that would occur if all intervals were of this length, and plots this rate against time.

The uterine contractions can also be recorded either externally by a transducer on the abdomen, or internally, by means of a catheter which is inserted through the cervical canal and either incorporates or is connected to a pressure transducer. Whichever method is used, uterine activity over time is plotted and can be compared with fetal heart rate. Both methods record the length of each contraction reliably, but only the internal method can measure the intrauterine pressure in absolute units (mmHg or kPa), which is of interest because too high a pressure between contractions can impede the placental blood flow.

The fetal heart-rate plots produced by cardiotocographs are examined for (1) two characteristics which are apparent between uterine contractions, namely the baseline rate and the variation around this baseline that the rate normally exhibits ('variability'), and (2) periodic changes in rate ('accelerations' and 'decelerations'), which are usually associated with uterine contractions and involve a considerable number of heartbeats. Three kinds of deceleration have been defined: 'early', 'late', and 'variable'. Early decelerations begin and end with uterine contractions and are attributed to pressure on the fetal head. Late decelerations start after the uterine contractions with which they are associated, and are thought to be a sign of utero-placental insufficiency, which leads to impaired maternal–fetal exchange during contractions. Variable decelerations vary more than the other types in three respects: their timing relative to uterine contractions, their amplitude, and their duration. They are thought to be caused by umbilical cord compression.[12]

Table 21.2   Definitions of abnormal and borderline cardiotocograph findings

		Heartbeats per minute	
Variable measured	Abnormality	Borderline values	Abnormal values
Baseline fetal heart rate[a]	Tachycardia	150–170,[b] 160–180[c,d]	> 170,[b] > 180[c,d]
	Bradycardia	100–110,[b,d] 100–120[c]	< 100[b,c,d]
Range of variability of fetal heart rate around baseline[a]	High variability	> 25[b,d]	
	Low variability	5–10 for >40 min,[b] 5–10[d]	< 5 for >40 min,[b] <5; no accelerations in absence of sedation[d]
Reduction in fetal heart rate	Late deceleration[e]	15–45[c]	>45[c]
	Variable deceleration	>60[e] (deceleration for <60 s),[d] <70[f] (deceleration for 30–60 s),[c] 70–80[f] (deceleration for >60 s)[c]	>60[e] (deceleration for > 60 s)[d], <70[f] (deceleration for >60 s)[c]

[a] Beats per minute.
[b] Herbst and Ingemarsson[13] (values termed borderline and abnormal above were termed suspicious and abnormal respectively by these authors).
[c] Kubli *et al.*[12] (values termed borderline and abnormal above were termed moderate and severe respectively by these authors).
[d] Westgate *et al.*[14] (borderline values for low variability and variable deceleration interpolated using Westgate's definitions of normal and abnormal values).
[e] Beats per minute *by* which fetal heart rate drops.
[f] Beats per minute *to* which fetal heart rate drops.

Interpretation

Accelerations and early decelerations are not generally believed to be grounds for concern about the possibility of hypoxia, but hypoxia can lead to abnormal baseline rates and variability, and to late and variable decelerations. Table 21.2 gives several definitions of borderline and abnormal cardiotocograph findings.

Procedure when the test is positive

If the fetal scalp is accessible, blood sampling from this site is widely advocated as the next step to be taken when a cardiotocogram is judged to show persistent abnormality. The purpose of fetal blood sampling is to measure fetal blood pH, which tends to fall with increasing hypoxia. If the fetal blood pH is both below 7.20 and at least 0.15 units less than the mother's, instrumental or Caesarean delivery is generally undertaken immediately. Following a fetal blood pH reading of 7.20–7.25, intervention of this kind or further sampling is carried out after a further period of observation if the fetal heartbeat remains abnormal.[14–17]

Although fetal blood sampling as a secondary screening test has gained in popularity during the 1990s, its place in clarifying fetal heart-rate patterns is a matter of debate.[5] The diversity of practice is illustrated by the 12 randomized trials of continuous intrapartum EFM that have been reported.[13,15–25] Fetal scalp blood sampling was not used in at least three of these 12 trials,[18,24,25] and the reports of two others made no mention of this procedure at all.[20,22] Even those who normally sample the fetal blood when the results of cardiotocography are abnormal cannot do so if the fetal scalp is not yet accessible, and may choose not to do so if the second stage of labour has already started.[16] The alternative to sampling the fetal blood when the results of cardiotocography are clearly abnormal for more than a few minutes is to proceed straight to instrumental or Caesarean delivery.

Problems

The problems with continuous EFM during labour as a screening procedure include the previously mentioned disagreements regarding (1) what constitutes a positive result (Table 21.2) and (2) whether immediate delivery should be effected in all cases in which EFM is positive (however defined) or only in those in which the fetal blood pH is found to be low. Other data also illustrate the difficulties experienced by obstetricians in using EFM to select cases for intervention. In a study of inter- and intra-observer variability, four experienced obstetricians who were given 50 cardiotocograms to evaluate did not agree on whether intervention was indicated in 39 of the 50; and when they re-examined the same cardiotocograms again after two months, their conclusions differed from those reached at the first examination in one-fifth of cases.[26] In another study, the staff in attendance did not respond appropriately to abnormal cardiotocograms in 33 of 38 deliveries in which the clinical outcome was severe asphyxia.[27] This study also included normal deliveries, and the assessment of cardiotocograms as normal or abnormal was made by three experienced obstetricians who did not know the clinical outcome.

These uncertainties of definition and strategy reflect the fact that the effectiveness of using EFM in the management of labour has not been demonstrated.

Predictive performance

When an EFM pattern is believed to be abnormal, intervention usually follows. This makes determining the performance of EFM in terms of detection rate and false-positive rate impossible. These rates can only be calculated if fetuses in which an adverse outcome would have occurred in the absence of EFM-based intervention can be distinguished from other fetuses. A recent study of the birth records of cases of CP and controls[6] has, however, provided a basis for estimating upper and lower limits for the performance of EFM as a screening test for CP in infants weighing at least 2500 g at birth. In this study, moderate or severe CP diagnosed by age three years was found to be significantly associated with EFM findings of decreased beat-to-beat variability and/or multiple late decelerations, with an odds ratio of 2.7 (95 per cent CI 1.4–5.4) after adjustment for other risk factors. No significant association with tachycardia or bradycardia was found. Table 21.3 shows the measures of performance yielded by the data on two alternative assumptions: that EFM-based management prevented no cases of CP and that EFM-based management prevented all cases of CP caused by asphyxia or trauma during labour.

Even if a policy of intervention when EFM findings were abnormal in mature fetuses would prevent all severe and moderate CP caused by damage during labour, the data in Table 21.3 imply that less than one per thousand recipients of intervention would benefit from this effect, since the estimated prevalence of CP caused by damage during labour (0.07/1000) is less than one-thousandth of the false-positive rate (93/1000).

Comparable data regarding the performance of EFM as a screening test for death during labour or the neonatal period are not available. However, one can estimate the highest possible odds of being affected by death or CP caused by problems during labour, given a positive result of screening. The highest odds are those that would occur if continuous EFM during labour detected 100 per cent of pregnancies in which asphyxia or trauma during labour would result in death or CP if EFM was not used. The estimated prevalence of these outcomes is 1/1000 births (p. 529). The false-positive rate would presumably be close to 93/1000 (Table 21.3). If so, even with a

Table 21.3 Estimated performance of EFM as a predictor of cerebral palsy (CP) in infants weighing at least 2500 g at birth, based on a case-control study[6]

Assumption	Prevalence of CP if EFM not used in management	Detection rate	False-positive rate	Odds of being affected given a positive result
Worst case: intervention if EFM is positive is not effective	0.67/1000[6]	26.9%[6]	9.3%[6]	1:516
Best case: intervention if EFM is positive prevents 9% of cases of CP[a]	0.74/1000[b]	33.8%[c]	9.3%[d]	1:372

[a] 9% is the proportion of CP estimated to be caused by asphyxia or trauma during labour (Table 21.1).
[b] 0.67 × 100/(100 − 9).
[c] [(0.67 × 0.269) + (0.74 − 0.67)]/0.74.
[d] {[(1000 − 0.67) × 0.093] − (0.74 − 0.67)}/(1000 − 0.74).

detection rate of 100 per cent the odds of being affected given a positive result would be no greater than 1:93.

Effectiveness in preventing adverse outcomes

The effectiveness of EFM during labour in preventing mortality and morbidity was tested in the 12 randomized controlled trials cited already. These have been reviewed by Thacker et al.[28] Continuous EFM and auscultation were compared in nine of these studies, of which one was based on nearly 13 000 pregnancies[16] and the other eight on fewer than 1000 pregnancies each[15,17-21,23,24]. The alternatives compared in the other three trials were:

(1) routine use of continuous intrapartum EFM versus its use in selected cases only (based on 34 995 pregnancies);[23]

(2) continuous versus intermittent EFM (4044 pregnancies);[14] and

(3) intermittent EFM versus auscultation (1255 pregnancies).[26]

Among the 12 trials, one included only pregnancies in which labour occurred when estimated length of gestation and fetal weight were 26–32 weeks and 700–1750 g respectively;[17] four were based on pregnancies classified as at increased risk of an adverse outcome for various reasons, e.g. medical or obstetric problems during present or previous pregnancy ('high-risk' pregnancies);[15,18,19,25] three were restricted to pregnancies without such risk factors ('low-risk' pregnancies);[13,20,21] and four included all 'low-risk' and most or all 'high-risk' pregnancies.[16,22-24]

Thacker et al.[28] estimated the relative risks (RRs) of intrapartum or neonatal death, low Apgar score, and neonatal seizures following continuous EFM during labour, by carrying out a cumulative meta-analysis of the nine trials of this procedure versus auscultation. Low Apgar score and neonatal seizures are of interest because infants in whom these findings occur are at increased risk of CP (see below). If, therefore, the relative risks of low Apgar score and neonatal seizures were reduced by using continuous EFM to guide the management of labour there would be grounds for hoping that this procedure would also reduce the risk of CP.

Table 21.4 Performance of low Apgar scores and neonatal seizures as predictors of moderate or severe cerebral palsy by age 7 years or death with CP between 1 and 7 years, in children alive at age 1 year. Estimated from results of the Collaborative Perinatal Project of the US National Institute of Neurological and Communicative Disorders and Stroke,[29] in which CP as defined occurred in 3/1000 births.

Predictor of cerebral palsy	Detection rate (DR)	False-positive rate (FPR)	Prevalence of cerebral palsy in those with specified predictor	Odds of being affected for those with specified predictor (0.003DR:0.997FPR)	Likelihood ratio (DR/FPR)
Apgar score:					
0–3 at 1 min	26%	4.7%	1.7%	1:60	5.5
0–3 at 5 min	14%	0.9%	5.1%	1:21	15.6
0–6 at 1 min	43%	18.4%	0.7%	1:142	2.3
0–6 at 5 min	26%	3.7%	2.2%	1:47	7.0
Neonatal seizures	23%	0.3%	18.1%	1:4.3	76.7

The Apgar score ranges from 0 to 10, and is obtained by adding together scores of 0 (worst) to 2 (best) for the infant's respiratory effort, muscle tone, cry, colour, and heart rate. Estimates of the performance of low Apgar score and of neonatal seizures as predictors of CP are shown in Table 21.4. According to these estimates, low Apgar scores and neonatal seizures are not found in a majority of neonates who if they survive will develop CP, and even when one of these findings is present the odds are against CP developing. However, according to the likelihood ratios yielded by the estimates, children with CP are between 2 and 16 times as likely as other children to have had the Apgar scores listed and nearly 80 times as likely to have had neonatal seizures (Table 21.4, last column).

The RRs according to Thacker's analysis of the nine trials of continuous intrapartum EFM versus auscultation are given in the first data column in Table 21.5. The magnitude of these problems in populations not screened by EFM is broadly indicated by the figures in the second data column in Table 21.5, which are based on the three trials which included both 'high-risk' and 'low-risk' pregnancies. The remaining data columns of Table 21.5 give comparable information for the trial in which the routine use of continuous intrapartum EFM was compared with its use in high-risk pregnancies only.[22] The results of this trial are of particular interest because it was much larger than the others, and therefore might more readily have detected any benefits from using continuous intrapartum EFM, provided that these benefits were not restricted to high-risk pregnancies.

The results for the various outcomes of these trials are reviewed in the following subsections.

Table 21.5   Results of randomised clinical trials of continuous electronic fetal monitoring (EFM) during labour

Outcome	Nine trials of continuous EFM, with auscultation in controls[15–21,23,24]		One trial of continuous EFM for all, with continuous EFM in control group restricted to 'high-risk' cases[22]	
	Relative risk (95% CI)[28]	Range of prevalence of specified outcome in general populations[a]	Relative risk (95% CI)	Prevalence of specified outcome in controls
Intrapartum or neonatal death	0.83 (0.55–1.25)	2–13/1000	1.03 (0.82–1.30)	8/1000
1 min Apgar score 0–3	0.82 (0.65–0.98)[b]	1–4%	1.01 (0.80–1.27)[c]	0.8%[c]
1 min Apgar score 0–6	1.02 (0.90–1.14)[b]	5–12%	0.97 (0.83–1.13)[c]	2%[c]
Neonatal seizures	0.50 (0.30–0.82)	0–4/1000	1.16 (0.78–1.73)	3/1000
Cerebral palsy diagnosed at 18 months	2.54 (1.10–5.86)[d]	8%[d]	–	–

[a] Based on control groups in the three general population trials.[16,23,24]
[b] Eight trials only.
[c] Apgar scores at 5 min.
[d] One trial, in infants weighing 700–1750 g at birth.[30]

Intrapartum and neonatal mortality

No evidence of an effect was found. The RRs of intrapartum or neonatal death were 0.83 (95 per cent CI 0.55–1.25) in the trials of continuous EFM versus auscultation and 1.03 (0.82–1.30) in the trial of routine EFM versus EFM for high-risk cases only. In the trial of continuous versus intermittent EFM[13] only one death occurred. This followed continuous EFM.

Apgar score

The results indicated no significant improvement in Apgar scores after continuous EFM, except for scores of 0–3 in the trials of continuous EFM versus auscultation. The reduction in prevalence of these scores was of marginal significance (RR 0.82; 95 per cent CI 0.65–0.98), and was not accompanied by any decline in the prevalence of scores of 0–6 at one minute (RR 1.02; 95 per cent CI 0.90–1.14). In the trial of routine EFM versus EFM for high-risk cases only, Apgar scores were measured at 5 minutes, and the relative risks of scores of 0–3 and 0–6 were both close to unity, with 95 per cent confidence intervals of about 0.8–1.3 and 0.8–1.1 respectively. In the trial of continuous versus intermittent EFM,[13] the RRs for scores of 0–3 and 0–6 at 1 minute were 1.24 (95 per cent CI 0.33–4.62) and 1.35 (95 per cent CI 0.95–1.91) respectively.

Neonatal seizures

The risk of neonatal seizures with *routine* continuous EFM was much lower than with routine auscultation (RR 0.50; 95 per cent CI 0.30–0.82)[28] but not lower than with continuous EFM in 'high-risk' pregnancies alone (RR 1.16; 95 per cent CI 0.78–1.73).[22] At first consideration, this suggests that 'high-risk' but not 'low-risk' pregnancies benefit from continuous EFM. However, this suggestion is not supported by a separate analysis of 'high-risk' and 'low-risk' pregnancies in the largest trial of continuous EFM versus auscultation[16] (a trial which included 70 per cent of all the subjects in the nine trials of this kind). In this trial, the risk of seizures after EFM was much lower than after auscultation in 'low-risk' pregnancies (RR 0.37; 95 per cent CI 0.15–0.87), and the reduction in 'high-risk' pregnancies was less extreme (RR 0.64; 95 per cent CI 0.21–1.97).

Therefore, a conflict of evidence exists between this trial of routine EFM versus auscultation[16] and the trial of routine EFM versus EFM for high-risk cases only.[22] In an assessment of overall quality,[29] the former trial scored much more highly than the latter. This observation suggests that although the reduction in the incidence of neonatal seizures after routine EFM found in the former trial was not confirmed by the latter, it may be genuine.

Cerebral palsy (CP)

The strongest evidence that the use of EFM in the management of labour affects the risk of CP comes from the trial of continuous EFM versus auscultation in infants born weighing 700–1750 g at 28–32 weeks of gestation.[30] In this trial the risk of CP was much *increased* in children born after continuous EFM. CP was diagnosed by age 18 months in 20 per cent of the children in this group and in 8 per cent of those born after auscultation. The relative risk was 2.54, with 95 per cent CI of 1.10–5.86 (Table 21.5).

Even in mature infants, no strong evidence exists that the use of EFM reduces the prevalence of CP. Its prevalence was not given in the reports of the clinical trials that included mature infants. Given that children with CP are 80 times as likely as others to have a history of neonatal seizures (Table 21.4), the evidence that seizures are only half as common after continuous EFM as after auscultation (Table 21.5) has encouraged the idea that CP also may be less common after EFM. However, the risk of CP in mature infants with neonatal seizures varies widely with other characteristics. According to the Collaborative Perinatal Project on which Table 21.4 is based, this risk ranges from 0.13 per cent (the same as in unaffected children) to more than 50 per cent depending on whether the seizures are combined with none, one, or both of two other sets of findings (5 minute Apgar scores of below 6, and any of a group of five other neonatal signs—decreased activity after the first day of life, need for incubator care for three or more days, feeding problems, poor suck, or respiratory difficulty).[9] Possibly the seizures prevented by EFM-based management are confined to ones that would not affect the risk of CP. Some support for this suggestion is provided by the largest of the nine trials of continuous EFM versus auscultation.[16] The two arms of this trial yielded equal numbers of cases of seizures in which major neurological defects including CP were found one year later, although other seizures were less common in the EFM arm of the trial. However, the numbers were too small for the difference between seizures with and without neurological complications to be significant.

Safety

The standard obstetric response to evidence that a fetus is endangered by intrapartum asphyxia is to shorten the labour, either by Caesarean delivery or by using instruments (forceps or ventouse) to assist vaginal delivery. By influencing obstetricians' judgement regarding the danger, the use of intrapartum EFM must lead them to allow labour to proceed naturally in some cases and to intervene operatively in others in which the alternative course would have been followed if EFM had not been used. The net effect on the frequency of operative deliveries was explored in the randomized clinical trials (Table 21.6). The operative vaginal delivery rate did not vary to a statistically significant extent with monitoring policy; but routine use of EFM was

Table 21.6 Frequency of operative deliveries in clinical trials of continuous electronic fetal monitoring during labour

Outcome	Nine trials of continuous EFM, with auscultation in controls[15–21,23,24]		One trial of continuous EFM for all, with continuous EFM in control group restricted to 'high-risk' cases[22]	
	Relative risk (95% CI)[28]	Range of prevalence of specified outcome in general populations[a]	Relative risk (95% CI)	Prevalence of specified outcome in controls
Caesarean delivery	1.21 (1.04–1.39)	2–9%	1.08 (1.01–1.14)[c]	10%
Operative vaginal delivery	1.11 (0.92–1.30)[b]	6–13%	0.93 (0.85–1.03)	4%

[a] Based on control groups in the three general population trials.[16,23,24]
[b] Eight trials only.
[c] Excluding repeat Caesarean deliveries.

associated with statistically significant increases in the Caesarean delivery rate, both in the nine trials of routine EFM versus auscultation (RR 1.21; 95 per cent CI 1.04–1.39)[28] and in the single large trial of routine EFM versus EFM in high-risk pregnancies only (RR 1.08; 95 per cent CI 1.01–1.14).[22] In the trial of continuous versus intermittent EFM (not shown in the table), the rates for both categories of operative delivery were higher following continuous EFM, but not to a statistically significant extent.[13]

The increase in the Caesarean delivery rate occasioned by continuous EFM has led to concern,[6] especially because the high false-positive rate when EFM is used to predict CP (Table 21.3) suggests that surgery is unnecessary in most of those on whom it is carried out in response to an EFM abnormality. If so, this not only wastes resources but also has adverse clinical implications. Both intraoperative and postoperative complications of Caesarean delivery are common. In one large study, the incidence of intraoperative complications was 11.6 per cent, including major complications (mainly haemorrhage) in 4.1 per cent of intrapartum cases;[31] and postoperative complications have been reported following 13 per cent-65 per cent of Caesarean deliveries[32].

CONCLUSIONS

Drawing firm conclusions regarding the value of continuous EFM during labour is impossible. No evidence exists that it reduces the number of deaths. The incidence of neonatal seizures was low following continuous EFM in the trials of EFM versus auscultation; but although children with neonatal seizures are at increased risk of CP, a reduction in the prevalence of CP after EFM has not been demonstrated. In one trial in pregnancies in which the onset of labour was premature, CP was significantly *more* common after EFM (Table 21.5).

The increased risk of CP after EFM in the last-mentioned trial was unexpected and unexplained, suggesting that a further trial in cases of premature labour is needed. Although caution is needed when generalizing from trials in such unrepresentative pregnancies, a trial in the general population appears to be ruled out by the numbers that would be needed. *At best*, EFM would be unlikely to prevent more than 4 per cent of perinatal deaths and cases of CP (i.e. half the 7 or 8 per cent of perinatal deaths and cases of CP that are estimated in Table 21.1 to be caused by birth hypoxia and trauma); and to detect a 4 per cent reduction in the 1 per cent of pregnancies that is followed by perinatal death or CP (Table 21.1), a trial of nearly a million pregnancies would be needed.

Even if EFM *were* to prevent 4 per cent of cases of perinatal death or CP, the management of about 200 false-positives would be modified unnecessarily for every one pregnancy in which perinatal death or CP was prevented, given the false-positive rate indicated in Table 21.3 (9.3 per cent), because 9.3/0.04 is approximately 200. The measures taken unnecessarily include Caesarean deliveries, the rate of which was increased by 10–20 per cent in the clinical trial pregnancies in which EFM was used (Table 21.6). The risks and financial costs of these Caesarean deliveries, and the costs of EFM itself, need to be set against any benefits that routine EFM may confer; and the only evidence of benefit is that the use of EFM appears to prevent some neonatal seizures (but not necessarily those seizures that cause lasting damage).

All these considerations cast considerable doubt on the value of continuous EFM during labour as a population screening test.

REFERENCES

1. Office for National Statistics (1999). *Mortality Statistics: childhood, infant and perinatal,* Series DH3, no.30 (Review of the Registrar General on deaths in England and Wales, 1997). The Stationery Office, London.
2. Stanley FJ and Blair E (1994). Cerebral palsy. In *The Epidemiology of Childhood Disorders* (ed. IB Pless), pp. 473–97. Oxford University Press, New York.
3. Nelson KB and Ellenberg JH (1986). Antecedents of cerebral palsy. Multivariate analysis of risk. *New England Journal of Medicine,* **315**, 81–6.
4. Blair EM and Stanley FJ (1988). Intrapartum asphyxia: a rare cause of cerebral palsy. *Pediatrics,* **112**, 515–519.
5. MacDonald D (1996). Cerebral palsy and intrapartum fetal monitoring. *New England Journal of Medicine,* **334**, 659–60.
6. Nelson KB, Dambrosia JM, Ting TY, and Grether JK (1996). Uncertain value of electronic fetal monitoring in predicting cerebral palsy. *New England Journal of Medicine,* **334**, 613–18.
7. Hagberg B, Hagberg G, and Olow I (1975). The changing pattern of cerebral palsy in Sweden 1954–70. *Acta Paediatrica Scandinavica,* **56**, 187–200.
8. Quilligan EJ and Paul RH (1975). Fetal monitoring: is it worth it? *Obstetrics and Gynecology,* **45**, 96–100.
9. Ellenberg JH and Nelson KB (1988). Cluster of perinatal events identifying infants at high risk for death and disability. *Journal of Pediatrics,* **113**, 546–52.
10. Susser M (1988). The quantification of risk factors in major neurodevelopmental disorders. In *Perinatal Events and Brain Damage in Surviving Children,* (ed. F Kubli, N Patel, W Schmidt, and O Linderkamp), pp. 12–27. Springer, Berlin.
11. Parer JT (1997). *Handbook of Fetal Heart Rate Monitoring,* 2nd edn. Saunders, Philadelphia.
12. Kubli FW, Hon EH, Khazin AF, and Takemura H (1969). Observations on heart rate and pH in the human fetus during labour. *American Journal of Obstetrics and Gynecology,* **104**, 1190–206.
13. Herbst A and Ingemarsson I (1994). Intermittent versus continuous electronic monitoring in labour: a randomised study. *British Journal of Obstetrics and Gynaecology,* **101**, 663–8.
14. Westgate J, Harris M, Curnow JSH, and Greene KR (1993). Plymouth randomized trial of cardiotocogram only versus ST waveform plus cardiotocogram for intrapartum monitoring in 2400 cases. *American Journal of Obstetrics and Gynecology,* **169**, 1151–60.
15. Haverkamp AD, Orleans M, Langendoerfer S, McFee J, Murphy J, and Thompson HE (1979). A controlled trial of the differential effects of intrapartum fetal monitoring. *American Journal of Obstetrics and Gynecology,* **134**, 399–408.
16. MacDonald D, Grant A, Sheridan-Pereira M, Boylan P, and Chalmers I (1985). The Dublin randomized controlled trial of intrapartum fetal heart rate monitoring. *American Journal of Obstetrics and Gynecology,* **152**, 524–39.

17. Luthy DA, Shy KK, van Belle G, Larson EB, Hughes JP, Benedetti TJ *et al.* (1987). A randomized trial of electronic fetal monitoring in preterm labor. *Obstetrics and Gynecology*, **69**, 687–95.

18. Haverkamp AD, Thompson HE, McFee JG, and Cetrulo C (1976). The evaluation of continuous fetal heart rate monitoring in high-risk pregnancy. *American Journal of Obstetrics and Gynecology*, **125**, 310–17.

19. Renou P, Chang A, Anderson I, and Wood C (1976). Controlled trial of fetal intensive care. *American Journal of Obstetrics and Gynecology*, **126**, 470–6.

20. Kelso IM, Parsons RJ, Lawrence GF, Arora SS, Edmonds DK, and Cooke ID (1978). An assessment of continuous fetal heart rate monitoring in labor. *Americal Journal of Obstetrics and Gynecology*, **131**, 526–32.

21. Wood C, Renou P, Oats J, Farrell E, Beischer N, and Anderson I (1981). A controlled trial of fetal heart rate monitoring in a low-risk obstetric population. *American Journal of Obstetrics and Gynecology*, **141**, 527–34.

22. Leveno KJ, Cunningham FG, Nelson S, Roark M, Williams ML, Guzick D *et al.* (1986). A prospective comparison of selective and universal electronic fetal monitoring in 34,995 pregnancies. *New England Journal of Medicine*, **315**, 615–19.

23. Neldam S, Osler M, Hansen PK, Nim J, Smith SF, and Hertel J (1986). Intrapartum fetal heart rate monitoring in a combined low- and high-risk population: a controlled clinical trial. *European Journal of Obstetrics, Gynecology and Reproductive Biology*, **23**, 1–11.

24. Vintzileos AM, Antsaklis A, Varvarigos I, Papas C, Safatzis I, and Montgomery JT (1993). A randomised trial of intrapartum electronic fetal heart rate monitoring versus intermittent auscultation. *Obstetrics and Gynecology*, **81**, 899–907.

25. Mahomed K, Nyoni R, Mulambo T, Kasule J, and Jacobus E (1994). Randomised controlled trial of intrapartum fetal heart rate monitoring. *British Medical Journal*, **308**, 497–500.

26. Nielsen PV, Stigsby B, Nickelsen C, and Nim J (1987). Intra- and inter-observer variability in the assessment of intrapartum cardiotocograms. *Acta Obstetrica et Gynecologica Scandinavica*, **66**, 421–4.

27. Murphy KW, Johnson P, Moorcroft J, Pattinson R, Russell V, and Turnbull A (1990). Birth asphyxia and the intrapartum cardiotocograph. *British Journal of Obstetrics and Gynaecology*, **97**, 470–9.

28. Thacker SB, Stroup DF, and Peterson HB (1995). Efficacy and safety of intrapartum electronic fetal monitoring: an update. *Obstetrics and Gynecology*, **86**, 613–20.

29. Nelson KB and Ellenberg JH (1979). Neonatal signs as predictors of cerebral palsy. *Pediatrics*, **64**, 225–32.

30. Shy KK, Luthy DA, Bennett FC, Whitfield M, Larson EB, van Belle G *et al.* (1990). Effects of electronic fetal-heart-rate monitoring, as compared with periodic auscultation, on the neurological development of premature infants. *New England Journal of Medicine*, **322**, 588–93.

31. Nielsen TF and Hokegard K-H (1984). *Acta Obstetrica et Gynecologica Scandinavica*, **63**, 103–8.

32. Nielsen TF (1995). Caesarean section. In *Reproductive Health Care for Mothers and Babies*, (ed. BP Sachs, E Papiernik, and C Russell), pp. 279–90. Oxford University Press, New York.

IV

Wider issues

22 *Ethics of antenatal and neonatal screening*

Nicholas Wald, Ian Leck, and J. A. Muir Gray

INTRODUCTION

The preface to the first edition of this book made the point that screening represents a radical departure from traditional medicine because it usually aims to detect disorders at an asymptomatic stage when they could not have prompted the patient to seek medical attention (p. xv). In spite of this, the ethics of screening are not fundamentally different from those applied in clinical practice. First, the aim in both clinical and screening practice is to maximize benefit and minimize harm and cost. Second, screenees and patients both have the right to be appropriately informed and counselled about the services provided, to choose whether to accept them, and to receive on-going support regardless of their choice. Third, access to the services should be equitable.

An ethical distinction is sometimes made between the duty in clinical practice to do whatever one can to help a patient, even if there is no effective remedy, and the duty in screening not to offer a test unless there is an effective remedy. This is a false distinction because in both clinical and screening practice performing a test or procedure without an expected benefit is unacceptable. The only difference is that benefits may be different for those who are patients and those who are not. For example, a patient with serious symptoms or signs would need a diagnosis regardless of the prognosis and the management of incurable conditions is an important part of clinical medicine. Benefits in screening are more narrowly defined.

BENEFITS AND HAZARDS

It is an expectation that any screening procedure should confer a benefit on the individual who is screened, and screening is only worthwhile for disorders that lend themselves to effective presymptomatic interventions. Unfortunately much screening fails to meet this requirement. Even recognizing that the identification of trivial or untreatable conditions may cause anxiety and have no useful result does not prevent the screening for such conditions.

When a diagnostic test or treatment is inexpensive and without risk, it can be offered to everyone, not only those at high risk, so screening to select those at high risk is pointless. When a diagnostic procedure is hazardous or expensive it is appropriate to limit access to the procedure by identifying, through screening, those at high enough risk of the disorder to justify the hazard and expense of diagnosis. Screening is a rational and fair way of limiting the hazard and cost of diagnosis (or treatment) to those who would stand to benefit most. Achieving this goal is dependent on being able to quantify the efficacy, safety, and cost of screening and diagnostic methods. Sensible and ethical judgments can then be made.

A screening programme should do more good than harm, but this begs the question of how *good* and *harm* are defined and balanced.

As an example, in a screening programme for Down's syndrome, identifying an affected pregnancy would be regarded as a benefit and the loss of an unaffected pregnancy due to an amniocentesis as a harm, but the two are incommensurable. One cannot be equated with the other numerically. A balance must be struck between the two to determine policy and to select a screening cut-off level. It is therefore important to know the relationship between the numbers of screened affected and unaffected pregnancies which lead to an amniocentesis (for example, that for every affected pregnancy there may be 50 unaffected ones—an OAPR of 1:50) even if the final balance is a difficult and subjective judgment.

Anxiety is widely regarded as a harmful consequence of screening, but this is an over-simplification. Screening necessarily causes anxiety because it identifies individuals with a high risk of a serious medical disorder. Anxiety is an appropriate response that can help focus attention on a difficult and important issue. Only when anxiety is excessive and distorts that focus does it become harmful. Distinguishing appropriate from inappropriate anxiety is difficult, but even if it cannot be formally quantified the distinction must be attempted so measures can be taken to avoid or relieve unnecessary anxiety. A pragmatic approach is to take note of couples' responses to offers of screening and diagnostic tests, to apply common sense, and to encourage feedback from couples on how screening services can be improved or modified.

CHOICES

The choice to be screened and undergo antenatal diagnosis

The purpose of antenatal screening is to *offer* screening so that couples can choose whether to take up screening, recognizing what is involved if the screening result is positive, and the implications of a positive diagnosis. In organizing a public health service, the goal is to provide the best screening service that is affordable, and then it is up to couples whether they choose to accept the offer of screening.

There may be a temptation to regard the provision of screening programmes as presupposing a societal goal. For example, Down's syndrome screening may be thought to mean a state preference for couples to avoid having babies with Down's syndrome. Such a state policy or preference would imply a eugenic perspective and would be unacceptable. In fact this is not the position, and to imply that it is would be a serious misrepresentation. A screening service, like most other services in society, is available for people to use as they choose. A screening service based on personal choice, with appropriate background information available, is not eugenic.

While a pregnant woman can choose to be screened, a diagnostic test would normally be offered to her only if the screening result indicated that the risk exceeded a collectively agreed level, making the consequences of screening predictable and affordable. A recent trend to allow patients more freedom of choice encourages the idea that instead of an agreed level of risk, each woman who is screened should be given her risk and then reflect on whether to have the diagnostic test. This would mean that all women would require counselling after their screening test and that screening might become uncontrollable, with resources, diagnostic tests, and therapeutic intervention provided simply on demand rather than according to high risk or need. We believe that the current practice of telling women with risks above a set level what these risks are, and restricting the invitation for diagnostic testing to these women, is better because diagnostic resources are limited and diagnostic procedures carry a risk that is felt to be too high in relation to the benefit to actively encourage women to take.

The choice to have a termination of pregnancy

Most western societies, regardless of their religious background, leave the choice to terminate a pregnancy with a severe fetal abnormality to the prospective parents. This, appropriately, leaves the decision in the hands of individuals rather than the state. There has been much debate over the rights of a fetus, the rights of parents, and whether a termination of pregnancy should be lawful. We do not offer philosophical or legal insights into this debate, but one practical fact stands out: the fetus is carried within a mother and any action that affects the fetus affects that mother. It is impossible to consider the interests of the fetus without also considering those of the mother. It is therefore reasonable that a mother can exercise a choice over termination of pregnancy that she cannot exercise over the life of the baby after birth. There are circumstances in which that choice reasonably can be restricted, for example, termination on the grounds of fetal sex. The choice is not an unfettered one. In practice, many countries treat terminations of pregnancy as unlawful, except in specified circumstances. For example, in Britain the Human Fertilisation and Embryology Act of 1990 made medical abortion illegal beyond the 24th week of pregnancy, unless there was a risk of grave permanent illness or death to the mother or a substantial risk of her offspring being seriously handicapped. The Act is consistent with the view that termination of pregnancy is a legitimate and acceptable way to avoid the birth of an infant who would otherwise be severely handicapped, and that the choice to terminate in these circumstances should be left to the couple concerned. Once it is accepted that the choice to terminate a pregnancy because of severe fetal abnormality should be made by the couple, it follows that the ethical duty of health professionals is to support that decision. Even in countries with more restrictive laws, the authorities often allow individuals, within certain limits, to exercise their own choice over termination.

In a society which accepts that couples should take these decisions, an appropriate course of action for doctors who do not agree (for example, those who regard termination for fetal abnormality as immoral) is to refer any couple who may wish to choose termination for a serious fetal abnormality to a colleague to whom this will be acceptable.

Substantial risk of serious handicap is the only fetal condition which English law regards as grounds for allowing a termination of pregnancy. In the UK and over much of the world there is wide agreement that couples who, for example, do not wish to have daughters should not be able to have a fetal sex determination and then a termination of pregnancy if the fetus is found to be female.

Even more complex is the issue of termination for a fetal abnormality that is not substantially disabling, for example, Turner's or Kleinfelter's syndrome. In spite of the absence of substantial disability and morbidity a termination of pregnancy is often carried out when such cases are identified *in utero*, although with abnormalities such as talipes almost no one would consider termination. Where should the line be drawn? A general consensus needs to be reached regarding practice in this area. Whatever the difficulty there is no disagreement that practice should be guided by reliable information about the disorder, its natural history, and the available interventions.

A non-legal but important limitation on patient choice is that doctors feel that it would be wrong to comply with certain patient requests—for example, for termination on account of minor abnormalities. The doctor–patient relationship involves both parties being satisfied over the ethics of what is being done. Currently, the rights of the public and the rights of patients are often regarded as paramount; the collective views of medical practitioners should, however, not be neglected.

INFORMATION

In screening, as in all parts of medicine, those for whom services are provided should be given the information that a reasonable person would need to decide whether to accept the service being offered. The information should be given in clear and plain language. In antenatal and neonatal screening, parents need to be given appropriate information when screening is offered, when the results of the screening are available, and when the diagnosis is made. Even informing a mother that a test is negative may not be entirely straightforward, because people who test negative need to be reminded that screening inevitably misses some cases. Otherwise, false expectations may be created and those responsible for screening will be blamed when a case is missed. This may lead to litigation and put pressure on screeners to reduce screening cut-off levels to improve detection, increasing the false-positive rate until the burden of work associated with the management of false-positives becomes unsustainable. The solution is not defensive medicine but education, particularly explaining the distinction between screening and diagnostic tests. The probabilistic nature of screening results, in which false-positives usually outnumber true-positives and in which missed cases (false-negatives) are an expected element in the screening strategy rather than a failure, should be explicit.

Before each screening test, the mother and if possible her partner should be informed of the nature and birth prevalence of the disorder for which her pregnancy or child is being screened, the detection rate of the test, the probability of being affected if the result is positive, the diagnostic test that would be offered following such a result, and the implications if the diagnostic test is also positive (for example that termination of pregnancy may be an option). The anxiety that the screening process may cause should be acknowledged. If termination of pregnancy is a possible outcome this should be made clear, because a woman who is committed to continuing with her pregnancy regardless of whether her fetus is abnormal may prefer not to be screened.

The main method of providing this information is by leaflets given out before screening backed up by information given orally. Leaflets may have to be available in different languages and should encourage women to consult their midwife or general practitioner if there are matters which they wish to discuss at this stage. The Appendix (pp. 552–5) shows a leaflet of this kind about second-trimester screening for Down's syndrome and neural tube defects, produced by the Antenatal Screening Service, St Bartholomew's and The Royal London School of Medicine and Dentistry. Similar material is needed for other screening approaches, including ultrasound and first-trimester serum testing. The idea of producing a general leaflet for nationwide use including all antenatal and neonatal screening procedures seems attractive in principle, but the difficulties involved in dealing with all screening programmes in one leaflet may make this impracticable.

If a screening result is positive, an appropriate health professional should check that the parents understand the information they have already been given, before asking them to make a further choice. Counselling should be offered at this stage, but its provision (considered below) is an aspect of the health service's duty to support patients, rather than of its information-giving function. This distinction between providing information about screening and counselling patients is not only of importance in the implementation of screening programmes, but also has considerable personal implications in how the service is perceived by those passing through it.

COUNSELLING

The purpose of offering couples counselling is to help them to reach their own decisions, with the support and understanding of the professional providing the counselling. To this end, counselling is non-judgmental and non-directive.

Counselling may be provided at any time in the screening process if requested, but it should be offered mainly when the results of screening or diagnosis are positive. Learning of a positive screening result, and that the risk of a disorder is increased although the odds are still against it, makes uncertainty explicit, and having to choose, for example, whether to have a diagnostic test that involves some risk will cause acute anxiety. Learning that the results of a diagnostic test are positive and needing to choose, for example, between termination of pregnancy and allowing a severely disabled child to be born, is a harrowing experience: the couple may feel guilty whichever choice they make. Couples who remain undecided after talking with the counsellor should not be pressured but encouraged to come back after talking the matter through on their own or with someone they know and respect.

AFTER-CARE

Many couples need support in coping with the consequences of their decisions. Those who opt for termination face a perinatal bereavement with the added stress of having themselves taken the decision to end the life of their unborn child. They may be helped by referral to support groups such as Antenatal Results and Choices (ARC, formerly called Support Around Termination for Abnormality). Those who decide against termination may also face special psychological problems, as well as needing the same medical and social support as other families with a disabled child.

Concern has been raised, particularly in the lay press, that screening programmes offering terminations for serious disorders will encourage the idea that individuals with these disorders should not be born, and so lead to reduced medical and social commitment to the care of these individuals. There is no evidence that this is the case. Even patients with disorders caused by their own behaviour (for example, many cases of lung cancer and trauma) are not denied health care that is available to other patients, and it is generally accepted that such discrimination would be unethical. To reduce the care of people with disabilities such as Down's syndrome and spina bifida because their births could have been prevented would be no less unacceptable. The concern about the threat to the care of people born with these disorders may originate from people whose real objection is to termination itself. This confuses two issues. If there are objections to termination of pregnancy on moral or ethical grounds, these should stand on their own and not be concealed behind such unsupported allegations.

EQUITY

As in all public health programmes, anyone who stands to gain from a screening programme should have access to it. Equity of access and equity in the quality of service provided are both important. It is unacceptable to have one form of screening available in one part of the country, but another form elsewhere, unless the risk of the disorder has regional differences. The whole population should be offered the screening service that is most effective and safe according to the available medical evidence, provided it is affordable and judged to be cost-effective compared with alternative screening methods. The service should provide for all components of screening—not just the screening test, but also patient information, staff education, counselling, diagnostic and treatment facilities, and monitoring arrangements. To provide a test without adequate resources for all these related activities is irresponsible; however, failure to introduce a screening service on the basis that it must achieve a level of perfection that is likely to be unattainable is also irresponsible. A balance is needed to ensure that existing resources can achieve a reasonable level of service. To meet these requirements, a national screening authority, responsible for providing screening services that meet the tests of choice, efficacy, safety, cost effectiveness, equity, and ongoing monitoring would be an advantage. Each screening service would also benefit from a quality assurance system, including: (1) quality standards; (2) arrangements for monitoring screening performance; and (3) managerial authority to take action if performance fails to meet the standards.

Quality standards

If the service offered is to be equitable across the whole country, the standards of good care ideally should be set nationally. If (as in most countries) this has not been done, there should at least be nationally available authoritative guidelines to set standards, and those responsible for commissioning or providing screening programmes should use these guidelines when determining standards. Consultation with the community served by the programme is also important when setting standards, particularly when a trade-off has to be made between detection and false-positive rates. The community has to understand that the price of a high detection rate may be a high false-positive rate.

To develop standards, it is necessary to set objectives for the programme, identify reliable measurements to indicate progress towards these objectives, and decide what values of these measurements are acceptable. As well as detection and false-positive rates, the aspects of screening programmes for which standards need to be set include uptake, informing and counselling parents, diagnostic testing, and outcome in affected fetuses or infants.

The monitoring of screening performance

All the aspects of screening programmes for which standards must be set also require monitoring. For any screening population, data collected should include the number of people eligible for screening; the number screened, classified into true-positives, false-positives, true-negatives, and false-negatives; and information about the experience of those who have been screened.

The prevalence at birth or later of the condition for which one is screening should also be monitored. No one questions this in screening programmes that are intended to prevent perinatal death following high maternal blood pressure, or dislocation of the hip following neonatal instability. However, there is sometimes a reticence to recognize the importance of monitoring the birth prevalence of conditions such as Down's syndrome, in which the aim of screening is to enable parents to choose whether affected pregnancies are terminated. This reticence arises from a perception that the authorities responsible for monitoring consider that it would be a benefit *per se* if the birth prevalence of Down's syndrome were to decline because of antenatal diagnosis and selective abortion. The perception is unjustified. Monitoring the birth prevalence is simply part of monitoring the programme as a whole. It could be of benefit if, for example, the uptake of screening and the birth prevalence of Down's syndrome were both found to be high, because this might point to a failure in the programme which could be corrected. However, such screening should still permit parental choice, so that any decline in the birth prevalence that follows is the result of the collective choices of individuals, not a collective expectation.

Managerial responsibility

When monitoring indicates that a screening programme is not reaching its target standards, a person or organization with the authority to investigate what is wrong should be informed and if possible should put it right. This authority is often lacking. Sometimes the fault may be traced to laboratory technique and be readily solved. However, sometimes the failure affects activities of staff over which the screening service has no managerial authority—medical activities that may fall within the scope of clinical freedom. To overcome these problems medical and nursing staff must work as teams, and team leaders need to be appointed.

COMMUNITY PERSPECTIVES

The suggestion that there is a community or state interest in population screening is sometimes seen as intrusive and threatening. There have been occasions (for example, in Hitler's Germany and Stalin's Russia) when the wishes and rights of individuals have been violated in what has been claimed to be the interests of the state. To avoid such conflicts, the interests of any community need to be seen as no more and no less than the collective interests of the individuals who form the community. The community needs to facilitate the personal choice of individuals and to maintain the other ethical principles discussed above. It is also important that the individual members of the community recognize that the health and social services, including screening, are *their* services rather than something imposed from outside. This is most likely to happen if the services are seen to embody fairness, avoidance of waste, and community involvement.

A collective concern for fairness is characteristic of society at its best, and this concern is reflected in the objectives of improving health, reducing pain, and alleviating suffering in an equitable manner. For society to achieve these goals it must either provide and fund health care (including screening services) itself or ensure that others are doing so. However, individuals should not be forced to take up these services to serve the collective societal interest or indeed even to serve their own interests if they choose not to, except in exceptional situations—if for example, their own ill-health poses a significant threat to the health of others, or if they are not competent to refuse or consent to treatment.

The avoidance of waste is an ethical consideration, because with waste there are fewer resources available for other needy services. It is important, therefore, to try to ensure that screening services are as cost-effective as possible, commensurate with achieving a particular detection rate.

Community involvement is important, both in the development of new screening programmes (including standard-setting, as noted earlier) and in on-going management. The organizations that plan and manage screening programmes have a duty to encourage this involvement by informing their communities and enabling them to share in choices about the services provided, just as health professionals have a duty to inform parents about screening programmes and to respect their choices when offered tests or terminations. Although sample surveys are sometimes useful, there is no easy way of obtaining the views of the community as a whole, and it is necessary to rely on representatives of the community or special interest groups. In the UK, representatives of the community sit on the Health Authorities which run the National Health Service (including screening) and on Community Health Councils which act as watchdogs on the community's behalf to ensure that Health Authorities act with propriety and equity. In discussion with community representatives and groups it is important that concepts such as effectiveness and quality, detection and false-positive rates, and the relationship between them, are understood. It is important to understand that it is impossible to have a screening test with no false-negatives or false-positives. There are trade-offs in screening just as there are trade-offs in determining the provision of health services in general.

APPENDIX: AN INFORMATION LEAFLET FOR PREGNANT WOMEN

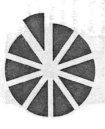

Antenatal Screening

MATERNAL SERUM SCREENING

FOR

DOWN'S SYNDROME

AND

OPEN NEURAL TUBE DEFECTS

Questions and Answers

Antenatal Screening Service
St Bartholomew's and the Royal London
School of Medicine and Dentistry

The maternal serum screening test is a blood test performed at about 16 weeks of pregnancy to screen for Down's syndrome and open neural tube defects. It is suitable for women of all ages. The blood test is a screening test and cannot determine on its own whether or not the baby has Down's syndrome or a neural tube defect.

The *screening* test identifies women who are in a higher risk group for having a pregnancy with either abnormality, so that they can be offered a diagnostic test (such as amniocentesis). The *diagnostic* test identifies women who actually have an affected pregnancy.

This leaflet answers some of the common questions women ask about the screening test. You are also encouraged to discuss the test with your midwife or doctor before you decide whether you would like to be screened.

If you would like to discuss any aspect of the screening test or your result with a screening counsellor at Bart's, we would be pleased to talk to you.

What is Down's syndrome?

Down's syndrome is caused by the presence of an extra chromosome number 21 in the cells of the developing baby. About 1 in every 700 (1.4 per 1000) babies are born with Down's syndrome. Usually it is not inherited and so a baby can be affected even if there is no history of Down's syndrome in the family.

Down's syndrome is the most common cause of severe mental handicap and is often associated with physical problems such as heart defects or difficulties with sight and hearing. It is not possible to assess the degree of handicap before the baby is born. 9 out of 10 babies with Down's syndrome will survive their first year and nearly half of these will reach 60 years of age.

What are open neural tube defects?

The two main kinds of neural tube defects (NTDs) are spina bifida and anencephaly.

Babies with spina bifida have an opening in the bones of the spine which can result

2

in damage to the nerves controlling the lower part of the body. This causes weakness and paralysis of the legs and sometimes bowel and bladder problems. Babies with spina bifida are also more likely to have a collection of fluid on the brain, called hydrocephalus, which can be treated surgically but may lead to mental handicap.

Babies with anencephaly have a large part of the skull missing and the brain is not properly formed. **They always die before or very soon after they are born.**

In about 1 in every 5 babies with spina bifida the spinal opening is covered with skin or thick tissue. This is called closed spina bifida and will not be detected by the blood test. This condition is usually less severe than open spina bifida.

What does the serum screening test involve?

A sample of your blood is taken between 15 and 22 weeks of pregnancy (16-18 weeks is the best time to screen for open neural defects). **The stage of pregnancy is best estimated by an ultrasound dating scan.** The levels of four substances in your blood will be measured and compared with the average levels for your stage of pregnancy. The substances are:

(i) alpha-fetoprotein (**AFP**)

(ii) unconjugated oestriol (**uE$_3$**)

(iii) inhibin-A (**inhibin**)

(iv) free ß human chorionic gonadotrophin (**free ß-hCG**).

The concentration of these four substances are used together with your age to estimate the risk of Down's syndrome in your pregnancy. The level of AFP is also used to determine if there is an increased risk of spina bifida or anencephaly.

What is a 'risk'?

A risk is the chance of an event occurring. For example, a risk of Down's syndrome of 1 in 100 means that if 100 women have this test result, we would expect that 1 of these women would have a baby with Down's syndrome and that 99 would not. This is the same as a 1% chance that the baby has Down's syndrome and a 99% chance that the baby does not.

How long does the result take?

Your result will usually be ready within one week of having your blood taken and will be sent to your antenatal clinic or General Practitioner.

The result will be either 'screen-negative' or 'screen-positive'.

What does a screen-negative result mean?

If the risk of Down's syndrome, based on your age and the levels of the four blood markers, is lower than 1 in 300 and the AFP level is not high, then the result is called 'screen-negative' and a diagnostic test would not usually be offered.

Although a **screen-negative means that you are not at high risk** of having a baby with Down's syndrome or a neural tube defect, *a screen-negative result does not rule out the possibility of a pregnancy with either of these abnormalities.*

Why do women with screen-negative results occasionally have babies with Down's syndrome or a neural tube defect?

It is unusual for a woman to have a baby with either of these abnormalities, and it is even more unusual for a woman with a screen-negative result, but it does sometimes happen. This is because the screening test cannot completely distinguish affected from unaffected pregnancies. However small the risk is, we cannot rule out the possibility of the baby having Down's syndrome or a neural tube defect.

What does a screen-positive result mean?

A screen-positive result means that you **are in a higher risk group** for having a baby with Down's syndrome or a neural tube defect. If your result is in this group, you will be offered a diagnostic test.

The result is called screen-positive if

i) the risk of Down's syndrome in your pregnancy is 1 in 300 or greater. About 1 in every 20 women screened will be in this risk group.

or

ii) the AFP level is more than two and a half times higher than the normal (median) level. About 1 in every 40 women screened will be in this risk group.

Most women with screen-positive results do not have a pregnancy with Down's syndrome or a neural tube defect. For example, of 50 women with screen-positive results for Down's syndrome, only one would actually have a pregnancy with Down's syndrome.

Can any other abnormalities be identified?

The risk of Trisomy 18 (a rare and usually fatal abnormality) can be estimated using AFP, uE$_3$ and free ß-hCG. In cases where the risk is high this is reported.

What further tests will I be offered if my result is screen-positive?

ULTRASOUND DATING SCAN

An ultrasound scan provides the best estimate of your gestation (i.e. how advanced your pregnancy is), and ideally should be carried out before the screening test. If you have a screen-positive result and have not already had a scan then this is normally carried out now.

If the result is screen-positive on account of an increased risk of Down's syndrome and the scan estimate of your gestation is within 17 days of the estimate by your 'dates' (time since the first day of your last menstrual period) then the result will remain screen-positive. If the scan indicates a difference of more than 17 days from your 'dates', then the screening result will need to be re-interpreted using the scan information.

If the result is screen-positive on account of a raised AFP level, suggesting an increased risk of a neural tube defect, then the result will need to be re-interpreted whatever the difference is between your scan and 'dates' estimates of your gestation.

If your final result is screen-positive, you will be offered a diagnostic test which will include an amniocentesis or chorionic villus sampling (CVS) and a detailed ultrasound scan. The diagnostic test will determine whether or not the pregnancy is actually affected.

AMNIOCENTESIS

What is amniocentesis?

An amniocentesis is a simple and widely used procedure which usually takes only a few minutes to perform. It involves collecting a small sample (about 4 teaspoons) of amniotic fluid from around the baby by passing a thin needle through the abdominal wall and into the uterus. The needle will be inserted under the guidance of an ultrasound scan. It does not usually involve a stay in hospital.

What will the amniocentesis tell me?

The amniotic fluid contains cells from the baby which can be used to tell you whether or not the baby has Down's syndrome. These cells must grow before they can be examined and so the results

can take up to 3 or 4 weeks. A diagnostic test for neural tube defects can also be performed on the amniotic fluid.

No test can guarantee that your baby will be free of all birth defects but if the result of the amniocentesis is negative it will almost certainly rule out Down's syndrome or another chromosome abnormality.

Is it safe to have an amniocentesis?

Amniocentesis is a procedure that has been offered for many years and over 15,000 are carried out in Britain each year. Its safety has been carefully studied and it is estimated that 1 in 100 women who have an amniocentesis will have a miscarriage as a result of the procedure.

Why do you measure the four substances in my blood?

In pregnancies with Down's syndrome, AFP and uE_3 levels tend to be low, inhibin and free β-hCG levels tend to be raised. By assessing how high or low your blood levels are, we can give a more accurate risk of Down's syndrome than we could by using your age alone.

In pregnancies with an open neural tube defect, the AFP level tends to be raised. The risk of a pregnancy being affected by a neural tube defect will increase if the AFP level is high.

In Trisomy 18 the levels of AFP, uE_3, and free β-hCG tend to be very low.

Why do you take age into account?

Any woman could have a baby with Down's syndrome, whatever her age, but the likelihood of this happening does increase as a woman gets older and so we use age as one of the factors when working out your risk of a pregnancy

Does the screening test detect all pregnancies with Down's syndrome or a neural tube defect?

No. Three out of four cases of Down's syndrome and four out of five cases of neural tube defects will be detected (classified as screen-positive). Therefore one out of four pregnancies with Down's syndrome and one out of five pregnancies with open spina bifida will have a screen-negative result and so will be missed. Nearly all cases of anencephaly are detected.

with Down's syndrome. It also means that an older woman is more likely to have a result in the higher risk group (screen-positive) and so be offered a diagnostic test. This is shown in the table below.

Maternal age group (years)	Probability of a screen-positive result for Down's syndrome	Proportion of Down's syndrome pregnancies detected (%)
Under 25	1 in 40	60%
25-29	1 in 30	65%
30-34	1 in 15	70%
35-39	1 in 5	85%
40-44	1 in 3	95%
45 and over	greater than 1 in 2	greater than 99%
All	1 in 20	75%

CHORIONIC VILLUS SAMPLING (CVS)

CVS is also a diagnostic test for Down's syndrome. This test is offered early in pregnancy in some hospitals (about 11 weeks) but may also be offered as an alternative to amniocentesis following a screen-positive result. CVS involves taking a sample of placental tissue, again by inserting a needle through the abdominal wall. It may not be necessary to grow the cells and so a result is usually ready within one week. At this stage of pregnancy the risk of miscarriage is thought to be the same as for amniocentesis.

DETAILED ULTRASOUND SCAN

Anencephaly and Spina bifida

Nearly all cases of anencephaly are detected by an ultrasound scan and over 90% of cases of spina bifida can be detected. The best detection of spina bifida is achieved by performing a detailed ultrasound scan and an amniocentesis together, although amniocentesis carries a risk of miscarriage.

Down's syndrome

It is not possible to make a diagnosis of Down's syndrome from an ultrasound scan. There are however certain physical features which may be associated with Down's syndrome and can be seen on an ultrasound scan between 18 and 20 weeks. If any of these features are seen this would be a further indication for a diagnostic test but the absence of these features could not rule out Down's syndrome.

If I do not have an affected pregnancy, how could I have a screen-positive result?

The screening result is based on your age and the blood marker levels. You are therefore more likely to have a screen-positive result if you are older, if your AFP or uE_3 are low, and if your inhibin or β-hCG levels are high. However, since the four markers also naturally vary between women, there is usually **no apparent reason** for women having either high or low levels and so most women with screen-positive results will **not** have an affected pregnancy.

A screen-positive result only indicates who is in a higher risk group so that we know who should be offered a diagnostic test.

What happens if my baby does have Down's syndrome or a neural tube defect?

Remember that the majority of amniocentesis results will show that the baby does **not** have Down's syndrome or a neural tube defect. If the baby did have one of these abnormalities, you would have the chance to discuss how your baby could be affected. If you decided to have a termination of pregnancy your doctor or midwife would be able to make arrangements for this. If you decided to continue with the pregnancy you could talk to someone about the special help and support you would receive to help you look after your baby.

For further information, please contact:

Antenatal Screening
Department of Environmental and Preventive Medicine
Wolfson Institute of Preventive Medicine
St Bartholomew's and the Royal London
School of Medicine and Dentistry
Charterhouse Square
London
EC1M 6BQ
Telephone: 0171-982-6293/4

23 *Conclusions*

Nicholas Wald and Ian Leck

In the first edition of this book, it was pointed out that it is the *purpose* for which a procedure is carried out that qualifies it as screening: with screening the intention is not to offer *therapeutic* intervention in the event of a positive result alone, but to carry out a diagnostic test or preventive action when a result is positive.

Over the 15 or so years since the publication of the first edition the distinction between screening and diagnostic tests has become better recognized. For example, there are few who would now regard amniocentesis as a screening test for Down's syndrome. Also, the use of simple enquiries that distinguish a high-risk from a low-risk group is now widely accepted as screening, even if it does not involve a special test such as an ultrasound examination or a blood test. For example, the determination of age is widely regarded as a screening test for Down's syndrome, and asking someone if they are an Ashkenazi Jew is the initial screening test for Tay–Sachs disease. Also, the assessment of screening tests from a quantitative perspective, rather than simply categorizing results qualitatively as positive and negative, has been accepted and better understood. What has not been as widely acknowledged as perhaps it should be is the need to demonstrate the efficacy of screening in terms of clear and measurable improvements in outcome. For example, screening for iron-deficiency anaemia (which is not in itself an adverse outcome) is still accepted instead of screening for the adverse outcomes that are due to iron-deficiency anaemia. The objective and quantitative evaluation of population screening still has a way to go before sound judgments can be reached on the selection of disorders for which screening can be judged to be worthwhile.

SUMMARY OF ANTENATAL AND NEONATAL SCREENING FOR CERTAIN DISORDERS

Tables 23.1–23.4 summarize our assessment of the performance of the screening tests presented in this book as they are used in the United Kingdom (UK). From the information given, readers should be able to judge the applicability to their own countries of these approaches to screening, provided that they know the local prevalence at birth of each relevant disorder, which affects the odds of being affected given a positive result (OAPR). Two groups of disorders considered earlier are not included in Tables 23.1–23.4: infectious diseases for which screening is not widely practised or recommended in the UK (see Table 7.3, p. 185–6), and most of the congenital defects observed at routine ultrasonography which are not the subjects of separate screening programmes (see Tables 18.2 and 18.12, pp. 444–5 and 463). Severe cardiac malformations are, however, included in spite of being in the latter category, in view of their numerical importance.

Tables 23.1 and 23.2 relate to disorders of the offspring which are not secondary to disease in the mother (although they may be caused by other maternal conditions, such as alloimmunization following exposure to a fetal red cell antigen during a previous pregnancy). These disorders can be divided into two groups—those for which screening is predominantly antenatal (see Table 23.1) and those screened for neonatally (see Table 23.2).

Table 23.3 relates to disorders of the offspring which are secondary to maternal disease. Screening for these disorders is largely antenatal, and may benefit the mother as well as the offspring; for example, screening by measuring the mother's blood pressure has a role in the prevention of maternal eclampsia as well as perinatal death. However, no attempt is made in Table 23.3 to measure the benefit of screening to the mother: the measures of performance given in this table, like those in Tables 23.1 and 23.2, assess the effectiveness of screening in identifying *fetuses* in whom the disorders listed would occur if measures to prevent them were not taken. For example, the OAPR given for hepatitis B shows the estimated odds that an individual whose mother tests positive for the hepatitis B surface antigen during pregnancy will, if untreated, develop clinical disease later as a result of vertical transmission of the virus at birth.

In each table, disorders are listed alphabetically. For each disorder, the relevant chapter is indicated, followed by the approximate natural prevalence of the disorder (i.e. the prevalence in the absence of intervention based on screening) and the extent of disability. In the column 'Can effective intervention be offered?', effective intervention includes both prevention or treatment and the abortion of affected fetuses. The next two columns indicate the primary and secondary screening tests used (primary tests being those applied to all pregnancies or infants and secondary tests those performed when a primary test is positive). Then follow the detection rate and false-positive rate for the primary screening test, and the odds of having a fetus or neonate with the specified disorder when the primary screening test is positive. Where a secondary screening test is specified, the next column gives the odds of being affected if primary and secondary tests are both positive.

The tables do not specify the various diagnostic tests available or the odds of screening given positive screening *and* diagnostic tests. For most of the tests considered these odds are very high and are given in the individual chapters concerned.

The last column attempts to answer the question: 'Is screening worthwhile?' This represents a judgment based on all the relevant factors including the prevalence and seriousness of the disorder, the discriminatory performance of screening, and the availability of an acceptable intervention. The final assessment is a judgment over which there may be legitimate differences of opinion.

As was indicated in Chapter 1 (pp. 4–5), there are a few screening tests in which all individuals with a positive result are defined as having a disorder; and when, as in

Table 23.1 Summary of antenatal screening in the UK for specific disorders which primarily affect the offspring

Disorder	Chapter	Approximate natural prevalence (per 10 000 births)	Disability (the more stars the greater the severity)	Can effective intervention be offered?	Primary screening test	Secondary screening test(s)	Detection rate (%)*	False-positive rate (%)†	Odds of being affected given a positive primary screening test	Odds of being affected given positive primary and secondary screening tests	Is screening worthwhile?
Anencephaly	3	10	***	Yes[1]	Ultrasound		100	0	1:0	—	Yes
Cystic fibrosis[2]	13	4	***	Yes[1]	Test for mutation in both parents		72	0.09	1:3	—	Yes
Down's syndrome[3]	4, 18	18	***	Yes[1]	1st and 2nd trimester integrated test		85	0.9	1:6	—	Yes
Duchenne muscular dystrophy	5	1	***	Yes[1]	Recognition of affected male relative (carrier detection)	Test for mutation in mother	32	0.03	1:5 if previous son affected	1:3	Probably
Fragile-X syndrome	5	2	Males:**/*** Females: *	Yes[1]	Polymerase chain reaction test in mother	Southern blot test in mother	100	20	1:1100	1:4	Possibly
Haemolytic disease of the fetus and newborn:[4]											
(a) anti-D	12	40[5]	**/***	Yes	Rh grouping and test for antibody in mother	Rh grouping of father; quantitation of maternal antibody	100[6]	16	1:31[5,6]	1:26[5,6]	Yes
(b) anti-K and anti-c	12	1	**	Yes	Test for antibodies in mother	Quantitation of maternal antibodies; Coombs' test in newborn	?	?	?	?	Probably

					Primary screening test						
Haemophilia	11	0.5	**	Yes[1]	Recognition of affected male relative (carrier detection)	Test for mutation in mother	55	<0.01	1:5 if previous son affected	1:3	Yes
Severe cardiac malformations	18	20	***	Yes[1]		Ultrasound	50	≤0.6	≥1:6	—	Yes
Spina bifida (open)[7]	3, 18	8.5	***	Yes[1]		Maternal serum α-fetoprotein assay	86	0.3	1:4	—	Yes
Tay-Sachs disease	6	0.035	***	Yes[1]	Ethnic origin enquiry (Ashkenazi Jew)	Hexoseaminidase assays in father, and in mother if positive in father	50	1	1:3 600	1:3	Yes
β thalassaemia[8]	11	6	*/***	Yes[1]	Red cell MCV or MCH in mother[9]	Hb A_2 assay in mother, and in father if positive in mother	89	7	1:125	1:3	Yes
X-linked retinitis pigmentosa	5	0.4	**	Yes[1]	Recognition of affected male relative (carrier detection)	Maternal retinal function assessment	75	0.02	1:3 if previous son affected	1:3	Possibly

* Proportion of affected (i.e. having a fetus with the specified disorder) individuals with positive primary screening test.

† Proportion of unaffected (i.e. having a fetus without the specified disorder) individuals with positive primary screening test.

1 Termination of affected pregnancies.

2 See Screening Brief in *Journal of Medical Screening*, 3, 55 (1996).

3 See Screening Brief in *Journal of Medical Screening*, 2, 56 (1995).

4 See Screening Brief in *Journal of Medical Screening*, 2, 232 (1995).

5 Assuming that 40 per cent of pregnancies are first, 40 per cent second, and 20 per cent third.

6 Performance of screening as a method of detecting women in their first or second pregnancy who would have affected offspring in next pregnancy if prophylaxis is not given.

7 See Screening Brief in *Journal of Medical Screening*, 5, 167 (1998).

8 See Screening Brief in *Journal of Medical Screening*, 5, 215 (1998).

9 MCV = mean cell volume. MCH = mean cell haemoglobin.

Table 23.2 Summary of neonatal screening in the UK for specific disorders which primarily affect the offspring

Disorder	Chapter	Approximate natural prevalence (per 10 000 births)	Disability (the more stars the greater the severity)	Can effective intervention be offered?	Primary screening test	Secondary screening test(s)	Detection rate (%)*	False-positive rate (%)†	Odds of being affected given a positive primary screening test	Odds of being affected given positive primary and secondary screening tests	Is screening worthwhile?
Congenital dislocation of hip[1]	16	13	**	Yes	Ortolani–Barlow test by junior paediatrician	Clinical examination (including Ortolani–Barlow test) by orthopaedic surgeon	75	1.6	1:16	1:9	Probably
Congenital hypothyroidism	15	3	***	Yes	T4 or TSH assay	TSH and repeat T4 assays[2]	100[2]	20[2]	1:668[2]	1:19[2]	Yes
Galactosaemia due to absence of transferase	14	0.15	***	Yes	Fluorometric test for transferase activity		100	0.08	1:53	–	Probably
Phenylketonuria[3]	14	1	***	Yes	Serum phenylalanine assay	Repeated serum phenylalanine assay	100	0.2	1:22	1:0.5	Yes

* Proportion of affected individuals with positive primary screening test.

† Proportion of unaffected individuals with positive primary screening test.

[1] See Screening Brief in *Journal of Medical Screening*, 2, 117 (1995).

[2] If T4 assay is the primary screening test.

[3] See Screening Brief in *Journal of Medical Screening*, 6, 113 (1999).

...screening in the UK for specific disorders of the offspring which are secondary to diseases in the mother

Disorder	Chapter	Approximate natural prevalence (per 10 000 births)	Disability (the more stars the greater the severity)	Can effective intervention be offered?	Primary screening test	Secondary screening test(s)	Detection rate (%)*	False-positive rate (%)†	Odds of being affected given a positive primary screening test	Odds of being affected given positive primary and secondary screening tests	Is screening worthwhile?
Congenital syphilis	7	0.2	***	Yes	VDRL test or flocculation test in mother	Specific treponemal test in mother	>90	0.2	1:100	1:50	Probably
Perinatal mortality	9	93	***	Yes	Maternal blood pressure measurement	Test for proteinuria	38	30	1:77	1:41	Yes
Perinatal mortality or cerebral palsy	21	110	***	Yes	Electronic fetal monitoring	Measurement of fetal scalp blood PH	10	10	1:100	?	Probably not
Rubella syndrome	7	0.12	***	Yes	Test for antibodies in mother		>90	1.6	<1:1300	–	Probably not
Sickle cell disease	11	3	**	Yes	Ethnic origin enquiry (black)	Sickling test; Hb electrophoresis in mother, and in father if positive in mother	99	3	1:100	1:3	Yes
Vertically transmitted hepatitis B[1]	7	1.4	**	Yes	ELISA test for HBsAg in mother (repeated if positive)		≥98	0.14	1:10	–	Yes
Vertically transmitted HIV[2]	7	1	***	Yes	ELISA test for IgG antibody in mother (repeated on same sample if positive)	ELISA test on repeat sample	99.9	0.13	1:13	1:<5	Yes

* Proportion of affected (i.e. having a fetus with the specified disorder) individuals with positive primary screening test.
† Proportion of unaffected (i.e. having a fetus without the specified disorder) individuals with positive primary screening test.
[1] See Screening Brief in Journal of Medical Screening, 5, 54 (1998).
[2] See Screening Brief in Journal of Medical Screening, 4, 177 (1997).

Table 23.4 Summary of antenatal screening in the UK for specific disorders of the mother which may put the fetus at risk

Disorder	Chapter	Approximate natural prevalence (per 10 000 women)	Effects on fetus		Primary screening test	Is screening worthwhile?
			Nature	Disability (the more stars the greater the severity)		
Hyperglycaemia	8	5 (undiagnosed non-insulin-dependent diabetes mellitus—WHO definition[1])	Perinatal death, congenital abnormalities, macrosomia	**/***	Oral glucose tolerance test	Uncertain
Iron-deficiency anaemia	10	4000–5000 (<11 gHb/dl)	Reduced iron stores. Possible retardation of prenatal growth and postnatal development	*	Haemoglobin measurement	Yes
Thrombocytopenia	10	760 (<150 × 10⁹ platelets/l)	Neonatal thrombocytopenia	*	Platelet count	No

[1] Plasma glucose >200 mg/dl, 2 hours after 75 g oral glucose.

these cases, a disorder is not defined independently of the relevant screening test, the performance of this test cannot be properly assessed. This problem applies to screening for maternal hypoglycaemia, iron-deficiency anaemia, and thrombocytopenia, for which it is therefore impossible to derive detection rates, false-positive rates, and odds of being affected given a positive test. Other information about these tests is given in Table 23.4. Firm quantitative evidence that their use can improve the offspring's health is lacking, even though the maternal attributes they measure may be related to the risks of certain disorders in the offspring.

SCREENING AS A METHOD OF REDUCING LATE-FETAL AND INFANT MORTALITY

Screening can lead to reductions in late-fetal and infant mortality by leading to the identification of two groups of disorders—firstly, severe congenital abnormalities which cannot be treated satisfactorily but in which termination of pregnancy is a valid option, and secondly, conditions in which early recognition sometimes enables life-saving measures to be taken. Of the disorders considered in Tables 23.1–23.3 which commonly lead to late-fetal and infant mortality, anencephaly, cystic fibrosis, Down's syndrome, severe cardiac malformations, and spina bifida fall into the first category; and the second category includes haemolytic disease of the newborn, vertically transmitted syphilis and HIV infections, and perinatal mortality due to hypertensive disease of pregnancy.

Table 23.5 summarizes the approximate reduction in late-fetal and infant mortality in the UK that would be expected from the screening methods described in this book.

Table 23.5   Estimate of late-fetal and infant mortality preventable by screening in the UK

Disorder	Preventable late-fetal and infant deaths (per 10 000 births)
Conditions in which termination of pregnancy is an option:	
Anencephaly	10
Cystic fibrosis	0.4[a]
Down's syndrome	1.7
Severe cardiac malformations	10
Spina bifida (open)	4.4
Subtotal	26
Conditions for which life-saving measures are available:	
Congenital syphilis	0.04
Haemolytic disease of the fetus and newborn	20
Perinatal mortality due to hypertensive disease of pregnancy	6
Vertically transmitted HIV infection	0.2
Subtotal	26
Totals:	
Conditions in which most deaths preventable by screening are being prevented[b]	40
Other conditions	12
Grand total	52

Observed late-fetal and infant mortality from all causes[c]: 110/10 000.
Estimates of all-cause late-fetal and infant mortality[d]:
i, in the absence of screening: $[110 + (0.75 \times 52)]/10\,000 = 149/10\,000$;
ii, if all deaths preventable by screening were being prevented:
$[110 - (0.25 \times 52)]/10\,000 = 97/10\,000$.
Deaths preventable by screening as a proportion of deaths that would occur in the absence of screening: $(149 - 97)/149 = 35$ per cent.
[a] Cases with meconium ileus.
[b] Anencephaly, spina bifida, congenital syphilis, haemolytic disease of the newborn, perinatal deaths due to hypertensive disease of pregnancy.
[c] Provisional figures for England and Wales in 1998.[1]
[d] Assuming that three-quarters of deaths preventable by screening are being prevented, as suggested by the above totals for conditions in which screening is already preventing most deaths (40/10 000) and for the other conditions listed (12/10 000).

It is estimated that these methods make it possible to prevent 52 late-fetal and infant deaths in every 10 000 births, and that the screening programmes that already exist are preventing three-quarters of these deaths (nearly all those that neural tube defects, congenital syphilis, haemolytic disease of the newborn, and hypertensive disease of pregnancy would otherwise cause, and a minority of the remainder). It follows from these estimates that in the UK one-third of all late-fetal and infant deaths are being or could be prevented by screening (Table 23.5).

SCREENING AS A METHOD OF REDUCING CHILDHOOD HANDICAP

The contribution which antenatal and neonatal screening can make to the prevention of disability in surviving children is estimated in Table 23.6. The conditions listed here include most of those listed as causes of mortality in Table 23.5, together with six additional disorders in which termination of pregnancy is a valid option and five in which treatment based on screening enables those affected to survive without handicap. The 11 additional disorders include the rubella syndrome, congenital dislocation of the hip, congenital hypothyroidism, and eight conditions of known genetic origin.

According to Table 23.6, screening by the methods shown prevents survival with a severe disability in 43/10 000 births. This estimate may be compared with a figure of 256/10 000 for the prevalence in young children of all severe disability due to defects which were congenital or arose at or shortly after birth. This figure was ascertained by a seven-year follow-up of 17 418 children born in Great Britain during one week of 1958.[2] Although there have been two more recent surveys of the prevalence of childhood disability in the UK, the range of conditions enumerated was too broad in one of these studies[3] and too narrow in the other[4] to be comparable.

At the time of the 1958 study, only a few of the screening tests described were carried out, and these only on a modest scale. We therefore estimate from the

Table 23.6 Estimate of severe childhood disability preventable by screening in the UK

Disorder	Preventable cases of handicap (per 10 000 births)
Conditions in which termination of pregnancy is an option:	
Cystic fibrosis	2.5
Down's syndrome	14
Duchenne muscular dystrophy	0.45
Fragile-X syndrome	1.2
Haemophilia	0.3
Rubella syndrome	0.03
Spina bifida (open)	3
Tay–Sachs disease	0.02
β thalassaemia	5
Subtotal	26
Conditions in which children can be enabled to survive without handicap:	
Congenital dislocation of hip	7
Congenital hypothyroidism	3
Congenital syphilis	0.15
Galactosaemia due to absence of transferase	0.15
Haemolytic disease of the fetus and newborn	2
Phenylketonuria	1
Sickle cell disease	3
Vertically transmitted HIV infection	0.6
Subtotal	17
Total	43*

* Represents approximately 17 per cent of severe childhood disability that would occur in the absence of screening (taken to be 256/10 000).[2]

prevalence of severe disability at that time that antenatal and neonatal screening can reduce this prevalence by 17 per cent (43/256).

It may at first sight seem surprising that the figure given in Table 23.6 for the proportion of infants in whom survival with a disability due to haemolytic disease is prevented by screening (2/10 000) is so much lower than our estimate of the natural prevalence of this disease (40/10 000, Table 23.1). The reason for the difference is that the lower figure does not include infants who in the absence of screening would either die (about half) or be saved from severe disability by measures such as exchange transfusion.

Apart from some specific haematological conditions and four other defects—Down's syndrome, open spina bifida, congenital dislocation of the hip, and hypothyroidism—most of the disorders for which antenatal and neonatal screening is effective contribute little to the total burden of childhood disability. The commonest of these other disorders are cystic fibrosis and the Fragile-X syndrome. Since the previous edition of this book, screening for cystic fibrosis in pregnancy has become possible, but has not been generally introduced into practice in spite of successful demonstration projects in Edinburgh and Maine. Recent advances in screening for Fragile-X may soon make it possible to offer antenatal screening for this disorder. Otherwise, there are no immediate prospects for antenatal and neonatal screening making further inroads into the prevention of disability.

Although Tables 23.1–23.6 relate specifically to recent experience in the United Kingdom, they may be useful as models for evaluating antenatal and neonatal screening in other parts of the world, where the pattern of disease and therefore the conclusions to be drawn about screening may be very different.

TAKING STOCK

Our analyses suggest that screening is capable of preventing about 35 per cent of late fetal and infant deaths that would otherwise occur. This corresponds to a rate of about five deaths per 1000, of which approximately 75 per cent are in fact being prevented in the UK. Also, about 17 per cent of severe childhood disability (four cases per 1000 births) is being or could be prevented by antenatal and neonatal screening. Preventing death or disability in close to 10/1000 or 1 per cent of children represents an important contribution to preventive medicine, although the fact that only a minority of deaths and disabilities can be prevented in this way underlines the importance of traditional postnatal medical services, notably the treatment of congenital orthopaedic and cardiac abnormalities. It is important that the ability to recognize these abnormalities *in utero* is not equated with worthwhile screening, since many can be treated effectively when recognized clinically after birth and do not benefit from being diagnosed earlier.

The contents of this book demonstrate how medical services can benefit from new technologies and scientific advances. But it is also clear that most of the benefits have arisen from the application of techniques that have been available for over 20 years, notably conventional laboratory techniques and ultrasound. Much progress has been the result of the better application and improvement in these techniques, the conduct of large-scale research into their application and a better application of existing knowledge. No single technique has revolutionized the field.

In the first edition of this book in 1984, one of us (NW) indicated that there was a risk that the practical application of molecular biology to antenatal screening might be exaggerated and that there was a need to avoid generating unreasonable expectations. The mapping of the human genome is continuing to fuel these expectations. In practice the position is little different from that described in 1984. Then there was concern that gene linkage analysis was of limited value. Now that gene-specific probes are being identified for an increasing number of disorders, problems with their application as general population screening tools are increasingly recognized. Often there are so many mutations responsible for a particular phenotype that DNA analysis is inappropriate. The situation with cystic fibrosis is an exception because only a few specific mutations happen to be responsible for most cases. The caution of 1984 was justified and applies as much now as it did then.

Terminology such as 'genetic screening' is unhelpful because it lacks specificity.[5] Even the most promising recent advances in screening rely on more firmly established methods, such as protein or steroid hormone measurements in a woman's blood coupled with the use of ultrasound visualization of abnormalities in the fetus. Although the screening strategy proposed for Fragile-X (Chapter 5) involves DNA analysis (polymerase chain reaction and/or Southern blotting) in all pregnant women, this is not entirely satisfactory, because half of the affected fetuses detected are females, and antenatal detection serves no useful purpose in them because most have little or no disability. This difficulty would be avoided if the relatively simple assessment of the sex of the fetus became the initial procedure in screening for Fragile-X, the DNA studies being carried out as a secondary screening test. The same arguments apply to screening for some other conditions. It may well be that outside the area of diagnosis, the main application of the newer molecular DNA techniques will be as secondary or ancillary screening tests.

A major disappointment is that, in the 15 or so years since the publication of the first edition of this book, little has been achieved in the organization of screening; health-care services are still insufficiently designed to cater for asymptomatic patients, with little attention paid to population screening. The screening services, including those for antenatal screening, but to a lesser extent for neonatal screening, have tended to be fragmented. There has been little consistency with respect to priorities, the specification of services needed, tests used, and monitoring the effectiveness of delivery. Although the need for improved organization is better recognized and committees have been set up to guide practice, this is not enough.

Above all, it is important that tests and procedures are judged on the basis of their efficacy and safety. Antenatal screening should not become a lottery of tests and investigations in which women in different parts of the country are offered different tests. Provided a screening approach is affordable, the most effective and safe one should be offered to all on an equitable basis. A process is needed to establish the preferred approach. A satisfactory system for achieving this goal has not yet been created, but a mechanism is needed that stimulates the necessary research and works within a framework of public confidence. The provision of screening in general, including antenatal and neonatal screening, needs to be coordinated within a responsible public health screening service so that all screening programmes are well chosen, effectively implemented, and continually researched. This is the greatest challenge in antenatal and neonatal screening.

REFERENCES

1. Anon. (1999). Report: Infant and perinatal mortality 1998: health areas, England and Wales. *Health Statistics Quarterly*, **03**, 62–5.
2. Davie, R., Butler, N., and Goldstein, H. (1972). *From Birth to Seven* (Second Report of the National Child Development Study: 1958 Cohort). Longman, London.
3. Bone, M. and Meltzer, H. (1989). *The Prevalence of Disability Among Children* (OPCS Surveys of Disability in Great Britain, Report 3). HMSO, London.
4. Bradshaw, J. (1980). *The Family Fund.* Routledge and Kegan Paul, London.
5. Wald, N. J. (1996). What is genetic screening anyway? *Journal of Medical Screening*, **3**, 57.

Glossary of terms

Abortion
In the UK, abortion is defined as expulsion or extraction from the uterus of a conceptus before 24 completed weeks of gestation. Before October 1992 the cut-off point was before 28 completed weeks of gestation. In some countries it is earlier (before 20 weeks in the US). A *spontaneous abortion* (also called a miscarriage) is one that occurs naturally. An *induced abortion* is one that occurs as a result of medical or other human intervention.

Affected individuals
Individuals who have the disorder being screened for.

Birth rate
The number of live births occurring in a given period (usually one year) divided by the total population, usually expressed per thousand.

Conceptus
All the products of conception at any stage of development from fertilization until birth.

Cut-off level
The value of a test variable which distinguishes positive from negative results. It is necessary to clarify whether a result exactly at the cut-off level is regarded as being positive or negative, for example by specifying that values greater than *or equal to* the cut-off level are positive.

Detection rate (DR) or sensitivity
The proportion of affected individuals with positive test results (usually expressed as a percentage). An advantage of 'detection rate' over the synonym 'sensitivity' is that it avoids confusion, as 'sensitivity' has a different meaning in analytical biochemistry (the minimum detectable amount in an assay). 'Detection rate' is sometimes used in a different sense in cancer screening—as the number of screen-positive individuals with cancer divided by the total number of people screened. This is better described as the prevalence of screen-positive cancers in the population.

Diagnostic test
A test which provides a diagnosis. (This does not imply that the diagnosis in question is always correct.) There is usually an intention to offer therapeutic intervention following a positive diagnostic test.

False-negatives
Affected individuals with negative test results.

False-positive rate (FPR)
The proportion of unaffected individuals with positive test results (usually expressed as a percentage). The false-positive rate, when so defined, is the complement of the specificity (the proportion of unaffected individuals with negative results), or the difference between 100 and the specificity expressed as a percentage. The advantages of using the false-positive rate rather than the specificity are that (1) it is more easily understood and remembered, (2) it focuses attention on the group that will be offered further medical intervention, (3) it conveys a better impression of the performance of the test, e.g. a 10 per cent false-positive rate is twice as bad as one of 5 per cent, whereas the corresponding specificity values (90 per cent and 95 per cent) conceal the difference.

False-positives
Unaffected individuals with positive test results.

Fetal death
Death of an unborn offspring prior to its complete expulsion or extraction from its mother.

Gestational age
The duration of an on-going or completed pregnancy, measured from the first day of the last menstrual period (usually about two weeks longer than the duration measured from conception). Gestational age is usually measured in completed weeks (e.g. a pregnancy between 16 weeks and 16 weeks 6 days duration counts as a 16 week pregnancy).

Gravidity
The total number of pregnancies that a woman has experienced (including the current one if she is pregnant), irrespective of duration.

Incidence or incidence rate
The number of new cases of a disorder which arise in a specified period of time and in a defined population. This is usually expressed as a rate per thousand per year. The incidence is thus the frequency with which *new* cases of a condition arise.

Infant mortality rate
The number of deaths in liveborn infants under one year of age divided by the number of live births in the same period (usually one year), usually expressed per thousand.

Likelihood ratio (LR)
The likelihood ratio for a population is the detection rate (DR) divided by the false-positive rate (FPR).

The likelihood ratio for an individual is the height of the relative frequency distribution of affected subjects at the value of the screening test variable observed in the individual, divided by the height of the relative frequency distribution of unaffected subjects at the same test value.

For both populations and individuals, LR × odds of being affected before test performed = odds of being affected given the test result.

Maternal mortality rate
The number of maternal deaths ascribed to causes related to pregnancy, childbirth, and the puerperium, divided by the number of live births during the same period (because the total number of women at risk is unknown), usually expressed per thousand.

Miscarriage
See Abortion.

Neonatal mortality rate
The number of deaths in the first 27 completed days of life divided by the number of live births during the same period, usually expressed per thousand.

Odds of being affected given a positive result (OAPR)
The ratio of the number of affected individuals to the number unaffected among those with positive results (i.e. true-positives:false-positives).

Another measure of the relationship between the numbers of true-positive and false-positive results of a screening test is the *positive predictive value* (PPV) of the test. PPV is the number of affected individuals with positive results divided by the total number of individuals with positive results, both affected and unaffected (true positives/(true positives + false positives)). The advantage of the OAPR over the PPV is that when these are high the OAPR conveys a clearer impression of the performance of the test. For example, if the odds of being affected for two tests are 20:1 and 50:1, the equivalent predictive values of 95 per cent and 98 per cent respectively tend to conceal the large difference.

Parity
The number of occasions on which a woman has given birth to living or stillborn infants. A pregnancy ending with multiple births is counted once only.

Perinatal mortality rate
The number of stillbirths and deaths in the first seven days after birth divided by the number of total births (i.e. live births plus stillbirths) during the same period, usually expressed per thousand.

Positive rate (PR)

The proportion of screened individuals with positive test results. For most screening procedures the PR is almost the same as the false-positive rate (FPR), because the disease being screened for is rare and false-positives outnumber true-positives by a large margin. In these circumstances the PR can be used as an approximation to the FPR. This is convenient because the PR can be calculated without needing to identify affected individuals. It is generally high enough to be reliable when calculated for a few hundred individuals screened, which means that it can be examined every few weeks when monitoring the performance of a screening programme locally.

Prevalence or prevalence rate

The number of cases of a disorder present at a point in time (point prevalence) or during a specified period (period prevalence). This is usually expressed as a rate per 1000.

When 'prevalence' is not preceded by 'point' or 'period', it usually means point prevalence. The point may be an actual or average point in calendar time, or the point at which a particular life event (e.g. birth) occurs. For example, the 'prevalence at birth' or 'birth prevalence' of a disorder is the proportion of infants in whom the disorder is present at the time of birth.

Screening

The systematic application of a test or inquiry, to identify individuals at sufficient risk of a specific disorder to benefit from further investigation or direct preventive action, among persons who have not sought medical attention on account of symptoms of that disorder.

Screening test

A test or inquiry to identify individuals at sufficient risk of a specific disorder to benefit from further investigation or direct preventive action, among persons who have not sought medical attention on account of symptoms of that disorder. The 'test' may take the form of a simple inquiry. For example, asking whether a woman is Jewish or has a Jewish parent is generally the initial screening test for Tay–Sachs disease. There is no intention to offer therapeutic intervention on the basis of a positive screening test alone.

Sensitivity

See Detection rate.

Specificity

See False-positive rate.

Stillbirth
In the UK, stillbirth is defined as the birth of a dead fetus after 24 completed weeks of gestation. The lower limit was set at 28 weeks in the UK until 1992, and is defined as 20 weeks in the US.

Stillbirth rate
The number of stillbirths divided by the number of total births (i.e. live births plus stillbirths) during the same period, usually expressed per thousand.

True-negatives
Unaffected individuals with negative test results.

True-positives
Affected individuals with positive test results.

Unaffected individuals
Individuals who do not have the disorder being screened for.

Index

Page numbers in **bold** refer to pages on which the only reference to the subject is in a table or illustration